BIOTECHNOLOGY IN MEDICAL SCIENCES

BIOTECHNOLOGY IN MEDICAL SCIENCES

Firdos Alam Khan
Manipal University
Dubai, UAE

CRC Press
Taylor & Francis Group
Boca Raton London New York

CRC Press is an imprint of the
Taylor & Francis Group, an **informa** business

CRC Press
Taylor & Francis Group
6000 Broken Sound Parkway NW, Suite 300
Boca Raton, FL 33487-2742

First issued in paperback 2017

ISBN-13: 978-1-4822-2367-5 (hbk)
ISBN-13: 978-1-138-07679-2 (pbk)

Library of Congress Cataloging-in-Publication Data

Khan, Firdos Alam, author.
Biotechnology in medical sciences / Firdos Alam Khan.
p. ; cm.
Includes bibliographical references and index.
Summary: "This book is a comprehensive overview of all the important aspects of medical biotechnology intended for interested, scientifically oriented laypersons, along, who want a relatively low level presentation of important biotechnology medical specialties such as bacteriology, immunology, recombinant DNA, molecular diagnostics, gene therapy, synthetic biology, tissue engineering, bioethics, IP issues, vaccines, and more"--Provided by publisher.
ISBN 978-1-4822-2367-5 (hardcover : alk. paper)
I. Title.
[DNLM: 1. Biomedical Technology. 2. Genetic Engineering. W 82]

R856
610.28--dc23 2014001503

Visit the Taylor & Francis Web site at
http://www.taylorandfrancis.com

and the CRC Press Web site at
http://www.crcpress.com

Contents

Preface

Over the past few decades, we have seen an exponential growth in biotechnology products especially in the medical and health care sectors. Most prominently the discovery of penicillin (an antibiotic), recombinant insulin, and cell-based therapy have completely revolutionized the field of medical diagnosis and treatments. Biotechnology is a field of applied biology that involves the use of living organisms with engineering tools to develop useful therapeutic products. Biotechnology has applications in four major industrial areas: health care (medical), crop production and agriculture, nonfood (industrial) uses of crops and other products (e.g., biodegradable plastics, vegetable oil, biofuels), and environmental uses. Among these, the medical aspects of biotechnology have been extensively used in the development of health products and diagnostic tools. In medicine, modern biotechnology finds promising applications in such areas as drug production, pharmacogenomics, gene therapy, and genetic testing. The field of medical biotechnology keeps growing with new discoveries and products. It becomes necessary to have a book that addresses the basic to the advanced level and from laboratory to clinic levels of medical biotechnology in a lucid and concise way.

There are many books available in the market that discuss the applications and fundamentals of biotechnology, but there is no single book available that deals with all aspects of medical biotechnology. Many times, students and researchers need to refer to various books to get a holistic view of the recent progress in medical biotechnology. In this book, I collate and discuss topics that are associated with medicine. The book consists of 15 chapters. Each chapter begins with a brief introduction of the topic followed by significances and applications, including colorful illustrations to explain the significance of particular topics. I have also included the names and brief contributions of important scientists and a chapter-focused bibliography at the end of each chapter to help the reader to learn each topic with great ease and interest. Chapter 1 deals with an introduction to biotechnology in medical sciences. Chapter 2 discusses human diseases and epidemiology. Chapter 3 focusses on bacteriology and antibiotics. Chapter 4 furnishes details with regard to virology and vaccines. Chapter 5 deals with immunology and monoclonal antibodies. Chapter 6 provides details on recombinant DNA technology and therapeutic proteins. Chapter 7 discusses stem cell technology. Chapter 8 covers tissue engineering. Chapter 9 includes molecular diagnostics and forensic science. Chapter 10 contributes to gene therapy. Chapter 11 focusses on synthetic biology and nanomedicine. Chapter 12 contributes to pharmacogenomics. Chapter 13 discusses bioethics. Chapter 14 deals with biobusiness and intellectual property rights. And Chapter 15 discusses career opportunities.

Acknowledgments

First and foremost, I am grateful to Almighty Allah who gave me the strength to write a second book on topics in biotechnology. I am thankful to CRC Press and especially to Dr. Michael J. Slaughter, executive editor, for having complete faith in me and giving yet another opportunity to write this book. My first book titled *Biotechnology Fundamentals* was published in 2011 and has been adopted as a textbook in the United States, Canada, and Finland. I am thankful to many people who helped me in producing this book, especially to Stephanie Morkert, project coordinator, and Ed Curtis, project editor, Taylor & Francis Group, for their valuable help in completing the book in record time. I am also thankful to Syed Mohamad Shajahan for copyediting and to the entire team of CRC Press/Taylor & Francis Group for making this book a reality.

I would like to thank the entire management team, faculty, and staff of Manipal University, India and Dubai, for their constant support. I am thankful to all my teachers and mentors, especially to Professor Nishikant Subhedar and the late Professor Obaid Siddiqi, FRS, for their training.

I am thankful to all my friends, well-wishers, and colleagues for their support and cooperation. I am grateful to all my family members, especially my father, the late Nayeemuddin Khan, and mother, Sarwari Begum; my brothers Aftab Alam Khan, Javed Alam Khan, Intekhab Alam Khan, and Dr. Sarfaraz Alam Khan; my sisters Sayeeda Khanum, Kausar Khanum, Kahkashan Khanum, and Aysha Khanum; my wife Samina Khan; my sons Zuhayr Ahmad Khan, Zaid Ahmad Khan, and Zahid Ahmad Khan; and my daughter Azraa Khan; father-in-law Abdul Qayyum Siddiqui; and mother-in-law Uzma Siddiqui for their constant support and prayers.

I welcome your comments and suggestions to make this book error-free and more thought-provoking in the future. You may send your comments to the address below.
Enjoy reading!

Firdos Alam Khan, PhD
Professor and Chairperson
School of Life Sciences
Manipal University Dubai Campus
P.O. Box 345050 Dubai
United Arab Emirates
Email: firdoskhan1969@gmail.com

Author

Firdos Alam Khan is a professor and chairperson in the School of Life Sciences, Manipal University Dubai Campus, Dubai, United Arab Emirates. He earned his doctorate from Nagpur University, India in 1997. He has more than 20 years of research and teaching experience.

Dr. Khan did his first postdoctoral research from the National Centre for Biological Sciences in Bangalore, India, where he worked on a World Health Organization sponsored research project titled Olfactory Learning in *Drosophila melanogaster.* In 1998, Dr. Khan moved to the United States and joined the Department of Brain and Cognitive Sciences, Massachusetts Institute of Technology, and worked on the research project titled Axonal Nerve Regeneration in Adult Syrian Hamster. In 2001, he returned to India and joined Reliance Life Sciences, a Mumbai-based biotechnology company, where he was associated with adult and embryonic stem cell research projects. Dr. Khan showed that both adult and embryonic stem cells have the ability to differentiate into neuronal cells. He also developed novel protocols to derive neuronal cells from both adult and embryonic stem cells.

Over the past 7 years, Dr. Khan has been associated with the Department of Biotechnology, Manipal University Dubai as chairperson. He teaches bioethics and biotechnology business courses to graduate and postgraduate students.

Dr. Khan's area of specialty in biotechnology includes stem cell technology, pharmacology, and neuroscience. He has written numerous articles in various national and international journals in the areas of neuroscience, neuropharmacology, and stem cell biology. He holds two US patents in the field of stem cell technology. He has been associated with various international scientific organizations such as the International Brain Research Organization, France, and Society for Neuroscience, USA. He has presented his research work at more than 23 different national and international conferences in India, Singapore, UAE, and the United States.

chapter one

Introduction to biotechnology in medical sciences

1.1 Introduction

The term medical biotechnology is the application of living organisms or cells or tissues to produce pharmaceutical and diagnostic products that help to treat and to prevent the progress of human diseases. One of the best-known examples of medical biotechnology is the production of antibiotics for treating various bacterial infections; these antibiotics are produced by using known microorganisms. Similarly, over the past few decades various other types of products have been produced, which include biopesticides, pest-resistant crops, and bioremediation techniques and many more. The most remarkable discovery made in recent times is the production of human proteins (insulin) outside of the human body, which has completely revolutionized the medical treatment modality. The synthesis of human insulin and growth hormones are considered to be the rewards of modern biotechnology. In both insulin and growth hormone production, scientists have used recombinant DNA technology to be administered in patients suffering from various incurable diseases such as diabetes and genetic disorders. It has been suggested that one of the major problems in treating patients with cancer and diabetes conditions is not being able to completely eradicate the disease. The only available option for any physician is to either go for drug therapy or surgical interventions to give symptomatic relief.

1.2 What is biotechnology all about?

The field of biotechnology has been in use for ages in various forms, which include the growing of better crops (agricultural biotechnology) and animal breeding (animal biotechnology). Similarly, the use of biotechnology has been around for thousands of years, especially the application of microorganisms in the production of cheese and yogurt (food biotechnology). In addition, the tools of biotechnology have been implied in animal husbandry, to develop pest-resistant crops, bioremediation (environmental biotechnology), as well as in bioethanol production. But the most promising application of biotechnology is found to be in the medical field by generations of biotherapeutics (insulin, growth hormones) and diagnostics tools (PCR, FISH, micro-array technique). Before we discuss various applications of medical biotechnology, let us briefly go through the historical aspects of biotechnology and this information will make you to understand the field better. It all began with the discovery made by Sir Alexander Fleming in the year 1918 where he observed that the mold *Penicillium* inhibited the growth of human skin disease-causing bacteria called *Staphylococcus aureus.* The discovery by Sir Alexander Fleming lead to the making of antibiotics that we use today. These antibiotics are highly recommended and extensively used medicinally for bacterial infections (Figures 1.1 and 1.2). These antibiotics are basically substances produced by microorganisms that normally inhibit the growth of

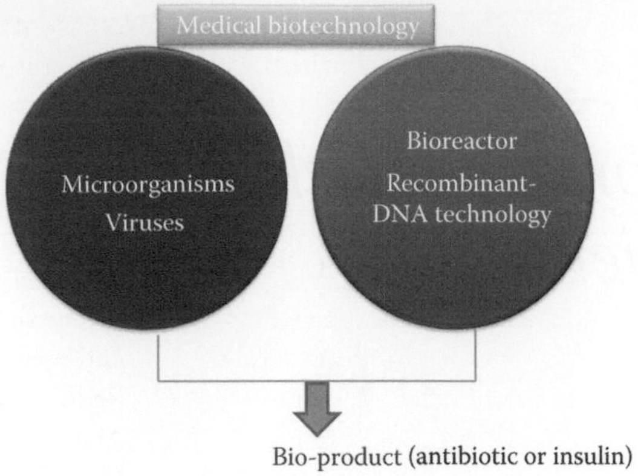

Figure 1.1 Application of microorganisms and viruses in making of medicine using bioreactor and recombinant DNA technology.

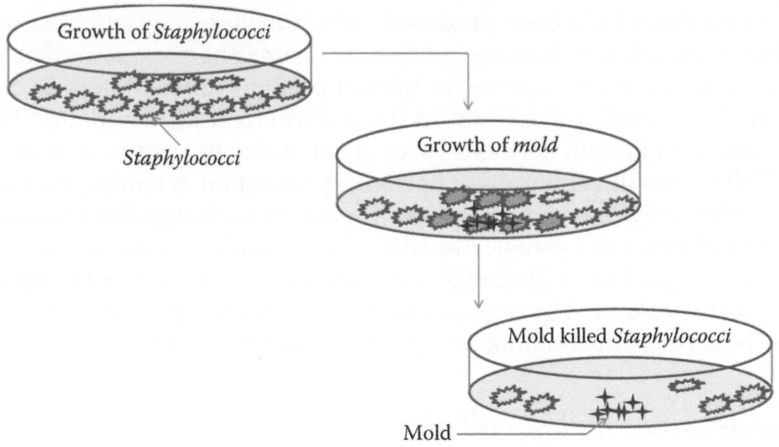

Figure 1.2 The pioneering experiment conducted by Dr. Alexander Fleming resulted in the discovery of the penicillin drug, an antibiotic drug.

other microorganisms. Later on, antibiotics became widely available as a drug for treating microbial infections in human beings, especially with the development of penicillin (Figure 1.3) as the most used antibiotic. Currently, a variety of microorganisms have been used to generate thousand liters of antibiotic drugs by using advanced biotechnology tools.

The field of biotechnology has taken a leap with the discovery of the double-helix structure of the deoxyribose nucleic acid (DNA) molecule and the credit goes to one research publication titled "This structure has novel features which are of considerable biological interest" authored by James Watson and Francis Crick in 1953, which claimed to discover the structure of the human DNA helix, the molecule that carries genetic information from one generation to the other. Nine years later, in the year 1962, they shared the Nobel Prize with Wilkins for cracking one of the most important of all biological puzzles. This discovery has led to the birth of genetic mapping, manipulation, and genetic engineering-type fields. Surprisingly, with the help of genetic engineering, the gene of interest can be cut and inserted into the genome of other living organisms (microorganisms and viruses) and

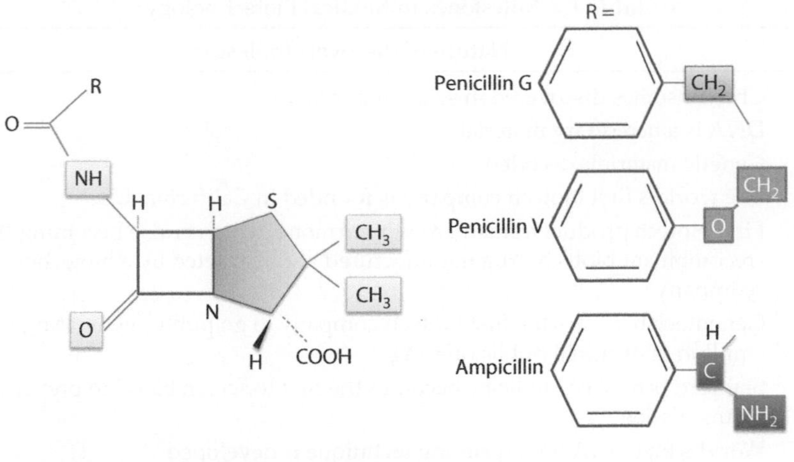

Figure 1.3 Structures of penicillin G, penicillin V, and ampicillin.

this process of gene insertion and manipulation is called recombinant DNA technology. Over the past few years recombinant DNA technology has been extensively employed to generate therapeutic products (insulin and growth hormones) for treating human diseases. With a rapid increase in the number of patient's worldwide, there has been a tremendous scope to identify and create medicine for various human diseases. Thankfully with the availability of biotechnology tools, now it is possible to develop therapy for various diseases. In Table 1.1, major biotechnology-related discoveries and milestones are listed to appreciate the contribution of biotechnology in human health care.

1.3 Medical products developed by using biotechnology tools

One of the salient features of medical biotechnology is the contribution of arrays of products, which include treatment of bacterial infections, diabetes, immune disorders, cancer, and degenerative conditions such as heart infarction and neurodegenerative diseases (i.e., Parkinson's disease, Alzheimer's disease, or stroke diseases). We have briefly discussed below some of the major biotechnology-based products which have been widely used around the world.

1.3.1 Antibiotics

Penicillin is one of the earliest discovered antibiotics which is basically derived from molds such as *Penicillium*. Penicillin was discovered by Scottish scientist and Nobel laureate Sir Alexander Fleming in 1928. It all started with a basic experiment where Sir Fleming noticed a Petri dish containing *Staphylococcus* plate culture which he had mistakenly left open was contaminated by blue-green mold, which had formed a visible growth. But surprisingly he also found that there was a circle of inhibited bacterial growth around the mold. Later on, Sir Fleming hypothesized that the mold was releasing a substance that was preventing the growth and could contain a substance with antibiotic properties. In order to prove his hypothesis, he grew a pure culture and discovered the first antibiotic substance from the Penicillium mold, known as *Penicillium notatum*. Sir Alexander showed that *P. notatum* when grown in the appropriate substrate caused the release of chemical substances and these chemical substances were named as antibiotics. He later on named

Table 1.1 Milestones in Medical Biotechnology

Year	Nature of discovery/milestone
1882	Chromosomes discovered in salamander larva
1944	DNA is a hereditary material
1963	Genetic materials decoded
1971	The world's first biotech company is founded in California, US
1979	First biotech product human growth hormone, which is also becoming the first recombinant biotech drug manufactured and marketed by a biotechnology company
1980	Genentech becomes the first biotech company to go public, generating $35 million in its initial public offering
1983	Stanford School of Medicine becomes the first to screen blood to prevent AIDS transmission
1984	World's first DNA fingerprinting technique is developed
1984	Chiron Corporation announced the first cloning and sequencing of the entire HIV virus genome
1984	Genentech obtains USFDA approval to market human growth hormone, the first recombinant product to be sold by a biotechnology company
1986	The USFDA awards Chiron Corporation, a license for the production of first recombinant vaccine to battle the hepatitis B virus
1988	The "Harvard Mouse" becomes the first mammal patented in the United States
1991	Cancer patients are treated with a gene therapy that produces the tumor necrosis factor, a natural tumor-fighting protein
1995	The first full gene sequence of a living organism other than a virus is completed for the bacterium hemophilic influenza
1997	A sheep named "Dolly" becomes the first mammal cloned
2002	First vaccine against cervical cancer development

that chemical substance as penicillin. Soon after this discovery, penicillin was considered to be the most effective drug against bacteria (Gram-positive bacteria), and not at all effective against Gram-negative bacteria. The discovery of penicillin marks the beginning of the antibiotic production and so far more than 200 different types of antibiotics have been produced (Figure 1.3).

1.3.2 *Recombinant insulin*

Another discovery which was made in the medical field was the recombinant DNA technology, which has completely revolutionized disease treatments especially in the Type 1 diabetes mellitus, where insulin-producing cells become dysfunctional and do not produce sufficient amount of insulin to regulate blood-sugar level. In a healthy human being, insulin regulates glucose metabolism in the body. In diabetic conditions, the level of insulin decreases which causes the elevation of the blood sugar level and this clinical condition is known as diabetes mellitus. One of the best treatments of diabetes mellitus is insulin injections, where insulin is injected into the patient's body and the insulin regulates the blood-sugar level. The insulin is either synthesized chemically or produced by recombinant DNA technology. These synthesized insulins are used medically to treat patients with Type 1 diabetes mellitus, whereas patients with Type 2 diabetes mellitus are insulin resistant.

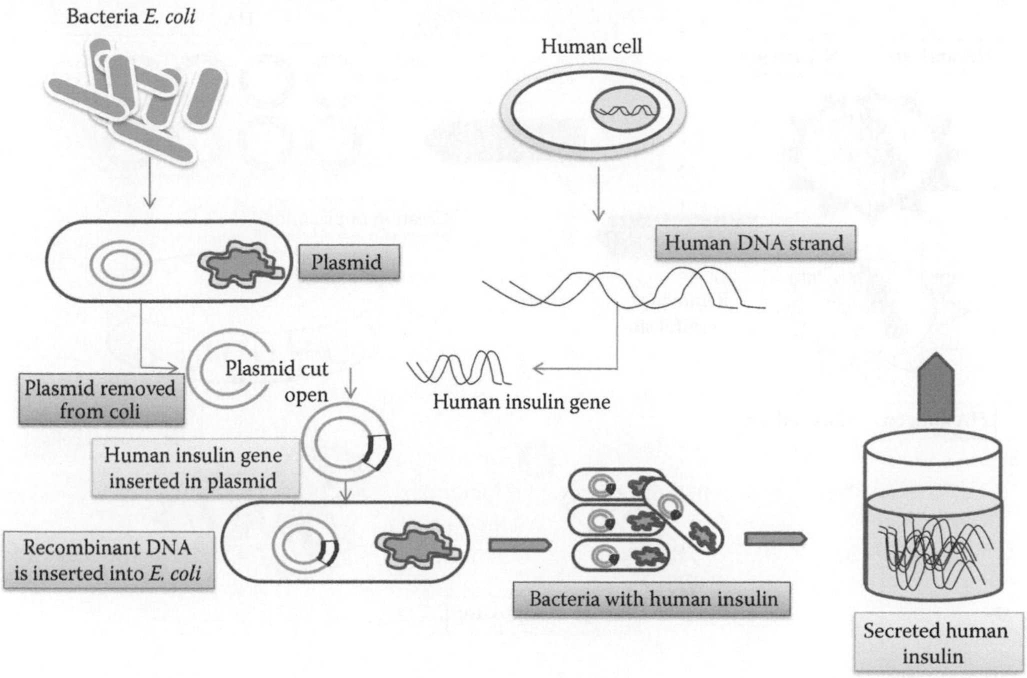

Figure 1.4 Making of human insulin by recombinant DNA technology.

However, some patients with Type 2 diabetes may eventually require insulin treatment if other medications fail to control blood glucose levels adequately, though this is somewhat uncommon. With the advent of recombinant DNA technology, it became possible to make insulin outside the human body and this biosynthetic insulin is now manufactured for widespread clinical use. More recently, scientists have succeeded in introducing human insulin gene into plants in order to produce human insulin in plants, and the safflower plant has been used for this purpose. In addition to recombinant DNA technology, there are other ways to synthesize human insulin outside the human body and they are usually referred to as insulin analogues and these analogues are chemically synthesized (Figure 1.4). One of the major hurdles in the diabetes treatment is the delivery of insulin, as insulin cannot be taken orally because it will not be absorbed properly and will lose its biological activity. In recent years, an attempt has been made to develop insulin which can be safely given through the oral route or sublingually. It has been reported that insulin can be taken as subcutaneous injections; few companies have also attempted to develop an oral form of insulin and trials are underway.

1.3.3 *Vaccines*

The vaccine is basically a biological preparation that improves the human immune defense system to fight diseases. The vaccines normally contain an agent that diligently resembles a disease-causing bacteria, and is frequently produced from debilitating or killed forms of the microorganisms. Upon injection into the human body, the vaccine can stimulate the body's immune system to recognize the agent as a foreign body, and recognize it, so that the immune system can recall and destroy or kill any of these microorganisms that later

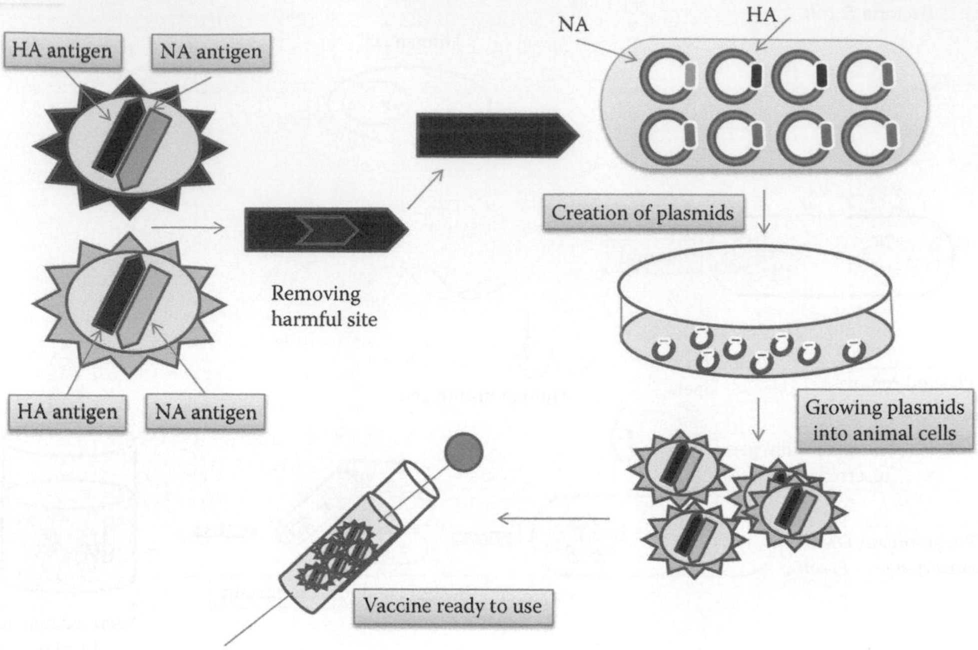

Figure 1.5 Making of vaccine.

infect the human body. In a simpler way, the vaccine basically trains the human body to defend or fight or kill the microorganisms. The vaccines are classified based on its application; the vaccines that are used to prevent the effects of an upcoming infection by any natural or wild pathogen are called prophylactic, and the vaccines which are used against cancer are called therapeutic vaccines (Figure 1.5).

The story of vaccine development dates back to the seventeenth century when Edward Jenner found a milkmaid infected with smallpox, and a few days later he took pus from the hand of the milkmaid with cowpox and inoculated an eight-year-old boy with it. After six weeks he found that the boy did not contract smallpox. After a few years, Sir Louis Pasteur adapted Jenner's idea of developing a rabies vaccine and, subsequently, vaccine development progress started and became a matter of national concern. After that obligatory vaccination laws were passed in various countries around the globe. During the twentieth century, we have seen an introduction of several successful vaccines against diseases such as diphtheria, measles, mumps, and rubella. Interestingly, the major achievement was done in the 1950s when the polio vaccine was made and clinically used; also vaccines were synthesized to eradicate smallpox.

1.3.4 Monoclonal antibodies

Another milestone achieved in the beginning of the twentieth century was the making of monoclonal antibodies, which was proposed by Paul Ehrlich. He suggested that drug compounds can be accurately, precisely, and specifically delivered along with monoclonal antibodies. Monoclonal antibodies are mono-specific antibodies as they are made by identical cells that are all clones of a distinctive parent cell (Figure 1.6). Currently, it is possible to produce monoclonal antibodies that specifically bind to that antigen and have a variety

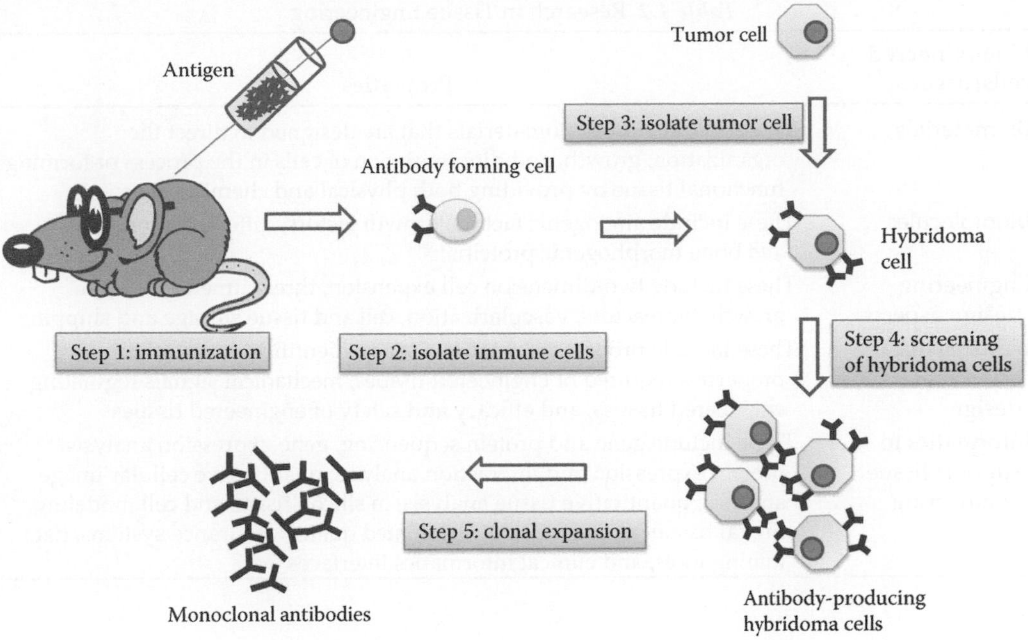

Figure 1.6 Making of monoclonal antibodies.

of applications, especially to detect or purify that substance (antigen), and has become an important tool in diagnostics and biomedical research.

In diagnostics and biomedical research, monoclonal antibodies are very useful tools. First, they are extremely specific; that is, each antibody binds to the specific site of the antigen. Second, some antibodies, once activated by the occurrence of a disease, continue to confer resistance against that disease; classic examples are the antibodies to the childhood diseases chickenpox and measles. Another important application of monoclonal antibodies is to develop vaccines against various diseases. As you are aware, a vaccine is made from bacteria or viruses either killed or inactivated. Upon introduction into the human body this vaccine stimulates the production of antibodies against the antigens to fight back the diseases. The production of monoclonal antibodies involves human and mouse hybrid cells and this technology is known as hybridoma technology. During monoclonal antibody production, tumor cells are merged with mammalian cells that produce an antibody against a particular antigen. The result of these merged tumors with mammalian cells is a called hybridoma, which can frequently produce antibodies. These antibodies are called monoclonal antibodies because they come from only one type of cell; whereas, the antibodies that are produced by conventional methods contain many kinds of cells and are called polyclonal antibodies.

1.3.5 *Bioengineered tissues*

Over the last decade, tissue engineering became the most fascinating medical field, especially in body-parts reconstruction or cosmetic surgery areas. The basic concept about tissue engineering is to make human tissues through in vitro methods under controlled laboratory conditions and the making of such tissues is called bioengineered tissues. The

Table 1.2 Research in Tissue Engineering

Bioengineered cells/tissues	Properties
Biomaterials	These include novel biomaterials that are designed to direct the organization, growth, and differentiation of cells in the process of forming functional tissue by providing both physical and chemical cues
Biomolecules	These include angiogenic factors, growth factors, differentiation factors, and bone morphogenic proteins
Engineering design aspects	These include two-dimension cell expansion, three-dimension tissue growth, bioreactors, vascularization, cell and tissue storage and shipping
Biomechanical aspects of design	These include properties of native tissues, identification of minimum properties required of engineered tissues, mechanical signals regulating engineered tissues, and efficacy and safety of engineered tissues
Informatics to support tissue engineering	These include gene and protein sequencing, gene-expression analysis, protein expression and interaction analysis, quantitative cellular image analysis, quantitative tissue analysis, in silicon tissue and cell modeling, digital tissue manufacturing, automated quality assurance systems, data mining tools, and clinical informatics interfaces

definition of tissue engineering covers a broad range of applications in the healthcare field, however, in practice the term tissue engineering closely relates to repair or replacing portions of, or whole, human body tissues which include neurons, cardiomyocytes, bone, and cartilage. The bioengineered tissues are constructed by integrating certain mechanical and structural properties for proper functioning in the human body, so one can say that bioengineering is basically the use of a combination of cells, engineering, and biocompatible materials, and is finally suitable to improve or replace biological functions (Table 1.2). The bioengineered field was once categorized as a sub-field of biomaterials, but having grown in scope and application it is considered as a field in its own right (Figure 1.7). Tissue engineering is an emerging multidisciplinary field involving biology, medicine, and engineering that is likely to revolutionize the ways we improve the health of millions of people worldwide by repairing, maintaining, or enhancing tissue and organ function. The tissue engineering can also have diagnostic applications where the human cells or tissues are used to test drug metabolism and drug uptake, toxicity, and pathogenicity.

1.3.6 *Adult stem cell therapy*

Over the last few years, there has been tremendous interest in adult stem cells for the autologous cell transplantation as these specialized cells have the potential ability to repair or restore the dysfunctional cells or tissues in the human body afflicted with various diseases that include blood cancer and neurological disorders. The stem cells are generally found in all multicellular organisms and they are characterized by the ability to renew themselves through cell division and differentiate into a varied range of specialized cell types. Moreover, mammalian stem cells may be broadly classified into two major types: adult stem cells and embryonic stem cells (ESCs) that are isolated from the inner cell mass of blastocysts.

One of the main roles of adult stem cells is that they remain in an undifferentiated state in the human body and multiply by cell division to replenish dying cells and restore damaged tissues and organs. The adult stem cells are also known as somatic stem cells;

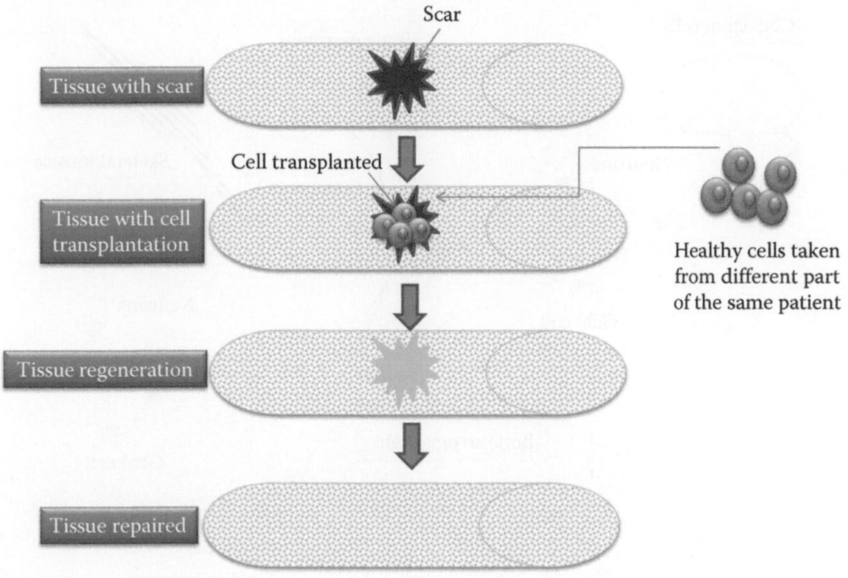

Figure 1.7 Tissue engineering.

these stem cells can be found in both juvenile and adult ages. Moreover, adult stem cells are specialized cells that have the capability to divide and generate all cell types of the organ from which they originate, and can also possibly regenerate the entire organ. Unlike ESCs, the use of adult stem cells is not contentious as they are derived from adult source or tissue rather than by killing human embryos. Moreover, adult stem cells have been in use for many years predominantly in the treatment of cancer (such as leukemia and related bone and blood cancers) employing bone marrow transplants. Interestingly, the majority of the government funding especially in the United States is confined to adult stem cell-based research. Among adult stem cells, hematopoietic stem cells (HSCs) and mesenchymal stem cells (MSCs) are found to be the most successful stem cells because they can be clinically used in patients. These stem cells can be directly injected or placed at the site of repair or injected through vascular delivery (Figure 1.8).

1.4 Emerging trends

In addition to above-mentioned fields, there are other fields which are emerging and are in the initial phase of development. These emerging fields will provide improved technology or tools to treat or diagnose various diseases.

1.4.1 Embryonic stem cells

Over the last few years ESCs have been a highly discussed and debated scientific topic at all levels which include public life, scientific forums, ethical, legal, and political platforms. Before we discuss the ethical or legal issues associated with ESCs, we will first learn what ESCs are all about. The ESCs are basically pluripotent stem cells isolated from the inner cell mass of the blastocyst, which is an early-stage embryo. Moreover, human embryos reach the blastocyst stage 4 to 5 days post fertilization, at which time they consist of about

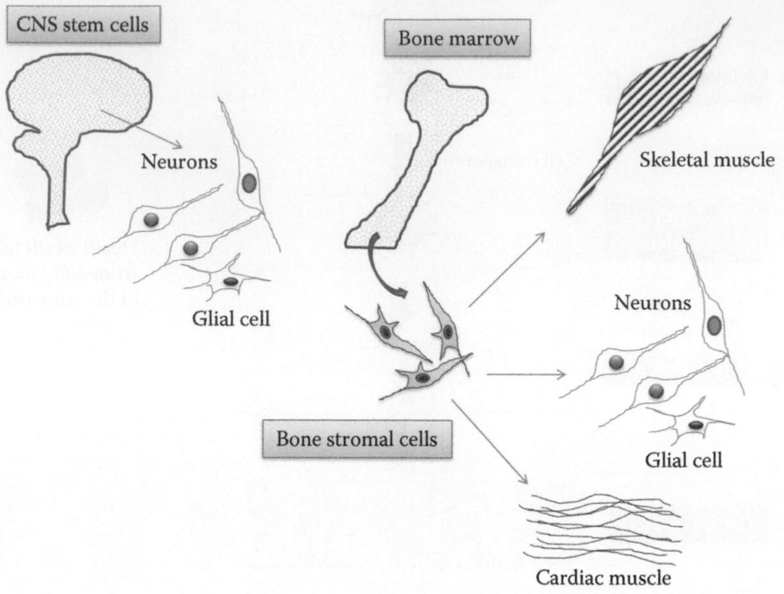

Figure 1.8 Adult stem cells.

50–150 cells. In addition to this, ESCs are adept at propagating themselves for an indefinite period under controlled culture situations. The culture and propagation of ESCs through in vitro methods is considered to be the best technology to culture human cells in large quantities and to be engaged as valuable tools for both research and cell-based therapy (Figure 1.9).

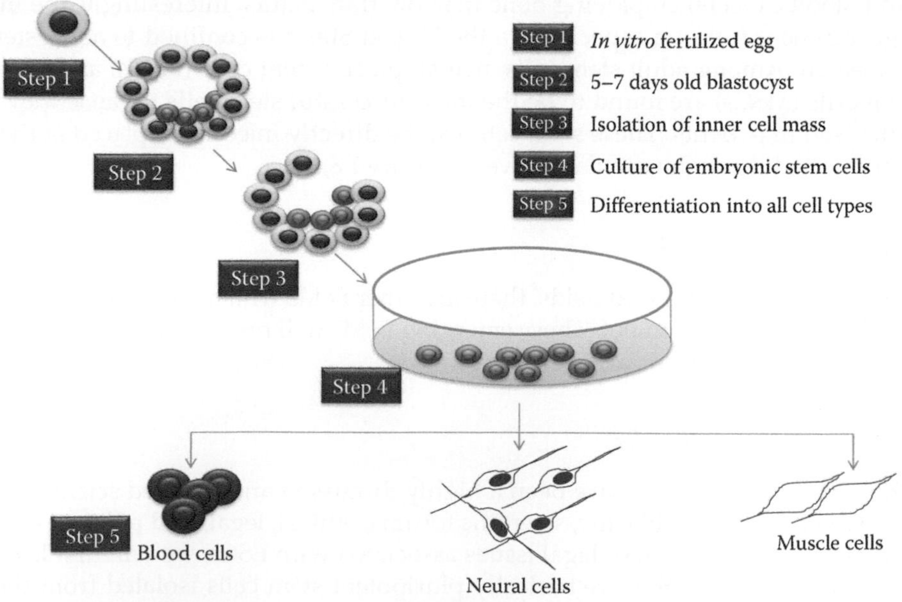

Figure 1.9 Embryonic stem cells.

One of the best applications of ESCs is to provide a large supply of required cells to be used as cell-based therapy and tissue replacement in patients who are suffering from degenerative diseases. Moreover, a number of diseases that could possibly be treated by ESCs are cancers, diabetes, Parkinson's disease, Alzheimer's disease, stroke, blindness, and spinal cord injuries. In contrast to its various therapeutic applications, the issues related to ESCs need to be resolved before making them useful for human use. These issues are the problem of immune rejection associated with allogeneic stem cell transplantation. These problems can be solved by using adult stem cells in autologous transplantation. Besides, cell-based therapy, the ESCs can be used as diagnostic tools to study an early human development and genetic disease, as well as in vitro drug testing. Other issues related to ESCs transplantation is that there is a possibility that transplanted stem cells could form tumors and have the possibility of becoming cancerous if cell division continues uncontrollably. Contrary to this, supporters of ESCs research argue that such research should be continued because the resultant research findings will have significant medical potential. The recent development of induced pluripotent stems cells (iPSc) has created tremendous interest among scientists, as adult stem cells can be converted into pluripotent stem cells and there is no need to kill the human embryos.

In spite of all controversies over ethical use of human ESCs, on January 23, 2009, Geron Corporation, USA, has received an approval from US Food and Drug Administration (FDA) to test ESCs in humans. The Phase 1 clinical trial for transplantation of a human-ES-derived cell population into spinal cord-injured individuals became the first human ES cell human trial. The Phase 1 clinical study was conducted on eight to ten paraplegic patients who have had their injuries no longer than two weeks before the trial began, and stem cells were injected before the formation of scar in the tissue. Nevertheless, the researchers are stressing that the injections are not expected to fully cure the patients and restore all mobility. The success of such clinical trials goes back to the experiments conducted by University of California, USA, and which was supported by Geron Corporation of Menlo Park (Biotechnology Company), California. The results of an animal study showed that there was functional improvement in locomotive recovery in spinal cord-injured rats after stem cell transplantation. Interestingly, the first trial is mainly for testing the safety of cell-based transplantation. However, the trial had been put on hold in August 2009 due to apprehensions made by the FDA regarding a small number of microscopic tumors found in several treated rat models, but the hold has been lifted since.

1.4.2 Human genome project

The Human Genome Project (HGP) was an international collaborative research project with a primary aim to decode the human DNA genome. The main objective of the HGP was to map about 20–25 k genes of the human genome from both a physical and functional perspective. The initial task of the project was to identify the full set of genetic instructions enclosed inside human DNA. The project began with the end of several years of work supported by the United States Department of Energy (DoE). It has been reported that the \$3-billion project was founded in 1990 by the DoE and the US National Institutes of Health. In addition to the United States, other countries also took part in the HGP, including the United Kingdom, France, Germany, Japan, China, and India. The team of scientists worked hard over the years and drafted a proposal for the genome project and the final sequencing of the human genome was done in 2006. Although the objective of the HGP is to understand the genetic organization of the human genome, the project has worked with other nonmammalian organisms.

1.4.2.1 *Significance of the genome project*

The reason for starting the HGP was to understand the role of genes in the development of diseases. There are reports that suggest more than 3000 genetic disorders known to be caused by genetic mutations. With the current treatment modalities, these genetic disorders cannot be cured without knowing the real cause. And to know the cause we have to know the role of genes in the diseases. Recent efforts have been made to find out the causes of cancer with genetic tools, but not much success was achieved. It has been recommended that information gained from the HGP would help to understand the genetic cause of the devastating illnesses, which include Parkinson's disease, schizophrenia, or Alzheimer's disease.

The genetic mutations play a role in many genetic diseases that include heart disease, diabetes, immune system disorders, and congenital defects. These diseases are thought to be the consequence from complex collaborations between genes and environmental factors. When genes for diseases have been identified, researchers can study how environmental factors, food, drugs, or pollutants can influence those genes. The location of the gene is important in identifying the type of protein which is produced by a particular gene. It has been reported that understanding the mechanism of a genetic disease is an important step in curing genetic diseases. It has been suggested that one day it may be possible to treat genetic diseases by gene therapy. Besides therapeutic applications, the information gained from the HGP can help to know the reason for the pluripotency nature of ESCs and how these ESCs can be differentiated into many different specialized cells such as muscle cell, neural cells, or hepatocytes.

1.4.3 *RNA interference technology*

The RNA interference (RNAi) is a natural process that cells dictate to turn down or go to a silent state; such activity cell is regulated by a specific gene known as RNAi. The RNAi technology provides excellent tools to study the role specific gene in the development, causes, and progression of particular diseases, and has taken the biomedical community by storm. It has been reported that RNAi was first noticed in the plant *Petunia* when plant biologists tried to develop the purple color of the flower by introducing a pigment-producing gene. Surprisingly, the gene which was introduced to intensify color in the plants was found to suppress the color. In the end the resulting flowers developed white patches or became completely white. Surprisingly, a few years later another group of researchers observed a similar kind of gene-silencing effect in *Caenorhabditis elegans*. Later on, it has been reported that the gene-silencing effect is caused by the presence of double-stranded RNA, and this double-stranded RNA is normally not found in healthy cells.

RNAi technology has been in use in various fields of biotechnology, particularly in the food plant engineering that produces lower levels of natural toxins.

No plant that uses RNAi technology has yet passed the experimental stage; however, research work has been known to effectively reduce the allergen levels in tomato plants and also is known to cut the cancer-causing agents in tobacco plants. Also, other plant characters that have also been bioengineered include the production of nonnarcotic natural products by using the opium plant, development of resistance to common plant viruses, and protection of plants with dietary antioxidants. Interestingly, bioengineered plants such as *FlavrSavr* tomatoes and two cultivars of *ring-spot*-resistant papaya were originally developed by employing antisense technology.

One of the pronounced applications of RNAi technology is its application in medicine. Over the past few years, efforts have been made to understand RNAi's role in normal and diseased cells, and also to use the RNAi technology for use in medical therapies. It has been suggested that human disease progression can be blocked by using RNAi-based therapies to turn down the activity of genes. Cancer, for example, is frequently caused by over-excited genes in the cells, and retarding their activities could stop the disease progression. Over the last few years, several pharmaceutical companies are using RNAi-based therapies to treat for various forms of cancer. In addition, viral infections can also be treated using RNAi-based therapies and this can be done by reducing the activity of key viral genes. It has been shown in the laboratory that human cells have successfully stopped the growth of HIV, polio, hepatitis C, and other viruses in human cell culture and RNAi-based therapies against HIV are under clinical trial stages. Moreover, the importance of RNAi technology has some beneficial effects in finding out the cause of the disease. Using RNAi technology, the activity of a particular gene can be knocked down which will help us to understand its role in the disease development and progression. For many years, researchers have been studying how proteins regulate gene activity. Now with the help of RNAi technology, it would be possible to discover the role of proteins in gene regulation.

1.4.4 *Phage therapy*

Phage therapy is generally to treat pathogenic infections caused by microorganisms and bacteriophages. Phages are basically viruses that enter bacterial cells and disturb bacterial metabolism causing the bacterium to lyse. It has been reported that phage therapy is very effective in special clinical conditions and is known to have some unique advantages over antibiotic treatments. Unlike antibiotics, phage therapies have special advantages for localized use in humans because they infiltrate deeper in the infected area and remove the infection from the source. Another interesting aspect of bacteriophage is that these phages stop reproducing once the specific bacteria they target are destroyed. It has been reported that phages do not develop secondary resistance, which happens quite often in antibiotic treatments. With the increasing incidence of antibiotic-resistant bacteria in humans, there is a need to apply phages in treating various kinds' of infections. In addition, phage therapy has many potential applications that include medicine, dentistry, veterinary science, and agricultural science. In addition, bacteriophages are found to be much more specific than antibiotics, and this bacteriophage do not cause any harmful effects on the host organism such as human, animal, or plant, but instead maintains a healthy relationship with beneficial bacteria in the body.

Over the last few years, it has been reported that phages are being used to treat bacterial infections in the patients and especially in those patients who do not respond to antibiotics. It has been found that these phage therapies tend to be more successful than antibiotics because there is a biofilm covered by a polysaccharide layer, which antibiotics typically cannot penetrate. In the West, no therapies are currently authorized for use on humans, although phages for killing food poisoning bacteria such as *Listeria* are now in use. On the contrary, there are some disadvantages of phage therapy because a phage will only kill a bacterium if it is a match to the specific strain of the bacterium and it will not kill non-specific strain of bacterium.

1.4.5 *Recombinant DNA technology*

Recombinant DNA (rDNA) technology is one of the most sought-after technologies that has completely revolutionized the current treatment modalities, especially the use of humanized insulin for diabetes treatment. The rDNA technology soon to be developed can also be used in the treatment of diseases such as diabetes, genetic disorders, cystic fibrosis, cancer, and sickle cell anemia. The organisms that have been developed by using rDNA technology will be used to produce new vaccines, monoclonal antibodies, enzymes, and hormones. It has been suggested that biotechnology be used to enhance breeding in plants and animals. In addition, rDNA technology can also be used to develop disease and herbicide-resistant plants, disease-resistant animals, seedless fruits, and quick-growing chickens.

1.4.6 *Biochips*

With the advent of information technology, it is possible to store biological information in a chip format which is called as a biochip. Biochip is a chip made of metal and designed to work inside the human body to treat and to diagnose the disease. There are various applications of biochips, which include biochips that can be implanted in the body and used for delivering precise amounts of drugs to the affected organs. Biochips can also be used as biosensors to monitor levels of enzymes, monoclonal antibodies, proteins in the human body, to detect hazardous substances, and to monitor blood components in the body.

1.4.7 *Gene therapy*

To treat genetic disorders, the default or dysfunctional gene can either be replaced with a new gene or repaired with gene therapy. In brief, the gene therapy involves correcting defects in genes and in this process a normal/healthy gene is introduced to replace a defective gene. Gene therapy is still under development stages and various clinical trials are underway around the world. Its success will be based on the successful cure of genetic diseases by gene therapy.

1.4.8 *Liposome-based drug delivery*

One of the major challenges of current drug therapy is to successfully transport the drugs to targeted sites in the human body. In recent times researchers have made efforts to develop a system to accurately and precisely release the drugs at the sites and one of the approaches is to transport the drug using liposomes as a vehicle. Liposomes are basically tiny vesicles made out of the same material as the human cell membrane. It has been suggested that liposomes can be packed with drug molecules and be used to deliver drugs in a precise and accurate manner to the affected regions of cells, especially in the treatment of cancer, without affecting the surrounding healthy cells.

1.4.9 *Bionanotechnology*

Bionanotechnology is a term that refers to the intersection of nanotechnology and biology. This discipline helps to indicate the merger of biological research in various fields of nanotechnology. The concepts that are enhanced through nanobiology include: nanodevices, nanoparticles, and nanoscale that occurs within the discipline of nanotechnology. Moreover, this technical method in biology allows scientists to imagine and create systems that can be used for biological research. Biologically inspired nanotechnology uses biological systems as the inspiration for technologies not yet created. The most important objectives that are frequently found in nanobiology involve applying nanotools to relevant medical or biological problems and refining these applications. Moreover, developing new tools for the medical and biological fields is another primary objective in nanotechnology.

Interestingly, new nanotools are often made by refining the applications of the nanotools that are already being used. The imaging of native biomolecules, biological membranes, and tissues is also a major topic for the nanobiology researchers. Other topics concerning nanobiology include the use of cantilever array sensors and the application of nanophotonics for manipulating molecular processes in living cells.

Recently, the use of microorganisms to synthesize functional nanoparticles have been of great interest. Microorganisms can change the oxidation state of metals. Moreover, these microbial processes have opened up new opportunities for us to explore novel applications, for example, the biosynthesis of metal nanomaterials. In contrast to chemical and physical methods, microbial processes for synthesizing nanomaterials can be achieved in aqueous phases under gentle and environmentally benign conditions. This approach has become an attractive focus on current green bionanotechnology research toward sustainable development.

The applications of bionanotechnology are extremely widespread and nanobiotechnology is best described as helping modern medicine progress from treating symptoms to generating cures and regenerating biological tissues. Three American patients have received whole cultured bladders with the help of doctors who use nanobiology techniques in their practice. Also, it has been demonstrated in animal studies that a uterus can be grown outside the body and then placed in the body in order to produce a baby. Furthermore, there is also funding for research into allowing people to have new limbs without having to resort to prosthesis. Artificial proteins might also become available to manufacture without the need for harsh chemicals and expensive machines. It has even been surmised that by 2055, computers may be made out of biochemical and organic salts. Another example of current nanobiotechnological research involves nanospheres coated with fluorescent polymers. Moreover, investigators are seeking to design polymers whose fluorescence are quenched when they encounter specific molecules. Different polymers would detect different metabolites. Interestingly, the polymer-coated spheres could become part of new biological assays, and the technology might someday lead to the particles which could be introduced into the human body to track down metabolites associated with tumors and other health problems. Another example, from a different perspective, would be an evaluation and therapy at the nanoscopic level, that is, the treatment of nanobacteria (25–200 nm sized) as is done by NanoBiotech Pharma.

Despite the fact that biological systems are inherently nano in scale, nanoscience must merge with biology in order to deliver biomacromolecules and molecular machines that are similar to the human body or organ. In the twenty-first century, scientists have developed the technology to artificially tap into nanobiology. This process is best described as organic merging with synthetic. Interestingly, colonies of live neurons can live together on a biochip device. The self-assembling nanotubes have the ability to be used as a structural system as they would be composed together with rhodopsins, which would help the optical computing process and also help with the storage of biological materials. The most fascinating aspects would be of DNA as the software for all living things, which can be used as a structural proteomics system—a logical component of molecular computing.

1.5 Summary

The term biotechnology generally refers to the integration of technology or engineering knowledge in biological science. The fundamental applications of biotechnology are to produce arrays of products which are beneficial for human consumptions and also for making our environment healthy and pollution free. In particular, the human body is very critical and requires proper care, diagnosis, and treatment. There are many diseases (malaria, typhoid, cold flu, fever, etc.) which are being treated by using synthetically designed medicines (tablets, capsules, syrups, etc.), but there are many diseases (diabetes, genetic disorders) that cannot be treated with synthetically designed medicines and require biotechnological interventions like insulin and gene therapy. Medical biotechnology primarily deals with providing solutions to major human diseases either in the form of diagnostic kits or in the form of vaccines, antibiotics, monoclonal antibodies, cell-based therapy, or gene therapy. One of the best examples of modern medical biotechnology is the development of antibiotics and vaccines, which in fact is experienced by almost every human being.

1.6 Scholar's achievement

Sir Alexander Fleming: Sir Alexander Fleming, FRSE, FRS, FRCS (Eng) (August 6, 1881 to March 11, 1955) was a Scottish biologist, pharmacologist, and botanist. He wrote many articles on bacteriology, immunology, and chemotherapy. His best-known discoveries are the enzyme lysozyme in 1923 and the antibiotic substance penicillin from the mold *Penicillium notatum* in 1928, for which he shared the Nobel Prize in Physiology or Medicine in 1945 with Howard Florey and Ernst Boris Chain.

James Watson and Francis Crick: Francis Crick and James D. Watson, the two scientists who discovered the structure of DNA in 1953. James Dewey Watson, KBE, ForMemRS (born April 6, 1928), is an American molecular biologist, geneticist, and zoologist, best known as a co-discoverer of the structure of DNA in 1953 by Francis Crick. Watson, Crick, and Maurice Wilkins were awarded the 1962 Nobel Prize in Physiology or Medicine "for their discoveries concerning the molecular structure of nucleic acids and its significance for information transfer in living material." Francis Harry Compton Crick, OM, FRS (June 8, 1916 to July 28, 2004) was an English molecular biologist, biophysicist, and a neuroscientist.

Edward Jenner: Edward Anthony Jenner, FRS (May 17, 1749 to January 26, 1823) was an English physician and scientist from Berkeley, Gloucestershire, who was the pioneer of smallpox vaccine. He is often called "the father of immunology," and his work is said to have "saved more lives than the work of any other man."

Sir Louis Pasteur: Louis Pasteur was a French chemist and microbiologist who was one of the most important founders of medical microbiology. He is remembered for his remarkable breakthroughs in the causes and prevention of diseases. His discoveries reduced mortality from puerperal fever, and he created the first vaccines for rabies and anthrax. His experiments supported the germ theory of disease. He was best known to the general public for inventing a method to treat milk and wine in order to prevent it from causing sickness, a process that came to be called pasteurization. He is regarded as one of the three main founders of microbiology, together with Ferdinand Cohn and Robert Koch. He worked chiefly in Paris.

Paul Ehrlich: Paul Ehrlich (March 14, 1854 to August 20, 1915) was a German physician and scientist who worked in the fields of hematology, immunology, and chemotherapy. He invented the precursor technique to Gram staining bacteria, and the methods he developed for staining tissue made it possible to distinguish between different types of blood cells, which led to the capability to diagnose numerous blood diseases. His laboratory discovered Arsphenamine (Salvarsan), the first effective medicinal treatment for syphilis, thereby initiating and also naming the concept of chemotherapy. Ehrlich popularized the concept of a "magic bullet." He also made a decisive contribution to the development of an antiserum to combat diphtheria and conceived a methodology for standardizing therapeutic serums. In 1908 he received a Nobel Prize in Physiology or Medicine for his contributions to immunology.

1.7 Knowledge builder

PCR: Polymerase chain reaction (PCR) enables researchers to produce billions of copies of a specific DNA sequence as shown in the picture. This automated process bypasses the need to use bacteria for amplifying DNA. Developed in 1983 by Kary Mullis, PCR is now a common and often indispensable technique used in medical and biological research labs for a variety of applications. The PCR technique was patented by Kary Mullis and assigned to Cetus Corporation, where Mullis worked when he invented the technique in 1983. The PCR techniques have mainly used to study DNA cloning for sequencing, DNA-based phylogeny, or functional analysis of genes; the diagnosis of hereditary diseases; the identification of genetic fingerprints (used in forensic sciences and paternity testing); and the detection and diagnosis of infectious diseases. In 1993, Mullis was awarded the Nobel Prize in Chemistry along with Michael Smith for his work on PCR.

FISH: Fluorescence in situ hybridization (FISH is a cytogenetic technique to detect and localize the presence or absence of specific DNA sequences on chromosomes. FISH uses fluorescent probes that bind to only those parts of the chromosome with which they show a high degree of sequence complementarity. FISH is frequently used for finding specific topographies in DNA for use in genetic counseling, medicine, and species identification. FISH can also be used to detect and localize specific RNA targets in tumor cells, and pathological tissue samples.

Microarray: A microarray, also known as a DNA chip or biochip, is basically a collection of microscopic DNA spots attached to a solid surface (see picture). Scientists use DNA microarrays to measure the expression levels of large numbers of genes simultaneously or to genotype multiple regions of a genome. The gene expression can be used to measure the difference between the normal and diseased tissues or samples to be able to find out the role of different genes in the development of disease.

Gram-positive bacteria: Gram-positive bacteria are those that are stained dark blue or violet by Gram staining. Gram-positive organisms are able to retain the crystal violet stain because of the high amount of peptidoglycan in the cell wall. The examples of Gram-positive bacteria are *Streptococcus* and *Staphylococcus*.

Gram-negative bacteria: Gram-negative bacteria are bacteria that do not retain the crystal violet dye in the Gram staining procedure because these bacteria contain an outer membrane. The Proteobacteria are a major group of Gram-negative bacteria, including *Escherichia coli, Salmonella, Shigella,* and other Enterobacteriaceae, *Pseudomonas, Moraxella, Helicobacter, Stenotrophomonas, Bdellovibrio,* acetic acid bacteria, *Legionella* and numerous others.

Micro-array technique: A DNA microarray (also commonly known as a DNA chip or biochip) is a collection of microscopic DNA spots attached to a solid surface. Scientists use DNA microarrays to measure the expression levels of large numbers of genes simultaneously or to genotype multiple regions of a genome. Each DNA spot contains picomoles (10 – 12 moles) of a specific DNA sequence, known as probes (or reporters or oligos). These can be a short section of a gene or other DNA element that is used to hybridize a CDNA or CRNA (also called antisense RNA) sample (called target) under high-stringency conditions. Probe–target hybridization is usually detected and quantified by detection of fluorophore-, silver-, or chemiluminescence-labeled targets to determine relative abundance of nucleic acid sequences in the target.

Recombinant DNA technology: Recombinant DNA (rDNA) molecules are DNA sequences that result from the use of laboratory methods (molecular cloning) to bring together genetic material from multiple sources, creating sequences that would not otherwise be found in biological organisms. Recombinant DNA is possible because DNA molecules from all organisms share the same chemical structure; they differ only in the sequence of nucleotides within that identical overall structure. Consequently, when DNA from a foreign source links to host sequences that can drive DNA replication, and then is introduced into a host organism, the foreign DNA is replicated along with the host DNA.

Hybridoma technology: Hybridoma technology is a technology of forming hybrid cell lines (called hybridomas) by fusing a specific antibody-producing B cell with a myeloma (B cell cancer) cell that is selected for its ability to grow in tissue culture and for an absence of antibody chain synthesis. The antibodies produced by the hybridoma are all of a single specificity and are, therefore, monoclonal antibodies (in contrast to polyclonal antibodies). The production of monoclonal antibodies was invented by Cesar Milstein and Georges J. F. Köhler in 1975.

Biocompatible materials: A biocompatible material (sometimes shortened to biomaterial) is a synthetic or natural material used to replace part of a living system or to function in intimate contact with living tissue. Biocompatible materials are intended to interface with biological systems to evaluate, treat, augment, or replace any tissue, organ, or function of the body. Biomaterials are usually nonviable, but may also be viable.

Autologous cell transplantation: Autologous stem cell transplantation is a medical procedure in which stem cells (cells from which other cells of the same type develop) are removed, stored, and later given back to the same person. Though most frequently performed with hematopoietic stem cells (blood forming), cardiac cells have also been used successfully to repair damage caused by heart attacks.

FDA: The Food and Drug Administration (FDA or USFDA) is a regulatory agency of the United States Department of Health and Human Services, belonging to the US federal executive departments. The FDA is responsible for protecting and promoting public health through the regulation and supervision of food safety, tobacco products, dietary supplements, prescription and over-the-counter pharmaceutical drugs, vaccines, biopharmaceuticals, blood transfusions, medical devices, electromagnetic radiation-emitting devices, and veterinary products.

Geron Corporation: Geron Corporation is a biotechnology company located in Menlo Park, California, USA, that focuses on the development and commercialization of products in three specific areas: therapeutic products for cancer treatment; pharmaceuticals that activate telomerase in tissues impacted by cell aging, injury, or degenerative diseases; and cell-based therapies derived from human ESCs for treatment of various chronic diseases.

Further reading

Allen R, Millgate A, Chitty J, Thisleton J et al. 2004. RNAi-mediated replacement of morphine with the nonnarcotic alkaloid reticuline in opium poppy. *Nat Biotechnol* 22 (12): 1559–1566. doi:10.1038/nbt1033. PMID 15543134.

Altman J and Das GD 1965. Autoradiographic and histological evidence of postnatal hippocampal neurogenesis in rats. *J Compar Neurol* 124 (3): 319–335. doi:10.1002/cne.901240303. PMID 5861717.

Alvarez-Buylla A, Seri B, and Doetsch F 2002. Identification of neural stem cells in the adult vertebrate brain. *Brain Res Bull* 57 (6): 751–758. doi:10.1016/S0361-9230(01)00770-5. PMID 12031271.

Bains WE 1993. *Biotechnology from A to Z*. Oxford, UK: Oxford University Press.

Barnhart BJ 1989. DOE Human Genome Program. *Human Genome Quarterly* 1: 1. http://www.ornl.gov/sci/techresources/Human_Genome/publicat/hgn/v1n1/01doehgp. html (retrieved 2005-02-03).

Barrilleaux B, Phinney DG, Prockop DJ, and O'Connor KC 2006. Review: Ex vivo engineering of living tissues with adult stem cells. *Tissue Eng* 12 (11): 3007–3019. doi:10.1089/ten.2006.12.3007. PMID 17518617.

Beachy PA, Karhadkar SS, and Berman DM 2004. Tissue repair and stem cell renewal in carcinogenesis. *Nature* 432 (7015): 324–331. doi:10.1038/nature03100. PMID 15549094.

Benton D 1996. Bioinformatics—Principles and potentials of a new multidisciplinary tool. *Trends Biotechnol* 14:261–72.

Bjornson CR, Rietze RL, Reynolds BA et al. 1999. Turning brain into blood: A hematopoietic fate adopted by adult neural stem cells in vivo. *Science* 283 (5401): 534–537. doi:10.1126/science.283.5401.534. PMID 9915700.

ter Brake O, Westerink JT, and Berkhout B. 2010. Lentiviral vector engineering for anti-HIV RNAi gene therapy. *Methods Mol Biol* 614: 201–213. doi: 10.1007/978-1-60761-533-0_14.

Bull ND and Bartlett PF 2005. The adult mouse hippocampal progenitor is neurogenic but not a stem cell. *J Neurosci* 25 (47): 10815–10821. doi:10.1523/JNEUROSCI.3249-05.2005. PMID 16306394.

Cavalieri D, McGovern PE, Hart DL, Mortimer R, and Polsinelli M 2003. Evidence for *S. cerevisiae* fermentation in ancient wine. *J Mol Evol* 57: S226–S232.

Centeno CJ, Busse D, Kisiday J, Keohan C et al. 2008a. Increased knee cartilage volume in degenerative joint disease using percutaneously implanted, autologous mesenchymal stem cells. *Pain Phys* 11 (3): 343–353. PMID 18523506. http://www.painphysicianjournal.com/linkout_vw.php?issn=1533-3159&vol=11&page=343.

Centeno CJ, Busse D, Kisiday J, Keohan C et al. 2008b. Regeneration of meniscus cartilage in a knee treated with percutaneous implanted autologous mesenchymal stem cells. *Med Hypoth* 71 (6): 900–908. doi:10.1016/j.mehy.2008.06.042. PMID 18786777.

Chaudhary PM and Roninson IB 1991. Expression and activity of P-glycoprotein, a multidrug efflux pump, in human hematopoietic stem cells. *Cell* 66 (1): 85–94. doi:10.1016/0092-8674(91)90141-K. PMID 1712673.

Chiang C, Wang J, Jan F, Yeh S, and Gonsalves D. 2001. Comparative reactions of recombinant papaya ringspot viruses with chimeric coat protein (CP) genes and wild-type viruses on CP-transgenic papaya. *J Gen Virol* 82 (Part 11): 2827–2836. PMID 11602796.

Cogle CR, Guthrie SM, Sanders RC, Allen WL, Scott EW, and Petersen BE 2003. An overview of stem cell research and regulatory issues. *Mayo Clinic Proc* 78 (8): 993–1003. doi:10.4065/78.8.993. PMID 12911047.

Covey S, Al-Kaff N, Langara A, and Turner D 1997. Plants combat infection by gene silencing. *Nature* 385: 781–782. doi:10.1038/385781a0.

DeLisi C. 2001. Genomes: 15 years later a perspective by Charles DeLisi, HGP Pioneer. *Human Genome News* 11: 3–4. http://genome.gsc.riken.go.jp/hgmis/publicat/hgn/v11n3/05delisi.html (retrieved 2005-02-03).

Dirar H. 1993. *The Indigenous Fermented Foods of the Sudan: A Study in African Food and Nutrition*. UK: CAB International

Doetsch F, Petreanu L, Caille I, Garcia-Verdugo JM, and Alvarez-Buylla A 2002. EGF converts transit-amplifying neurogenic precursors in the adult brain into multipotent stem cells. *Neuron* 36 (6): 1021–1034. doi:10.1016/S0896-6273(02)01133-9. PMID 12495619.

Dontu G, Jackson KW, McNicholas E, Kawamura MJ et al. 2004. Role of Notch signaling in cell-fate determination of human mammary stem/progenitor cells. *Breast Cancer Res* 6 (6): R605–R615. doi:10.1186/bcr920. PMID 15535842.

Ecker JR and Davis RW 1986. Inhibition of gene expression in plant cells by expression of antisense RNA. *Proc Natl Acad Sci USA* 83 (15): 5372–5376. doi:10.1073/pnas.83.15.5372. PMID 16593734.

Fermented fruits and vegetables. 2007. A global perspective. FAO Agricultural Services Bulletins—134. http://www.fao.org/docrep/x0560e/x0560e05.htm (retrieved on 2007-01-28).

Fischer UM, Harting MT, Jimenez F et al. June 2009. Pulmonary passage is a major obstacle for intravenous stem cell delivery: The pulmonary first-pass effect. *Stem Cells Dev* 18 (5): 683–692. doi:10.1089/scd.2008.0253. PMID 19099374.

Gardner RL March 2002. Stem cells: Potency, plasticity and public perception. *J Anat* 200 (Part 3): 277–282. doi:10.1046/j.1469-7580.2002.00029.x. PMID 12033732.

Gavilano L, Coleman N, Burnley L, Bowman M, Kalengamaliro N et al. 2006. Genetic engineering of *Nicotiana tabacum* for reduced nornicotine content. *J Agric Food Chem* 54 (24): 9071–9078. doi:10.1021/jf0610458. PMID 17117792.

Gimble JM, Katz AJ, and Bunnell BA 2007. Adipose-derived stem cells for regenerative medicine. *Circ Res* 100 (9): 1249–1260. doi:10.1161/01.RES.0000265074.83288.09. PMID 17495232.

Guo S and Kemphues K 1995. Par-1, a gene required for establishing polarity in C. elegans embryos, encodes a putative Ser/Thr kinase that is asymmetrically distributed. *Cell* 81 (4): 611–620. doi:10.1016/0092-8674(95)90082-9. PMID 7758115.

Kruger GM, Mosher JT, Bixby S, Joseph N et al. 2002. Neural crest stem cells persist in the adult gut but undergo changes in self-renewal, neuronal subtype potential, and factor responsiveness. *Neuron* 35 (4): 657–669. doi:10.1016/S0896-6273(02)00827-9. PMID 12194866.

Le L, Lorenz Y, Scheurer S, Fötisch K, Enrique E, Bartra J et al. 2006. Design of tomato fruits with reduced allergenicity by dsRNAi-mediated inhibition of ns-LTP (Lyc e 3) expression. *Plant Biotechnol J* 4 (2): 231–242. doi:10.1111/j.1467-7652.2005.00175.x. PMID 17177799.

Lewis PD 1968. Mitotic activity in the primate subependymal layer and the genesis of gliomas. *Nature* 217 (5132): 974–975. doi:10.1038/217974a0. PMID 4966809.

Liu S, Dontu G, and Wicha MS 2005. Mammary stem cells, self-renewal pathways, and carcinogenesis. *Breast Cancer Res* 7 (3): 86–95. doi:10.1186/bcr1021. PMID 15987436.

Maggie F (Reuters) 2006. U.S. firm says it made stem cells from human testes. *Washington Post*. http://www.washingtonpost.com/wp-dyn/content/article/2006/04/01/AR2006040101145.html.

Marshall GP, Laywell ED, Zheng T, Steindler DA, and Scott EW 2006. In vitro-derived neural stem cells function as neural progenitors without the capacity for self-renewal. *Stem Cells* 24 (3): 731–738. doi:10.1634/stemcells.2005-0245. PMID 16339644.

Matzke MA and Matzke AJM 2004. Planting the seeds of a new paradigm. *PLoS Biol* 2 (5): e133. doi:10.1371/journal.pbio.0020133. PMID 15138502.

Mol JNM and van der Krol AR 1991. *Antisense Nucleic Acids and Proteins: Fundamentals and Applications*. pp. 248. New York: Marcel Dekker.

Murrell W, Féron F, Wetzig A et al. 2005. Multipotent stem cells from adult olfactory mucosa. *Dev Dynam* 233 (2): 496–515. doi:10.1002/dvdy.20360. PMID 15782416.

Napoli C, Lemieux C, and Jorgensen R 1990. Introduction of a chimeric chalcone synthase gene into *Petunia* results in reversible co-suppression of homologous genes in trans. *Plant Cell* 2 (4): 279–289. doi:10.1105/tpc.2.4.279. PMID 12354959.

Niggeweg R, Michael A, and Martin C 2004. Engineering plants with increased levels of the antioxidant chlorogenic acid. *Nat Biotechnol* 22 (6): 746–754. doi:10.1038/nbt966. PMID 15107863.

Nora S 2008. A source of men's stem cells—Stem cells from human testes could be used for personalized medicine. *Technol Rev*. http://www.technologyreview.com/biomedicine/21487/.

Pederson RA 1999. Embryonic stem cells for medicine. *Sci Am* 280: 68–73.

Phinney DG and Prockop DJ 2007. Concise review: Mesenchymal stem/multipotent stromal cells: The state of transdifferentiation and modes of tissue repair—Current views. *Stem Cells* 25 (11): 2896–2902. doi:10.1634/stemcells.2007-0637. PMID 17901396.

Ratajczak MZ, Machalinski B, Wojakowski W, Ratajczak J, and Kucia M 2007. A hypothesis for an embryonic origin of pluripotent Oct-4(+) stem cells in adult bone marrow and other tissues. *Leukemia* 21 (5): 860–867. doi:10.1038/sj.leu.2404630. PMID 17344915.

Ratcliff F, Harrison B, and Baulcombe D 1997. A similarity between viral defense and gene silencing in plants. *Science* 276: 1558–1560. doi:10.1126/science.276.5318.1558.

Reynolds BA and Weiss S 1992. Generation of neurons and astrocytes from isolated cells of the adult mammalian central nervous system. *Science* 255 (5052): 1707–1710. doi:10.1126/science.1553558. PMID 1553558.

Rick W 2006. Embryonic stem cell success. *Washington Post*. http://www.washingtonpost.com/wp-dyn/content/article/2006/03/24/AR2006032401721.html.

Rob W 2008. *Testicle Stem Cells Become Bone, Muscle in German Experiments.Bloomberg*. http://www.bloomberg.com/apps/news?pid=20601124&sid=aNmiXs8SPp4w&refer=home.

Romano N and Macino G 1992. Quelling: Transient inactivation of gene expression in *Neurospora crassa* by transformation with homologous sequences. *Mol Microbiol* 6 (22): 3343–3353. doi:10.1111/j.1365-2958.1992.tb02202.x. PMID 1484489.

Rose D 2008. Claudia Castillo gets windpipe tailor-made from her own stem cells. *The Times*. London: The Times Newspapers Ltd. http://www.timesonline.co.uk/tol/life_and_style/health/article5183686.ece (retrieved 2008-2011).

Sanders R and Hiatt W 2005. Tomato transgene structure and silencing. *Nat Biotechnol* 23 (3): 287–289. doi:10.1038/nbt0305-287b. PMID 15765076.

Shi S, Bartold PM, Miura M, Seo BM, Robey PG, and Gronthos S 2005. The efficacy of mesenchymal stem cells to regenerate and repair dental structures. *Orthod Craniofac Res* 8 (3): 191–199. doi:10.1111/j.1601-6343.2005.00331.x. PMID 16022721.

Sieber-Blum M and Hu Y 2008. Epidermal neural crest stem cells (EPI-NCSC) and pluripotency. *Stem Cell Rev* 4 (4): 256–260. doi:10.1007/s12015-008-9042-0. PMID 18712509.

Siritunga D and Sayre R 2003. Generation of cyanogen-free transgenic cassava. *Planta* 217 (3): 367–373. doi:10.1007/s00425-003-1005-8. PMID 14520563.

Sugihara TF 1985. Microbiology of breadmaking. In *Microbiology of Fermented Foods*, ed. B.J.B. Wood, UK: Elsevier Applied Science Publishers.

Sunilkumar G, Campbell L, Puckhaber L, Stipanovic R, and Rathore K 2006. Engineering cotton seed for use in human nutrition by tissue-specific reduction of toxic gossypol. *Proc Natl Acad Sci USA* 103 (48): 18054–18059. doi:10.1073/pnas.0605389103. PMID 17110445.

Takahashi K and Yamanaka S 2006. Induction of pluripotent stem cells from mouse embryonic and adult fibroblast cultures by defined factors. *Cell* 126 (4): 663–676. doi:10.1016/j.cell.2006.07.024. PMID 16904174.

Van Blokland R, Van der Geest N et al. 1994. Transgene-mediated suppression of chalcone synthase expression in *Petunia* hybrida results from an increase in RNA turnover. *Plant J* 6: 861–877. doi:10.1046/j.1365-313X.1994.6060861.x/abs/. http://www.blackwell-synergy.com/links/doi/10.1046/ j.1365-313X.1994.6060861.x/abs/.

Wakitani S, Nawata M, Tensho K, Okabe T, Machida H, and Ohgushi H 2007. Repair of articular cartilage defects in the patello-femoral joint with autologous bone marrow mesenchymal cell transplantation: Three case reports involving nine defects in five knees. *J Tissue Eng Regen Med* 1 (1): 74–79. doi:10.1002/term.8. PMID 18038395.

Zadeh A and Foster G 2004. Transgenic resistance to tobacco ringspot virus. *Acta Virol* 48 (3): 145–152. PMID 15595207.

chapter two

Human diseases

Causes and reasons

2.1 Introduction

The human body has an intrinsically controlled system, also called an immune defense system, to fight back disease and its infections and in case the body is unable to control infection or deficiency on its own, it then gives the signals to patients in the form of pain, fever, and/or distress. These symptoms become indicator for the development of disease. Therefore, disease can be defined as an abnormal condition affecting the body of an organism. It is often interpreted to be a medical condition associated with specific symptoms and signs. Diseases can also be caused by external factors, for example, in the case of food poisoning caused by consuming bacterial contaminated food. Disease can also be caused by internal factors, for example, in the case of infectious disease, such as autoimmune diseases, where the body's own defense system works against itself. Moreover, human disease is often used to refer to the condition that causes pain, dysfunction, suffering, and social problems. In a broader sense, the disease sometimes includes injuries, disabilities, disorders, syndromes, infections, whereas isolated symptoms and irregular behaviors may be considered distinguishable categories. There is another type of disease condition, which is not about the dysfunction of a particular organ but the psychology of the affected person, which may be included as depression and anxiety-like conditions.

2.2 Human disease

To understand the human disease comprehensively, it is very important to know how diseases are caused and its mode of transmission. The human gets disease a number of ways that include an infection caused by a microorganism, deficiencies due to low levels of certain biochemicals in the body, or genetic alteration or mutation of gene(s) in the body's cells. All these diseases have different implications on a patient's health and status. We have classified human diseases in various subtypes based on their actions on the human body (Figure 2.1).

2.2.1 Infection

One of the main types of disease in humans is infection which is usually caused by microorganism's assault in the human body. This term, infection, broadly refers to any abnormal condition of the human body that impairs normal function of the body. Generally, this term is used to denote specific infectious diseases, which are clinically evident diseases resulting from the presence of pathogenic microorganisms such as viruses, bacteria, fungi, protozoa, multicellular parasites, and also due to aberrant proteins known as prions. The infection that does not produce any clinically evident impairment of normal functioning is not considered a disease. Diseases which are caused by noninfectious means are called

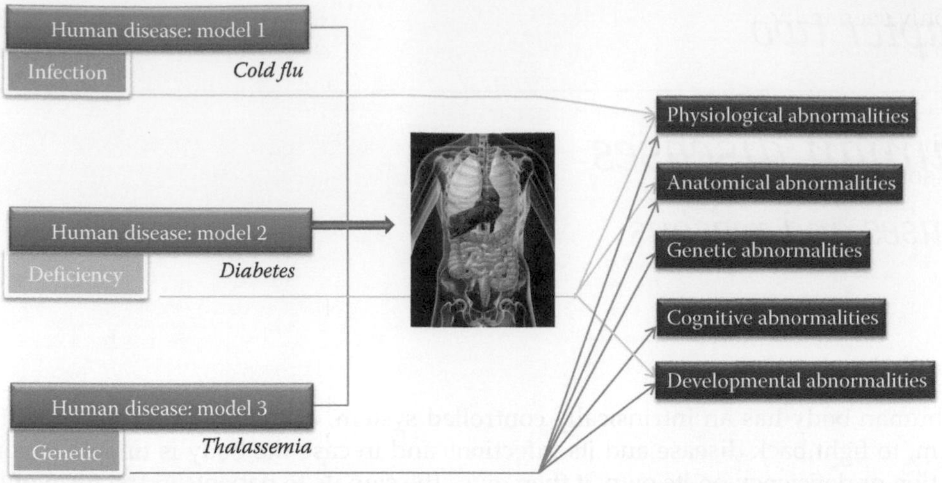

Figure 2.1 Human body and disease.

anoninfectious disease which includes cancer, heart disease, and genetic disease as a few examples.

2.2.2 *Illness*

Another prominent feature of human disease is about the patient's personal experience of his or her disease. In this condition, it is possible for a person to be diseased without showing any symptoms such as fever and pain. Illness is often not due to infection, but a collection of complex responses that include lethargy, depression, anorexia, sleepiness, hyperalgesia, and the inability to concentrate.

2.2.3 *Disorder*

Disorder is another type of disease that has been associated with a functional abnormality or disturbance of physiological or metabolic functions of the human body. Clinical disorders can be categorized into mental disorders, physical disorders, genetic disorders, emotional and behavioral disorders. The word disorder is often considered less branding than the word disease and, therefore, is preferred terminology in some medical situations. In neurological conditions, the term mental disorder is used as a way of recognizing the complex interaction of biological and psychological factors. However, the term disorder is also used in many other fields of medicine, primarily to identify physical disorders that are not caused by infectious organisms.

2.2.4 *Medical condition*

There is another condition in which a patient gets physical or accidental injuries known as a medical condition. Medical conditions also include normal health situations like pregnancy. Though the term medical condition generally includes mental illnesses, in some circumstances the term is also used specifically to denote any illness, injury, or disease, except mental illnesses. All mental or brain-related disorders used the *Diagnostic and Statistical Manual of Mental Disorders* for describing the illness and this practice is also commonly seen in the neurological literature. With regard to health insurance companies, they do have a set of policies which define a medical condition as any illness, injury, or disease except for psychiatric illnesses. For example, the term medical condition is sometimes preferred by people with health issues that they do not consider being injurious, such as pregnancy. On the other hand, by emphasizing the medical nature of the condition, this term is sometimes rejected by supporters of the autism rights movement.

2.2.5 *Morbidity*

Morbidity is, in general terms, another condition which refers to a un-well state, disability, or poor health due to any cause. This term is normally used to refer to the existence of disease or to the degree that the health condition affects the patient. In severe medical medications, the level of morbidity is often measured by intensive care unit (ICU) scoring systems. In addition, comorbidity is the simultaneous presence of two medical conditions in the same patient such as having Alzheimer's disease and Parkinson's disease together. In the epidemiology field, the word morbidity can refer to either the incidence ratio or the prevalence of a disease or medical condition.

2.2.6 *Other classifications*

In addition to above-mentioned diseases and health conditions, human diseases can also be classified based on the occurrence and progression in the body such as localized disease, disseminated disease, and systemic disease. A localized disease is an infectious process that initiates in and is confined to one organ system or general area in the body, such as a twisted ankle, or a swelling of the hand. Moreover, localized cancer that has not extended beyond the margins of the organ involved can also be defined as localized disease, while cancers that extend into other tissues are termed as nonlocalized. Localized diseases can be differentiated from disseminated diseases and systemic diseases. In addition, some diseases are capable of changing from local to disseminate diseases. Pneumonia, for example, is generally confined to one or both lungs, but can become disseminated through sepsis, in which the microbe responsible for the pneumonia the bloodstream or lymphatic system and is transported to distant sites in the body. When that occurs, the process cannot be referred as a localized disease, but rather as a disseminated disease. In humans, disseminated disease refers to a diffuse disease process, generally either infectious, but occasionally also referring to a connective tissue disease. A disseminated infection, for example, is one that has extended beyond its origin and involved the bloodstream to migrate to other areas of the body. Correspondingly, metastatic cancer can be viewed as a disseminated infection in that it has extended into the bloodstream or the lymphatic system to migrate to distant sites in the patient. A systemic disease is one that affects multiple organs and tissues of a patient.

2.3 *Classification of diseases*

As we have learned in the previous sections about clinical or medical conditions arising due to various diseases, you may find a great deal of overlapping in the different types of diseases. Nevertheless, we can broadly classify diseases into two different types: infectious and noninfectious. Infectious diseases are those that are caused by parasites, bacteria, and virus or fungus, and noninfectious diseases are those which are caused by nutrient deficiency, genetic, or environmental factors.

2.3.1 Infectious diseases

In simple form, an infectious disease is a disease caused by bacteria, viruses, fungus, or protozoans. Nevertheless, some infectious diseases are not transmissible, while others may be transmitted from animal to person; for example, bird flu and cat scratch disease or from person to person such as sexually transmitted or blood transfused diseases. Infectious diseases are also named as communicable diseases or transmissible diseases due to their transmission from one person or species to another species by a replicating agent. Moreover, transmission of an infectious disease may occur through one or more of diverse passages including physical contact with infected individuals. The infections can also be transmitted through liquids, food, body fluids, contaminated objects, or airborne inhalation. It has been found that infectious diseases usually require a more specialized path of an infection, such as transmission through a vector, and more importantly, blood or needle transmission, or sexual transmission, are usually regarded as contagious diseases.

2.3.1.1 Bacterial diseases

The bacterial infections are the most common type of infections among humans that are caused by microorganisms. These tiny microorganisms cannot be seen without a microscope and these microorganisms include viruses, fungi, and some parasites as well as bacteria. The bacteria can be beneficial as well as harmful to the human body. You might be surprised to know that the vast majority of bacteria do not cause disease and many microorganisms are actually helpful and even necessary for good health. In addition, millions of bacteria normally live on the skin and in a human body such as the intestines, genitalia, or armpit. Bacterial diseases are caused by harmful bacteria which get into an area of the body that is normally germfree, such as the bladder. Additionally harmful bacteria, also called as pathogenic, include *Neisseria meningitides,* which causes meningitis; *Streptococcus pneumonia,* which causes pneumonia; and *Staphylococcus aureus,* which causes a variety of infections. Other common pathogenic bacteria include *Helicobacter pylori,* which cause gastric ulcers, and *Escherichia coli,* and *Salmonella,* which both cause food poisoning (Figure 2.2). It has been found that pathogenic bacteria can enter the body through a variety of means, through nose and lungs, food, or through sexual contact. As soon as bacteria enter the body, a healthy immune system can recognize the bacteria as foreign invaders and try to kill or stop the bacteria from reproducing. Nevertheless, even in a healthy person with a healthy immune system, the body is not always able to fight the bacteria from multiplying and spreading. For instance, harmful bacteria reproduce and many emit toxins substances which can damage the cells of the body.

When the patient is infected with bacterial infections, which may result in increased body temperature or pains; occasionally bacterial infections can lead to serious, even life-threatening complications such as sepsis, kidney failure, toxic shock syndrome, and finally death. People at risk for bacterial diseases and its complications include those who have had a significant exposure to pathogenic bacteria, such as *Neisseria meningitides,* or *Streptococcus pneumonia.* In addition, other risks factors which are associated with bacterial infections are compromised immune system or combined immune deficiencies. People who occasionally take certain medications, such as corticosteroids, are also at risk for infectious bacterial diseases because corticosteroids are known to suppress the body's natural immune response. Additional risk factors for being infected with bacterial infection include undernourishment, high stress levels, and having a genetic susceptibility to bacterial infection.

The first step toward treating an individual who is suffering from bacterial infections, is to know the cause of such infection and it is generally done by diagnostic tests beginning with taking a thorough personal and family medical interventions. The kinds

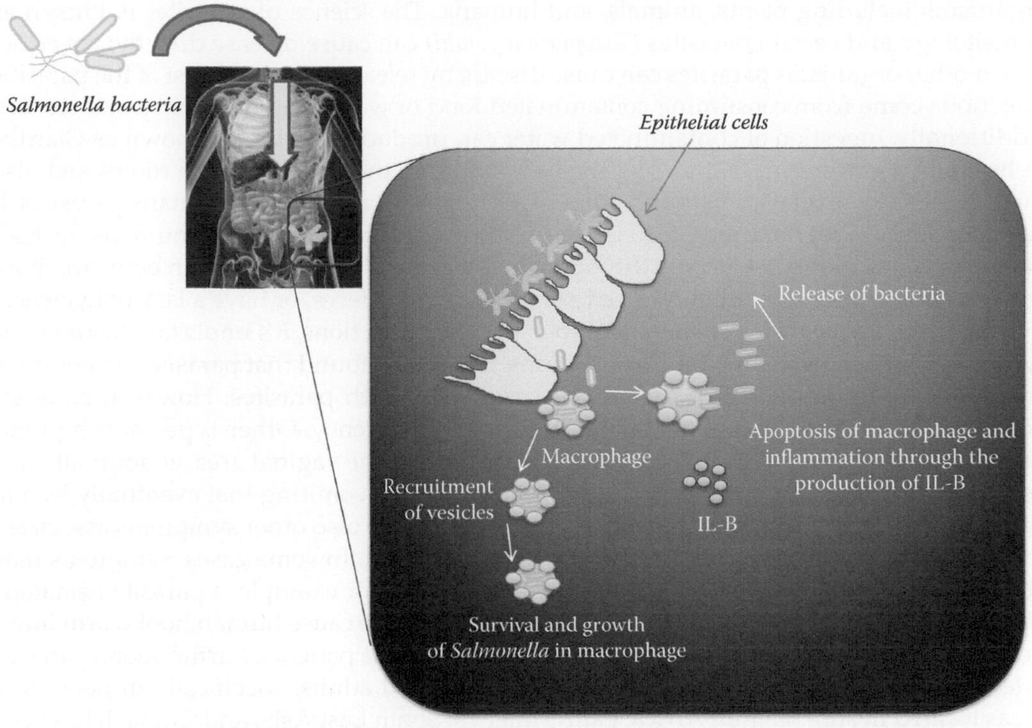

Figure 2.2 Food poisoning by *Salmonella*.

of diagnostic testing performed for a so-called bacterial disease varies depending on the symptoms. A complete blood count is a blood test that is generally done to know the bacterial infections. In addition, a complete blood count measures the number of different types of blood cells that include white blood cells (WBCs). There is an increase in the number of different types of WBCs in the infected person. In addition to this, a culture and sensitivity test can be accomplished as this test requires taking a small sample (blood) from the patient that is suspected to be infected with a bacterial infection and grows the sample in a culture. This test decides the type of bacteria causing a bacterial disease as well as which antibiotic drugs would be most effective in treating that specific bacteria.

In addition, sample can also be collected using lumbar puncture of the spinal cord which involves extracting a small amount of cerebro-spinal fluid (CSF) with a sterile needle. The sample of CSF is tested for WBCs and other symptoms of bacterial diseases that may be in the central nervous system. In addition, x-rays can be performed to assist in the diagnosis of some type of bacterial diseases. This may include taking a chest x-ray and computed tomography (CT) scan for further investigation. Additional tests can be recommended by the physician in order to confirm other diseases that may complement bacterial diseases, such as diarrhea or neck stiffness. It is possible that a diagnosis of bacterial diseases can be overlooked or delayed because some symptoms, such as fever, headache, and nausea and vomiting are similar to symptoms of other diseases.

2.3.1.2 *Parasitic diseases*

Like bacteria, many parasites are harmless and do not cause diseases, however there some parasites which cause disease in humans. Also parasitic diseases can affect almost all living organisms including plants, animals, and humans. The science of parasites is known as parasitology and certain parasites (*Toxoplasma gondii*) can cause disease directly; nevertheless in other organisms parasites can cause disease by releasing toxins. Most of the parasitic infections come from consuming contaminated food or water, bug bites, or sexual contact. Additionally, ingestion of contaminated water can produce the disease known as Giardia. In humans, parasites normally enter the body through the skin or mouth routes and also through close contact with pets and animals, as dogs and cats are host to many parasites. It has been found that hundreds of diseases can be spread from animals to humans through parasites. Some of the risk factors through which parasites enter the human body are those who walk bare feet, do not maintain adequate disposal of feces, or have a lack of hygiene.

Before considering the treatment of such parasitic infections, it's important to know the symptoms associated with parasitic infections. It has been found that parasites do not show any specific symptoms which can be only associated with parasites. However, parasites do show few symptoms like anemia or a hormone deficiency. Other types of symptoms caused by parasites include itching affecting the anus or the vaginal area, abdominal pain, bowel obstructions, increased appetite, and diarrhea and vomiting that eventually lead to dehydration, weight loss, and sleeping problems. There are also other symptoms associated that include the presence of worms in the vomit or stools. In some cases, symptoms may also be misdiagnosed as pneumonia or food poisoning. For example, a parasite nematode *Necator americanus* and *Ancylostoma duodenale* are known to cause human hookworm infection, which leads to anemia and protein malnutrition in the patients. Furthermore, parasitic infection can affect more than 700 million children and adults, specifically in poor rural areas located in sub-Saharan Africa, Latin America, South East Asia, and China. It has been further stated that chronic hookworm in children leads to impaired physical and mental development and also effects learning capabilities. Pregnant women affected by a hookworm infection can also develop anemia which results in negative outcomes both for the mother and the infant. The parasitic infections can be treated with the drugs Albendazole and Mebendazole, which can be administered to affected and nonaffected populations to control hookworm infection. It has been found that for many parasitic diseases there is no treatment and in the case of serious situations, medication to remove the parasite is administered, while in some cases, a symptom relief medication is used.

2.3.1.3 Viral diseases

Similar to bacterial infection, a viral infection is a type of disease caused by a virus. A viral infection occurs when a virus enters the body through breathing air contaminated with a virus, eating contaminated food, or by having intercourse with a person who is infected with a virus. Additionally a viral infection can also be caused by an insect bite. It's important to know the process of viral infections in order to use any treatment modalities. The infection starts with an entry of the virus in the human body's cells and the virus then spreads to other cells by replication. The infection results in a variety of different characters that depends on the type of viral infection and individual factors. The most common symptoms of a viral infection include body pain, fatigue, flu-like symptoms, and fever. Many types of viral infections, such as a cold or flu are time bounded that means that the viral infection causes illness for a period of time, then it resolves and the symptoms disappear. Nevertheless, some patients are at risk for developing serious complications of viral infection. In addition, certain types of viral infections are not self-limiting and cause serious complications and are eventually fatal. Additionally, there are many types of viruses that cause a wide variety of viral infections, for example, there are over 200 different viruses that can cause a cold. In addition, there are other common viruses including

Table 2.1 List of Diseases Caused by Pathogenic Bacteria

Name of disease	Name of bacteria
Food poisoning	*Escherichia coli*
Strep throat	*Streptococcus pyrogenes*
Tuberculosis	*Mycobacterium tuberculosis*
Legionnaire's disease	*Legionella pneumonia*
Cholera	*Vibrio cholerae*
Syphilis	*Treponema pallidum*
Gonorrhea	*Neisseria gonorrhea*
Anthrax	*Bacillus anthracis*
Leprosy	*Mycobacterium leprae*
Bubonic plague	*Yersinia pestis*
Tetanus	*Clostridium tetani*
Pneumonia	*Streptococcus pneumoniae*
Influenza	*Haemophilus influenzae*
Pneumonia	*Klebsiella pneumoniae*
Septicemia	*Pseudomonas aeruginosa*
Respiratory tract infections	*Moraxella catarrhalis*
Pneumonia	*Chlamydophila pneumoniae*
Walking pneumonia	*Mycoplasma pneumoniae*
Pneumonia	*Legionella pneumophila*
Whooping cough	*Bordetella pertussis*
Lyme disease	*Borrelia burgdorferi*
Gas gangrene	*Clostridium perfringens*
Tularemia	*Francisella tularensis*
Leprosy	*Mycobacterium leprae*

the influenza virus, which can cause influenza or the flu. In addition, the Epstein–Barr virus and the cytomegalovirus can also cause infectious mononucleosis.

The diagnosis of a viral infection begins with taking a thorough medical examination. Diagnosing some viral infections, such as seasonal influenza, may be made based on a history and physical examination. Generally, blood tests which include complete blood count (CBC) may be done to check the viral infections. Moreover, a complete blood count generally measures the numbers of different types of blood cells, including WBCs. Different types of WBCs increase in number in distinctive ways during an infectious process. A culture test may also be performed and as this test requires a small sample from the body area (throat, blood, saliva, or sputum) that is suspected to be infected with a virus. The virus can be further cultured in a sterile laboratory to determine the type of microorganism causing illness. The list of diseases caused by pathogenic bacteria is shown in the Table 2.1.

2.3.2 *Noninfectious diseases*

In humans, diseases are also caused by noninfectious ways. There are many varieties of noninfectious diseases which are caused by the environment, nutritional deficiencies, lifestyle choices, or genetic inheritances. Unlike infectious diseases, noninfectious diseases are not communicable or contagious, even though some kind of infectious diseases can be passed down genetically to the children of a carrier. It has been found that infectious diseases were the main cause of death in the world and, undeniably, in some developing regions of the world this may still be the case. With the development of antibiotics and vaccinations, infectious disease is no longer the prominent cause of death in the world especially in the developed countries. In contrast, noninfectious diseases are now accountable as the prominent reasons of death in both developed and some developing countries. Particular medical conditions are not infectious in nature and are also not normally classified with noninfectious diseases. These include physiological malfunction, brain illnesses, aging, and obesity.

The noninfectious diseases can be categorized into two types, which include genetically inherited disease and environmentally induced disease. The genetic disorders are caused by mutation in genetic information that produces diseases in the affected people. Furthermore, these genetic mutations may be caused due to (i) a change in the chromosome numbers, (ii) a defect in a single gene caused by mutation, and (iii) a rearrangement of genetic information. Cystic fibrosis is an example of an inherited disease that is caused by a genetic mutation. In cystic fibrosis the faulty gene impairs the normal movement of sodium chloride within the cell, which causes the mucus-secreting organs to produce abnormally thick mucus. In cystic fibrosis disease, the gene is found to be in a recessive mode, which means that a person can have two copies of the faulty gene for them to develop the disease. In cystic fibrosis disease, the body organs known to be affected include the respiratory, digestive, reproductive systems, and sweat glands. The environmentally induced, noninfectious disease is caused by external factors such as sunlight, food, pollution, and lifestyle. Examples of environmentally induced disease include cardiovascular disease, chronic obstructive pulmonary disease caused by smoking tobacco, diabetes mellitus type 2, and skin cancer caused by harmful radiation from the sun.

2.3.2.1 Necrosis

The body cells do degenerate and eventually die throughout the human life; such premature or accidental death of living cells is called necrosis. Additionally, necrosis is caused by external factors to the cell or tissue, such as an infection or toxins. The cell death in necrosis is different from apoptosis, which is basically a programmed cell death. Although apoptosis often provides beneficial effects to the organism, necrosis has been almost always harmful and can be serious (Figure 2.3). Moreover, cells that die due to necrosis do not usually send the same signals to the immune system that cells undergoing apoptosis do. This prevents nearby phagocytes from locating and engulfing the dead cells, leading to a build-up of dead tissue and cell debris at or near the site of the cell death. The different types of necrosis are shown in Table 2.2.

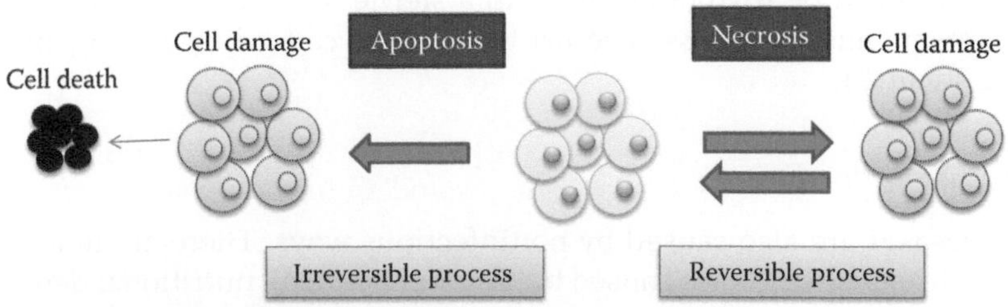

Figure 2.3 Cell damage and recovery process.

Table 2.2 Types of Necrosis

Types of necrosis	Pathology
Coagulative necrosis	It is typically seen in low-oxygen environments, such as an infection.
Liquefactive necrosis	It is usually associated with cellular destruction and pus formation such as pneumonia.
Gummatous necrosis	It is restricted to necrosis involving spirochaetal infections such as syphilis.
Hemorrhagic necrosis	It is due to obstruction of the venous drainage of an organ or tissue.
Caseous necrosis	It is caused by mycobacteria such as tuberculosis, fungi, and some foreign substances.
Fatty necrosis	This results from the action of lipases on fatty tissues.
Fibrinoid necrosis	It is caused by immune-mediated vascular damage.

The process of necrosis usually begins with certain morphological changes such as cell swelling, chromatin digestion, and disruption of the plasma membrane and organelle membranes. Moreover, late necrosis are generally characterized by extensive DNA hydrolysis, vacuolation of the endoplasmic reticulum, organelle breakdown, and cell damage. In necrosis, inflammation causes a release of intracellular content. Treatment of necrosis typically involves two different processes. Usually, the underlying cause of the necrosis can be treated before the dead tissue itself can be dealt with. For example, a snake bite victim receives an antivenom medicine to stop the spread of the toxins, while an infected patient can also receive antibiotics. In spite of halting an initial cause of the necrosis, the necrotic tissue will persist in the body. Furthermore, the body's immune response to apoptosis is not triggered by necrotic cell death. The standard therapy of necrosis is surgical removal of necrotic tissue and, depending on the severity of the necrosis and removal, could be a small part of skin or removal of an organ (Figure 2.4).

2.3.2.2 Apoptosis

Unlike necrosis, an apoptosis is the natural way of cell death, also known as programmed cell death, that can occur in multicellular organisms. Apoptosis generally begins with biochemical changes in the cell leading to morphological changes and to final death. These changes include loss of cell membrane morphology, cell shrinkage, nuclear fragmentation, chromatin condensation, and chromosomal DNA fragmentation. The process of apoptosis is controlled by a diverse range of cell signaling pathways, which may originate either extracellular or intracellular sources. Extracellular signals may include toxins, hormones, growth factors, nitric oxide, or cytokines that can either cross the plasma membrane or transducer to affect a response. These signals may produce positive or negative effects on apoptosis. In addition, binding and subsequent initiation of apoptosis by a molecule (e.g., a drug) is termed as positive induction, while an inhibition of apoptosis by a molecule is termed negative induction. Moreover, a cell which initiates an intracellular apoptotic signaling in response to a stress can also trigger cell death pathway. The binding of nuclear receptors by glucocorticoids, heat, radiation, nutrient deprivation, viral infection, hypoxia, and increased intracellular calcium concentration can all trigger the release of intracellular apoptotic signals by a damaged cell (Figure 2.3).

Before the actual process of cell death is being initiated, apoptotic proteins need to activate to initiate the apoptosis pathway because this step allows apoptotic signals to cause cell death. There are several regulatory proteins involved in the apoptosis pathway; however, two main methods of regulation have been reported which target mitochondria

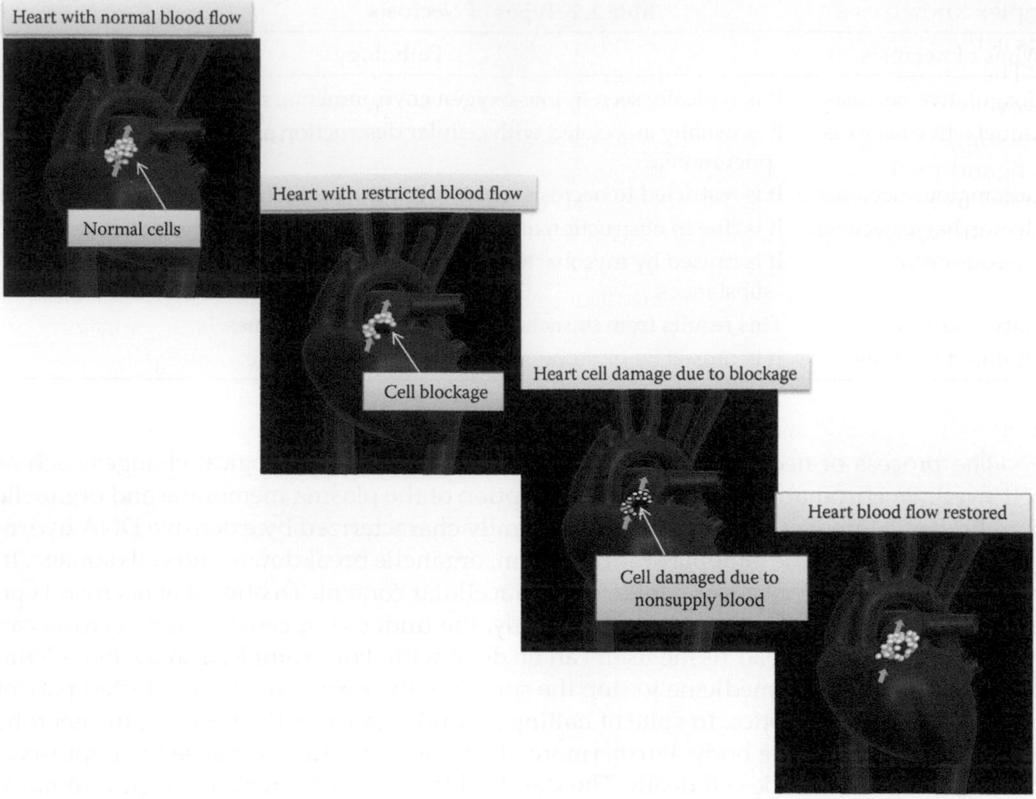

Figure 2.4 Cell damage by necrosis.

functionality. As you are aware, mitochondria is a powerhouse of the cell and known to create energy for the cell. The process of creating cell energy is known as cellular respiration and most of the chemical reactions involved in cellular respiration take place in the mitochondria. In the absence of functional mitochondria, a cell ceases to respire aerobically and quickly dies. In the case of apoptosis, mitochondria get affected by different pathways, for example, on the onset of apoptosis, mitochondrial swell through the formation of membrane pores, which may lead to an increase in the penetrability of the mitochondrial membrane. Furthermore, there are also reports which suggest that nitric oxide can induce apoptosis by helping to disintegrate the membrane potential of mitochondria and therefore make it more permeable.

During the apoptosis induction, mitochondria are known to release certain proteins which are known as second mitochondria-derived activator of caspases (SMAC). These SMAC are released into the cytosol following an increase in permeability during apoptosis. These SMAC also bind to inhibitors of apoptosis proteins (IAPs) and deactivate them, consequently allowing apoptosis to progress. Moreover, IAP normally suppresses the activity of a group of cysteine proteases, called caspases, which carry out the degradation of the cell. Furthermore, cytochrome c is also released from mitochondria due to the formation of a channel, mitochondria-derived activator of caspases (MAC) in the outer mitochondrial membrane. Once cytochrome c is released, it binds with apoptotic protease activating factors such as Apaf-1 and ATP, which then bind to pro-caspase-9 site to generate a protein complex known as an apoptosome. Furthermore, this apoptosome cleaves the pro-caspase to its active form of caspase-9, which in turn activates the effector caspase-3.

The mechanism behind the initiation of apoptotic pathways is not clearly understood; however, two theories have direct initiation of apoptotic mechanisms in mammals has been suggested. They are the TNF-induced (tumor necrosis factor) model and the Fas-Fas ligand-mediated model, both involving receptors of the TNF receptor (TNFR) family coupled to extrinsic signals. TNF which is also a cytokine is generally produced by activated macrophages, and most cells in the human body have two types of TNF receptors such as TNFR1 and TNFR2. The binding of TNF to TNFR1 has been reported to initiate the pathway that leads to caspase activation via the intermediate membrane proteins TNF receptor-associated death domain (TRADD) and Fas-associated death domain protein (FADD). Furthermore, the binding of this receptor can indirectly lead to the activation of transcription factors that are involved in cell survival. There has been a link between TNF and apoptosis because there is an abnormal production of TNF in several human diseases, especially in autoimmune diseases.

2.3.2.3 Nutritional deficiency diseases

Food-based nutrition is essential for normal and healthy body function and not taking the required amount of nutrition may lead to a deficiency in the body. These nutritional deficiencies may cause the development of a disease, such as rickets or scurvy. These diseases are due to insufficient intake, digestion, absorption, or utilization of a nutrient. It has been shown that nutrient deficiency diseases occur when there is an absence of essential nutrients in the body. One of the major reasons of nutritional deficiencies is the lack of food. Another cause for a deficiency disease may be due to biological imbalance in the metabolic system of an individual. There are more than 50 known nutrients in food which enable body tissues to grow and maintain themselves and these nutrients contribute to the energy requirements of the individual organism to regulate the processes of the body function. Among several nutrients, carbohydrates, fats, and proteins generally provide the body with energy. Besides the water and fiber content of food, which is also important for their role in nutrition, the nutrients can be classified into four different groups: proteins, vitamins, fats, and minerals. Furthermore, there are approximately 25 mineral elements in the body and those which appear in large quantities are called macro minerals, whereas those that are in small amounts are micro minerals. These essential minerals are cobalt, copper, fluorine, iodine, iron, sodium, chromium, calcium, phosphorous, and tin, whereas aluminum, lead, and mercury are not as essential. The various diseases caused by nutritional deificiences are listed in Table 2.3.

Table 2.3 Diseases Caused by Nutritional Deficiencies

Name of disease	Causes	Symptoms
Scurvy	Vitamin deficiency	Hemorrhage marks
Beriberi	Lacking Vitamin B1	Fatigue, loss of appetite
Pellagra	Lacking Vitamin B3	Reddened dermatitis
Rickets	Lacking Vitamin D	Anatomical abnormalities of bone
Night blindness	Lacking Vitamin D	Night blindness
Kwashiorkor	Protein deficiency	Characterized by edema, irritability, anorexia, and an enlarged liver with fatty infiltrates
Sideropenia or hypoferremia	Iron deficiency	Iron-deficiency anemia

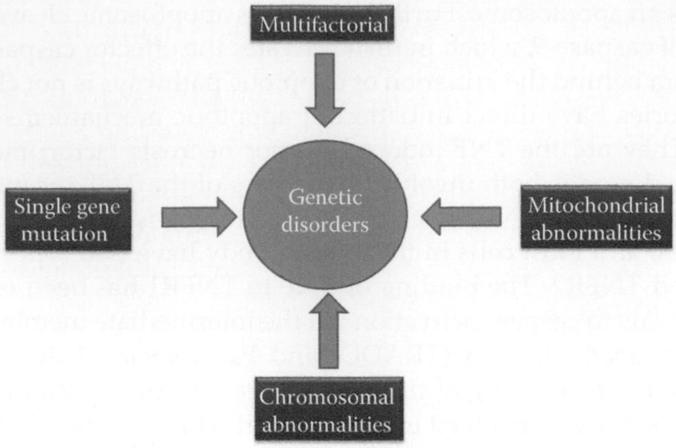

Figure 2.5 Types of genetic disorders.

2.4 *Genetic diseases*

A genetic disorder is a disease caused by abnormalities in an individual's genetic material. There are different types of genetic disorders identified in humans which are described briefly (Figure 2.5).

2.4.1 *Single-gene disorder*

The genetic disorder in which a single gene gets mutated is called as a single-gene disorder. As you know each gene is responsible for making special type of proteins which in turn regulate the body function. When a gene is mutated so that its protein product cannot carry out its normal body function, it leads to the development of a disorder. Additionally, there are more than 6000 known single-gene disorders in humans that occur in about 1 out of every 200 births. Some examples of single-gene disorder are cystic fibrosis, sickle cell anemia, Marfan syndrome, Huntington's disease, and hereditary hemochromatosis. There are three kinds of single-gene disorders described briefly.

2.4.1.1 *Autosomal dominant disorder*

The autosomal dominant disease is caused due to mutation of one gene and each affected person usually has one affected parent. In humans, there is a 50% chance that a child will inherit the mutated gene. The prevalence of autosomal dominant often has low penetrance, which means that although only one mutated copy is needed, a relatively small fraction of those who inherit that mutation go on to develop the disease. There are various examples of autosomal dominant disorder such as Huntington's disease, neurofibromatosis type 1, Marfan syndrome, and colorectal cancer. Moreover, birth defects are also called congenital anomalies (Figure 2.6).

2.4.1.2 *Autosomal recessive disorder*

In humans, autosomal recessive disorder is caused due to mutation in two copies of the gene. An affected person carrying a single copy of the gene (mutated) is referred to as a carrier. Furthermore, two unaffected people who each contains one copy of the mutated gene have about 25% chance with each pregnancy of having a child affected by this disorder. There are various examples of the types of disorder including cystic fibrosis, sickle-cell

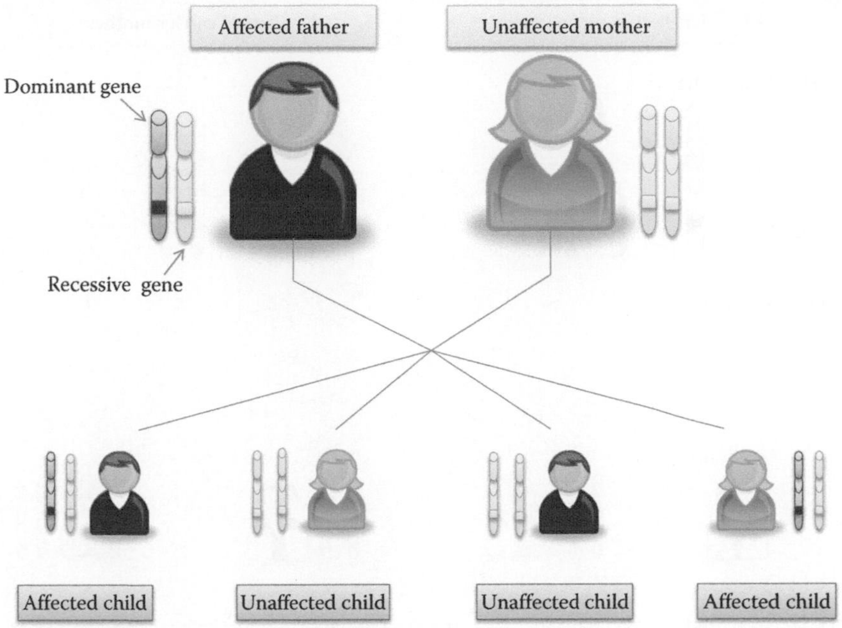

Figure 2.6 Autosomal dominant disorder.

disease (also partial sickle-cell disease), Tay–Sachs disease, Niemann–Pick disease, spinal muscular atrophy, Roberts's syndrome, and dry earwax (Figure 2.7).

2.4.1.3 X-linked dominant disorder

The X-linked dominant disorders are caused by mutations in genes located on the X chromosome. There are however, only a few disorders that have been known to be associated with X-linked dominant disorder. Besides both males and females are known to be affected by these disorders, with males typically being more severely affected than females. Furthermore, there are some X-linked dominant conditions such as Rett syndrome and Aicardi syndrome that are usually fatal in males. There are a few exceptions such as Klinefelter syndrome (47, XXY) where boys also inherit an X-linked dominant condition and exhibit symptoms more similar to those of a female in terms of disease severity. Furthermore, the chance of passing on X-linked dominant disorder traits differs between men and women as the sons of a man with an X-linked dominant disorder will all be unaffected, whereas his daughters will all inherit the condition. Furthermore, a woman with an X-linked dominant disorder has about 50% chance of having an affected fetus with each pregnancy.

2.4.1.4 X-linked recessive disorder

The X-linked recessive conditions are also caused by mutations in genes on the X chromosome. Additionally, men are more frequently affected than women, and the chance of passing on the disorder differs between men and women. The sons of a man with an X-linked recessive disorder will not get the disease, whereas his daughters will carry one copy of the mutated gene. A woman who is a carrier of an X-linked recessive disorder has a 50% chance of having sons who are affected and a 50% chance of having daughters who carry one copy of the mutated gene and are therefore carriers. X-linked recessive conditions include serious diseases Hemophilia A, Duchenne muscular dystrophy, and Lesch–Nyhan syndrome

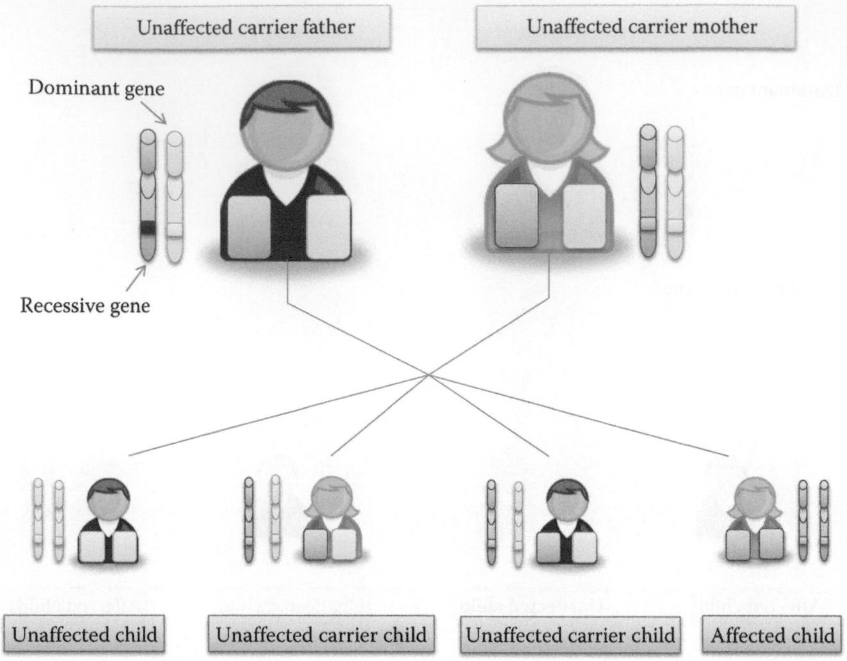

Figure 2.7 Autosomal recessive disorder.

as well as common and less serious conditions such as male pattern baldness and red-green color blindness. Furthermore, X-linked recessive conditions are sometimes marked in females due to skewed X-inactivation or monosomy X (Turner syndrome) (Figure 2.8).

2.4.1.5 *Y-linked disorder*

Y-linked disorders are caused by mutations on the Y chromosome. Y-linked disorder is basically a male-associated disorder; every son of an affected father will be affected by this disease. Interestingly, females inherit an X chromosome from their fathers, so daughter will not get affected by such disease. It has been shown that the Y chromosome is relatively small in size and contains very few genes. The main symptoms associated with such a disease are infertility.

2.4.1.6 *Multifactorial disorder*

It has been shown that this type of disease is caused by a combination of environmental factors and mutations in multiple genes, for example, different genes that influence breast cancer susceptibility have been found on chromosomes number 6, 11, 13, 14, 15, 17, and 22. Furthermore, some of the most common chronic disorders are due to multifactorial gene disorders. There are several examples of multifactorial gene disorders including Alzheimer's disease, arthritis, diabetes, cancer, heart disease, high blood pressure, and obesity. Additionally multifactorial inheritance is associated with heritable traits such as height, eye color, and skin color.

2.4.2 *Chromosomal abnormalities*

The chromosomes are carriers of genetic material in humans. There are possibilities of the addition, deletion, or structural change of chromosomes and such conditions are known as

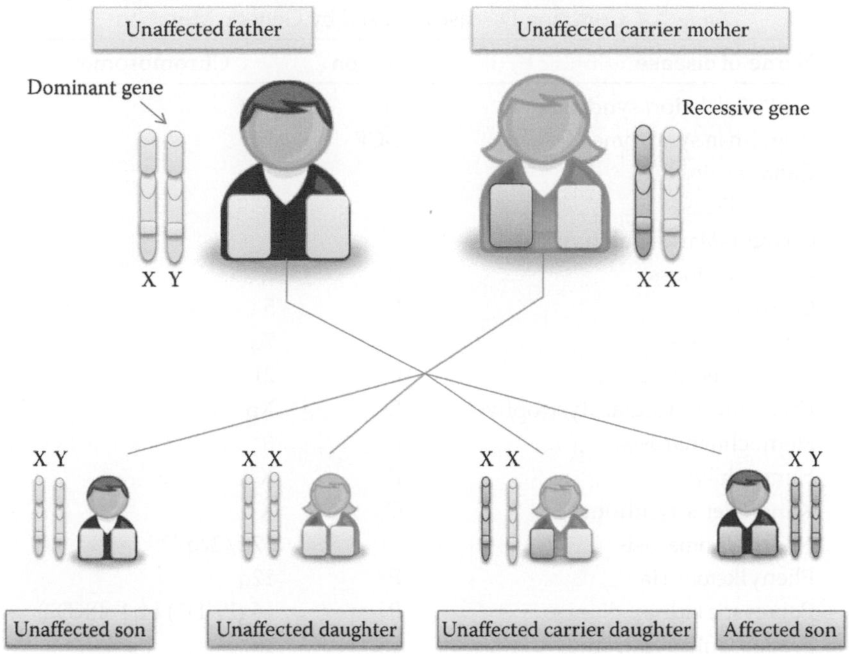

Figure 2.8 X-linked recessive disorder.

chromosomal abnormalities. Such abnormalities in chromosome structure and numbers can result in chromosomal disease. There are various types of chromosomal abnormalities associated that include syndrome or trisomy 21, which is a common disorder occurring when a person has three copies of chromosome 21. The common diseases which are caused by genetic mutation are listed in Table 2.4.

2.4.3 Mitochondrial disorders

These are a relatively rare type of genetic disorder caused by mutations in the nonchromosomal DNA of mitochondria. As you know, mitochondria are small rod-like organelles involved in cellular respiration and found in the cytoplasm of both plant and animal cells and, moreover, each mitochondrion contains 5–10 circular pieces of DNA.

2.5 Autoimmune disease

Autoimmune diseases are caused by an overactive immune response of the body against substances and tissues normally present in the body. Sometimes the immune system acts differently and attacks the body's own defense system leading to the development of an autoimmune disease. Furthermore, the immune system mistakes some part of the body as a pathogen and attacks it; this can be restricted to few organs or tissue in different places of the human body. In case of autoimmunity, the patient's immune system is activated against the body's own proteins, whereas in the case of inflammatory diseases, it is the overreaction of the TNF or IFN which causes problems. It has been projected that autoimmune diseases are among the 10 leading causes of death among women. The autoimmune disease can be categorized into two types which include systemic autoimmune disease

Table 2.4 Common Diseases Caused by Genetic Mutation

Name of disease	Mutation	Chromosome
22q11.2 deletion syndrome	D	22q
Angelman syndrome	DCP	15
Canavan disease		17p
Celiac disease		
Charcot–Marie–Tooth disease		
Color blindness	P	X
Cri du chat	D	5
Cystic fibrosis	P	7q
Down syndrome	C	21
Duchenne muscular dystrophy	D	Xp
Hemochromatosis	P	6
Hemophilia	P	X
Klinefelter's syndrome	C	X
Neurofibromatosis		17q/22q/?
Phenylketonuria	P	12q
Polycystic kidney disease	P	16 (PKD1) or 4 (PKD2)
Prader–Willi syndrome	DC	15
Sickle-cell disease	P	11p
Tay–Sachs disease	P	15
Turner syndrome	C	X

and organ-specific disease. In the case of systemic autoimmune disease, the immune system attacks many different body organs, tissues, and cells of the body (Table 2.5).

2.6 *Disease transmission*

Most of the infectious diseases are generally spread through various ways including air, water, blood, and so on. The disease is generally communicated from an infected host or patient to some other individual, regardless of whether the other individual was previously infected or not. Transmission can also be indirect; some vectors such as tapeworm in pigs can be transmitted to humans who ingest inadequately cooked pork flesh. The disease can also spread through an indirect transmission by other organisms such as rats and dogs. In a broader sense, disease that can be transmitted from one individual to another in the same generation is called horizontal transmission. Horizontal transmission can occur by either direct contact which includes licking, touching, biting, or indirect contact through air—cough or sneeze. The disease which is passed through parent to offspring is called vertical or perinatal transmission.

2.6.1 *Transmission through droplet contact*

The disease transmission through droplet contact is a typical mode of transmission among many infectious agents. The disease transmission begins when an infected person coughs or sneezes on another person; the microorganisms in the form of droplets generally penetrate the body through the nose, mouth, or eye body surfaces. Additionally influenza A viruses

Table 2.5 List of Autoimmune Diseases

Name of disease	Affected organ
Alopecia areata	Skull hair
Ankylosing spondylitis	Spinal cord
Crohn's disease	Inflammatory bowel disease
Coeliac disease	Small intestine
Dermatomyositis	Muscles and skin
Diabetes mellitus type 1	Beta cells of the pancreas
Endometriosis	Uterine cavity and ovaries
Goodpasture's syndrome	Lung
Graves' disease	Thyroid gland
Guillain–Barré syndrome	Peripheral nervous system
Hashimoto's thyroiditis	Thyroid gland
Hidradenitis suppurativa	Skin (sweat gland)
Kawasaki disease	Blood vessels, skin, mucous membranes, and lymph nodes
IgA nephropathy	Kidney
Idiopathic thrombocytopenic purpura	Blood cells
Interstitial cystitis	Urinary bladder
Lupus erythematosus	Skin, kidneys, blood cells, heart, and lungs
Mixed connective tissue disease	Connective tissues
Multiple sclerosis	Brain and spinal cord
Myasthenia gravis	Neuromuscular junction
Narcolepsy	Sleep disorder
Pemphigus vulgaris	Skin
Perniciousanemia	Gastric cells
Psoriasis	Skin
Psoriatic arthritis	Skin
Polymyositis	Skin and muscles
Primary biliary cirrhosis	Liver
Relapsing polychondritis	Cartilage
Rheumatoid arthritis	Bone joints
Sjogren's syndrome	Exocrine gland
Temporal arteritis	Blood vessels
Ulcerative colitis	Intestine
Vasculitis	Blood vessels
Wegener's granulomatosis	Blood vessels

spread in the population through tiny droplet nuclei. When viruses are shed by an infected person through cough and sneeze into the air, the liquid coating on the virus starts to fade away. As soon as this mucus secretion vaporizes, the remaining virus starts penetrating other individuals. The mucus secretion rate is determined by the temperature and humidity inside the room or vicinity. The lower the humidity, the quicker the mucus shell evaporates hence permitting the droplet nuclei to stay airborne and not drop to the ground. Various diseases spread by coughing or sneezing includes measles, common cold, influenza, mumps, rubella, chickenpox, strep throat, tuberculosis, or whooping cough, and bacterial meningitis.

2.6.2 Fecal–oral transmission

The infectious disease can also be transmitted through human or animal excreta touch and also with contamination of fecal materials with drinking water. In this type of transmission, foodstuffs or water become contaminated due to unhygienic ways of food preparation or drinking water is being contaminated with untreated sewage water. The examples of this typical mode of transmission are hepatitis A, polio, rotavirus, cholera, or salmonella.

2.6.3 Sexual transmission

Infectious diseases can also be transmitted through sexual activity with multiple partners or having sex with an infected person. Transmission is either directly between surfaces in contact during intercourse or from secretions which carry infectious agents that get into the partner's bloodstream through tiny tears in the penis or vagina. Sexually transmitted diseases (STDs) such as HIV and hepatitis B are thought to not normally be transmitted through mouth-to-mouth contact, although it is conceivable to transmit some STDs between the genitals and the mouth during oral sex. In HIV patients this possibility has been established. It is also responsible for the increased incidence of herpes simplex virus 1 in genital infections and the increased incidence of the type 2 virus in oral infections. Some diseases transmissible by the sexual route include gonorrhea, hepatitis B, syphilis or herpes, HIV/AIDS, chlamydia, and genital warts.

2.7 Epidemiology of diseases

After learning about various diseases and their definitions, classifications, types, and transmission, we also need to know how diseases are spread globally and its nature and frequency of spread. The science to study the distribution and determinants of health-related states or events including disease, and the application of this study to the control of diseases and other health problems is called epidemiology. It is the keystone method of public health research and helps inform evidence-based medicine the identifying risk factors for disease and determining optimal treatment at a global level. In communicable and noncommunicable disease-based studies, epidemiologists are generally involved in outbreak study. Epidemiologists rely on a number of other scientific disciplines such as biology to better understand disease processes, whereas biostatisticians analyze the current statistical data available.

The history behind epidemiology goes back to the sixteenth century when Greek physician Hippocrates examined the relationships between the occurrence of disease and environmental influences. He later on coined the terms endemic (for diseases usually found in some places) and epidemic (for disease that are seen at some times). Dr. John Snow showed for the first time the clusters of cholera cases in the London epidemic of 1854. Dr. Snow was famous for his investigations into the causes of the nineteenth century cholera epidemics. Later on he began noticing the significantly higher death rates in two areas which were supplied by a particular water company. Furthermore, his identification of a disease-outbreak is considered the classic example of epidemiology. To clean the infected area, he used chlorine to clean the water and thus causing the end of the outbreak. This had been perceived as a major event and is regarded as the founding event of the science of epidemiology.

2.8 Diseases diagnosis

To treat a particular disease, it is very important to know the cause of the disease and it can be found out by using diagnostic tools. Normally, a person with certain symptoms will

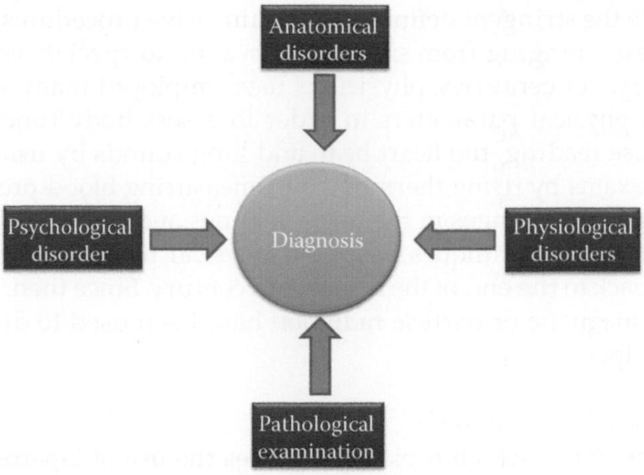

Figure 2.9 Diagnosis of human diseases.

consult a physician who will obtain a medical history of the patient's illness and perform a physical examination for signs of any disease. The physician can formulate a hypothesis of likely diagnoses and in many cases can obtain further testing to confirm the diagnosis before providing treatment. Also medical tests which are commonly performed include measuring urine tests, fecal tests, saliva tests, blood tests, medical imaging, electrocardiogram, hydrogen breath test, and, infrequently, biopsy. There are four basics of diagnostic testing: anatomy, physiology, pathology, and psychology. Once the physicians know what is normal, s/he can then determine the patient's particular departure from homeostasis and the degree of difference which in the medical field is called a diagnosis. Apart from the fact that there are differing theoretical views toward mental conditions and there are few laboratory tests available for various major disorders, a casual examination with respect to symptomatology associated with the disease is not always possible (Figure 2.9).

2.8.1 *Types of diagnosis tests*

There are various types of diagnostic tests available that include disease diagnosis, measuring the progress or recovery from disease, and to confirm that a person is free from disease. Medical tests can be classified into three categories: invasive, minimally invasive, and noninvasive.

2.8.1.1 *Invasive tests*

An invasive test is a surgical procedure or operative procedures in which skin or connective tissue is incised in the patients. The invasive tests include biopsy, excision, or deep cryotherapy for malignant lesions, extensive multiorgan transplantation, and all procedures in the surgery section. There are other surgical procedures being used, such as percutaneous transluminal angioplasty and cardiac catheterization; these are minimally invasive procedures involving biopsies.

2.8.1.2 *Noninvasive tests*

A diagnostic test where the test is conducted without hurting the patient physically is normally called a noninvasive test, for example, deep palpation and percussion is noninvasive, but a rectal examination is invasive. Similarly, examination of the ear drum or inside the nose fall outside the stringent definition of noninvasive procedures. There are various noninvasive processes, ranging from simple observation to specialized forms of surgery, such as radiosurgery. For centuries, physicians have employed many simple noninvasive methods based on physical parameters in order to assess body function in health and disease such as pulse reading, the heart beat, and lung sounds by using the stethoscope, body temperature exams by using thermometers, measuring blood pressure by using the sphygmomanometer, and changes in the body volumes audiometry. The discovery of the first modern noninvasive techniques based on physical methods—electrocardiography and x-rays—dates back to the end of the nineteenth century. Since then, noninvasive methods such as electromagnetic or particle radiation have been used to diagnose the disease rather than by a scalpel.

2.8.1.3 Minimal invasive tests

This is another type of test which typically involves the use of laparoscopic devices and remote control manipulation of instruments. This method is performed with an endoscope and is carried out through the skin or a body cavity. The benefits of such tests are that patients do not have a long hospital stay. Furthermore, a minimally invasive procedure is distinct from a noninvasive procedure, for example, external imaging instead of exploratory surgery. When there is minimal damage of biological cells, tissues, or organs by a surgical instrument the procedure is called minimally invasive.

2.8.2 Diagnostic laboratories

Clinical laboratories are the diagnostic services that apply laboratory techniques to the diagnosis and management of patients. Furthermore in the United States these services are managed by a recognized pathologist. The personnel that work in these medical laboratories are technically trained staff who do not hold medical degrees, but who usually hold an undergraduate medical technology degree or diploma in medical laboratory; who actually perform the tests, assays, and procedures needed for providing the specific services. The clinical laboratories consist of cellular pathology, clinical chemistry, hematology, clinical microbiology, and clinical immunology sections.

2.8.2.1 Pathology laboratory

Pathology as another branch of laboratory testing that deals with the study of diseases by examining the morphological and physiological changes. Furthermore, pathology can be considered the basis of modern laboratory diagnosis and plays an important role in evidence-based diagnosis. There are many advanced laboratory tests such as flow cytometry, polymerase chain reaction (PCR), immunohistochemistry, cytogenetic, gene rearrangements studies, and fluorescent *in situ* hybridization (FISH) fall within the domain of pathology.

2.8.2.2 Radiology laboratory

The radiology laboratory mainly deals with imaging of the human body for identifying cellular or morphological abnormalities by using x-rays, x-ray computed tomography (CT), ultrasonography, and nuclear magnetic resonance tomography techniques.

2.8.2.3 Nuclear medicine laboratory

Nuclear medicine is the science of studying human organ systems by administering radiolabeled pharmaceuticals into the body, which can then be viewed or imaged by using special machine such as a gamma camera or positron emission tomography (PET) scanner. Additionally, each radiopharmaceutical is made of two components, the tracer (to track the neurotransmitter pathway, metabolic pathway, blood flow) and a radionuclide. Furthermore, there is a degree of similarity between nuclear medicine (to treat disease) and radiology (to diagnose the disease).

2.8.2.4 Clinical neurophysiology laboratory

The neurophysiology laboratory is specially related to testing the physiology or function of the central and peripheral nervous system and these kinds of tests can be done by using a special kind of recording machine. These machines record the electrical impulse generated by the patients nervous system. The electrical impulses can be divided into spontaneous or continuously running electrical activity, or stimulus-induced responses. Furthermore, these electrical impulses can be sub-classified into electroencephalography, electromyography, evoked potential, and nerve conduction study.

2.9 Diagnostics tools

Over the last few decades, we have seen tremendous growth in various diagnostic tools and applications which in fact has helped the physician make precise and accurate decisions on various pathological conditions. We have discussed a few techniques that are extensively used in clinical laboratories to identify the progression and development of diseases.

2.9.1 Molecular tools

The disease can be accurately diagnosed with molecular biological techniques which include mapping of the genes associated with diseases.

2.9.1.1 Polymerase chain reaction technique

The PCR is the most powerful technique to amplify patients DNA into a million fold, by constant replication in a short period of time. The method employs DNA isolated from patients' blood and set of primers and the design of the primers is dependent upon the sequences of the DNA that is desired to be analyzed. The technique is carried out through 20–50 cycles of melting the template at high temperature, allowing the primers to anneal to complementary sequences within the template (patient DNA sample) and then replicating the template with DNA polymerase. The process can be automated with the use of thermo-stable DNA polymerases. During the first round of replication, a single copy of DNA is converted into two copies and so on resulting in a constant increase in the number of copies of the sequences targeted by the primers. After 20 cycles, a single copy of DNA is amplified over 2 million copies (Figure 2.10). Besides its applications in disease diagnosis, the PCR technology has also been employed in genetic fingerprinting and in the forensic science to identify a person by comparing DNAs through different PCR-based methods. Some PCR fingerprints methods have the high discriminative power and can be used to identify genetic relationships between individuals, such as parent–child or between siblings, and are used in paternity testing. Furthermore, this technique can be used in the analysis of disease genes by detecting small amounts of specific DNA fragments. The examples of inherited diseases which can be detected by the PCR is listed in Table 2.6.

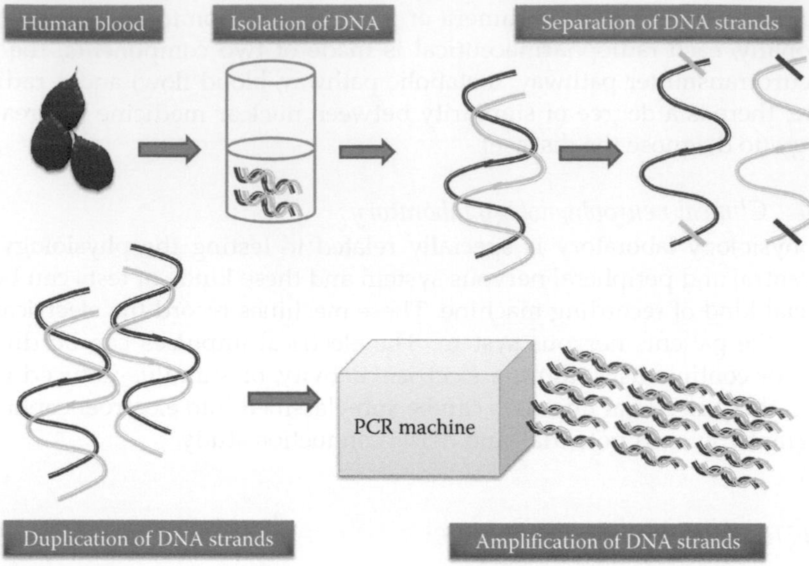

Figure 2.10 Polymerase chain reaction machine.

Table 2.6 Examples of Inherited Disorders Detectable by PCR

Disease	Affected gene region
Severe-combined immunodeficiency, SCID	Adenosine deaminase (ADA)
Lesch–Nyhan syndrome	Hypoxanthine-guanine phosphoribosyltransferase (HGPRT)
α1-Antitrypsin deficiency	α1-Antitrypsin
Cystic fibrosis	Cystic fibrosis transmembrane conductance (CFTR) protein
Fabry disease	α-Galactosidase
Gaucher disease	Acid β-glucosidase (glucocerebrosidase)
Sandhoff disease	Hexosaminidase A and B
Tay–Sachs disease	Hexosaminidase A
Familial hypercholesterolemia (FH)	LDL receptor
Glucose-6-phosphate dehydrogenase deficiency	Glucose-6-phosphate dehydrogenase
Maple syrup urine disease	Branched-chain α-keto acid dehydrogenase
Phenylketonuria (PKU)	Phenylalanine hydroxylase
Ornithine transcarbamylase deficiency	Ornithine transcarbamylase
Retinoblastoma (Rb)	RB gene product, pRB
Sickle-cell anemia	Point mutation in β-globin
β-Thalassemia	Mutations in β-globin gene that result in loss of synthesis of protein
Hemophilia A	Factor VIII
Hemophilia B	Factor IX
von Willebrand disease	von Willebrand factor (vWF)

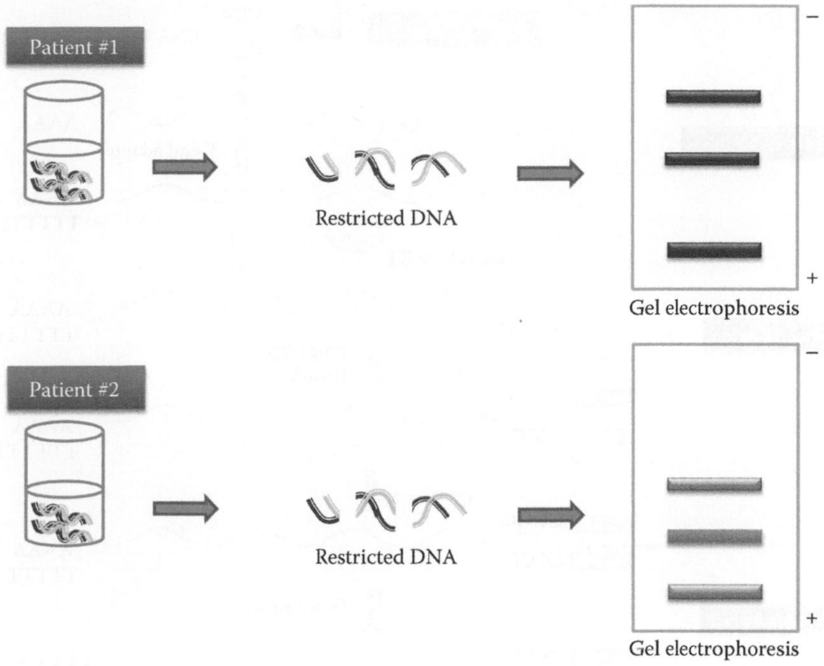

Figure 2.11 Restriction fragment-length polymorphism analysis.

2.9.1.2 *Restriction fragment-length polymorphism analysis*

The genetic disease can be diagnosed by using the RFLP method which is basically to identify genetic variability at a particular gene. Interestingly, sickle cell anemia is a classic example of a disease detectable by RFLP method. Furthermore, sickle cell anemia results from a single-nucleotide change (adenosine to thymine) at codon 6 within the β-globin gene. This genetic alteration causes a change from a glutamine (G) to valium (V) amino acid position, whereas at the same time abolishing an MstII restriction site. As a result of this alteration, a β-globin gene probe can be used to detect the different MstII restriction fragments. Furthermore, it can be recalled that there are two copies of each gene in all human cells; consequently, RFLP analysis detects both copies of the affected allele and the unaffected allele (Figure 2.11).

2.9.1.3 *Reverse transcription-PCR*

Reverse transcription-PCR (RT-PCR) is a rapid and quantitative procedure for the analysis of the level of expression of genes associated with diseases. This technique utilizes the ability of reverse transcriptase (RT) to convert RNA into single-stranded cDNA and couples it with the PCR-mediated amplification of specific types of cDNAs present in the RT reaction. The cDNAs that are produced during the RT reaction represent a pattern screen that genes are being expressed at the time the RNA was extracted. In brief, RT-PCR reactions can be achieved by first extracting total cellular RNA from cells. After that RNA is primed using random primers and RT reaction is then added to a PCR reaction containing primers specific to the gene sequences. Finally, the products of the RT-PCR can then be visualized through the computer screen (Figure 2.12).

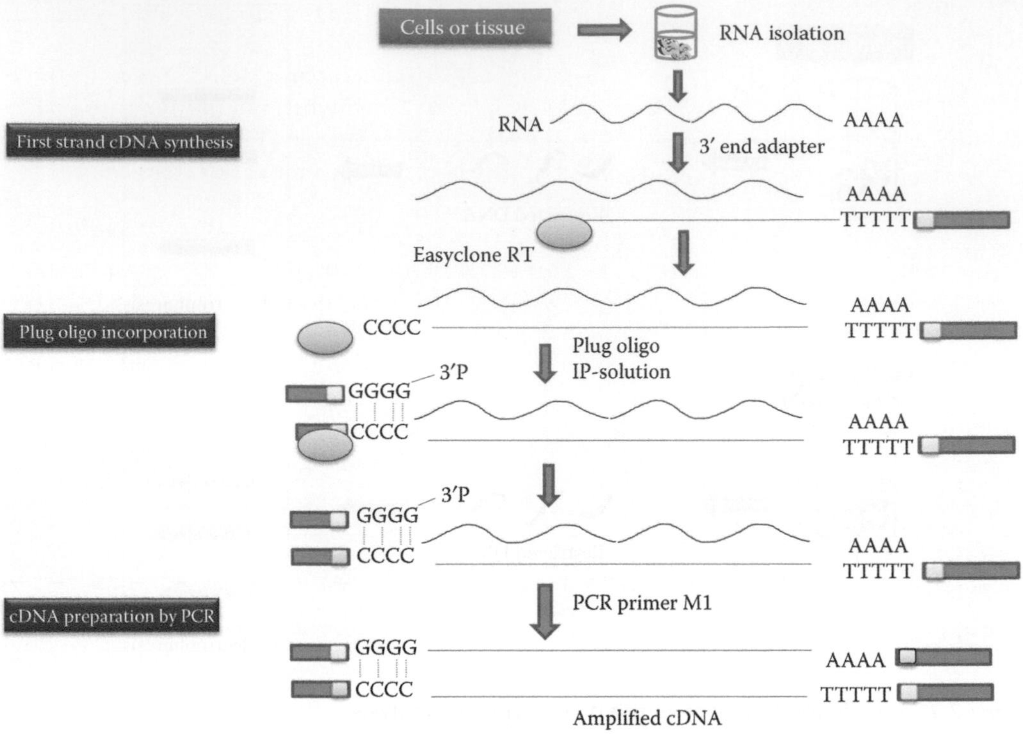

Figure 2.12 Reverse transcriptase polymerase chain reaction.

2.9.1.4 *Single-strand conformation polymorphism-PCR*

Single-strand conformation polymorphism (SSCP)-PCR or SCP-PCR technique can be used to detect single mutation in the genes. For that purpose specific PCR primers are made that span the sequences of a given disease gene where a mutation is known to exist and the region amplified by PCR and in the same region of the wild-type gene is PCR also amplified. After running the gel, the two strands of wild-type PCR products can be migrated differently than the two strands of mutant PCR product. Henceforth, to accurately visualize the PCR products either the primers are radio-labeled are incorporated into the PCR products. Finally, the PCR products are separated on a polyacrylamide gel and visualized by exposure of the gel to x-ray film. The gel picture will tell us the difference between wild-type and mutant gene samples as homozygous wild type will exhibit two distinct bands in the gel as will those individuals that are homozygous mutants, whereas heterozygous wild type will exhibit a pattern consisting of all four bands (Figure 2.13).

2.9.1.5 *Ligase chain reaction*

The ligase chain reaction (LCR) is a technique that allows detection of single point mutations in disease-associated genes. In a general sense, this technique employs a thermostable DNA ligase to ligate together perfectly neighboring oligos. Additionally, two sets of oligos are designed to anneal to one strand of the gene, a second set of two oligos anneals to the other strand of the gene. The oligos are designed in such way that they can completely anneal to the wild-type sequences only. For example, in sickle-cell mutation, the three nucleotides of one logo in each pair are found to be mismatched. Interestingly, this mismatch prevents the annealing of the oligos directly adjacent to each other; consequently,

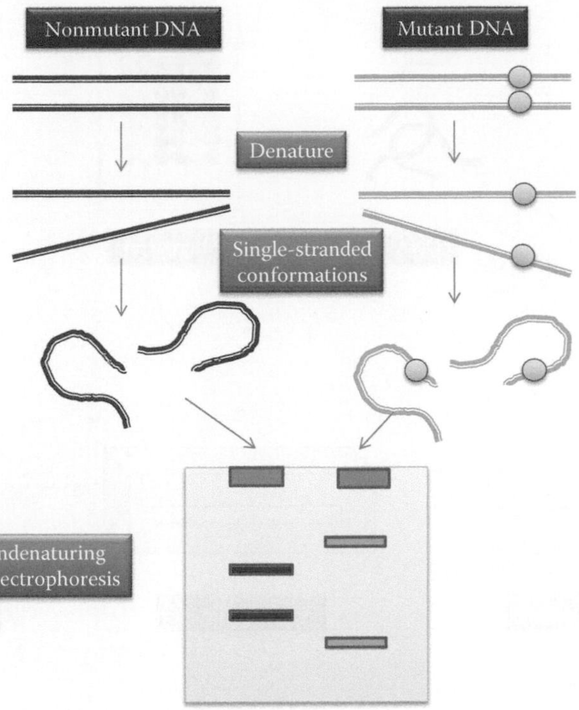

Figure 2.13 Single-strand conformation polymorphism PCR.

DNA ligase cannot ligate the two oligos of each pair together. With the wild-type sequence the oligo pairs that are ligated together become targets for annealing the oligos and, hence, this results in an exponential amplification of the wild-type target. The LCR technique can be utilized for the diagnosis of the presence of a mutant allele in high-risk patients.

2.9.1.6 Microarray analysis

With the rapid advancements in molecular tools, it becomes possible to map several genes through one technique called microarray. In brief, the microarray technique involves the use of gene chips to define the expression of a large set of genes in a single experiment. These gene chips are commercially available and can be bought from different companies, such as Affymetrix, or they can also be customized in the laboratories with the proper equipment. Furthermore, gene chips are created through the covalent attachment of synthetically designed oligos to a small surface. In general, there are about 20 or more different kinds of oligos that can be fixed on the chip corresponding to different regions of each gene to be analyzed. In addition to this, a set of oligos that each contain a nucleotide mismatch are considered as negative sample for each gene. Additionally, thousands of different genes can be analyzed by using single chip with an approximate size of 2 cm^2 (Figure 2.14).

2.9.1.7 Fluorescence in situ hybridization technique

FISH (fluorescence *in situ* hybridization) is a cytogenetic technique used to study the presence or absence of specific DNA sequences located on the chromosomes which are associated with diseases. In brief, the FISH technique involves the use of fluorescent probes that bind the parts of the chromosome with which they show a high degree of sequence

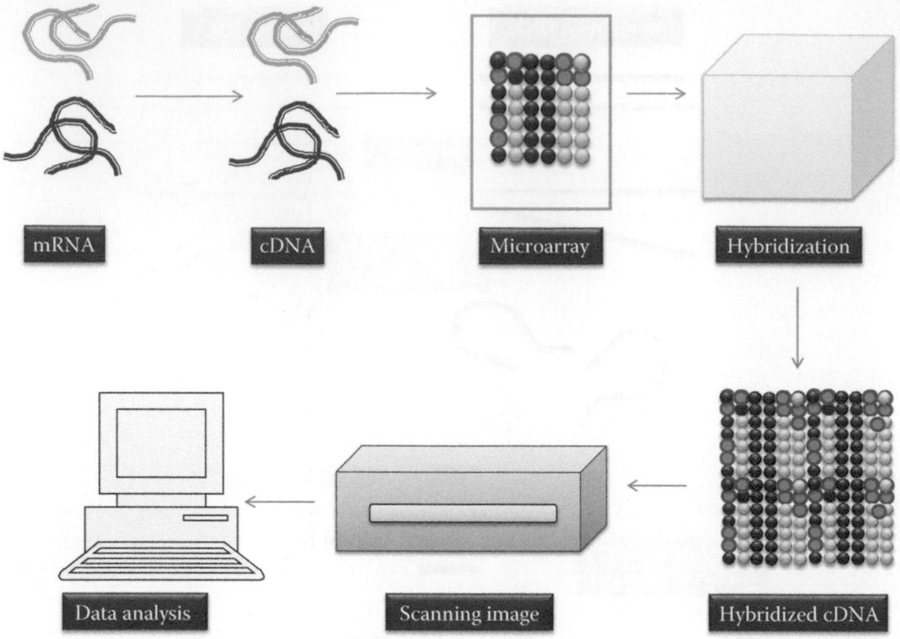

Figure 2.14 Microarray analysis.

resemblance. To visualize where the fluorescent probe bound to the chromosomes, the fluorescence microscopy is being used. There are various applications of the FISH technique in the diagnostics field, which include its use in finding out specific structures in DNA for use in genetic counseling or species identification. In addition, FISH can also be used to detect and localize specific mRNAs within tissue samples.

There are several examples of diseases that are diagnosed by using the FISH technique, including Angelman syndrome, 22q13 deletion syndrome, Prader–Willi syndrome, chronic myelogenous leukemia, Velocardiofacial syndrome, Down syndrome, acute lymphoblastic leukemia, and Cri-du-chat. Furthermore, the FISH technique is often used in clinical studies. For example, if a patient is infected with a suspected pathogen, a sample which contains bacteria can be obtained from the patient, which is typically grown on agar to determine the identity of the pathogen. However, many bacteria, even well-known species, do not grow well under laboratory conditions and in this kind of condition, FISH technique can be used to directly detect the presence of bacteria.

2.9.2 *Biochemical techniques*

In the medical diagnosis, the biochemical techniques are most widely used as diagnostic tools which basically involve the determination of the level of chemical components in body fluids and tissues. Besides human body fluids such as blood contain thousands of different biomolecules, which include glucose, ions, hormones, toxins, and large numbers of different proteins.

2.9.2.1 *Blood analyzer*

A blood test is performed on a blood sample that is usually taken from the patients. Blood tests are used to determine physiological and biochemical status of body biomolecules.

There are various kinds of blood tests available which include simple glucose content analyzer used to monitor blood sugar levels. There are portable instruments used to analyze the levels of certain minerals, amino acids, and metabolites in the bloodstreams of athletes. This is a type of blood testing common among coaches, especially those who work with professional and Olympic-level competitive athletes. In addition to this, there are an extensive variety of diagnostic procedures, which involve analysis of white and red blood cells, hemoglobin content, and the structure of other proteins and enzymes.

2.9.2.2 Enzyme-linked immunosorbent assay

Enzyme-linked immunosorbent assay (ELISA) also known as an enzyme immunoassay (EIA) is a technique used to detect the presence of an antibody or an antigen in a sample. In brief, performing an ELISA involves at least one antibody with specificity for a particular antigen and after that a sample with an unknown amount of antigen is immobilized on a polystyrene microtiter plate. Later on, the antigen is immobilized and the detection antibody is added which basically form an antigen–antibody complex. The antigen–antibody complex can be visualized by an enzyme or by secondary antibody which is linked to an enzyme through bio-conjugation. After several washes, the plate is developed by adding an enzyme to produce a visible signal, which indicates the quantity of antigen in the sample.

2.9.3 Histopathology

Histopathology refers to the microscopic examination of tissues or cells received from patients in order to study the manifestations of disease. In brief, histopathological examination of tissues starts with surgery, biopsy, or autopsy. The first step is to remove tissue from the body and immersed in a fixative which stabilizes the tissues to prevent deterioration. The most common type of fixative is formalin or paraformaldehyde. In the diagnostic labs, the histological slides are examined under a microscope by a pathologist, a medically qualified specialist.

2.9.3.1 Immunohistochemistry

Immunohistochemistry technique is the localization of antigens in cells or tissue sections by the use of labeled antibody generated against respective antigens that are visualized by fluorescent dye or enzyme, or radioactive element or colloidal gold. The immunohistochemistry technique involves specific antigen–antibody reactions; it has the apparent advantage over conventionally used special enzyme staining techniques that identify only a limited number of proteins, hormones, and enzymes. In recent times, immunohistochemistry technique has become a crucial technique in many medical research laboratories as well as clinical diagnostics. The immunohistochemistry method is an excellent detection technique and has the tremendous advantage of being able to show exactly where an anticipated protein is located within the tissue examined. It is also an effective way to examine the tissues and over the past few years, this has made it a widely used technique in the neurosciences, embryology, and stem cells research fields. It has a major disadvantage, unlike immunoblotting techniques where staining is checked against a molecular weight ladder, it is difficult to show in immunohistochemistry that the staining corresponds with the protein of interest and for this reason primary antibodies must be well checked in a Western blot or similar procedure. The name of the disease with their immunological markers are listed in Table 2.7.

Table 2.7 Antibodies as Markers for Several Diseases

Name of antibodies	Tissue
Carcinoembryonic antigen (CEA)	Marker for adenocarcinoma
Cytokeratins	Marker carcinomas but may also be expressed in some sarcomas
CD15 and CD30	Marker for Hodgkin's disease
Alpha fetoprotein	Marker for yolk sac tumors and hepatocellular carcinoma
CD117 (KIT):	Marker for gastrointestinal stromal tumors (GIST)
CD10 (CALLA):	Marker for renal cell carcinoma and acute lymphoblastic leukemia
Prostate specific antigen (PSA)	Marker for prostate cancer
CD20	Marker for identification of B-cell lymphomas
CD3	Marker for identification of T-cell lymphomas

2.10 *Current challenges of human diseases*

The world keeps contracting new forms of diseases caused by viruses and bacteria, posing difficult challenges for patient diagnosis and treatment and for public health responses. There were approximately 1400 infectious pathogens recognized in 2005; about 180 met the criteria for emerging pathogens. Additionally, many different factors contributed to their emergence, which included societal changes, population health, and hospital and medical procedures. Most emerging infectious diseases are caused by zoonotic pathogens originating from animal sources. It has been found that many of these infections emerged in and around the equator, such as tropical Africa, Latin America, and much of Asia; nevertheless, new zoonotic pathogens also emerged in the southern US. Besides this, there is an emergence of antibiotic-resistant bacteria around the globe, as some drug-resistant bacteria keep causing clinical infection. Interestingly, the emergence of a hyper-virulent strain of *Clostridium difficile* is a particularly difficult problem to tackle. As it has been found only in patients previously treated with antibiotics, *Clostridium difficile* is now appearing in other groups as well. Furthermore, food and waterborne infections continue to pose a major danger to human health. In developing countries, better water sanitation techniques could enhance controlling these pathogens. Furthermore, hepatitis B and C virus and malaria also continue to threaten large segments of the world population.

2.11 *Summary*

Human disease is a malfunction of the normal functioning of the body that normally has a specific cause and identifiable symptoms. It is frequently interpreted to be a medical condition associated with specific symptoms and signs. In humans, disease is frequently used to refer to any condition that causes pain, dysfunction, suffering, or social psychological problems. In a general sense, it sometimes includes body injuries, disabilities, disorders, syndromes, and infections. Throughout our history epidemics and diseases have caused the extinction of whole populations. Over the last century, man has discovered many microorganisms that cause diseases in humans, and has learned how to protect himself from them by either prevention or treatment. In this chapter we have discussed the prevalence of different types of human diseases and have also discussed cellular and molecular pathogenesis associated with them.

2.12 Knowledge builder

Protozoans: Protozoa are a diverse group of unicellular eukaryotic organisms, many of which are motile. Originally, protozoa had been defined as unicellular protists with animal-like behavior, for example, movement. Protozoa were regarded as the partner group of protestors to Protophyta, which have plant-like behavior, for example, photosynthesis.

Cerebrospinal fluid: Cerebrospinal fluid (CSF) is a clear colorless bodily fluid produced in the choroid plexus of the brain. It acts as a cushion or buffer for the cortex, providing a basic mechanical and immunological protection to the brain inside the skull and serves a vital function in cerebral autoregulation of cerebral blood flow.

Computed tomography: X-ray computed tomography, also computed tomography (CT scans), computed axial tomography or computer-assisted tomography (CAT scan) is a medical imaging procedure that uses computer-processed x-rays to produce tomographic images or "slices" of specific areas of the body. These cross-sectional images are used for diagnostic and therapeutic purposes in various medical disciplines. Digital geometry processing is used to generate a three-dimensional image of the inside of an object from a large series of two-dimensional x-ray images taken around a single axis of rotation.

Complete blood count: A complete blood count (CBC), also known as full blood count or full blood exam or blood panel, is a test panel requested by a doctor or other medical professional that gives information about the cells in a patient's blood. A scientist or lab technician performs the requested testing and provides the requesting medical professional with the results of the CBC.

Mitochondria-derived activator of caspase (SMAC): Mitochondria is a protein that in humans is encoded by the DIABLO gene which is also referred to as second mitochondria-derived activator of caspase. SMAC is a mitochondrial protein that promotes cytochrome-c-dependent activation by eliminating the inhibition via IAP—a protein that negatively regulates apoptosis or programmed cell death.

Inhibitor of apoptosis proteins: The inhibitors of apoptosis (IAP) are a family of functionally and structurally related proteins, which serve as endogenous inhibitors of programmed cell death (apoptosis).

Mitochondria-derived activator of caspases: Diablo homolog, mitochondrial is a protein that in humans is encoded by the DIABLO gene. DIABLO is also referred to as second mitochondria-derived activator of caspases or SMAC. SMAC is a mitochondrial protein that promotes cytochrome-c-dependent activation by eliminating the inhibition via IAP—a protein that negatively regulates apoptosis or programmed cell death. SMAC is normally a mitochondrial protein but is found in the cytosol when a cell is primed for apoptosis by the final execution step of caspase activation. SMAC is the second protein in the apoptosis link, along with cytochrome c, that promotes apoptosis by activating caspases.

Apaf-1: Apoptotic protease-activating factor-1, a key regulator of the mitochondrial apoptosis pathway.

ATP: Adenosine-5′-triphosphate (ATP) is a nucleoside triphosphate used in the cells as a coenzyme. It is often called the "molecular unit of currency" of intracellular energy transfer. ATP transports chemical energy within cells for metabolism.

Apoptosome: The apoptosome is a large quaternary protein structure formed in the process of apoptosis. Its formation is triggered by the release of cytochrome c from the mitochondria in response to an internal or external cell death stimulus.

Tumor necrosis factor: Tumor necrosis factors (or the TNF family) refers to a group of cytokines whose family can cause cell death.

Fas-Fas ligand-mediated model: Fas/Fas ligand (FasL)-mediated apoptosis or programmed cell death.

Most restriction sites: The site of DNA which is cut by the Most II enzyme is useful for prenatal diagnosis.

cDNAs: In genetics, complementary DNA (cDNA) is DNA synthesized from a messenger RNA (mRNA) template in a reaction catalyzed by the enzymes reverse transcriptase and DNA polymerase. cDNA is often used to clone eukaryotic genes in prokaryotes.

DNA ligase: In molecular biology, DNA ligase is a specific type of enzyme, a ligase (EC 6.5.1.1) that facilitates the joining of DNA strands together by catalyzing the formation of a phosphodiester bond. It plays a role in repairing single-strand breaks in duplex DNA in living organisms, but some forms (such as DNA ligase IV) may specifically repair double-strand breaks (i.e., a break in both complementary strands of DNA).

Oligos: Oligonucleotides are short, single-stranded DNA or RNA molecules that have a wide range of applications in genetic testing, research, and forensics.

Further reading

Agarwal KS, Morgan R, Dahlbeck D, Borsani O, Villegas A et al. 2006. A pathogen-inducible endogenous siRNA in plant immunity. *Proc Natl Acad Sci USA* 103 (47): 18002–18007. doi:10.1073/pnas.0608258103. PMID 17071740.

Ahlquist P 2002. RNA-dependent RNA polymerases, viruses, and RNA silencing. *Science* 296 (5571): 1270–1273. doi: 10.1126/science.1069132. PMID 12016304.

Allen R, Millgate A, Chitty J, Thisleton J, Miller J et al. 2004. RNAi-mediated replacement of morphine with the nonnarcotic alkaloid reticuline in opium poppy. *Nat Biotechnol* 22 (12): 1559–1566. doi:10.1038/nbt1033. PMID 15543134.

Anantharaman V, Koonin E, and Aravind L 2002. Comparative genomics and evolution of proteins involved in RNA metabolism. *Nucleic Acids Res* 30 (7): 1427–1464. doi:10.1093/nar/30.7.1427. PMID 11917006.

Bagasra O and Prilliman KR 2004. RNA interference: The molecular immune system. *J Mol Histol* 35 (6): 545–553. doi:10.1007/s10735-004-2192-8. PMID 15614608. http://www.kluweronline.com/art.pdf?issn=1567–2379&volume=35&page=545.

Bartlett JM and Stirling D 2003. A short history of the polymerase chain reaction. *Methods Mol Biol* 226: 3–6.

Bass B. 2000. Double-stranded RNA as a template for gene silencing. *Cell* 101 (3): 235–238. doi:10.1016/S0092-8674(02)71133-1. PMID 10847677.

Bass B. 2002. RNA editing by adenosine deaminases that act on RNA. *Annu Rev Biochem* 71: 817–846. doi:10.1146/annurev.biochem.71.110601.135501. PMID 12045112.

Baulcombe D. 2007. Molecular biology. Amplified silencing. *Science* 315 5809: 199–200. doi:10.1126/science.1138030. PMID 17218517.

Berkhout B and Haasnoot J 2006. The interplay between virus infection and the cellular RNA interference machinery. *FEBS Lett* 580 (12): 2896–2902. doi:10.1016/j.febslet.2006.02.070. PMID 16563388.

Bernstein E, Caudy A, Hammond S, and Hannon G 2001. Role for a bidentate ribonuclease in the initiation step of RNA interference. *Nature* 409 6818: 363–366. doi:10.1038/35053110. PMID 11201747.

Bing DH, C Boles, FN Rehman, M Audeh, M Belmarsh, B Kelley, and CP Adams. 1996. Bridge amplification: A solid phase PCR system for the amplification and detection of allelic differences in single copy genes. *Genetic Identity Conference Proceedings, Seventh International Symposium on Human Identification*. Scottsdale, Arizona, USA. http://www.promega.com/geneticidproc/ussymp7proc/ 0726.html

Blevins T, Rajeswaran R, Shivaprasad P, Beknazariants D et al. 2006. Four plant Dicers mediate viral small RNA biogenesis and DNA virus induced silencing. *Nucleic Acids Res* 34 (21): 6233–6246. doi:10.1093/nar/gkl886. PMID 17090584.

Boutros M, Kiger A, Armknecht S, Kerr K, Hild M et al. 2004. Genome-wide RNAi analysis of growth and viability in Drosophila cells. *Science* 303 5659: 832–835. doi:10.1126/science.1091266. PMID 14764878.

ter Brake O, Westerink JT, Berkhout B 2010. Lentiviral vector engineering for anti-HIV RNAi gene therapy. *Methods Mol Biol* 614:201–213. doi: 10.1007/978-1-60761-533-0_14.

Brummelkamp T, Bernards R, and Agami R. 2002. A system for stable expression of short interfering RNAs in mammalian cells. *Science* 296 5567: 550–553. doi:10.1126/science.1068999. PMID 11910072.

Buchon N and Vaury C 2006. RNAi: A defensive RNA-silencing against viruses and transposable elements. *Heredity* 96 (2): 195–202. doi:10.1038/sj.hdy.6800789. PMID 16369574.

Carrington J and Ambros V 2003. Role of microRNAs in plant and animal development. *Science* 301 5631: 336–338. doi:10.1126/science.1085242. PMID 12869753.

Cerutti H and Casas-Mollano J 2006. On the origin and functions of RNA-mediated silencing: From protists to man. *Curr Genet* 50 (2): 81–99. doi:10.1007/s00294-006-0078-x. PMID 16691418.

Check, E. 2007. RNA interference: Hitting the on switch. *Nature* 448 7156: 855–858. doi:10.1038/448855a. PMID 17713502.

Cheng S, Fockler C, Barnes WM, and Higuchi R 1994. Effective amplification of long targets from cloned inserts and human genomic DNA. *Proc Natl Acad Sci USA*, 91 (12): 5695–5699. doi:10.1073/pnas.91.12.5695. PMID 8202550.

Chiang C, Wang J, Jan F, Yeh S, and Gonsalves D 2001. Comparative reactions of recombinant papaya ringspot viruses with chimeric coat protein (CP) genes and wild-type viruses on CP-transgenic papaya. *J Gen Virol* 82 (Part 11): 2827–2836. PMID 11602796.

Chien A, Edgar DB, and Trela JM 1976. Deoxyribonucleic acid polymerase from the extreme thermophile *Thermus aquaticus*. *J Bacteriol* 174 (3): 1550–1557. PMID 8432.

Covey S, Al-Kaff N, Lángara A, and Turner D 1997. Plants combat infection by gene silencing. *Nature* 385: 781–782. doi:10.1038/385781a0.

Cullen B 2006. Is RNA interference involved in intrinsic antiviral immunity in mammals? *Nat Immunol* 7 (6): 563–567. doi:10.1038/ni1352. PMID 16715068.

Cullen L and Arndt G 2005. Genome-wide screening for gene function using RNAi in mammalian cells. *Immunol Cell Biol* 83 (3): 217–223. doi:10.1111/j.1440-1711.2005.01332.x. PMID 15877598.

DaRocha W, Otsu K, Teixeira S, and Donelson J 2004. Tests of cytoplasmic RNA interference (RNAi) and construction of a tetracycline-inducible T7 promoter system in *Trypanosoma cruzi*. *Mol Biochem Parasitol* 133 (2): 175–186. doi:10.1016/j.molbiopara.2003.10.005. PMID 14698430.

David, F and Turlotte, E, 1998. An isothermal amplification method. *CR Acad Sci Paris Life Science* 321 (1): 909–914.

Don RH, Cox PT, Wainwright BJ, Baker K, Mattick JS 1991. Touchdown' PCR to circumvent spurious priming during gene amplification. *Nucl Acids Res* 19 (14): 4008. doi:10.1093/nar/19.14.4008. PMID 1861999. PMC 328507. http://www.pubmedcentral.nih.gov/pagerender.fcgi?artid=328507&pageindex=1.

Drinnenberg IA, Weinberg DE, Xie KT, Nower JP et al. 2009. RNAi in budding yeast. *Science* 326 (5952): 544–550. doi:10.1126/science.1176945. PMID 19745116.

Ecker JR and Davis RW 1986. Inhibition of gene expression in plant cells by expression of antisense RNA. *Proc Natl Acad Sci USA* 83 (15): 5372–5376. doi:10.1073/pnas.83.15.5372. PMID 16593734.

Fortunato A and Fraser A 2005. Uncover genetic interactions in *Caenorhabditis elegans* by RNA interference. *Biosci Rep* 25 (5–6): 299–307. doi:10.1007/s10540-005-2892-7. PMID 16307378.

Fritz J, Girardin S, and Philpott D 2006. Innate immune defense through RNA interference. *Sci STKE* 2006 (339): pe27. doi:10.1126/stke.3392006pe27. PMID 16772641.

Gavilano L, Coleman N, Burnley L, Bowman M, Kalengamaliro N et al. 2006. Genetic engineering of *Nicotiana tabacum* for reduced nornicotine content. *J Agric Food Chem* 54 (24): 9071–9078. doi:10.1021/jf0610458. PMID 17117792.

Ge G, Wong G, and Luo B 2005. Prediction of siRNA knockdown efficiency using artificial neural network models. *Biochem Biophys Res Commun* 336 (2): 723–728. doi:10.1016/j.bbrc.2005.08.147. PMID 16153609.

Geldhof P, Murray L, Couthier A, Gilleard J, McLauchlan G et al. 2006. Testing the efficacy of RNA interference in *Haemonchus contortus*. *Int J Parasitol* 36 (7): 801–810. doi:10.1016/j.ijpara.2005.12.004. PMID 16469321.

Geldhof P, Visser A, Clark D, Saunders G, Britton C, Gilleard J. et al. 2007. RNA interference in parasitic helminths: Current situation, potential pitfalls and future prospects. *Parasitology* 134 (Part 5): 1–11. doi:10.1017/S0031182006002071. PMID 17201997.

Gregory R, Chendrimada T, Cooch N, and Shiekhattar R 2005. Human RISC couples microRNA biogenesis and posttranscriptional gene silencing. *Cell* 123 (4): 631–640. doi:10.1016/j.cell.2005.10.022. PMID 16271387.

Gregory R, Chendrimada T, Shiekhattar R 2006. MicroRNA biogenesis: Isolation and characterization of the microprocessor complex. *Methods Mol Biol* 342:33–47. doi:10.1385/1-59745-123-1:33. PMID 16957365.

Grimm D, Streetz K, Jopling C, Storm T, Pandey K, Davis C et al. 2006. Fatality in mice due to oversaturation of cellular microRNA/short hairpin RNA pathways. *Nature* 441 (7092): 537–541. doi:10.1038/nature04791. PMID 16724069.

Gu S and Rossi J 2005. Uncoupling of RNAi from active translation in mammalian cells. *RNA* 11 (1): 38–44. doi:10.1261/rna.7158605. PMID 15574516.

Guo S and Kemphues K 1995. par-1, a gene required for establishing polarity in C. elegans embryos, encodes a putative Ser/Thr kinase that is asymmetrically distributed. *Cell* 81 (4): 611–620. doi:10.1016/0092-8674(95)90082-9. PMID 7758115.

Hammond S, Bernstein E, Beach D, and Hannon G. 2000. An RNA-directed nuclease mediates post-transcriptional gene silencing in *Drosophila* cells. *Nature* 404 (6775): 293–296. doi:10.1038/35005107. PMID 10749213.

Hart BL 1988. Biological basis of the behavior of sick animals. *Neurosci Biobehav Rev.* 12: 123–137.

Haslam DW, James WP 2005. Obesity. *Lancet* 366 (9492): 1197–1209. doi:10.1016/S0140-6736(05)67483-1. PMID 16198769.

Henschel A, Buchholz F, Habermann B 2004. DEQOR: A web-based tool for the design and quality control of siRNAs. *Nucleic Acids Res* 32 (Web Server issue): W113–120. doi:10.1093/nar/gkh408. PMID 15215362.

Herman JG, Graff JR, Myohanen S, and Nelkin BD 1996. Methylation-specific PCR: A novel PCR assay for methylation status of CpG islands. *Proc Natl Acad Sci USA* 93 (13): 9821–9826. doi:10.1073/pnas.93.18.9821. PMID 8790415.

Holmquist G and Ashley T 2006. Chromosome organization and chromatin modification: Influence on genome function and evolution. *Cytogenet Genome Res* 114 (2): 96–125. doi:10.1159/000093326. PMID 16825762.

Hu L, Wang Z, Hu C, Liu X, Yao L et al. 2005. Inhibition of measles virus multiplication in cell culture by RNA interference. *Acta Virol* 49 (4): 227–234. PMID 16402679.

Huesken D, Lange J, Mickanin C, Weiler J, Asselbergs F et al. 2005. Design of a genome-wide siRNA library using an artificial neural network. *Nat Biotechnol* 23 (8): 995–1001. doi:10.1038/nbt1118. PMID 16025102.

Humphreys DT, Westman BJ, Martin DI, and Preiss T 2005. MicroRNAs control translation initiation by inhibiting eukaryotic initiation factor 4E/cap and poly(A) tail function. *Proc Natl Acad Sci USA* 102 (47): 16961–16966. doi:10.1073/pnas.0506482102. PMID 16287976.

Innis MA, Myambo KB, Gelfand DH, and Brow MA. 1988. DNA sequencing with *Thermus aquaticus* DNA polymerase and direct sequencing of polymerase chain reaction-amplified DNA. *Proc Natl Acad Sci USA* 85 (24): 9436–4940. doi:10.1073/pnas.85.24.9436. PMID 3200828.

Irvine D, Zaratiegui M, Tolia N, Goto D, Chitwood D, Vaughn M et al. 2006. Argonaute slicing is required for heterochromatic silencing and spreading. *Science* 313 (5790): 1134–1137. doi:10.1126/science.1128813. PMID 16931764.

Isenbarger TA, Finney M, Ríos-Velázquez C, Handelsman J, Ruvkun G 2008. Miniprimer PCR, a new lens for viewing the microbial world. *Appl Environ Microbiol* 74 (3): 840–849. doi:10.1128/AEM.01933-07. PMID 18083877.

Izquierdo M 2005. Short interfering RNAs as a tool for cancer gene therapy. *Cancer Gene Ther* 12 (3): 217–227. doi:10.1038/sj.cgt.7700791. PMID 15550938.

Jakymiw A, Lian S, Eystathioy T, Li S, Satoh M, Hamel J, Fritzler M, and Chan E 2005. Disruption of P bodies impairs mammalian RNA interference. *Nat Cell Biol* 7 (12): 1267–1274. doi:10.1038/ncb1334. PMID 16284622.

Janitz M, Vanhecke D, and Lehrach H 2006. High-throughput RNA interference in functional genomics. *Handb Exp Pharmacol* 173 (173): 97–104. doi:10.1007/3-540-27262-3_5. PMID 16594612.

Jia F, Zhang Y, and Liu C 2006. A retrovirus-based system to stably silence hepatitis B virus genes by RNA interference. *Biotechnol Lett* 28 (20): 1679–1685. doi:10.1007/s10529-006-9138-z. PMID 16900331.

Jiang M and Milner J. 2002. Selective silencing of viral gene expression in HPV-positive human cervical carcinoma cells treated with siRNA, a primer of RNA interference. *Oncogene* 21 (39): 6041–6048. doi:10.1038/sj.onc.1205878. PMID 12203116.

Jones L, Ratcliff F, and Baulcombe DC 2001. RNA-directed transcriptional gene silencing in plants can be inherited independently of the RNA trigger and requires Met1 for maintenance. *Curr Biol* 11 (10): 747–757. doi:10.1016/S0960-9822(01)00226-3.

Jones-Rhoades M, Bartel D, and Bartel B 2006. MicroRNAS and their regulatory roles in plants. *Annu Rev Plant Biol* 57:19–53. doi:10.1146/annurev.arplant.57.032905.105218. PMID 16669754.

Kamath R and Ahringer J 2003. Genome-wide RNAi screening in *Caenorhabditis elegans*. *Methods* 30 (4): 313–321. doi:10.1016/S1046-2023(03)00050-1. PMID 12828945.

Kelley KW, Bluthe RM, Dantzer R, Zhou JH, Shen, WH, Johnson RW, and Broussard SR 2003. Cytokine-induced sickness behavior. *Brain Behav Immun* 17 (Suppl 1): S112–118.

Khan Z, Poetter K, and Park DJ 2008. Enhanced solid phase PCR: Mechanisms to increase priming by solid support primers. *Anal Biochem* 375 (2): 391–393. doi:10.1016/j.ab.2008.01.021. PMID 18267099.

Kleppe K, Ohtsuka E, Kleppe R, Molineux I, and Khorana HG 1971. Studies on polynucleotides. XCVI. Repair replications of short synthetic DNA's as catalyzed by DNA polymerases. *J Mol Biol* 56 (2): 341–361. doi:10.1016/0022-2836(71)90469-4.

Kusov Y, Kanda T, Palmenberg A, Sgro J, and Gauss-Müller V 2006. Silencing of hepatitis A virus infection by small interfering RNAs. *J Virol* 80 (11): 5599–5610. doi:10.1128/JVI.01773-05. PMID 16699041.

Lawyer FC, Stoffel S, Saiki RK, Chang SY, Landre PA, Abramson RD, and Gelfand DH 1993. High-level expression, purification, and enzymatic characterization of full-length *Thermus aquaticus* DNA polymerase and a truncated form deficient in 5′ to 3′ exonuclease activity. *PCR Methods Appl* 2 (4): 275–287. PMID 8324500.

Le L, Lorenz Y, Scheurer S, Fötisch K, Enrique E et al. 2006. Design of tomato fruits with reduced allergenicity by dsRNAi-mediated inhibition of ns-LTP (Lyc e 3) expression. *Plant Biotechnol* J 4 (2): 231–242. doi:10.1111/j.1467-7652.2005.00175.x. PMID 17177799.

Lee R, Feinbaum R, and Ambros V 1993. The *C. elegans* heterochronic gene lin-4 encodes small RNAs with antisense complementarity to lin-14. *Cell* 75 (5): 843–854. doi:10.1016/0092-8674(93)90529-Y. PMID 8252621.

Lee Y, Nakahara K, Pham J, Kim K, He Z et al. 2004. Distinct roles for *Drosophila* Dicer-1 and Dicer-2 in the siRNA/miRNA silencing pathways. *Cell* 117 (1): 69–81. doi:10.1016/S0092-8674(04)00261-2. PMID 15066283.

Leuschner P, Ameres S, Kueng S, Martinez J 2006. Cleavage of the siRNA passenger strand during RISC assembly in human cells. *EMBO Rep* 7 (3): 314–320. doi:10.1038/sj.embor.7400637. PMID 16439995.

Li C, Parker A, Menocal E, Xiang S, Borodyansky L, and Fruehauf J 2006. Delivery of RNA interference. *Cell Cycle* 5 (18): 2103–2109. PMID 16940756.

Li LC, Okino ST, Zhao H, Pookot D, Place RF et al. 2006. Small dsRNAs induce transcriptional activation in human cells. *Proceedings of the National Academy of Sciences, USA* 103(46): 17337–42. PMID 17085592.

Lian S, Jakymiw A, Eystathioy T, Hamel J et al. 2006. GW bodies, microRNAs and the cell cycle. *Cell Cycle* 5 (3): 242–245. PMID 16418578.

Liu Q, Rand T, Kalidas S, Du F, Kim H et al. 2003. R2D2, a bridge between the initiation and effector steps of the Drosophila RNAi pathway. *Science* 301 5641: 1921–1925. doi:10.1126/science.1088710. PMID 14512631.

Luciano D, Mirsky H, Vendetti N, and Maas S 2004. RNA editing of a miRNA precursor. *RNA* 10 (8): 1174–1177. doi:10.1261/rna.7350304. PMID 15272117.

Lucy A, Guo H, Li W, and Ding S 2000. Suppression of post-transcriptional gene silencing by a plant viral protein localized in the nucleus. *EMBO J* 19 (7): 1672–1680. doi:10.1093/emboj/19.7.1672. PMID 10747034.

Makarova K, Grishin N, Shabalina S, Wolf Y, and Koonin E 2006. A putative RNA-interference-based immune system in prokaryotes: Computational analysis of the predicted enzymatic machinery, functional analogies with eukaryotic RNAi, and hypothetical mechanisms of action. *Biol Direct* 1: 7. doi:10.1186/1745-6150-1-7. PMID 16545108.

Matranga C, Tomari Y, Shin C, Bartel D, and Zamore P 2005. Passenger-strand cleavage facilitates assembly of siRNA into Ago2-containing RNAi enzyme complexes. *Cell* 123 (4): 607–620. doi:10.1016/j.cell.2005.08.044. PMID 16271386.

Matzke M.A and Matzke A.J.M. 2004. Planting the seeds of a new paradigm. *PLoS Biol* 2 (5): e133. doi:10.1371/journal.pbio.0020133. PMID 15138502.

McGinnis K, Chandler V, Cone K, Kaeppler H et al. 2005. Transgene-induced RNA interference as a tool for plant functional genomics. *Methods Enzymol* 392:1–24. doi:10.1016/S0076-6879(04)92001-0. PMID 15644172.

Morita T, Mochizuki Y, and Aiba H 2006. Translational repression is sufficient for gene silencing by bacterial small noncoding RNAs in the absence of mRNA destruction. *Proceedings of the National Academy Sciences, USA* 103 (13): 4858–4863. doi:10.1073/pnas.0509638103. PMID 16549791.

Mueller PR and Wold B 1988. *In vivo* foot printing of a muscle specific enhancer by ligation mediated PCR. *Science* 246 4931: 780–786. doi:10.1126/science.2814500. PMID 2814500.

Mullis K. 1990. The unusual origin of the polymerase chain reaction. *Scientific American* 262 (4): 56–61, 64–5. doi:10.1038/scientificamerican0490-56.

Myrick KV and Gelbart WM 2002. Universal fast walking for direct and versatile determination of flanking sequence. *Gene* 284 (1–2): 125–131. doi:10.1016/S0378-1119(02)00384-0. PMID 11891053.

Naito Y, Yamada T, Ui-Tei K, Morishita S, and Saigo K 2004. siDirect: Highly effective, target-specific siRNA design software for mammalian RNA interference. *Nucleic Acids Res* 32 (Web Server issue): W124–129. doi:10.1093/nar/gkh442. PMID 15215364.

Nakayashiki H, Kadotani N, and Mayama S 2006. Evolution and diversification of RNA silencing proteins in fungi. *J Mol Evol* 63 (1): 127–135. doi:10.1007/s00239-005-0257-2. PMID 16786437.

Napoli C, Lemieux C, and Jorgensen R 1990. Introduction of a chimeric chalcone synthase gene into petunia results in reversible co-suppression of homologous genes in trans. *Plant Cell* 2 (4): 279–289. doi:10.1105/tpc.2.4.279. PMID 12354959.

Newton CR, Graham A, Heptinstall LE, Powell SJ et al. 1989. Analysis of any point mutation in DNA. The amplification refractory mutation system (ARMS). *Nucleic Acids Res* 17 (7): 2503–2516. doi:10.1093/nar/17.7.2503. PMID 2785681.

Niggeweg R, Michael A, and Martin C 2004. Engineering plants with increased levels of the antioxidant chlorogenic acid. *Nat Biotechnol* 22 (6): 746–754. doi:10.1038/nbt966. PMID 15107863.

Nishikura K 2006. Editor meets silencer: Crosstalk between RNA editing and RNA interference. *Nat Rev Mol Cell Biol* 7 (12): 919–931. doi:10.1038/nrm2061. PMID 17139332.

Noma K, Sugiyama T, Cam H, Verdel A, Zofall M, Jia S et al. 2004. RITS acts in cis to promote RNA interference-mediated transcriptional and post-transcriptional silencing. *Nat Genet* 36 (11): 1174–1180. doi:10.1038/ng1452. PMID 15475954.

Ochman H, Gerber AS, and Hartl DL 1988. Genetic applications of an inverse polymerase chain reaction. *Genetics* 120 (3): 621–623. PMID 2852134.

Okamura K, Ishizuka A, Siomi H, and Siomi M 2004. Distinct roles for Argonaute proteins in small RNA-directed RNA cleavage pathways. *Genes Dev* 18 (14): 1655–1666. doi:10.1101/gad.1210204. PMID 15231716.

Paddison P, Caudy A, and Hannon G 2002. Stable suppression of gene expression by RNAi in mammalian cells. *Proceedings of the National Academy of Sciences, USA* 99 (3): 1443–1448. doi:10.1073/pnas.032652399. PMID 11818553.

Pak J and Fire A. 2007. Distinct populations of primary and secondary effectors during RNAi in *C. elegans*. *Science* 315 (5809): 241–244. doi:10.1126/science.1132839. PMID 17124291.

Palatnik J, Allen E, Wu X, Schommer C et al. 2003. Control of leaf morphogenesis by microRNAs. *Nature* 425 (6955): 257–263. doi:10.1038/nature01958. PMID 12931144.

Palauqui J, Elmayan T, Pollien J, and Vaucheret H 1997. Systemic acquired silencing: Transgene-specific post-transcriptional silencing is transmitted by grafting from silenced stocks to non-silenced scions. *EMBO J* 16 (15): 4738–4745. doi:10.1093/emboj/16.15.4738. PMID 9303318.
Parker G, Eckert D, and Bass B 2006. RDE-4 preferentially binds long dsRNA and its dimerization is necessary for cleavage of dsRNA to siRNA. *RNA* 12 (5): 807–818. doi:10.1261/rna.2338706. PMID 16603715.
Pavlov AR, Pavlova NV, Kozyavkin SA, and Slesarev AI 2004. Recent developments in the optimization of thermostable DNA polymerases for efficient applications. *Trends Biotechnol* 22 (5): 253–260. doi:10.1016/j.tibtech.2004.02.011. PMID 15109812.
Sambrook J and Russel DW 2001. Molecular cloning: A laboratory manual (3rd ed.). Cold Spring Harbor, NY: Cold Spring Harbor Laboratory Press. ISBN 0-87969-576-5. Chapter 8: *In vitro* amplification of DNA by the polymerase chain reaction.
Takeshita F, Ochiya T 2006. Therapeutic potential of RNA interference against cancer. *Cancer Sci* 97 (8): 689–696. doi:10.1111/j.1349-7006.2006.00234.x. PMID 16863503.

chapter three

Bacteriology and antibiotics

3.1 Introduction

A microbe is a microscopic small living creature and the science of microbes is called microbiology. Furthermore, the field of microbiology includes parasitology, bacteriology, virology, mycology, and other branches. Microorganisms can be of various types such as bacteria, fungi, archaea, green algae, plankton, and planarian. Moreover, some microbiologists also consider viruses as a microorganism, but then others consider them as nonliving organisms. Furthermore, most of the microorganisms are generally unicellular or single-cell organism. This is not universal; it has been observed that some of the multicellular organisms are microscopic, whereas some unicellular protists and bacteria, such as *Thiomargarita namibiensis*, are macroscopic and visible to the naked eye.

3.2 Microorganism: Historical perspective

In the late sixteenth century, scientist Antonie van Leeuwenhoek had observed for the first time the structure of a microorganism using a microscope. Leeuwenhoek's discovery, along with subsequent observations by Lazzaro Spallanzani and Louis Pasteur, ended the prolonged belief that life spontaneously appeared from nonliving substances during the process of spoilage. Lazzaro Spallanzaniper performed research to confirm that boiling broth should kill microorganism; however, he interestingly found the appearance of new microorganisms on the cold broth. Later on, Louis Pasteur expanded upon Spallanzani's findings by exposing boiled broths to the air, in vessels that contained a filter to prevent all particles from passing through to the growth medium, and also in vessels with no filter at all, with air being admitted through a bent tube that would not allow dust particles to come in contact with the broth. Finally, he concluded that living organisms came from the outside as spores on dust, rather than spontaneously generated within the broth. The Luis Pasteur research finding completely ridiculed the theory of spontaneous generation and supported germ theory.

There had been tremendous research on microbe's anatomy, physiology, and its functionality. In 1876, scientist Robert Koch established that microbes can cause disease in animals and humans. During his research he found that blood from cattle that were infected with anthrax always had large numbers of *Bacillus anthracis*. Later on, Koch transmitted anthrax from one animal (infected one) to another (healthy one) by taking a small sample of blood and later on found that the healthy animal did get sick. This experiment proved that microbes are living organisms that can be easily transmitted between two species and also cause the disease. He also found that he could grow the bacteria in a nutrient-filled culture, inject it into a healthy animal, and cause illness.

3.3 Classification of microorganisms

Microorganisms can be classified based on their color appearance. Bacteria are colored blue, eukaryotes are red, and archaea are green in color. Microorganisms can be found

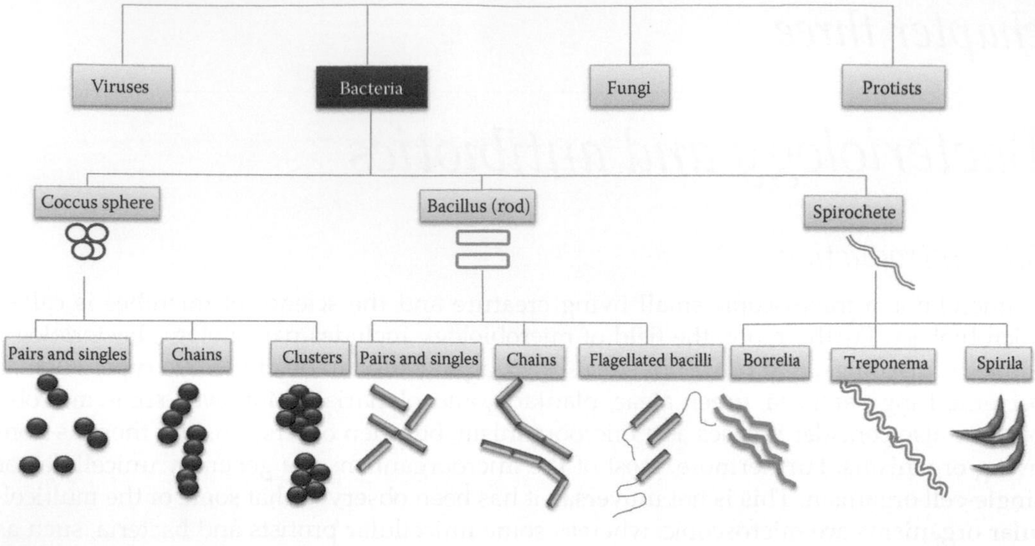

Figure 3.1 Microorganisms.

almost anywhere on earth. It has been observed that bacteria and archaea are mostly microscopic, whereas a number of eukaryotes such as protists and some fungi are also microscopic (Figure 3.1). Among microorganisms, the prokaryotes are organisms that lack a cell nucleus and other membrane-bound organelles; they are always unicellular. Additionally, some species of prokaryotes, such as myxobacteria have complex structures. Also prokaryotes are the most dissimilar and abundant group of microorganisms on the face of the earth and these small creatures inhabit practically all environments where some water is available and they can also survive under extreme temperatures. Furthermore, prokaryotes are found in sea water, soil, air, inside the animal's stomach, hot springs, and even deep beneath the earth's crust in rocks.

3.4 *Organization of bacteria*

Bacteria are a large group of single-celled prokaryote microorganisms. Normally, the size of these bacteria are few micrometers. Additionally, bacteria have a wide variety of shapes, extending from spheres to rods and spirals. Moreover, bacteria are abundant in all types of habitat on the face of earth and can grow and survive in soil, radioactive waste, sea water, acidic hot springs, and deep in the earth's crust.

3.4.1 *Structure of bacterium*

Bacteria exhibit a wide diversity of shapes and sizes. Bacterial cells are about one-tenth the size of eukaryotic cells and normally 0.5–5 μm in length. However, quite a few species of bacteria, for example, *Thiomargarita namibiensis* and *Epulopiscium fishelsoni,* have size ranges up to 0.5 μm long and can be seen without using a microscope. The genus *Mycoplasma* is among the smallest bacteria, which measures only 0.3 μm and some bacteria can be even smaller. Morphologically, most bacterial species are either spherical or rod-shaped. Furthermore, there are some rod-shaped bacteria, called vibrio, that are slightly comma-shaped, whereas others are spiral-shaped (spirilla), or tightly coiled (spirochaete).

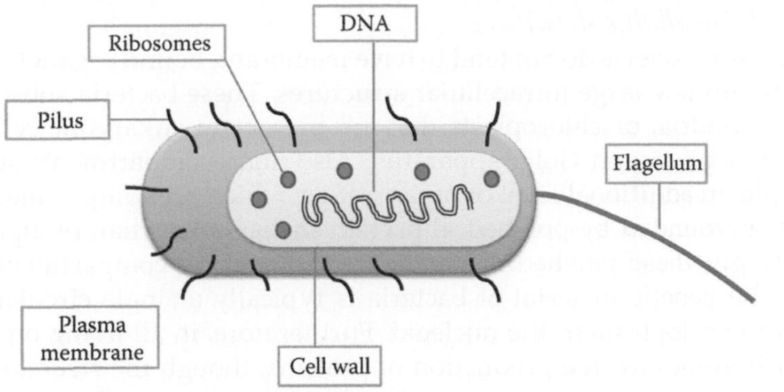

Figure 3.2 Structure of prokaryotes.

Moreover, a small number of species even has tetrahedral or cuboidal-shaped structure (Figure 3.2).

More recently, bacteria were discovered deep under the soil's crust that can grow as long rods with a star-shaped cross section. Moreover, the huge surface area gives these bacteria an advantage in nutrient-deficient environments. A wide variety of shapes determined by the bacterial cell wall and the cytoskeleton are important because it affects the ability of bacteria to obtain nutrients, attach to surfaces, swim through liquids, and escape from predators. Moreover, many bacterial species exist as a single-cell colony, while others exist in groups, for example, *Streptococcus* forms chain-like structures and *Neisseria* forms diploid structures. Additionally, bacteria often attach to surfaces and form dense collections of cells called biofilms. These biofilms can range from a few micrometers in thickness to up to half a meter in depth, and may contain multiple species of bacteria, protists, and archaea. Also, bacteria living in biofilms show a complex arrangement of cells to enable better dissemination of nutrients (Figure 3.3).

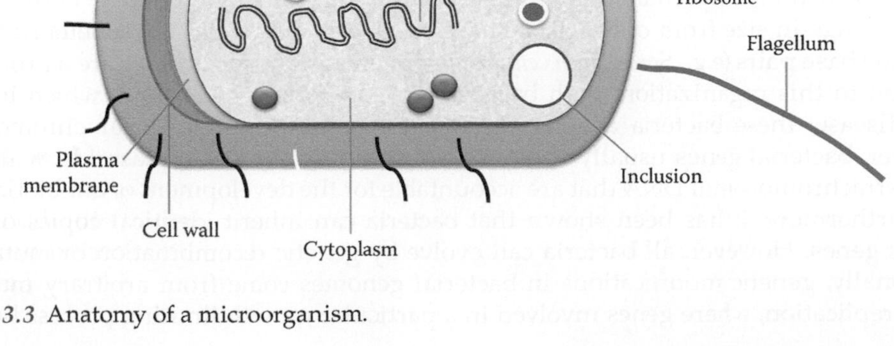

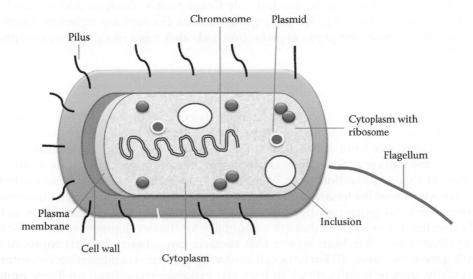

Figure 3.3 Anatomy of a microorganism.

3.4.1.1 *Intracellular structures*

Unlike eukaryotes, bacteria do not tend to have membrane-bound organelles in their cytoplasm and contain few large intracellular structures. These bacteria subsequently lack a nucleus, mitochondria, or chloroplasts that are present in eukaryotic cells, such as the endoplasmic reticulum and Golgi apparatus. Also microcompartments such as carbonxysome provide an additional level of organization, which are compartments within bacteria that are surrounded by polyhedral protein shells, rather than by lipid membranes. More interestingly, these polyhedral organelles localize and compartmentalize bacterial metabolism. The genetic material of bacteria is typically a single circular chromosome positioned in the cytoplasm in the nucleoid. Furthermore, in all living organisms, bacteria contains ribosomes for the production of proteins, though the structure of the bacterial ribosome is different from those of eukaryotes and archaea. There are some bacteria that produce intracellular nutrient storage granules such as glycogen and poly phosphate. There are certain bacterial species, such as the photosynthetic cyanobacteria, that produce internal gas vesicles, which they use to move up or down into water layers with different light intensities and nutrient planes.

3.4.1.2 *Extracellular structures*

The bacterial cell walls are normally made of peptidoglycan, which are polysaccharide chains cross linked by peptides enclosing D-amino acids. Also, bacterial cell walls are different from the plant cell walls and fungal cell walls, which are made of cellulose and chitin-like chemicals, respectively. Moreover, the cell wall of bacteria is also distinct from that of archaea, which do not contain peptidoglycan. The cell wall is crucial to the survival of many bacterial organisms and there are two different types of cell walls in bacteria, called Gram-positive and Gram-negative. Gram-positive bacteria keep a thick cell wall containing many layers of peptidoglycan and teichoic acids, whereas in the case of Gram-negative bacteria, the cell is thin and contains few layers of peptidoglycan enclosed by lipopolysaccharides and lipoproteins. Additionally, most bacteria have the Gram-negative cell wall; only the *Firmicutes* and *Actinobacteria* have the alternative Gram-positive organization. These differences in cell structure can produce differences in antibiotic vulnerability; for example, vancomycin can kill only Gram-positive bacteria and is found to be ineffective against Gram-negative pathogens, such as *Haemophilus influenza*. Lastly, cell wall provides chemical and physical protection and can act as a macromolecular diffusion barrier (Figure 3.4).

3.4.2 *Bacterial genetics*

One of the most interesting things in bacteria is its genetic code, which are not only very simple but also equally challenging. Most bacteria have a single circular chromosome that can range in size from only 160,000 base pairs (e.g., *Candidatus* Carsonella ruddii) to 12,200,000 base pairs (e.g., *Sorangium cellulosum*). Interestingly, spirochetes are a prominent exception to this organization, with bacteria such as *Borrelia burgdorferi*, which induces Lyme disease; these bacteria are also known to contain a single linear chromosome. Moreover, bacterial genes usually contain a single unbroken DNA, plasmids, which are small extrachromosomal DNA that are accountable for the development of antibiotic resistant. Furthermore, it has been shown that bacteria can inherit identical copies of their parent's genes. However, all bacteria can evolve by genetic recombination or mutations. Additionally, genetic modifications in bacterial genomes come from arbitrary mutation during replication, where genes involved in a particular growth limiting process have an

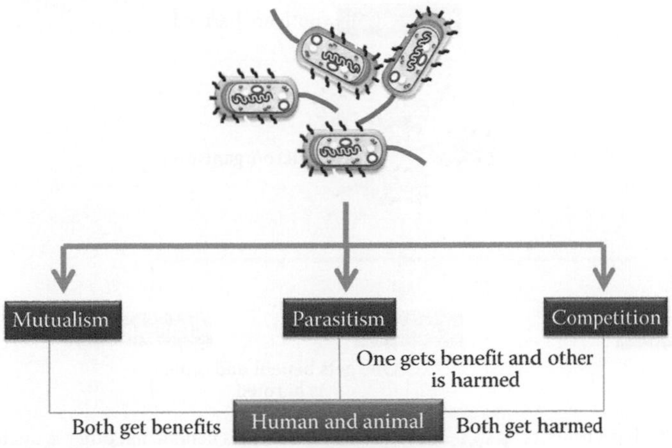

Figure 3.4 Bacterial life cycle.

increased mutation rate. In addition, there are few bacterial species that transfer genetic material between each other in three different ways. In the first situation, bacteria can take up exogenous DNA from their environment, and this process is called *transformation;* in the second case, genes can be transferred by the process of *transduction;* and the third way of gene transfer is where DNA is transferred through direct cell contact known as *conjugation.*

3.4.3 Nomenclature of bacteria

In order to distinguish one bacterium from another bacterium, numerous methods have been used through which bacteria can be classified on the basis of cell structure, cellular metabolism, or differences in cell constituents such as DNA, fatty acids, antigens, and quinones. Interestingly, the International Committee on Systematics of Prokaryotes maintains international rules for the description of bacteria. Moreover, identification of bacteria is particularly relevant in medicine, where the exact treatment is examined by the bacterial species causing an infection or disease. Subsequently, the need to recognize human pathogens is a major motivation for the development of techniques to identify bacteria. Over the last few years, identification of bacteria is done using molecular tools such as PCR methods due to their specificity and speedy result.

3.4.4 Bacteria: Friends or foes

One of the interesting aspects of the bacterial life cycle is their association with other organisms because bacteria can form complex associations with both animals and humans. There are three types of association reported: mutualism, competition, and parasitism.

3.4.4.1 Parasitism

It is a type of reciprocal association between two dissimilar organisms, where the parasite benefits at the expense of the host (human). One parasite passes on its life stages in various hosts; these are called macroparasites, typically protozoa and helminths. Additionally, parasites also include microparasites, which are viruses and bacteria typically smaller in size, which can be directly transmitted between humans. Many adult end parasites reside

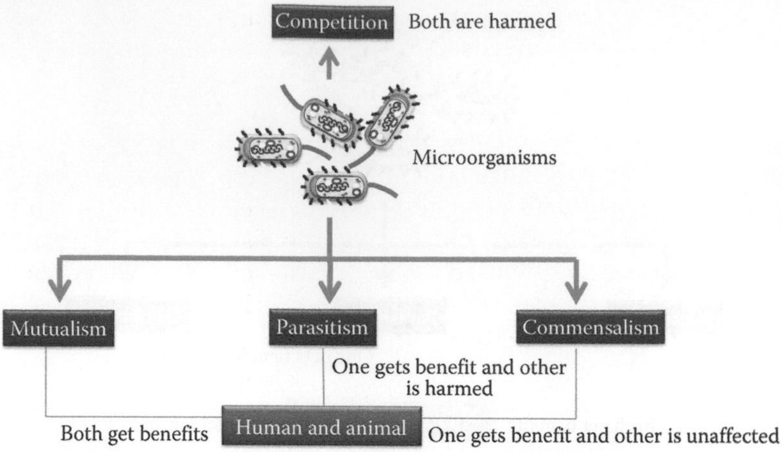

Figure 3.5 Types of bacterial relation with humans and animals.

in the host's gastrointestinal tract, where the offspring can be shed along with host excreta (Figure 3.5).

3.4.4.2 *Mutualism*

In this kind of association, bacteria live with a host that is essential for their survival for both bacteria and host, for example, the presence of over thousands of bacterial species in the human gut flora of the intestines can enhance gut immunity, and also the ability to synthesize vitamins (folic acid, vitamin K, and biotin) and convert milk protein to lactic acid. Moreover, the presence of these bacteria also prevents the growth of possibly pathogenic bacteria. These beneficial bacteria are subsequently sold as probiotic dietary supplements.

3.4.4.3 *Commensalism*

Commensalism is a type of association between two organisms where one organism benefits but the other is not affected. There are a large number of bacteria that live in a healthy human and do not cause any harmful effects on humans. They are called commensal bacteria and such a relationship is called commensalism. There are millions of bacteria living in the human gut alone and many of these bacteria have mutualistic or even potential pathogenic relationships with their human hosts. Some of the most common commensal bacterial reported in humans are *Staphylococcus epidermidis, Mycobacteria, Propionibacterium, Corynebacterium.*

3.4.5 *Pathogenic bacteria*

In addition to some of the harmless bacteria, there are some bacteria that cause diseases in humans and are known as pathogenic bacteria. Tuberculosis is a bacterial disease that kills about two million people a year, mostly in African countries. This disease is caused by the bacterium *Mycobacterium tuberculosis*. Pneumonia is caused by bacteria such as *Streptococcus* and *Pseudomonas*, and food-borne illnesses are caused by bacteria such as *Shigella, Campylobacter,* and *Salmonella*. Furthermore, pathogenic bacteria are also known to cause infections such as typhoid fever, diphtheria, syphilis, tetanus, and leprosy. There are some bacteria under certain conditions that can cause the disease, for example,

Staphylococcus or *Streptococcus* are also part of the normal human flora and usually occur on the skin and they do not cause any diseases (Figure 3.5).

3.5 Applications of microbes

Besides having both harmful and beneficial effects on the human body, bacteria have been found to be most effective in various other applications. There are various benefits of bacteria, especially in food biotechnology. Bacteria (*Lactobacillus* and *Lactococcus*) combined with yeasts and molds are efficiently used in the preparation of fermented foods such as sauce, cheese, vinegar, pickles, soy, and yogurt. Interestingly, the capability of bacteria to destroy a variety of organic compounds is remarkable and has been used in bioremediation of industrial toxic wastes. In addition, bacteria are capable of digesting the hydrocarbons in petroleum and are often used to clean up oil spills. Bacteria (*Bacillus thuringiensis*) can also be employed in biological pest control.

One of the remarkable features of bacteria is that they grow quickly and their genetic materials can be easily manipulated. Moreover, bacterial DNA has been extensively used in understanding the function of genes, enzymes, and metabolic pathways in bacteria, and this knowledge has then been applied to animals and humans. Over the last few decades, the knowledge of bacterial genetics was used for the production of therapeutic proteins, such as growth hormones, growth factors, antibodies, and insulin. There are various therapeutic applications of bacteria, which include the use of bacteria in making recombinant DNA products, therapeutic proteins, next-generation antibiotics, and diagnostics tools and kits.

3.5.1 Antimicrobial drugs

One of the most remarkable features of microbes is their ability to kill microbes. These capabilities have been extensively exploited by biotechnology and pharmaceutical companies to produce tons of antibiotics. An antibiotic or antibacterial is a substance or compound that kills bacteria or inhibits their growth. Moreover, antibiotics belong to the broader group of antimicrobial compounds, which are used to treat infections caused by bacteria, fungi, and protozoa. The word antibiotic was first coined by Selman Waksman in 1942 to describe any substance produced by bacteria that retards the growth of other microorganisms. However, this original definition does not include naturally occurring substances that kill bacteria. With rapid advances in the field of medicinal chemistry, most antibiotics are basically semisynthetic in nature are derived from original compounds found in nature, for example, beta-lactams, which include the penicillins, produced by fungi in the genus *Penicillium*. Interestingly, some antibiotics are still produced and isolated from living bacteria, such as aminoglycosides, and others have been created through purely synthetic means such as sulfonamides, oxazolidinones, and quinolones. In addition, antibiotic drugs can be classified into natural, semisynthetic, and synthetic based on their effects on the microorganisms (Tables 3.1 and 3.2).

3.5.1.1 Classification of antibiotics

Antibiotic drugs can also be divided into two types: those that kill bacteria, known as bactericidal agents, and those that only impair bacterial growth, known as bacteriostatic agents. Furthermore, antibiotics are commonly classified based on their chemical structure and mechanism of action on the bacteria. It has been shown that most of the antibiotics generally target bacterial functions or growth. Antibiotics (penicillin and cephalosporins) that target the bacterial cell wall or cell membrane are usually bactericidal in nature and

Table 3.1 Antibiotics Produced by Microorganisms

Microorganism	Antibiotics	Applications
Bacillus brevis	Tyrothricin (G+, G–)	Mouth and throat infection
Bacillus polymyxa	Polymyxin B (AT)	UTI, gastroenteritis
Bacillus subtilis	Bacitracin (G+)	Dermatitis, superficial pyogenic infection, dysentery
Streptococcus cremates	Nisin (G+)	In cheese, food preservation (nonmedical use)

Table 3.2 Microorganisms and Their Biological Products

	Microbial products			
Microorganisms	Primary metabolites (1)	Secondary metabolites (2)	Enzymes (3)	Others (4)
		Bacteria		
Acetobacter aceti	Acetic acid			
Acetobacterirum woodii	Acetic acid			
Bacillus brevis		Gramicidin		
Bacillus polymyxa		Polymyxin B	Amylase	
Bacillus popilliae		Endotoxin		
Bacillus subtilis		Bacitracin		
Bacillus buringiensis		Endotoxin		
Clostridium aceticum	Acetic acid			
Gluconobacter suboxidans	Vinegar			
Methylophilus methylotrophus	Glutamic acid			
Pseudomonas denitrificans	Vitamin B12			Yogurt
		Actinomycetes		
Micromonosporsa purpurea		Gentamicin		
Nocardia mediterranei		Rifamycin		

antibiotics (aminoglycosides, macrolides, and tetracycline) that target protein synthesis are usually bacteriostatic in nature. Interestingly, there is a further categorization of antibiotics based on their target specificity; for example, antibiotics will work differently for both Gram-negative and Gram-positive bacteria, respectively. There are broad-spectrum antibiotics known to affect a wide range of bacteria. In the last few years, three new classes of antibiotics have been brought into clinical use. These new antibiotics are cyclic lipopeptides (brand name: daptomycin), glycylcyclines (brand name: tigecycline), and oxazolidinones (brand name: linezolid) (Figure 3.6).

3.5.2 *Antibiotic production*

It is equally important to know how these antibiotics are manufactured or produced in large quantity in the industrial level and penicillin antibiotics are historically significant because they are the first drugs that were manufactured and produced to supply to the different parts of the world (Figure 3.7).

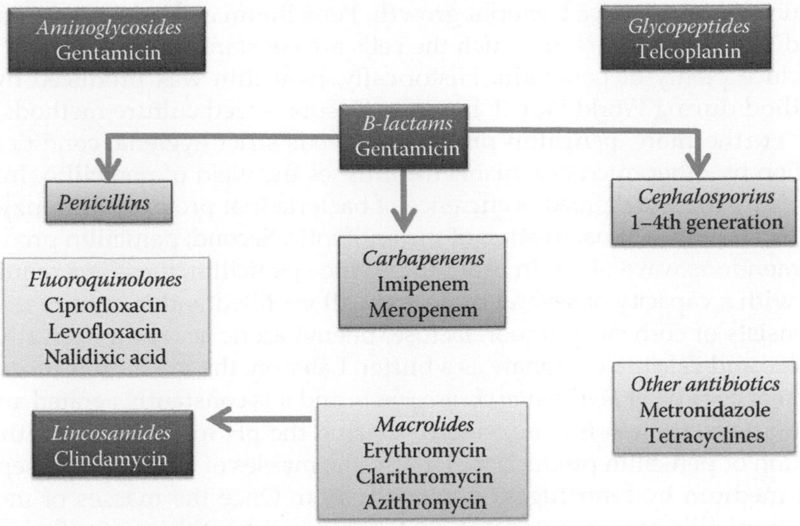

Figure 3.6 Classification of antibiotics.

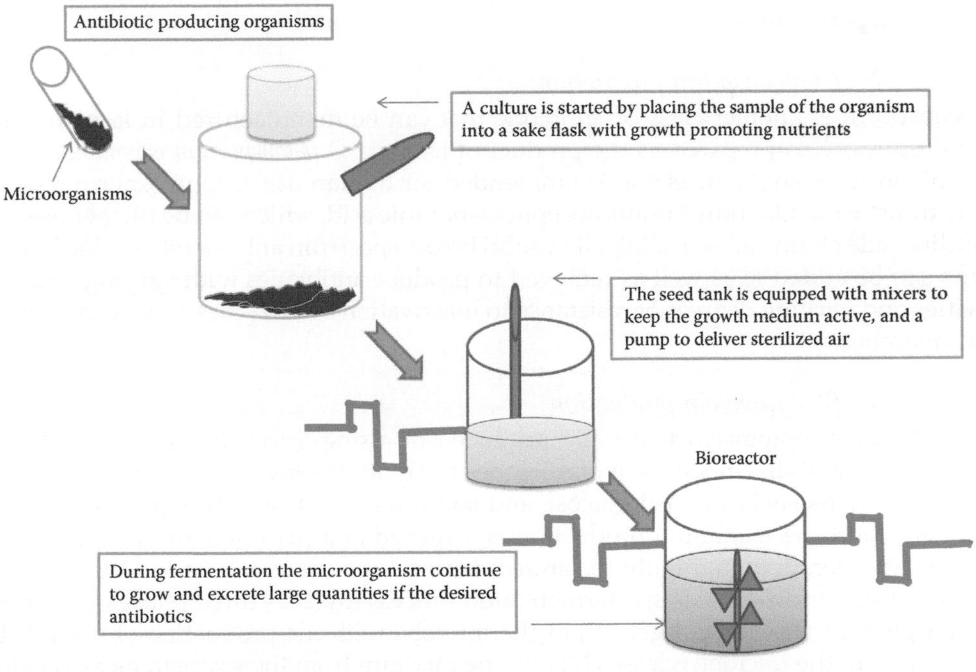

Figure 3.7 Making of antibiotics.

3.5.2.1 *Penicillin production*

In order to understand the production of penicillin, let us first learn how penicillin is made through natural ways, because that would allow one to become familiar with the chemical pathway involved in its production. Penicillin is basically a secondary metabolite of fungus. Penicillin is produced when the growth of *Penicillium* is inhibited by stress and it is not produced during active bacterial growth. Penicillium cells are grown using a technique called fed-batch culture, in which the cells are constantly subjected to stress condition to produce plenty of penicillin. Historically, penicillin was produced by a surface culture method during World War II, but in 1943, submerged culture methods were used exclusively. Furthermore, penicillin production needs strict hygienic conditions because contamination by other microorganisms diminishes the yield of penicillin. Interestingly, this is caused by the widespread occurrence of bacteria that produces the enzyme *penicillinase*, which can cause an inactivation of the antibiotic. Second, penicillin production also needs a tremendous wave of air. In order to produce penicillin, there is a requirement for fermenters with a capacity of several thousand gallons filled with a culture medium. The medium consists of corn steep liquor, lactose, phenyl acetic acid or a derivative, glucose, nutrient, salts, and calcium carbonate as a buffer. Later on, the medium is inoculated with a suspension of conidia of *Penicillium chrysogenum* and it is constantly aerated and agitated. After about 7 days, growth is completed by raising the pH to 8.0 or above, thus causing the completion of penicillin production. Finally, the masses of mold growth separate from the culture medium by centrifugation and filtration. Once the masses of mold growth that contain penicillin are separated, the next step is to extract the penicillin in pure form. The purification method involves organic solvents and crystallization process. In order to check the effectiveness of the penicillin, the potency of a batch of penicillin is determined by a bioassay in which the unknown is compared with a standard preparation of crystalline sodium penicillin G.

3.5.2.2 Cephalosporin production

Cephalosporin is another class of antibiotic that can be manufactured in large quantity. Cephalosporin C is prepared as the product of bacteria *Cephalosporium acremonium*; however, this form of antibiotic is not recommended for human use. Cephalosporin molecule can be transformed to form 7-α-aminocephalosporanic acid, which can be further modified by adding side chains to form clinically useful broad-spectrum antimicrobials. Various side chains can be added to as well as removed to produce antibiotics with varying spectra of activities and varying degrees of resistance to inactivation by enzymes produced by pathogenic microbes.

3.5.2.3 Streptomycin production

The antibiotic streptomycin is usually produced by using *Streptomyces griseus*. The process is started with the inoculation of microbes to obtain the mycelia biomass. The culture medium contains soybean meal glucose and sodium chloride and this process is carried out at 28°C and the maximum production is achieved at a pH range of 7.6–8.0. The high agitation and aeration are highly recommended and the process lasts for about 10 days. It has been shown that the classic fermentation process involves three phases, and during the first phase, there is rapid growth of the microbe with the production of mycelia biomass. Later on, the microbe releases NH_3 to the medium from the soybean meal, causing a rise in pH value, and during this initial fermentation phase, there is a slight production of streptomycin. Moreover, during the second phase, there is little production of mycelium, but the secondary metabolite accumulates in the form of streptomycin in the medium. The glucose and NH_3 released are spent during this phase. In the third and final phase, when carbohydrates become exhausted, streptomycin production stops and the microbial cells begin to lyse and pH value increases, which finally lead to the ends of the process. After the process is complete, mycelium is separated from the broth by the filtration method and the antibiotic recovered in the crude form. The crude antibiotic is then purified by the activated charcoal method and eluted with acid alcohol. The antibiotic is then precipitated with chemical solvent (acetone) and additionally purified by the use of column chromatography.

3.5.2.4 *Synthesis of vitamin B12 using microbes*

Vitamins are very important for the normal development and health of individuals and have been supplemented with many antibiotic drugs. The production of vitamins, especially B12, generally requires a wide range of bacteria and streptomycetes, though not to the same extent by yeasts and fungi. While over 100 fermentation processes have been described for the production of vitamin Bl, only half a dozen have apparently been used on a commercial scale. The processes using the *Propionibacterium* species are the most productive and are now widely used commercially. It is important to select microbial species that produce the 5,6-dimethyl benzimidazolylcobamid exclusively. Several manufacturers have been led astray by organisms that gave high yields of the related cobamides including pseudo-vitamin Bu (adeninylcobamide). The natural form of the vitamin is Barker's coenzyme where a deoxyadenosyl residue replaces the cyano group found in the commercial vitamin. Practically all of the cobamides formed in the fermentation are retained in the cells, and the first step is the separation of the cells from the fermentation medium. Large high-speed centrifuges are used to concentrate the bacteria to a cream, while filters are used to remove streptomycete cells. The vitamin B12 activity is released from the cells by acid, heating, cyanide, or other treatments. The addition of cyanide solutions decomposes the coenzyme form of the vitamin and results in the formation of the cyanocobalamin. The cyanocobalamin is adsorbed on ion exchange resin or charcoal, and is eluted. It is then purified further by partitions between the phenolic solvents and water. The vitamin is finally crystallized from aqueous acetone solutions. The crystalline product often contains some water of crystallization.

3.5.2.5 *Production of enzymes by using microbes*

The enzymes can be extracted from the tissues of higher organisms; however, it is easier and economical to obtain the enzymes from microorganisms. The first industrial production of enzymes from microorganisms dates back to 1894 when *Fungal diastase* was produced in the United States to be employed as a pharmaceutical agent for digestive disorders. These enzymes have found a variety of applications in medicine, food industries, textiles, and leather industries and also in analytical processes. Most commercialized microbial enzymes come from a small number of fungi and bacteria. *Aspergillus, Fusarium, Trichoderma,* and *Humicola* all belong to the ascomycetes class. *Mucor* and *Rhizomucor* belong to zygomyctes, which are the fungi from which biocatalysts are retrieved. *Bacillus* and *Pseudomonas* are the bacterial strains employed for the production of enzymes. The most important industrially produced microbial enzymes are alpha-amylase, proteases, and lipases. Three different molecular techniques are adopted for the largescale production of microbial enzymes; they are an expression cloning, molecular screening, and protein engineering.

3.6 Microbial biotransformation

Biotransformation is the process of the modification of an organic compound into a recoverable product of simple chemical reactions, catalyzed by cellular enzymes. Both the substrate and the product are not involved in the primary or secondary metabolism of the organism concerned. They are not at all synonymous with the metabolites as discussed earlier, produced by the complex pathways of primary and secondary metabolism of the

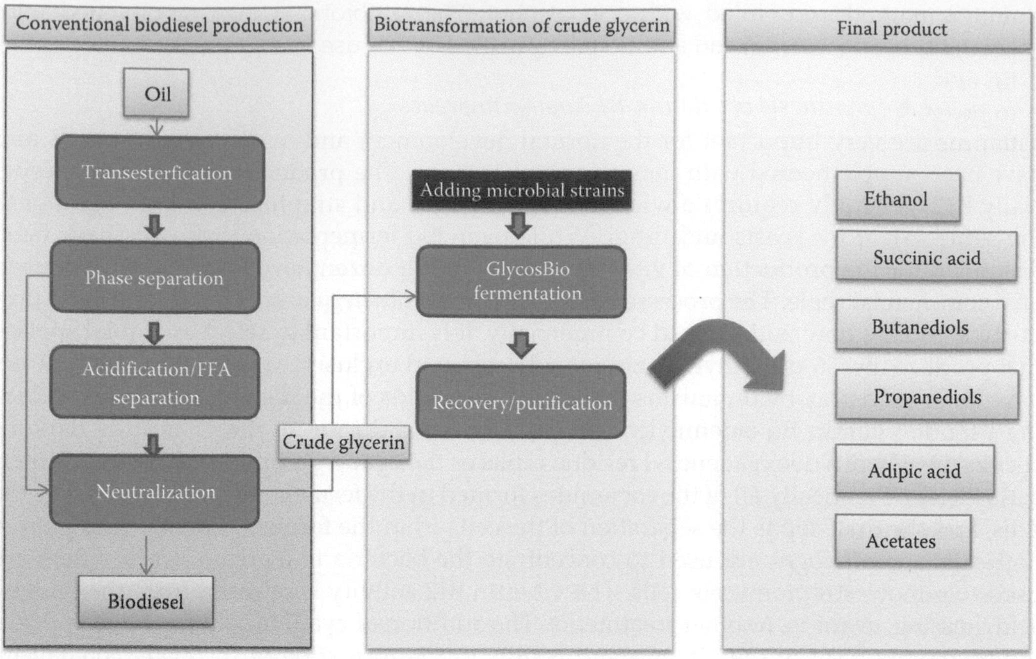

Figure 3.8 Biotransformation using microorganisms.

organism. Plant cells and animal cells as well as microbes are capable of performing biotransformation. But owing to the rapid microbial growth and high metabolic rates of microorganisms, a microbial process of biotransformation is far more efficient and economical. Transformations were practiced as early as 5000 BC in Babylonia to convert wine to vinegar. Nonetheless, it was only in 1864 that Pasteur showed that the process was mediated by microbes. By the beginning of the nineteenth century, several bioconversions were known that included conversion of deoxycorticosterone of corticosterone by ox adrenals as the first commercial biotransformation. This biotransformation is now more efficiently achieved by a microbial process especially used in the making of biofuels and biochemicals (Figure 3.8).

3.6.1 *Biotransformation of* D*-sorbitol to* L*-sorbose*

The commercial production of ascorbic acid involves the chemical conversion of glucose to D-sorbitol, which is then biotransformed by *Acetobacter suboxydans* to L-sorbose. L-Sorbose produces ascorbic acid again by chemical transformation. It has been reported that for biotransformation and production of L-sorbose, 15–30% D-sorbitol is supplemented to the medium and *A. suboxydans* is inoculated at 300°C. Thereafter, vigorous aeration and agitation is provided in the culture medium and approximately 90–95% conversion occurs in 1–2 days. The culture media is then filtered in vacuum and the concentrated powder is then allowed to cool. With this method, about 65% of L-sorbose can be recovered.

3.6.2 *Biotransformation of antibiotics*

New antibiotics are found to be more effective than the existing ones and they have always been the aim of scientists. Several microbial-mediated transformations have been achieved with remarkable success. Biotransformation is now routinely employed for the commercial production of several useful antibiotics, for example, production of semisynthetic penicillin and cephalosporins. Naturally produced penicillin G and penicillin V are deacylated to produce the penicillin nucleus 6-aminopenicillanic acid. It is then chemically modified to produce semisynthetic penicillin and cephalosporin.

3.6.3 Biotransformation of steroids

Biotransformation of steroids is the second important microbial process to produce pharmaceuticals. With the help of biotransformation steroids, adrenocortical hormones such as corticosterone, cortisone, and hydrocortisone, and their therapeutically superior derivatives, for example, prednisone, prednisolone, triamcinolone, and so on, can be successfully produced. Progesterone is a steroid hormone active during pregnancy. It acts as a precursor for the industrial production of at least four products using microorganisms. These conversions involve hydroxylation and dehydrogenation. Hydroxylation as well as dehydrogenation gives the compound better efficiency as hormones, for example, the oxygen at C-11 is essential for the anti-inflammatory effect of cortisone. Steroid hormones can also be produced from sterol precursors, which are cheap. For example, diosgenin from *Dioscorea*; beta-sitosterol, campesterol, and stigmasterol from soybean; and cholesterol from wool grease are employed as hormone precursors. All these sterols have the same sterane nucleus and one or more side chains and biotransformation involves the removal of these side chains.

3.7 Food microbiology

Food microbiology is the science of microorganisms that evaluates food quality and food contamination. One of the major concerns faced by any food outlet or food manufacturing company is to maintain contamination-free food for long periods of time, especially under storage conditions.

3.7.1 Food pathogens

In a general sense, food infection generally refers to the presence of bacteria or other microbes in food, which causes sickness in humans. Food poison denotes the ingestion of toxins contained within the food. Most cases of food-related infections are caused by a range of pathogenic bacteria, viruses, and parasites that contaminate food, rather than chemical or natural toxins. Additionally, bacteria are a common cause of foodborne illness, which mainly include *Salmonella* and *Escherichia coli*. There are various symptoms associated with bacterial infections, which include diarrhea, vomiting, body and stomach aches, and fever. Some of the common food pathogens are listed in Table 3.3. Furthermore,

Table 3.3 List of Foodborne Pathogens

Most common bacteria	Other common bacteria	Less common bacteria
Campylobacter jejuni	*Bacillus cereus*	*Brucella* spp.
Clostridium perfringens	*Escherichia coli*	*Corynebacterium ulcerans*
Campylobacter jejuni	*Listeria monocytogenes*	*Coxiella burnetii*
Salmonella species	*Staphylococcus aureus*	*Plesiomonas shigelloides*
Escherichia coli	*Streptococcus*	

some foodborne illnesses are also caused by exotoxins, which are generally excreted by the bacterial cells. Exotoxins can cause illness even when the microbes that produced them have been exterminated. There are various symptoms associated with exotoxin-related infections; typically, a symptom appears after a couple of hours depending on the amount of toxin consumed. *Clostridium botulinum, Clostridium perfringens, Staphylococcus aureus,* and *Bacillus cereus* are known to produce exotoxins. Furthermore, *Staphylococcus aureus* produces a toxin that causes intense vomiting in patients.

3.7.2 Problems of food pathogens

In recent times, the rapid globalization of food production and trade marketing has increased the potential of food contamination and many eruptions of food-borne diseases that were once contained within a small community may now take place on a global level. More recently, food safety authorities all over the world have recognized that safeguarding food safety must not only be undertaken at the national level but also through closer relations among food safety authorities at the international level. This is vital for swapping routine information on food safety issues and to have quick access to information in case of emergencies. Furthermore, it is difficult to guess the global occurrence of foodborne disease; nevertheless, many of these cases have been ascribed to contamination of food and drinking water. Furthermore, diarrhea is considered a major cause of malnutrition in infants and children. The food pathogen-related illnesses in the United States are given in Table 3.4. About 30% of the population living in developed countries have been reported to suffer from food-borne diseases every year. In the United States alone, around 76 million cases of foodborne diseases were reported, and 325,000 hospitalizations and 5000 deaths are estimated to occur each year due to foodborne diseases. With reference to developing countries in particular, they are the worst affected by food-borne illnesses caused by microbes and parasites. In 1994, an outbreak of salmonellosis due to contaminated ice cream occurred in the United States, affecting an estimated 224,000 persons. In 1988, hepatitis A resulting from the consumption of contaminated clams affected more than 300,000 individuals in China. Besides the occurrence of diseases related to food pathogens, food pathogens also affect the food industry, especially in the United States, with a total loss of US $35 billion annually as per 1997 reports.

3.8 Challenges of treating microbial infections

One of the greatest challenges for current medical fields is the development of drug resistance in various microbial diseases. Drug resistance is basically a reduction of drug

Table 3.4 Causes of Foodborne Illness in the United States (1999)

	Cause	Annual cases	Rate (per 100,000 inhabitants)
1	Norwalk-like viruses	20,000 cases	7.3
2	*Salmonella*	15,608 cases	5.7
3	*Campylobacter*	10,539 cases	3.9
4	*Toxoplasma gondii*	2500 cases	0.9
5	*Listeria monocytogenes*	2298 cases	0.8
	Total	60,854 cases	22.3

effectiveness in treating a disease or condition. Over a period of time, the microbes generally develop a resistance against the drug, which leads to the antimicrobial drug becoming ineffective. Furthermore, the term "drug resistance" is used in the background of resistance acquired by pathogens (bacteria) and when an organism is resistant to more than one drug; it is believed to be multidrug resistant. There are a number of reasons for the microbes to develop drug resistance and one of the most widely known could be the extensive use of antibiotics. Furthermore, in some countries, antibiotics are sold over the counter in a pharmacy shop without a valid prescription from doctors or physicians, which also leads to the creation of bacteria resistance. There are other reasons contributing toward resistance, including the addition of antibiotics to the feed of livestock such as chickens and goats.

In addition to the above, the dosages of antibiotics prescribed are a major issue in increasing the rates of bacterial resistance, as a single dose of antibiotics may lead to a greater risk of developing resistance against that antibiotic treatment. In addition, the use of nonspecific antibiotics has also been accredited to a number of causes of drug resistance. Another issue that needs to be mentioned is that people, for example, believe that antibiotics are effective for common cold and flu, and a large number of patients do not complete a course of antibiotics primarily due to that fact that they start to feel better. Considering all these issues, it has now been recommended that compliance with one daily dose of antibiotics is better than with twice daily antibiotics. Additionally, taking antibiotic doses less than those recommended by doctors/physicians can also increase rates of drug resistance, and interestingly, shortening the duration of an antibiotic course may actually decrease the rates of resistance. Finally, poor maintenance of hygiene in the clinic and hospital staff has been linked to the spread of resistant organisms (Figure 3.9).

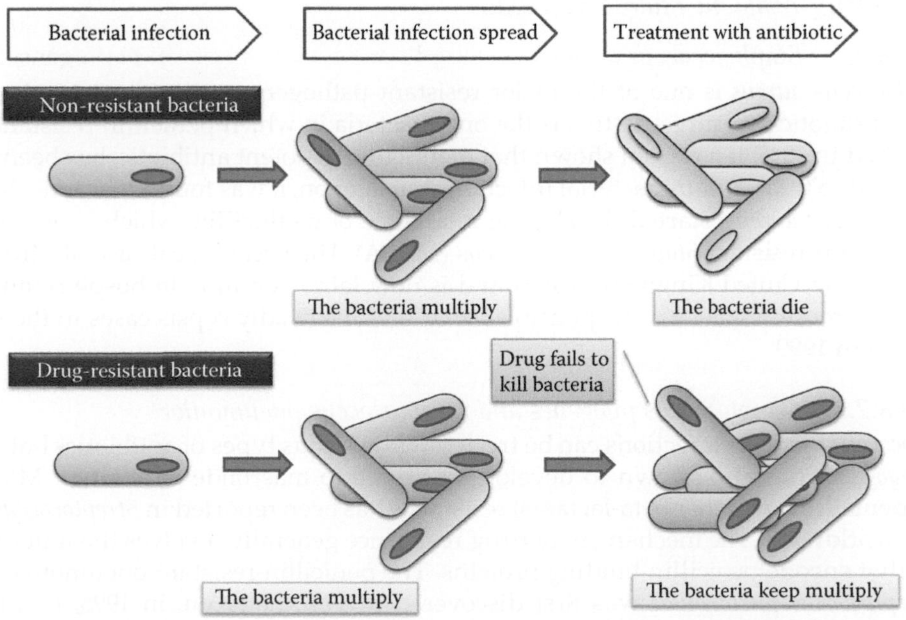

Figure 3.9 Bacterial drug resistance.

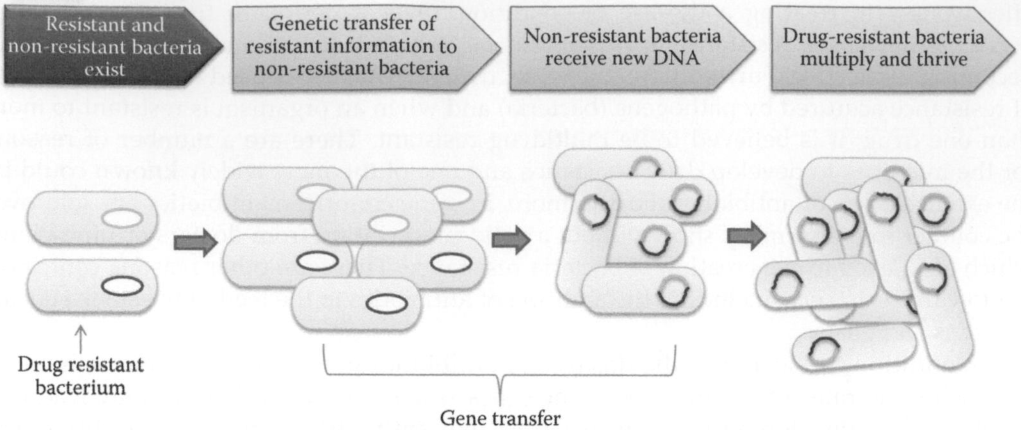
Resistant and non-resistant bacteria exist
Genetic transfer of resistant information to non-resistant bacteria
Non-resistant bacteria receive new DNA
Drug-resistant bacteria multiply and thrive
Drug resistant bacterium
Gene transfer

Figure 3.10 Mechanism of bacterial drug resistance by gene transfer.

3.8.1 Mechanism of drug resistance

There are four main mechanisms by which microorganisms exhibit resistance to antimicrobials which are (i) drug inactivation or modification, (ii) alteration of the target site, (iii) alteration of metabolic pathway, and (iv) reduced drug accumulation. The fluoroquinolone is found to be resistant by bacteria. Also, in Gram-negative bacteria, plasmid-mediated resistance genes produce proteins that can bind to DNA gyrase, shielding it from the action of quinolones. Consequently, mutations at key sites in DNA gyrase can decrease their binding affinity to quinolones, decreasing the drug's effectiveness. Furthermore, antibiotic resistance can also be presented artifcially in bacteria (Figure 3.10).

3.8.2 Drug-resistant microorganisms

3.8.2.1 Staphylococcus aureus

Staphylococcus aureus is one of the major resistant pathogens and it is extremely adaptable to antibiotic pressure and this is the only bacteria in which penicillin resistance was established in 1947. It has been shown that methicillin, a potent antibiotic, has been extensively used to treat various bacterial infections but later on, it was found that some bacteria (*Staphylococcus aureus*) started developing resistance of methicillin, which is now known as methicillin-resistant *Staphylococcus aureus* (MRSA). The first clinical case of MRSA was noticed in the United Kingdom in 1961 and is now fairly common in hospitals and clinics. Furthermore, MRSA was responsible for 37% of the deadly sepsis cases in the United Kingdom in 1999.

3.8.2.2 Streptococcus pyogenes and Streptococcus pneumoniae

Streptococcus pyogenes infections can be treated with various types of antibiotics but strains of *S. pyogenes* are also known to develop resistance to macrolide antibiotics. Moreover, drug (penicillin and other beta-lactams) resistance has been reported in *Streptococcus pneumoniae* worldwide. The mechanism of drug resistance generally involves the mutations in genes that encode penicillin-binding proteins. The penicillin-resistant pneumonia caused by *Streptococcus pneumoniae* was first discovered in 1967. Later on, in 1993, *E. coli* were found to be resistant to five fluoro-quinolone drugs. Moreover, *Mycobacterium tuberculosis* has been usually resistant to isoniazid and rifampin drugs.

3.8.2.3 *Pseudomonas aeruginosa*

P. aeruginosa is a highly widespread pathogen; one of the most frustrating characteristics of this organism is its low antibiotic vulnerability. Additionally, *P. aeruginosa* can easily acquire resistance either by a mutation process or by the horizontal gene transfer of antibiotic resistance elements. Some recent studies have shown that phenotypic resistance bacteria are associated with biofilm formation in the response to antibiotic treatment.

3.8.2.4 *Clostridium difficile*

C. difficile is a pathogen that causes diarrhea worldwide and in various parts of the United States. *C. difficile* develops clindamycin resistance. Additionally, the outbreaks of *C. difficile* strains were found to be resistant to fluoro-quinolone antibiotic drugs.

3.8.2.5 *Salmonella and E. coli*

E. coli and *Salmonella* are also known to cause food contamination and more than 80% of the *E. coli* and *Salmonella* are resistant to one or more antibacterial drugs. Additionally, *E. coli* and *Salmonella* cause bladder infections that are found to be resistant to antibiotics.

3.8.3 *Solution for drug-resistant microorganisms*

In view of the growing rate of drug resistance problems associated with microorganisms, there has been a surge of research to control this problem. There is a common saying that prevention is better than cure and it can also imply in the case of drug-resistant microorganisms. The minimum use of antibiotics may reduce the chances of developing antibiotic-resistant bacteria. Besides, vaccines do not undergo the problem of resistance because a vaccine enhances the body's natural immunity, while an antibiotic kills bacterial cells. While idealistic, antistaphylococcal vaccines have shown limited efficacy because of the immunological disparity between *Staphylococcus* species, and the limited duration of efficiency of the antibodies produced. Moreover, proteins synthesized in the animal body after a disease are not antibiotics so they do not contribute to the antibiotic resistance problem. Additionally, studies based on using cytokines have shown that they enhance the growth of animals without using antibiotics. Moreover, cytokines can achieve the animal growth rates conventionally without the contribution of antibiotic resistance.

An alternative approach through which drug resistance problems can be accomplished is phage therapy. Phage therapy can be used to treat pathogenic bacterial infections. Furthermore, phage therapy has been extensively investigated and utilized as a therapeutic agent for many years, especially in the former Soviet Union. Phage therapy (Figure 3.11) was widely used in the United States until the discovery of antibiotics. Unlike antibiotics, phage treatments have some disadvantages as phages must be frozen until used, and a physician's/healthcare professionals needs special training in prescribing and handling phages. The effectiveness of phage therapy becomes a disadvantage when the precise species of infecting bacteria is not known. It has been recommended that phages should be tested in the laboratory prior to application in the patients, making phages less suitable for critical cases where time is not available.

3.9 *Summary*

Bacteriology is the study of bacteria that comprises the identification, classification, and characterization of bacterial species. Bacteria are identified by their properties, for

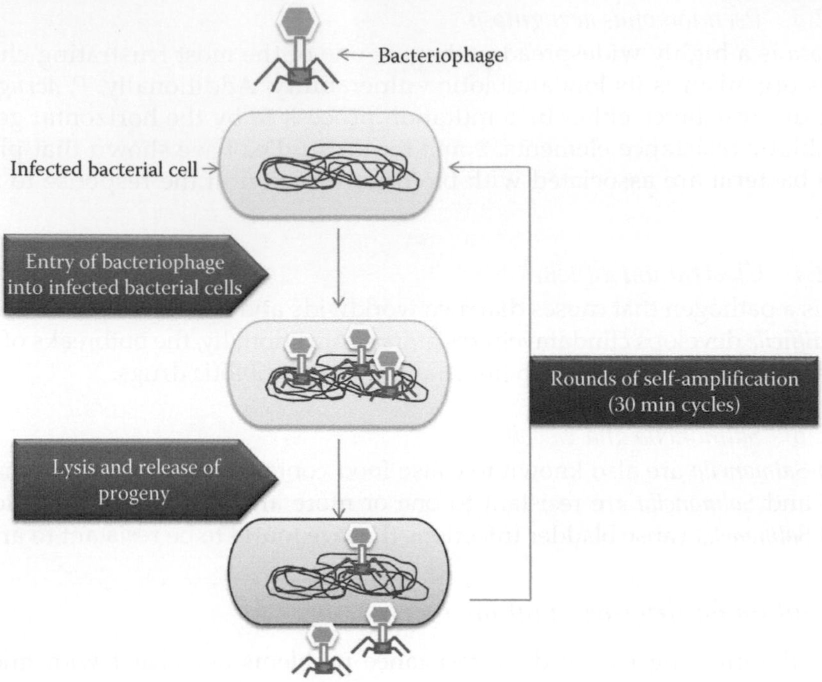

Figure 3.11 Bacteriophage therapy.

example, their looks, what nutrients they can grow on or not grow on, what temperature they require for growth, what substances they produce, and so on. The morphology and internal organization of bacteria is studied by using a microscope. Microbes are the oldest form of life on the earth and some types have been in existence for billions of years. These tiny microbes live in the water you drink, the food you eat, and the air you breathe. Right now, billions of microbes are swimming in your belly and crawling on your skin and skull. Surprisingly, over 95% of microbes are harmless, only the remaining 5% could be dangerous to your health. These microbes can be classified into categories such as beneficial microbes and harmful microbes. However, microbes do have various useful applications and over the past few decades, these microbes have been exploited by people in biotechnology, both in the making of traditional food and beverage and in modern technologies based on genetic engineering. In this chapter, we discussed the general characteristics of microbes and explained how these microbes are harmful and useful to humans.

3.10 Scholar's achievements

Antonie van Leeuwenhoek: Antonie Philips van Leeuwenhoek (October 24, 1632–August 26, 1723) was a Dutch tradesman and scientist from Delft, Netherlands. He is commonly known as "the father of microbiology," and considered to be the first microbiologist. He is best known for his work on the improvement of the microscope and for his contributions toward the establishment of microbiology.

Lazzaro Spallanzani: Lazzaro Spallanzani (10 January 1729–12 February 1799) was an Italian Catholic priest, a biologist, and physiologist who made important contributions to the experimental study of bodily functions, animal reproduction, and essentially animal echolocation.

Louis Pasteur: Louis Pasteur (December 27, 1822–September 28, 1895) was a French chemist and microbiologist who was one of the most important founders of medical microbiology. He is remembered for his remarkable breakthroughs in the causes and preventions of diseases. His discoveries reduced mortality from puerperal fever, and he created the first vaccines for rabies and anthrax.

Robert Koch: Robert Heinrich Herman Koch (December 11, 1843–May 27, 1910), considered to be the founder of modern bacteriology, is known for his role in identifying the specific causative agents of tuberculosis, cholera, and anthrax and for giving experimental support for the concept of infectious disease.

3.11 Knowledge builder

Plankton: Plankton (singular plankter) are any organisms that live in the water column and are incapable of swimming against a current. They provide a crucial source of food for many larger aquatic organisms, such as fish and whales.

Planarian: A planarian is one of many nonparasitic flatworms of the Turbellaria class. It is also the common name for a member of the genus *Planaria* within the family Planariidae. Sometimes, it also refers to the genus *Dugesia*.

International Committee on Systematics of Prokaryotes (ICSP): The ICSP, formerly the International Committee on Systematic Bacteriology (ICSB), is the body that oversees the nomenclature of prokaryotes, determines the rules by which prokaryotes are named and whose Judicial Commission issues opinions concerning taxonomic matters, revisions to the Bacteriological Code, and so on. The ICSB was established by the International Association of Microbiological Societies.

Biotransformation: Biotransformation is the chemical modification made by an organism on a chemical compound. Biotransformation means chemical alteration of chemicals such as (but not limited to) nutrients, amino acids, toxins, and drugs in the body. It is also needed to render nonpolar compounds polar so that they are not reabsorbed in renal tubules and are excreted. Biotransformation of xenobiotics can dominate toxicokinetics and the metabolites may reach higher concentrations in organisms than their parent compounds.

Bacteriostatic agent: Bacteriostatic agent or bacteriostatic, abbreviated Bstatic, is a biological or chemical agent that stops bacteria from reproducing, while not necessarily harming them otherwise. Depending on their application, bacteriostatic antibiotics, disinfectants, antiseptics, and preservatives can be distinguished. Upon removal of the bacteriostatic, the bacteria usually start to grow again.

DNA gyrase: DNA gyrase, often referred to simply as gyrase, is an enzyme that relieves strain while double-stranded DNA is being unwound by helicase. This causes negative supercoiling of the DNA. Bacterial DNA gyrase is the target of many antibiotics, including nalidixic acid, novobiocin, and ciprofloxacin.

Fluoro-quinolone: The quinolones are a family of synthetic broad-spectrum antibacterial drugs. The first generation of the quinolones began with the introduction of nalidixic acid in 1962 for the treatment of urinary tract infections in humans. Nalidixic acid was discovered by George Lesher and coworkers in a distillate during an attempt at chloroquine synthesis.

Further reading

Albrich WC, Monnet DL, and Harbarth S 2004. Antibiotic selection pressure and resistance in *Streptococcus pneumoniae* and *Streptococcus pyogenes*. *Emerg Infect Dis* 10 (3): 514–517. PMID 15109426. http://www.cdc.gov/ncidod/eid/vol10no3/03-0252.htm.

Arias CA and Murray BE 2009. Antibiotic-resistant bugs in the 21st century a clinical super-challenge. *N Engl J Med* 360 (5): 439–443. doi:10.1056/NEJMp0804651. PMID 19179312.

Arnold SR and Straus SE 2005. Interventions to improve antibiotic prescribing practices in ambulatory care. *Cochrane Database Syst Rev* 19 (4): CD003539.

Baker R 2006. Health management with reduced antibiotic use—The U.S. experience. *Anim Biotechnol* 17 (2): 195–205. doi:10.1080/10495390600962274. PMID 17127530.

Bearden DA, Allen GP, and Christensen JM 2008. Comparative *in vitro* activities of topical wound care products against community-associated methicillin-resistant *Staphylococcus aureus*. *J Antimicrob Chemother* 62 (4), 769–772.

Belland R, Ouellette S, Gieffers J, and Byrne G 2004. Chlamydia pneumoniae and atherosclerosis. *Cell Microbiol* 6 (2): 117–127. doi:10.1046/j.1462-5822.2003.00352.x. PMID 14706098.

Bengtsson B and Wierup M 2006. Antimicrobial resistance in Scandinavia after ban of antimicrobial growth promoters. *Anim Biotechnol* 17 (2): 147–156. doi:10.1080/10495390600956920. PMID 17127526.

Boyle-Vavra S and Daum RS 2007. Community-acquired methicillin-resistant *Staphylococcus aureus*: The role of Panton-Valentine leukocidin. *Lab Invest* 87 (1): 3–9. doi:10.1038/labinvest.3700501. PMID 17146447.

Bozdogan BL, Esel D, Whitener C, Browne FA, and Appelbaum PC 2003. Antibacterial susceptibility of a vancomycin-resistant *Staphylococcus aureus* strain isolated at the Hershey Medical Center. *J Antimicrob Chemother* 52: 864. doi:10.1093/jac/dkg457.

Castanon JI 2007. History of the use of antibiotic as growth promoters in European poultry feeds. *Poult Sci* 86 (11): 2466–2471. doi:10.3382/ps.2007-00249. PMID 17954599.

Chanishvili T, Tediashvili M, and Barrow PA 2001. Phages and their application against drug-resistant bacteria. *J Chem Technol Biotechnol* 76: 689–699. doi:10.1002/jctb.438. http://cat.inist.fr/?aModele=afficheN&cpsidt=1096871.

Cirz RT, Chin JK, Andes DR, de Crécy-Lagard V, Craig WA, and Romesberg FE 2005. Inhibition of mutation and combating the evolution of antibiotic resistance. *PLoS Biol* 3 (6): e176. doi:10.1371/journal.pbio.0030176. PMID 15869329. PMC 1088971. http://biology.plosjournals.org/perlserv/?request=get-document&doi=10.1371/journal.pbio.0030176.

Ferber D 2002. Livestock Feed Ban Preserves Drug' Power. *Science* 295 (5552): 27–28. doi:10.1126/science.295.5552.27a. PMID 11778017.

Fish DN 2002. Optimal antimicrobial therapy for sepsis. *Am J Health Syst Pharm* 59 (Suppl 1): S13–S19. PMID 11885408. http://www.ajhp.org/cgi/pmidlookup?view=long&pmid=11885408.

Frost F, Craun GF, and Calderon RL 1998. Increasing hospitalization and death possibly due to Clostridium difficile diarrheal disease. *Emerg Infect Dis* 4 (4): 619–625. doi:10.3201/eid0404.980412. PMID 9866738. PMC 2640242. http://www.cdc.gov/ncidod/eid/vol4no4/frost.htm.

Gerding DN, Johnson S, Peterson LR, Mulligan ME, and Silva J Jr. 1995. Clostridium difficile-associated diarrhea and colitis. *Infect Control Hosp Epidemiol* 16: 459–477.

Girou E, Legrand P, Soing-Altrach S et al. 2006. Association between hand hygiene compliance and methicillin-resistant *Staphylococcus aureus* prevalence in a French rehabilitation hospital. *Infect Control Hosp Epidemiol* 27 (10): 1128–1130. doi:10.1086/507967. PMID 17006822.

Goossens H, Ferech M, Vander Stichele R, and Elseviers M 2005. Outpatient antibiotic use in Europe and association with resistance: A cross-national database study. *Lancet* 365 (9459): 579–587. doi:10.1016/S0140-6736(05)17907-0. PMID 15708101.

Heise E 1982. Diseases associated with immunosuppression. *Environ Health Perspect* 43: 9–19. doi:10.2307/3429162. PMID 7037390. PMC 1568899. http://jstor.org/stable/3429162.

Johnson S, Samore MH, and Farrow KA 1999. Epidemics of diarrhea caused by a clindamycin-resistant strain of Clostridium difficile in four hospitals. *N Engl J Med* 341 (23): 1645–1651.

doi:10.1056/NEJM199911253412203. PMID 16322602. http://content.nejm.org/cgi/content/full/341/22/1645.

Kardas P 2007. Comparison of patient compliance with once-daily and twice-daily antibiotic regimens in respiratory tract infections: Results of a randomized trial. *J Antimicrob Chemother* 59 (3): 531–536. doi:10.1093/jac/dkl528. PMID 17289766.

Khachatourians GG 1998. Agricultural use of antibiotics and the evolution and transfer of antibiotic-resistant bacteria. *CMAJ* 159 (9): 1129–1136. PMID 9835883. PMC 1229782. http://www.cmaj.ca/cgi/pmidlookup?view=reprint&pmid=9835883.

Kuijper EJ, van Dissel JT, and Wilcox MH 2007. *Clostridium difficile*: Changing epidemiology and new treatment options. *Curr Opin Infect Dis* 20 (4): 376–383. doi:10.1097/QCO.0b013e32818be71d. PMID 17609596.

Kyong SY, Deok HK, Joseph P, Craig S et al. 2008. Biochemical and molecular analysis of deltamethrin resistance in the common bed bug (Hemiptera: Cimicidae). *J Med Entomol*, 45 (6), 1092–1101. doi:10.1603/0022-2585(2008)45[1092:BAMAOD]2.0.CO;2

Larsson DG and Fick J 2009. Transparency throughout the production chain—A way to reduce pollution from the manufacturing of pharmaceuticals. *Regul Toxicol Pharmacol* 53 (3): 161. doi:10.1016/j.yrtph.2009.01.008. PMID 19545507.

Li JZ, Winston LG, Moore DH, and Bent S 2007. Efficacy of short-course antibiotic regimens for community-acquired pneumonia: A meta-analysis. *Am J Med* 120 (9): 783–790. doi:10.1016/j.amjmed.2007.04.023. PMID 17765048.

Li X and Nikadio H 2009. Efflux-mediated drug resistance in bacteria: An update. *Drug* 69 (12): 1555–1623. doi:10.2165/11317030-000000000-00000. PMID 19678712.

Loo V, Poirier L, and Miller M 2005. A predominantly clonal multi-institutional outbreak of *Clostridium difficile*-associated diarrhea with high morbidity and mortality. *N Engl J Med* 353 (23): 2442–2449. doi:10.1056/NEJMoa051639. PMID 16322602.

Maree CL, Daum RS, Boyle-Vavra S, Matayoshi K, and Miller LG 2007. Community-associated methicillin-resistant *Staphylococcus aureus* isolates causing healthcare-associated infections. *Emerg Infect Dis* 13 (2): 236–242. doi:10.3201/eid1302.060781. PMID 17479885. PMC 2725868. http://www.cdc.gov/eid/content/13/2/236.htm?s_cid=eid236_e.

Mathew AG, Cissell R, and Liamthong S 2007. Antibiotic resistance in bacteria associated with food animals: A United States perspective of livestock production. *Foodborne Pathog Dis* 4 (2): 115–133. doi:10.1089/fpd.2006.0066. PMID 17600481.

Mathur MD, Vidhani S, and Mehndiratta PL 2003. Bacteriophage therapy: An alternative to conventional antibiotics. *J Assoc Physicians India* 51 (8): 593–596. doi:10.1258/095646202760159701. PMID 12194741.

McCusker ME, Harris AD, Perencevich E, and Roghmann MC 2003. Fluoroquinolone use and *Clostridium difficile*-associated diarrhea. *Emerg Infect Dis* 9 (6): 730–733. PMID 12781017. http://www.cdc.gov/ncidod/eid/vol9no6/02-0385.htm.

McDonald L 2005. *Clostridium difficile*: Responding to a new threat from an old enemy (PDF). *Infect Control Hosp Epidemiol* 26 (8): 672–675. doi:10.1086/502600. PMID 16156321. http://www.cdc.gov/ncidod/dhqp/pdf/infDis/Cdiff_ICHE08_05.pdf.

McNulty CA, Boyle P, Nichols T, Clappison P, and Davey P 2007. The public's attitudes to and compliance with antibiotics. *J Antimicrob Chemother* 60 (Suppl 1): i63–i68. doi:10.1093/jac/dkm161. PMID 17656386.

Mead PS et al. 1999. Food-related illness and death in the United States. *Emerg Infect Dis* 5 (5): 607–625. doi:10.3201/eid0505.990502. PMID 10511517. PMC 2627714. http://www.cdc.gov/ncidod/EID/vol5no5/mead.htm. 10.3201/eid0505.990502.

Mukhopadhyay J, Das K, Ismail S, Koppstein D, Jang M et al., 2008. The RNA polymerase "switch region" is a target for inhibitors. *Cell* 135 (2): 295–307. doi:10.1016/j.cell.2008.09.033. PMID 18957204.

Muto CA, Jernigan JA, Ostrowsky BE, Richet HM, Jarvis WR et al. 2003. SHEA guideline for preventing nosocomial transmission of multidrug-resistant strains of *Staphylococcus aureus* and enterococcus. *Infect Control Hosp Epidemiol* 24 (5): 362–386. doi:10.1086/502213. PMID 12785411.

Nelson JM, Chiller TM, Powers JH, and Angulo FJ 2007. Fluoroquinolone-resistant *Campylobacter* species and the withdrawal of fluoroquinolones from use in poultry: A public health success story. (PDF). *Clin Infect Dis* 44 (7): 977–980. doi:10.1086/512369. PMID 17342653. http://www.journals.uchicago.edu/doi/pdf/10.1086/512369.

Pechère JC, Hughes D, Kardas P, and Cornaglia G 2007. Non-compliance with antibiotic therapy for acute community infections: A global survey. *Int J Antimicrob Agents* 29 (3): 245–253. doi:10.1016/j.ijantimicag.2006.09.026. PMID 17229552.

Poole K 2004. Efflux-mediated multiresistance in Gram-negative bacteria. *Clin Microbiol Infect Offic Publ Eur Soc Clin Microbiol Infect Dis* 10 (1): 12–26. PMID 14706082.

Robicsek A, Jacoby GA, and Hooper DC 2006. The worldwide emergence of plasmid-mediated quinolone resistance. *Lancet Infect Dis* 6 (10): 629–640. doi:10.1016/S1473-3099(06)70599-0. PMID 17008172. http://linkinghub.elsevier.com/retrieve/pii/S1473-3099(06)70599-0.

Saiman L 2004. Microbiology of early CF lung disease. *Paediatr Respir Rev* 5 (Suppl A): S367–S369. doi:10.1016/S1526-0542(04)90065-6. PMID 14980298. http://linkinghub.elsevier.com/retrieve/pii/S1526054204900656.

Sapkota AR, Lefferts LY, McKenzie S, and Walker P 2007. What do we feed to food-production animals? A review of animal feed ingredients and their potential impacts on human health. *Environ Health Perspect* 115 (5): 663–670. doi:10.1289/ehp.9760. PMID 17520050.

Schneider K and Garrett L 2009. Non-Therapeutic Use of Antibiotics in Animal Agriculture, Corresponding Resistance Rates, and What Can be Done About It. http://www.cgdev.org/content/article/detail/1422307/.

Shand RF and Leyva KJ 2008. Archaeal antimicrobials: An undiscovered country. In: *Archaea: New Models for Prokaryotic Biology*, Paul Blum Beadle (ed.). Lincoln, USA: Caister Academic Press. ISBN 978-1-904455-27-1.

Singh G, Kapoor IP, Pandey SK, Singh UK, and Singh RK 2002. Studies on essential oils: Part 10; antibacterial activity of volatile oils of some spices. *Phytother Res* 16 (7): 680–682. doi:10.1002/ptr.951. PMID 12410554.

Soulsby EJ 2005. Resistance to antimicrobials in humans and animals. *BMJ* 331 (7527): 1219–1220. doi:10.1136/bmj.331.7527.1219. PMID 16308360. PMC 1289307. http://www.bmj.com/cgi/content/full/331/7527/1219.

Stermitz FR, Lorenz P, Tawara JN, Zenewicz LA, and Lewis K 2000. Synergy in a medicinal plant: Antimicrobial action of berberine potentiated by 5′-methoxyhydnocarpin, a multidrug pump inhibitor. *Proc Natl Acad Sci USA* 97 (4): 1433–1437. doi:10.1073/pnas.030540597. PMID 10677479. PMC 26451. http://www.pnas.org/cgi/content/full/97/4/1433.

Swoboda SM, Earsing K, Strauss K et al. 2004. Electronic monitoring and voice prompts improve hand hygiene and decrease nosocomial infections in an intermediate care unit. *Crit Care Med* 32 (2): 358–363. doi:10.1097/01.CCM.0000108866.48795.0F. PMID 14758148.

Tacconelli E, De Angelis G, Cataldo MA, Pozzi E, and Cauda R 2008. Does antibiotic exposure increase the risk of methicillin-resistant *Staphylococcus aureus* (MRSA) isolation? A systematic review and meta-analysis. *J Antimicrob Chemother* 61 (1): 26–38. doi:10.1093/jac/dkm416. PMID 17986491. http://jac.oxfordjournals.org/cgi/content/full/61/1/26.

Thomas JK, Forrest A, Bhavnani SM et al. 1998. Pharmacodynamic evaluation of factors associated with the development of bacterial resistance in acutely ill patients during therapy. *Antimicrob Agents Chemother* 42 (3): 521–527. PMID 9517926.

Thuille N, Fille M, and Nagl M 2003. Bactericidal activity of herbal extracts. *Int J Hyg Environ Health* 206 (3): 217–221. doi:10.1078/1438-4639-00217. PMID 12872531.

Vonberg R-P 2009. Clostridium difficile: A challenge for hospitals. European Center for Disease Prevention and Control. Institute for Medical Microbiology and Hospital Epidemiology. http://www.ihe-online.com/feature-articles/clostridium-difficile-a-challenge-for-hospitals/trackback/1/index.html (retrieved July 27, 2009).

Wallace RJ 2004. Antimicrobial properties of plant secondary metabolites. *Proc Nutr Soc* 63 (4): 621–629. doi:10.1079/PNS2004393. PMID 15831135.

Weber-Dabrowska B, Mulczyk M, and Gorski A 2003. Bacteriophages as an efficient therapy for antibiotic-resistant septicemia in man. *Transplant Proc* 35 (4): 1385–1386. doi:10.1016/S0041-1345(03)00525-6. PMID 12826166. http://linkinghub.elsevier.com/retrieve/pii/S00411345 03005256.

Wichelhaus TA, Boddinghaus B, Besier S, Schafer V, Brade V, and Ludwig A 2002. Biological cost of rifampin resistance from the perspective of *Staphylococcus aureus*. *Antimicrob Agents Chemother* 46 (11): 3381–3385. doi:10.1128/AAC.46.11.3381-3385.2002. PMID 12384339.

Yonath A and Bashan A 2004. Ribosomal crystallography: Initiation, peptide bond formation, and amino acid polymerization are hampered by antibiotics. *Annu Rev Microbiol* 58:233–251. doi:10.1146/annurev.micro.58.030603.123822. PMID 15487937.

chapter four

Virology and vaccines

4.1 Introduction

A virus is basically a small organism that cannot be seen by the naked eye and requires special tools such as microscopes to know its structure. The study of virus science is called virology. The elements of virus, known as virions, mainly contain about two or three parts, which include the genetic material present in the form of DNA or RNA. The shapes of viruses can range from simple helical to icosahedral forms and more complex arrangements; the size of an average virus is about one 100th the size of an average bacterium.

4.2 Discovery of viruses

There is an interesting story behind the discovery of viruses and it all started with Louis Pasteur's work in 1870s, who was unable to find a fundamental agent for rabies and guessed about a pathogen too small to be identified by the microscope. Later on, in 1884, the French microbiologist Chamberland invented a filter process with pores smaller than bacteria to isolate viruses and similarly, in 1892, a Russian biologist D. I. Ivanovsky employed this filter to isolate the tobacco mosaic virus and showed that wrinkled leaf extracts of infected tobacco plants stay infectious even after the filtration process. Later on, Ivanovsky suggested that the infection could be caused by a toxin produced by bacteria, but he did not pursue the idea. However, in 1898, the Dutch microbiologist M. W. Beijerinck performed these experiments repeatedly, convinced that the filtered solution contained a new form of organisms. He also observed that these organisms multiplied only in cells that were dividing. Nevertheless, his experiments did not show any form of virus structure. In 1899, Friedrich August Johannes Loeffler and Paul Frosch conducted an experiment and passed the culture agent of foot-and-mouth disease through a similar filter and excluded the likelihood of a toxin because of the reduced concentration; they did still find the replication by the viral agent.

Later on, the English bacteriologist F. W. Twort discovered a group of viruses called bacteriophages that infect bacteria and another scientist Felix d'Herelle described in his experiment that viruses when added to bacteria on agar can produce areas of killed bacteria. Moreover, he also accurately diluted a suspension of these viruses and discovered that the highest dilutions of virus can kill almost all the bacteria. By the end of the nineteenth century, viruses were considered an infectious organism. It has been shown that viruses can be grown only in plants and animals. However, in 1906, Ross Granville Harrison developed a method for growing tissue in lymph, and in 1913, scientists, namely, Steinhardt, Israeli, and Lambert, used this method to grow the vaccine virus in guinea pig corneal tissue. Moreover, in 1928, scientists Maitland and Maitland grew the vaccine virus in suspensions of hen's kidneys. Furthermore, another breakthrough came in 1931 when the American pathologist E. W. Good grew influenza and several other viruses in fertilized chicken's eggs. Later on, in 1949, Enders, Weller, and Robbins grew the polio virus in cultured human embryonic cells. This was the first method to grow viruses without using solid animal tissue, which enabled Jonas Salk to make an effective polio vaccine.

The second half of the twentieth century is considered the golden age of virus discovery as there were 2000 different types of animal, plant, and bacterial viruses discovered. Furthermore, hepatitis B virus was discovered by scientist Baruch Blumberg in 1963.

4.3 Anatomy of virus

The first image of the virus was obtained by using electron microscopy in 1931 by the German engineers Ernst Ruska and Max Knoll, and later on, in 1935, American biochemist and virologist W. M. Stanley studied the tobacco mosaic virus and found that viruses were completely made of protein (Figure 4.1). The structure of the tobacco mosaic virus was also described by using crystallography and the first x-ray diffraction images of the crystallized virus were obtained in 1941. On the basis of this image, scientist Rosalind Elsie Franklin discovered the complete structure of the DNA of the virus in 1955. Under microscopic observation, these viruses display a wide diversity of shapes and sizes, which is known as morphology. In a general sense, viruses are much smaller than bacteria and most viruses have a diameter between 10 and 300 nm; some *filoviruses* have a total length of up to 1400 nm with 80 nm diameters. Viruses can also be seen by using scanning electron microscope and transmission electron microscopes, and under a microscope the structure of the virus appears to have a lipid envelope derived from the host cell membrane. This envelope is known as a capsid and is made from proteins encoded by the viral DNA. The shape of each serves as the basis for morphological peculiarity from other viruses. Interestingly, the capsid is made of code protein subunits and proteins, which are associated with nucleic acid called nucleoproteins. The connection of viral capsid proteins with viral nucleic acid is called nuclear capsid. The capsid and entire virus structure can be mechanically examined through atomic force microscopy. In general form, there are four main morphological virus types, which are described below.

4.3.1 Helical-shaped viruses

This type of virus is generally in a helical shape composed of a single type of capsomer to form a helical structure and can have a hollow tube and this arrangement results in rod-shaped or filamentous virus. The genetic material of a helical-shaped virus is generally

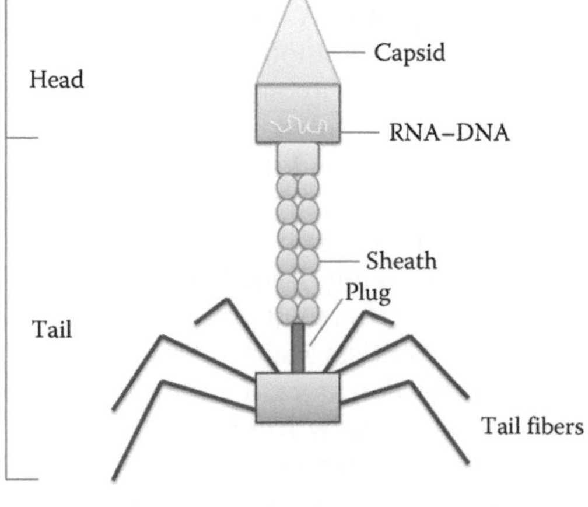

Figure 4.1 Microorganisms.

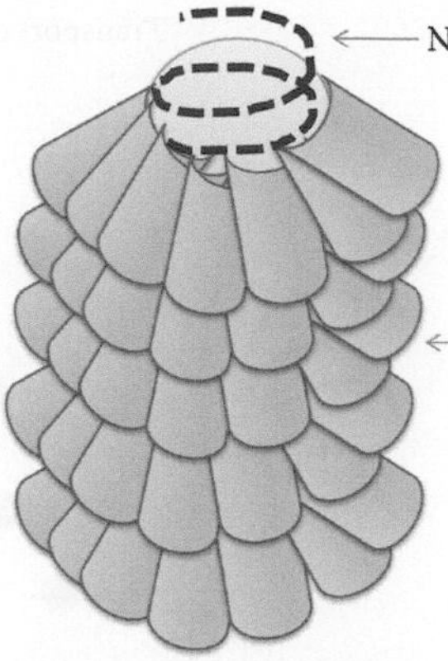

Figure 4.2 Helical-shaped virus (tobacco mosaic virus).

single-stranded RNA, and overall, the length of a helical capsid is connected to the length of the nucleic acid contained within it. Additionally, tobacco mosaic virus is an example of a helical virus (Figure 4.2).

4.3.2 *Icosahedral-shaped viruses*

Most of the animal viruses are icosahedral in shape. This kind of virus is generally has 12 identical capsomers, each composed of five identical subunits. Many viruses, including rotavirus, have more than 12 capsomers and appear spherical and they retain this symmetry. It has been found that the capsomers at the peaks are surrounded by five other capsomers that are called pentons (Figure 4.3).

4.3.3 *Enveloped viruses*

There are some species of viruses that create an envelope from the outside by modifying cell membranes. Furthermore, cell membranes are generally studded with proteins coded

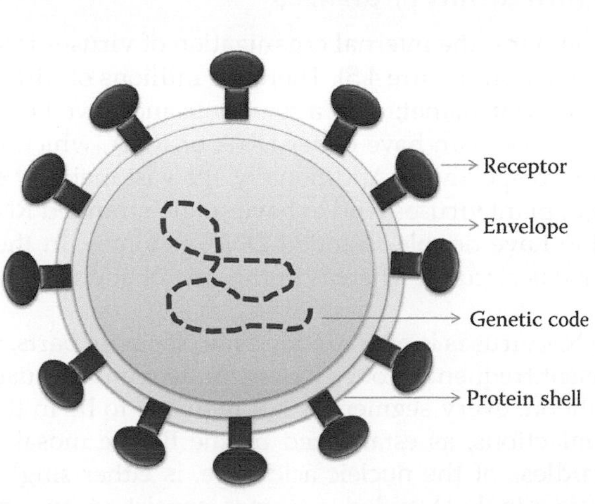

Figure 4.3 Icosahedral-shaped viruses.

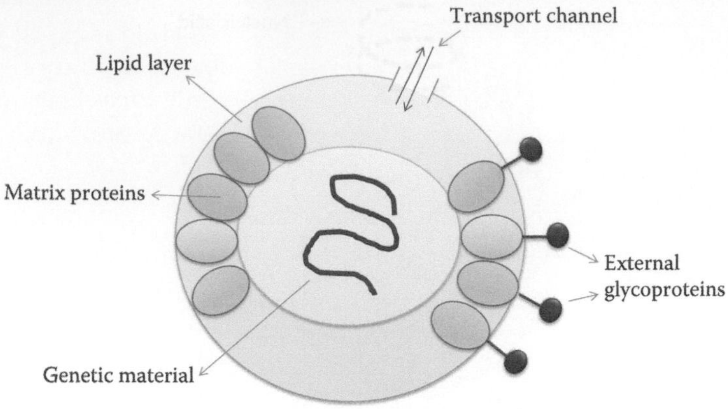

Figure 4.4 Complex viruses.

by the viral genome and host genome. The influenza virus and human immunodeficiency virus (HIV) are known to have enveloped shape and most enveloped viruses are dependent on the envelope in order to infect the host cells.

4.3.4 *Complex viruses*

In these types of viruses, it is a capsid that is neither completely helical nor completely icosahedral, and that can possess extra structures such as protein tails. Some bacteriophages, such as *Enterobacteria phage T4,* have a complex structure consisting of an icosahedral head connected to a helical tail, which may have a hexagonal base plate with bulging protein tail fibers. It has been found that this tail structure acts like a syringe that can adhere to the bacterial host in order to inject the viral genome into the cell. In this kind of virus, the outer wall is covered with a thick layer of protein studded over its surface and the whole virus is ovoid to brick shaped (Figure 4.4).

4.4 *Internal organization of viruses*

Unlike animals and humans, the internal organization of viruses is simple and accessible for any kind of manipulation (Figure 4.5). There are millions of different kinds of viruses known to be present on our planet; only a few thousand have been described so far in detail. Anatomically, viruses can have either DNA or RNA, which is also called a DNA virus or an RNA virus, respectively. Additionally, the vast majority of viruses have RNA genomes. Interestingly, plant viruses tend to have single-stranded RNA genomes whereas bacteriophages tend to have double-stranded DNA genomes. In the case of polyomaviruses, the viral genome is circular, whereas in the case of adenoviruses, the viral genome is linear in shape.

The genome of RNA viruses is often divided into separate parts, which are called segments and each segment frequently codes for one protein and are usually placed together in one capsid. In addition, every segment is not required to be in the same virus for the overall virus to be infectious, as established by the Brome mosaic virus. Additionally, a viral genome, regardless of the nucleic acid type, is either single stranded or double stranded. Furthermore, single-stranded genomes consist of an unpaired nucleic acid, whereas double-stranded genomes consist of two complementary paired nucleic acids.

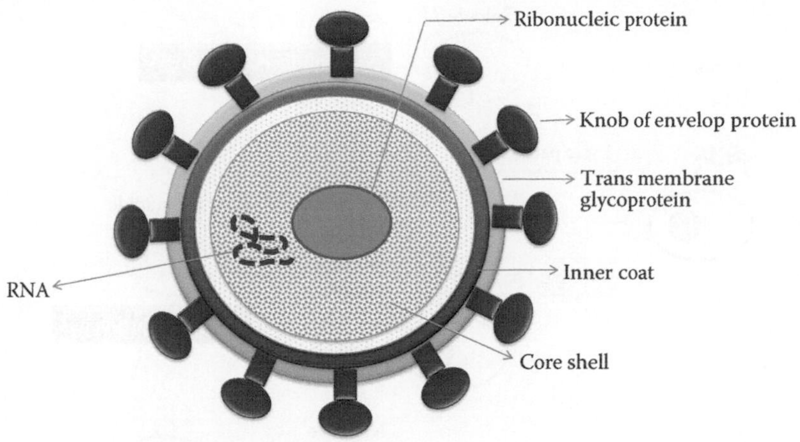

Figure 4.5 Internal organization of virus.

Interestingly, some viruses, such as those belonging to the family Hepadnaviridae do contain a genome that is partially double stranded and partially single stranded.

There are viruses with RNA or single-stranded DNA. The strands are said to be either positive-sense, also called the plus-strand, or negative-sense, also called the minus-strand, depending on whether it is complementary to the viral messenger RNA (mRNA). Positive-sense viral RNA is identical to viral mRNA and, consequently, can be immediately translated by the host cell. The negative-sense viral RNA is complementary to mRNA, which can be converted to positive-sense RNA by an RNA polymerase before translation. Additionally, DNA nomenclature is similar to RNA nomenclature, in that the coding strand for the viral mRNA is complementary to its negative end, and the noncoding strand is a copy of its positive end.

In a virus, the size of the genome varies greatly between species as the smallest viral genomes code for only four proteins and have a mass of about 106 Da, whereas the largest genomes have a mass of about 108 Da and code for over 100 proteins. Moreover, RNA viruses generally have smaller genomes than DNA viruses because of a higher error rate while replicating, and have a maximum upper size limit. In contrast to RNA viruses, DNA viruses generally have larger genomes because of the high dependability of their replication enzymes. Viruses are generally undergoing genetic change/alteration through several mechanisms and such a process is called genetic drift where individual bases in the DNA or RNA mutate/change to other bases. Moreover, most of these point mutations are quiet; they do not change the protein that the gene encodes. Moreover, antigenic shift occurs when there is a major change in the genome of the virus, which can be a result of recombination that may finally cause a pandemic situation.

4.5 Human diseases caused by viruses

The most common type of diseases caused by viruses in humans is the common cold, influenza, chickenpox, and cold sores. Many serious diseases such as avian influenza, severe acute respiratory syndrome (SARS), Ebola, and acquired immunodeficiency syndrome (AIDS) are caused by viruses. Moreover, viruses have different mechanisms by which they produce disease in an organism, which largely depends on viral types. The basic effect is generally at the cellular level, which includes cell lysis and subsequent death

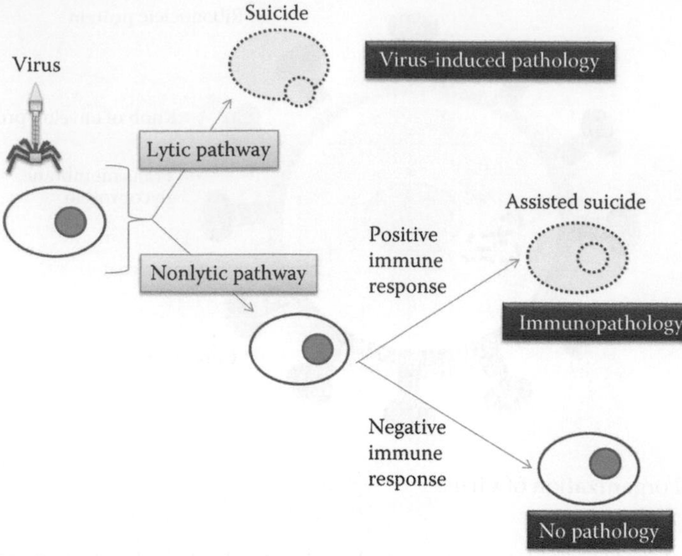

Figure 4.6 Viral-induced diseases.

of the cell. It has been observed that viruses can cause disruption of healthy homeostasis, resulting in disease and these viruses remain harmless within an organism. One example is cold sores, where herpes simplex virus, which causes cold sores, remains in a latent state within the human body. This kind of infection is called latency and is a characteristic of the herpes viruses, the Epstein-Barr virus (causes glandular fever), and varicella zoster virus (causes chickenpox). It has been observed that most people have been infected with these types of herpes virus. Nevertheless, the influence of latent viruses sometimes is beneficial, as the presence of the virus can increase the immunity against bacterial pathogens (Figure 4.6).

4.5.1 *Epidemiology of viral-induced diseases*

Viral epidemiology is the branch of health science that deals with the transmission and control of virus infections in humans. The process of viral transmission can be of two types: vertical transmission is basically from mother to child while horizontal transmission is from one person to another person. There are various examples of vertical transmission, which include hepatitis B virus and HIV. Another example is varicella zoster virus, which although causes relatively mild infections in humans, can be fatal to the fetus and newborn baby. Furthermore, horizontal transmission is the most common mechanism of viruses spreading in human populations (Table 4.1).

The speed of viral transmission depends on factors that include population, the number of vulnerable individuals, the quality of health care, and the weather circumstances. Control measures are generally taken to stop the further transmission of the disease in the population. The first step in this direction is to find the source of the outbreak and to identify the virus. As soon as the virus identity is established, the chain of transmission can sometimes be destroyed by using vaccines. Regularly infected people are isolated from the rest of the community and those that have been exposed to the virus are normally placed in quarantined rooms. In 2001, to control the outbreak of foot-and-mouth disease in cattle,

Table 4.1 Diseases Caused by Viruses

Disease	Causes
HIV	Body fluids are exchanged during sexual activity
Hepatitis C	Blood is exchanged by contaminated transfusion or needle sharing
Hepatitis B	A child is born to an infected mother
Epstein-Barr virus	Exchange of saliva by mouth
Norovirus	Contaminated food or water is ingested

thousands of cattle were slaughtered. It has also been noticed that most viral infections in humans and other animals have incubation periods, during which the infection causes no signs or symptoms in the body. Incubation periods can be from a few days to weeks, but there is a period of transmission, a time when an infected individual or animal is infectious and can infect another person or animal.

4.5.2 *Epidemic caused by viruses*

The epidemic is an outbreak of a contagious disease that spreads rapidly and widely. The list of diseases that are caused by viruses in various part of the world is depicted in Table 4.2.

4.5.3 *Pandemic caused by viruses*

Recently, it has been shown that viral diseases that spread through humans across a globe is called a pandemic. Flu pandemics do not include seasonal flu, except the flu of the season is a pandemic. In the past, the world has seen a number of pandemics such as smallpox and tuberculosis and, more recently, the occurrence of the HIV and flu pandemics. Based on the research survey, the World Health Organization (WHO) has formed a six-stage classification of viral disease that describes the process by which a novel influenza virus caused a pandemic-like situation. The process starts with animals or humans getting infected with a viral disease, then it moves to the stage where the virus begins to spread directly among the population. It has been clarified that a disease is not a pandemic merely because it is widespread or kills many people worldwide; it must also be infectious. For instance, cancer is accountable for many deaths but is not considered a pandemic because the disease is not infectious.

4.5.4 *Oncovirus*

Viruses can cause cancer in humans and other species, including animals. Interestingly, viral cancers only occur in a minority of people who are infected. Additionally, cancer viruses derive from a range of virus families, which include both RNA and DNA viruses. The progress of cancer is examined by a variety of factors such as host immunity and mutations in the host organism. There are various types of viruses that are known to cause cancers in human, including human papillomavirus (HPV), hepatitis B virus, hepatitis C virus, Epstein-Barr virus, Kaposi's sarcoma-associated herpesvirus, and human T-lymphotropic virus. Recently, it has been found that a human cancer virus (polyomavirus) which causes a rare form of skin cancer called Merkel cell carcinoma and hepatitis viruses can develop into a chronic viral infection that subsequently leads to liver cancer. Moreover, infection by human T-lymphotropic virus can lead to adult T-cell leukemia.

Table 4.2 List of Diseases Caused by Viruses: Global Scenario

Region	Years	Species
World	165–180	Smallpox
World	251–270	Smallpox
World	541–542	Bubonic plague
World	1300–1400	Bubonic plague
World	1501–1587	Typhus
World	1732–1733	Influenza
World	1775–1776	Influenza
World	1816–1826	Cholera
World	1829–1851	Cholera
World	1847–1848	Influenza
World	1852–1860	Cholera
World	1855–1950	Bubonic plague
World	1857–1859	Influenza
World	1863–1875	Cholera
World	1889–1892	Influenza
World	1899–1923	Cholera
World	1918–1920	Influenza virus A
World	1957–1958	Influenza virus A
World	1968–1969	Influenza virus A
World	1950–1960	Cholera
World	1980–present	HIV
World	2009–2010	Influenza virus A
Palestine	639	Bubonic plague?
China	1334	
Mecca	1349	
China	1353–1354	
China	1641–1644	Plague
Baghdad	1801	Plague
Persia	1829–1835	Plague
Yemen	1853	Plague
Iraq	1867	Plague
Russian Empire	1877	Plague
India	1903	Plague
China	1946	Bubonic plague
India	1974	Smallpox
India	1994	Plague
Asia	2002–2003	SARS coronavirus
Indonesia	2004	Dengue fever
Bangladesh	2004	Cholera
Afghanistan	2004	Leishmaniasis
Singapore	2005	Dengue
India	2006	Malaria
India	2006	Dengue
Philippines	2006	Dengue fever

Table 4.2 (continued) List of Diseases Caused by Viruses: Global Scenario

Region	Years	Species
Pakistan	2006	Dengue
India	2006	Chikungunya
Iraq	2007	Cholera
India	2007	Cholera
Vietnam	2007	Cholera
Cambodia	2008	Dengue fever
China	2008	Foot-and-mouth diseases
Philippines	2008	Dengue fever
Vietnam	2008	Cholera
India	2009	Hepatitis B (Gujarat hepatitis outbreak)
India	2009	Swine flu

Furthermore, HPVs are known to cause cancers of the skin, anus, cervix, and penis. The Epstein-Barr virus is known to cause Burkitt's lymphoma, Hodgkin's lymphoma, B lymphoproliferative disorder, and nasopharyngeal carcinoma.

4.5.5 *Avian flu*

In 2009, bird or avian flu created a tremendous impact on large areas of the world as a new strain of H1N1 influenza virus, often referred to as swine flu, affected thousands of people worldwide. Interestingly, unlike most strains of influenza, H1N1 does not unreasonably infect adults older than 60 years; this was an uncommon characteristic feature of the H1N1 pandemic. Moreover, healthy persons will develop viral pneumonia or acute respiratory distress syndrome. Additionally, manifestation of the disease typically occurs 3–6 days after initial onset of flu symptoms. The structure and nomenclature of flu virus H3N2 are illustrated in Figure 4.7 to show how the naming is done with regard to various trains of flu viruses. The outbreak of swine flu initiated in Mexico with evidence that there had been

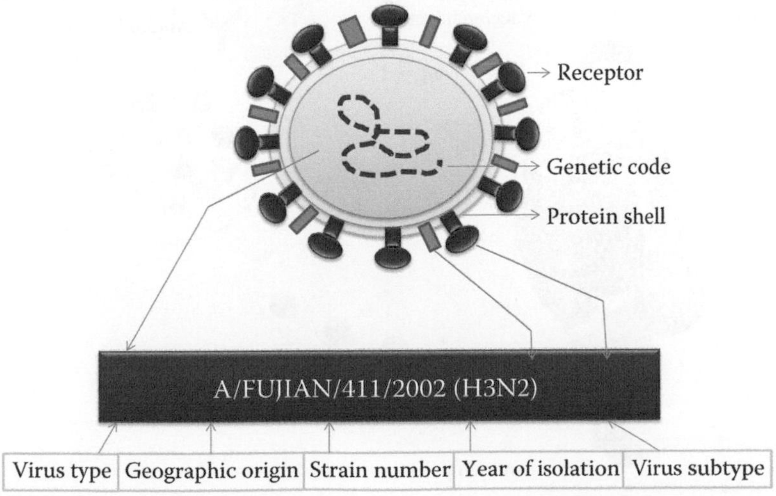

Figure 4.7 Nomenclature of H3N2 virus.

a continuing epidemic for months before it was officially recognized as swine flu. Later on, the Mexican government shut most of public and private facilities in an attempt to enclose the spread of the virus; however, the virus persistently spread globally. In June 2009, the WHO and US Centers for Disease Control (CDC) had declared the outbreak as a pandemic. The swine flu, and the H1N1 flu virus cannot be spread by eating pork, whereas influenza viruses are typically contracted through respiratory droplets. The influenza virus can be controlled by using antiviral drugs such as oseltamivir or zanamivir.

4.5.5.1 How to diagnosis viral infection

One of the best ways to control viral infection is to conduct the diagnosis as quickly as possible. The viral diagnosis of pandemic H1N1 flu requires testing of a nasopharyngeal, nasal tissue swab from the patient. Real-time RT-PCR is the recommended test as others are unable to differentiate between pandemic H1N1 and regular seasonal flu. Nevertheless, most people with flu symptoms do not need a test for pandemic H1N1 flu specifically, since the test results typically do not change the course of treatment. The US CDC recommends testing only for people who are hospitalized with assumed flu. Moreover, the diagnosis of influenza is widely available, which include rapid influenza diagnostic tests (RIDT) that can be completed within 30 min, whereas direct and indirect immunofluorescence assays can take 2–4 h. Under severe conditions, a definitive determination of infection with influenza virus is required by using RT-PCR technique and test results are available in 4 h with 96% accuracy.

4.6 Prevention strategy for viral infections

Viruses use vital metabolic pathways within host cells to replicate; they are very difficult to eradicate without using antiviral drugs. The most effective medical approaches to viral diseases are vaccinations, which provide immunity against viral infection (Figure 4.8), and antiviral drugs that selectively interfere with viral replication. Before we discuss antiviral drugs and vaccines in controlling viral infections, let us first find out how viral

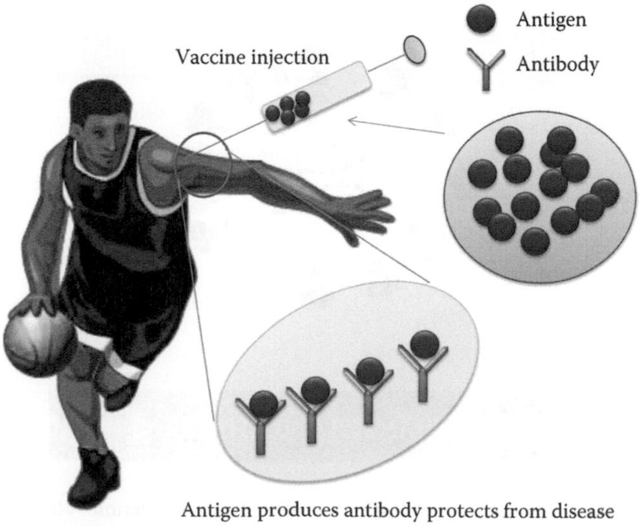

Figure 4.8 Treatment of viral disease.

infections can be prevented and controlled. The human body has an immune defense system to fight back any infection, and the immune defense system is composed of cells and other mechanisms that defend the host from infection in a nonspecific manner. This means that the cells of the innate system recognize and respond to pathogens in a common way, but unlike the adaptive immune system, it does not recognize protective immunity to the host. Furthermore, RNA interference is an important innate defense against viruses and many viruses have a replication strategy that involves double-stranded RNA (dsRNA). Once such a virus infects a cell, it releases its RNA molecules, which immediately bind to a protein complex called Dicer that cuts the RNA into smaller pieces. Later on, a biochemical pathway called the RISC complex is activated, which degrades the virus mRNA and the host cell survives the infection.

With regard to an adaptive immune system in vertebrate, upon viral action, the immune defense system produces specific antibodies that bind to the virus and make viruses noninfectious. The production of antibodies against the virus is called humoral immunity. There are two types of antibodies that are important for immunity; first, antibodies that are called immunoglobulin M (IgM) are highly effective at neutralizing the virus's effects, but are only produced by the cells for a few weeks: the second antibodies are called immunoglobulin G (IgG) and are produced indefinitely in the body. The presence of IgM in the blood is used to test for acute infection, whereas the level of IgG in the blood indicates an infection sometime in the past. Besides IgM and IgG, interferon plays an important role in defending the human against any kind of infection. Interferon is basically a hormone produced by the body when viruses are attacked or invade the host body. Although the role of interferon is not yet confirmed, it ultimately stops the viruses from reproducing/replicating by killing the infected cell. It has been found that not all virus infections can be controlled by the production of interferon; there are some viruses such as HIV that evades the immune system by constantly changing the structure of the amino acid sequence of the proteins.

4.7 *Antiviral drugs*

It is very difficult to completely get rid of the viruses in the human body because they use vital metabolic pathways within host cells to replicate. In addition, most antiviral drugs are also known to cause toxic effects to host cells in general. The most effective medical approaches to viral diseases are vaccinations to provide immunity to infection. In this section, we will discuss various treatments to control viral infection.

Almost all antiviral drugs are a class of medication used specifically for treating viral infections. There are drugs such as antibiotics that are used for treating bacterial infections; there are also some specific antiviral drugs that are used for treating specific virus infection. Most antiviral drugs do not destroy their target pathogen; instead they inhibit their development activity and growth. It has been claimed that antiviral drugs are antimicrobial, antifungal, and antiparasitic in action and are relatively harmless to the host cells, and therefore can be used to treat infections. There are various ways through which antiviral drugs can be used to treat viral infections.

4.7.1 *Targeting cell surface*

One of the most widely used sites for any antiviral drug is to attack the viral cell membrane. The antiviral drugs should target the viral cell membrane instantly before they can enter the host cells. The viral cell surface can also be attacked by using agents that can mimic the cellular receptor located on the surface of the virus and can also bind to the virus-associated protein (VAP). These types of drugs include anti-VAP antibodies, receptor anti-idiotypic antibodies, extraneous receptor, and synthetic receptor mimics. However, these strategies of designing drugs are expensive, and since the process of generating anti-idiotypic antibodies are partly based on trial and error, it can be a comparatively time-consuming process until the final drug is produced.

4.7.2 *Entry inhibitor*

One of the earliest treatments of any viral infection is to completely block the entry of the viruses into the host cells. A number of entries-inhibiting or entry-blocking drugs are being developed to fight HIV. HIV generally targets helper T cells of the immune systems and identifies these target cells through T-cell surface receptors designated as CD4 and CCR5. Moreover, blocking these receptors might stop the HIV to infect the helper T cells; nevertheless, research work is going on to develop blockers of CCR5 receptors.

4.7.3 *Uncoating inhibitor*

Antiviral drugs such as *amantadine* and *rimantadine* have been reported to combat influenza viruses and these agents act when the virus starts penetrating or during the uncoating phase of attack. Furthermore, there is another drug called *pleconaril* that also works against rhinoviruses, which are known to cause the common cold, by inhibiting a pocket on the surface of the virus that controls the uncoating process. Furthermore, these viral pockets are similar in most strains of rhinoviruses and enteroviruses, which are known to cause meningitis, conjunctivitis, diarrhea, and encephalitis.

4.7.4 *Viral synthesis*

Another approach to treating viruses is to target the processes that synthesize virus components after a virus invades a host cell. It can be done by developing nucleotide or nucleoside analogs that look like the building blocks of RNA or DNA, but deactivate the enzymes that synthesize the RNA or DNA of the virus once the analog is incorporated into the host cells. The first successful antiviral drug created by this technology is known as *Acyclovir,* which is basically a nucleoside analog and is effective against herpes virus infections. The first antiviral drug approved for treating HIV, *Zidovudine,* is also a nucleoside analog. Furthermore, researchers have gone further ahead and developed inhibitors that do not look like nucleosides, but can still block reverse transcriptase. Another target being considered for HIV antiviral drugs include RNase-H, which is a constituent of reverse transcriptase that splits the synthesized DNA from the original viral RNA.

4.7.5 *Integrase*

Another strategy to treat viral infection is to target integrase, which splices the synthesized DNA into the host cell genome. As soon as the virus enters the host cells, the virus genome becomes operational and generates messenger RNA (mRNA) molecules that lead to the synthesis of viral proteins. The production of mRNA is initiated by proteins known as transcription factors and several antiviral drugs are now being developed to block the attachment of transcription factors to viral DNA. These antiviral drugs are known as antisense-antiviral drugs. Furthermore, a phosphorothioate antisense drug named *fomivirsen* has been introduced that can be used to treat cytomegalovirus, which causes eye infections in AIDS patients.

4.7.6 Translation or ribozymes

Over the last few years, efforts have been made to make antiviral drugs based on ribozymes. The ribozymes are enzymes that will separately cut viral RNA or DNA at particular sites. In a normal situation, ribozymes are used as part of the viral manufacturing sequence; these synthetic designed ribozymes can cut RNA and DNA and make them nonfunctional. The ribozyme based-antiviral drugs that deal with hepatitis C has been suggested, whereas ribozyme antivirals are being developed to deal with HIV.

4.7.7 Protease inhibitors

There are enzymes in the body that are known as protease that can cut viral protein chains apart so they can be assembled into their final configuration. Over the last few years, considerable research has been performed to find how protease inhibitors can attack and control HIV infection. There are quite a few protease inhibitor-based drug under the developmental stage.

4.7.8 Challenges of antiviral drugs

Most of the antivirals now available are designed to help deal with HIV, herpes viruses, and hepatitis B and C viruses, which can cause liver cancer, and influenza A and B viruses. Additionally, there are a number of antiviral drugs available on the market for different kinds of pathogens. Designing safe and effective antiviral drugs is difficult, because viruses use the host's cells to replicate. It is a challenge to develop a drug that on the one hand kills the viruses, but at the same time does not cause any harmful effects on the health of neighboring cells. The emergence of antiviral drugs is a product of an expanded knowledge of the genetic and molecular function of organisms, allowing researchers to understand the structure and function of different types of viruses. This molecular information of the viruses would certainly help the researchers to make an effective therapy. Like antibiotics, almost all antiviral drugs are subject to drug resistance as the pathogens mutate over time, becoming less effective for the treatment. Furthermore, there is the development of antiviral drugs that can identify viral proteins, or parts of proteins, which can make them (viruses) disabled or dysfunctional. Additionally, these targets should be common across many strains of a virus, so a single drug can have strong effects.

4.8 Significance of vaccines

A vaccine is a biological preparation that improves human immunity to a particular disease. Moreover, a vaccine basically contains an agent that resembles a disease-causing microorganism, and is often made from weakened or killed forms of the microorganism or its toxins. Upon injecting these vaccines in humans, the vaccine molecules stimulate the body's immune system to recognize the agent as foreign, destroy it, and memorize it, so that the immune system can more effortlessly familiarize with it and destroy any of these microorganisms that it later encounters. The story behind vaccine development started with the research work done by Edward Jenner in the late 1700s. Jenner took pus from the hand of a milkmaid with cowpox, inoculated an 8-year-old boy with it, and 6 weeks later variolated the boy's arm with smallpox, afterwards observing that the boy did not catch smallpox. Later on, more experimentation was performed to demonstrate the efficacy of the procedure in infants. Interestingly, Louis Pasteur generalized Edward Jenner's idea by developing what he called a rabies vaccine, now termed an antitoxin, which caused an extensive development of vaccines around the globe and obligatory vaccination laws were passed. Furthermore, researcher Maurice Hilleman was the most successful developer of vaccines in the twentieth century. Vaccines became more common among all populations of the world; however, vaccines remain elusive for many important diseases, including malaria and HIV.

4.8.1 *Type of vaccines*

Vaccines are produced by either dead or inactivated organisms and there are four main ways to develop vaccines: (i) live attenuated vaccines contain bacteria or viruses that have been altered so they cannot cause disease, (ii) killed vaccines contain killed bacteria or inactivated viruses, (iii) toxoid vaccines contain toxins (or poisons) produced by the germ that have been made harmless, and (iv) component vaccines contain parts of the whole bacteria or viruses.

4.8.1.1 *Live attenuated vaccines*

The live attenuated or weakened vaccines can be created from the naturally occurring microorganisms; however, microorganisms used in this vaccine development can still infect people, but they rarely cause severe disease. Viruses are weakened by growing them over and over again in cell culture conditions. Furthermore, the procedure of growing a virus under cell culture conditions is known to decrease their disease-causing capabilities. There are various examples of live attenuated vaccines that include measles vaccine (as found in the MMR vaccine), rubella (German measles) vaccine (MMR vaccine), oral polio vaccine (OPV), mumps vaccine (MMR vaccine), and varicella (chickenpox) vaccine.

4.8.1.2 *Inactivated vaccines*

Inactivated vaccines cannot cause an infection, but they still can stimulate a protective immune response. Moreover, viruses can be inactivated with chemicals such as formaldehyde. One example of an inactivated vaccine is the inactivated polio vaccine (IPV), which is the shot form of the polio vaccine, inactivated influenza vaccine.

4.8.1.3 *Toxoid vaccines*

There are some kinds of vaccines that can be made by treating them with toxins (formalin) produced by microorganisms, to destroy their ability to cause illness. Additionally, toxoids do not cause disease; in fact, they stimulate the body to produce protective immunity. There are several examples of toxoid-based vaccines such as diphtheria toxoid vaccine, which may be given alone or as one of the components in association with DTP, and furthermore, tetanus toxoid vaccine can be given alone or as part of the DTP.

4.8.1.4 *Component vaccines*

Some vaccines are made by using only parts of the viruses or bacteria. These vaccines cannot cause disease; nevertheless, these vaccines can stimulate the body to create an immune response that protects against viral infection with the whole germ. So far, four vaccines have been produced by using this method that includes hemophilic influenza type b (Hib) vaccine, hepatitis B (Hep B) vaccine, hepatitis A (Hep A) vaccine, and pneumococcal conjugate vaccine.

4.8.1.5 Other vaccines

Recently, various efforts have been made to make vaccines in different ways. An immune response can be achieved by introducing a protein subunit rather than introducing an inactivated or attenuated microorganism. Examples include the subunit vaccine against hepatitis B virus that is composed of only the surface proteins of the virus (previously extracted from the blood serum of chronically infected patients, but now produced by recombination of the viral genes into yeast), the virus-like particle (VLP) vaccine against HPV that is composed of the virus capsid protein, and the hemagglutinin and neuraminidase subunits of the influenza virus.

The vaccine can also be prepared by conjugating certain bacteria that have polysaccharide outer coats that are poorly immunogenic. Moreover, by connecting these outer coats to proteins, for example, toxins, the immune system can be led to recognize the polysaccharide as if it were a protein antigen. Interestingly, this approach is used in the *Haemophilus influenzae* type B vaccine development. Furthermore, by similar methods, dendritic cell vaccines can also be made by combining dendritic cells with antigens in order to present the antigens to the body's white blood cells, thus stimulating an immune reaction. These vaccines have shown certain positive preliminary results for treating brain tumors. Moreover, vaccines can be monovalent or univalent or multivalent in nature. A monovalent vaccine can immunize against a single antigen or single microorganism, whereas a multivalent vaccine is developed to immunize against two or more strains of the same microorganism, or against two or more microorganisms, respectively. In certain cases, it has been observed that a monovalent vaccine may be preferable for rapidly developing a strong immune response. In recent years, a new type of vaccine called DNA vaccination has been created from infectious patient's DNA; however, DNA vaccination is still in the experimental stage.

4.8.2 Production of vaccines

Owing to high demands from different parts of the world, vaccines need to be produced in large quantities, especially in epidemic situations; hence, it becomes very important to have technology ready for producing large quantities of vaccines. Moreover, vaccines can be produced from the killed or inactivated disease-causing microorganisms. In a general sense, the first step is to isolate or create an organism and this can be done in many ways. One way is to kill the organism using chemical toxin such as formalin; vaccines produced by this method are called inactivated or killed vaccines. The most commonly used killed vaccines are the typhoid vaccine and the Salk poliomyelitis vaccine.

The second method to produce a vaccine is to use only the antigenic part of the disease-causing microorganism, for example, the flagella and the capsule; these types of vaccines are known as cellular vaccines. An example of a cellular vaccine is the *Haemophilus influenzae* B vaccine. It has been found that cellular vaccines exhibit some similarities to killed vaccines. In addition, neither killed nor acellular vaccines can cause disease in humans and, therefore, are considered to be safe for use in immunocompromised patients.

A third way of producing a vaccine is to attenuate or weaken a live microorganism by an aging process or by altering its growth conditions or status. Vaccines that are made with this method are often the most effective vaccines, probably because they multiply in the body by causing a large immune response. Nevertheless, attenuated vaccines also bring the greatest hazard because they can mutate back to the virulent form at any time. Such mutation would result in induction of the disease rather than protection against it and for this reason, attenuated vaccines are not recommended for use in immunocompromised patients. Examples of attenuated vaccines are those that protect against mumps, rubella, and measles.

Another method of making a vaccine is to use other microorganisms, which are similar to the virulent organism, but that does not pose serious disease. An example of this type of vaccine is the BCG vaccine used to protect against *Mycobacterium tuberculosis*. The BCG vaccine currently in use is an attenuated strain of *Mycobacterium bovis* and requires boosters every 3–4 years. In addition, the tools of genetic engineering techniques have been used to produce subunit vaccines, which means only parts of vaccines are used to stimulate a strong immune response. In order to create a subunit vaccine, researchers first isolate the gene or genes that code for appropriate subunits from the genome of the infectious agent. Then, genetic material is placed into bacterial host cells, which produce large quantities of subunit molecules by transcribing and translating the inserted foreign DNA. Here, it is important to note that these subunit molecules of vaccines are encoded by genetic material from the infectious agent, not from the host cell's genetic material. Hepatitis B vaccine is an example of this type of vaccine and subunit vaccines are safe for immunocompromised patients because they cannot cause the disease.

4.8.3 Delivery of vaccines

The success of preventing any viral diseases is dependent on the mode of vaccine delivery. There are several new delivery system developments that can make vaccines more efficient to deliver. The vaccines can be delivered through the use of liposomes. The current developments have made it possible to deliver vaccine orally. One example is the polio vaccine, which has been given to children orally in different parts of the world and the success rate is very high in controlling the disease. It has been further found that oral vaccines are safe as there is no risk of blood contamination. Another advantage of oral vaccines is that they can be formulated as a solid form, which can be stored a long time without freezing. Lastly, a microneedle approach, which is still in developmental stages, appears to be the vaccine of the future. The micro needle has pointed projections fabricated into arrays that can create vaccine delivery pathways through the skin. Moreover, the use of plasmids has been validated in animal studies as a protective vaccine strategy for cancer and infectious diseases. However, the crossover application into human studies has been met with weak results based on the inability to provide clinically relevant benefit. The overall usefulness of plasmid DNA immunization depends on increasing the plasmid's immunogenicity while also correcting for factors involved in the specific activation of immune effector cells.

4.9 Vaccines controversies

Besides having so many clinical benefits of the vaccines, there are some issues related to vaccines that need to be discussed to get a fair idea of the usefulness of the vaccines. The process of vaccination began in the late eighteenth century; opponents have claimed that vaccines do not work, that they are dangerous, and that individuals should rely on personal hygiene instead; vaccinations violate individual rights or religious principles. Since then, successful campaigns against vaccination have been initiated by ethical groups. Issues related to vaccines such as side effects and effectiveness of the vaccine for a long period of time are still debatable.

4.9.1 Effectiveness of vaccines

Mass vaccination programs really helped to eradicate smallpox from the face of the planet, which once killed as many as one in every seventh child in Europe. Later on, vaccination has almost eradicated polio in many parts of the world. Furthermore, the incidence of invasive disease with *Haemophilus influenzae*, a major cause of bacterial meningitis and other serious disease in children, have been continuously decreased by over 99% in the United States. Moreover, the complete vaccination plan in the United States, has been reported to save more than 33,000 lives and prevented an estimated 14 million infections. In contrast to the benefits of vaccines, some vaccine critics claim that vaccines do not have any useful benefits to public health. They argue that all the reduction of communicable diseases due to high level of hygienic condition and good foods, because they said these communicable diseases were due to overcrowding, poor sanitation, and almost nonexistent hygiene. Moreover, other critics argue that immunity given by vaccines is only short-term and needs boosters, whereas those who survive the disease become permanently immune.

4.9.2 *Safety of vaccines*

In the medical field, medicine is given to a person who has some disease, but in the case of a vaccine, it is given to healthy people. It has been shown that immunization programs decreases the incidence of disease in various parts of the world. Moreover, adverse effects ascribed to vaccines typically have an unknown origin. Controversies in this area revolve around the question of whether the risks of these perceived adverse events following immunization offset the benefits of preventing effects of common diseases. For example, in rare cases, immunizations can cause adverse events, such as the oral polio vaccine that may cause paralysis and autism.

4.9.2.1 *Vaccine overdose*

Vaccine overload is the notion that giving many vaccines at once may overwhelm or weaken a child's immune system and lead to adverse effects. Although scientific evidence does not support and even contradicts this idea, many parents of autistic children firmly believe that vaccine overload causes autism, and it has caused many parents to delay or avoid immunizing their children. Such parental misperceptions are major obstacles toward children's immunization. The idea of vaccine overload is considered flawed for several reasons as vaccines do not substitute the body's own immune system; the only thing a vaccine does is expose the immune system to a variety of viruses to enable it to remember and fight back in the future. Furthermore, vaccines constitute only a tiny portion of the pathogens naturally encountered by a child in a typical year and common juvenile circumstances such as fevers and middle ear infections pose a much greater challenge to the immune system than vaccines do. In addition, studies have shown that vaccinations, and even multiple synchronized vaccinations, do not weaken the immune system or compromise overall immunity. Lastly, there is no evidence of an immune system role in autism.

4.10 *Development of new vaccines*

Over the last few years, tremendous efforts have been made to develop vaccines for major diseases and many of the diseases are being eradicated with the use of vaccines. Although vaccines are not available for all diseases, current research is going on to develop vaccines. In addition, efforts have also been made to develop vaccines against diseases of global as well as a regional threat posed by meningococcal meningitis serogroup A (Men A), which causes recurrent epidemics and high rates of death and disability in African countries.

Also, efforts are being made to make vaccines for AIDS, malaria, tuberculosis, dengue, leishmaniasis, and enteric diseases.

4.10.1 Vaccine against rotavirus

Additionally, acute diarrhea is accountable for millions of deaths every year in children and rotavirus is responsible for as much as one-fourth of these casualties, mostly in developing countries. GlaxoSmithKline (GSK), a biotechnology company, developed a vaccine named RotaRix to control rotavirus diarrhea, which has been clinically used and now licensed in many countries. These vaccines are not only available in the private market but also in the public sector immunization programs of several countries. Furthermore, vaccines, namely, RotaTeq (a rotavirus diarrhea vaccine developed by Merck Company, USA) is licensed and has been introduced in the immunization program of Nicaragua.

4.10.2 Vaccine against pneumococcal disease

Acute lower respiratory infections are caused by *Streptococcus pneumoniae* (pneumococcus). So far, seven different types of conjugate vaccine are developed known as Prevnar or Prevenar that are designed to act against seven strains of pneumococcal disease. These vaccines are developed by Wyeth Vaccines and are licensed in the United States and over 70 other countries. In the United States, the use of this vaccine has led to a dramatic decline in rates of pneumococcal disease, not only in immunized children but also in the unimmunized population through reduced transmission. Wyeth Vaccines have also completed an evaluation of a nine-valent conjugate vaccine, including serotypes 1 and 5. A Phase III trial of the vaccine involving 40,000 people was completed in South Africa in 2002, and a Phase III trial with 17,437 subjects was concluded in the Gambia in 2004. In the South African trial, the vaccine reduced invasive diseases caused by the relevant serotypes by 83% in HIV-uninfected children and by 65% in HIV-infected children. Results from the Gambia trial show the vaccine is 77% effective in preventing infections caused by the relevant stereotypes; that resulted in 37% fewer cases of pneumonia confirmed by chest x-rays as compared with a control group; that recipients experienced a 16% reduction in overall mortality. Vaccines containing 10 or 13 stereotypes are expected to be submitted for licensure within the next few years. In addition, vaccine manufacturers in developing countries have initiated the development of conjugate vaccines. Vaccines based on common protein antigens of pneumococcus are also in the pipeline.

It can be difficult to establish the extent of pneumococcal disease as developing countries often lack the laboratory facilities, expertise, and resources to do so. As a result, public health decision makers are often unaware of the prevalence of the disease and of the toll it exacts in death and disability. Because of the scarcity of data from developing countries, there is concern over the appropriate serotype valency for developing countries. Concerns remain—although results to date are encouraging—that prevention of some serotypes of pneumococcal disease may be offset by an increase in incidence of disease due to other serotypes. The price of the vaccine, although still to be set for developing countries, may be too high for them to afford without special financing arrangements.

4.10.3 Human papillomavirus

Sexually transmitted HPV is the major cause of cervical cancer and the most common cause of cancer deaths among women in developing countries. About 500,000 cases occur each year, 80% of them in developing countries. Cervical cancer kills some 240,000 women annually. Gardasil, an HPV vaccine recently licensed by Merck, covers four types of HPV, including the cancer-causing types 16 and 18 and types 6 and 11 for noncancerous genital warts. In 2007, a second vaccine, developed by GSK which covers HPV types 16 and 18. HPV types 16 and 18 cause around 70% of HPV cervical cancers globally, but the vaccines in development will not cover the 30% of cancers attributed to other HPV types. Because these other types are numerous and individually only contribute a small percentage, significantly expanding vaccine coverage against them may present technical challenges for manufacturers. The duration of the immunity conferred by the vaccines is not yet known, and only time and follow-up studies will provide this critical information. Other clinical studies are planned that will look at alternative schedules and possibly lowering the age of vaccination. Because HPV is spread by sexual contact, and the high-risk years for infection are roughly from ages 18 to 25, the best subjects for vaccination will likely be preadolescents or adolescents, unlike for traditional vaccination programs, which are aimed mostly at infants and pregnant women. Access to the vaccines is likely to be an issue in developing countries due to limited resources for the implementation of vaccination programs. Discussions are ongoing about collecting the necessary data for introducing the vaccines into developing countries.

4.10.4 Meningococcal meningitis A

The African meningitis belt that includes all or parts of 21 countries stretching south of the Sahara desert from Senegal to Ethiopia is the site of frequent epidemics, usually caused by serogroup A meningitis. Over the past decade, more than 700,000 cases have been reported. Roughly 10–20% of persons infected die, and one out of five survivors is likely to suffer from a permanent disability such as hearing loss, mental retardation, or paralysis. The rate of meningitis epidemics in the region has increased in recent years. Polysaccharide vaccines are currently in use, but are not very effective at protecting young children, do not create long-lasting immunity, and do not confer a "herd effect," that is, do not prevent the spread of the disease in nonvaccinated people through the reduction of the carriage of the infectious agent by vaccinated people during epidemics. Because of these shortcomings, immunization with polysaccharide vaccines is usually undertaken only after the onset of an epidemic. To provide greater and more efficient protection, a public–private effort called the Meningitis Vaccine Project (MVP) is developing a Men A conjugate vaccine. This vaccine is intended to have long-lasting effect, to create immunity in infants, and to allow protection to be conferred in advance through mass immunization programs. Toxicology studies and animal studies have been successfully completed, and the animal studies suggest the conjugate vaccine is highly immunogenic—that is, stimulates high levels of antibodies against Men A infection. Phase I trials were conducted in India and Phase II trials are ongoing in Mali and the Gambia. Recruitment has been completed and preliminary results have been completed in 2007. Phase II and III trials are being prepared in the same sites, in addition to in Ethiopia and Senegal. A Phase II infant study is planned in Ghana. Other conjugate vaccines, including a heptavalent vaccine (DTP) covering serogroups A and C, are being developed by the private sector; and a tetravalent vaccine has recently been licensed by Sanofi-Pasteur in the United States and Canada.

4.11 Summary

Unlike microbes that cause infections in humans without entering into living (host) cells, a virus is a small communicable agent that can replicate only inside the living (host) cells. It has been a known fact that most of the viruses cannot be seen without the help of a microscope and these viruses can infect all living organisms, including human, animals, plants, and bacteria. After the discovery of the tobacco mosaic virus in 1898, more than 5000 viruses have been described so far. Viruses are known to spread in many ways such as air route, water routes, and blood route, and in animal, viruses can be carried by blood-sucking insects. Remarkably, influenza viruses can be spread by coughing and sneezing, whereas the norovirus and rotavirus, which cause viral gastroenteritis condition, are transmitted by the fecal–oral route or through food or water. Another type of virus that can be transmitted through sexual contact is HIV. Moreover, it is seemingly very difficult to control the infection caused by viruses, because viruses use vital metabolic pathways within host cells to replicate and survive, and they are very difficult to eliminate without using drugs or vaccines. The most effective medical approaches to viral diseases are vaccinations that provide immunity against infections. In this chapter, we have discussed the characteristics of viruses and how these viruses cause various diseases in humans and we have explained the prevention and treatment modalities of viral infections.

4.12 Scholar's achievements

Dmitri Iosifovich Ivanovsky: Dmitri Iosifovich Ivanovsky (1864–1920) was a Russian botanist, one of the discoverers of the filterable nature of viruses (1892), and thus one of the founders of virology.

Martinus Willem Beijerinck: Martinus Willem Beijerinck (March 16, 1851–January 1, 1931) was a Dutch microbiologist and botanist. He is considered one of the founders of virology. In 1898, he published results on the filtration experiments demonstrating that tobacco mosaic disease is caused by an infectious agent smaller than a bacterium. His results were in accordance with a similar observation made by Dmitri Ivanovsky in 1892.

Friedrich August Johannes Loeffler and Paul Frosch: Friedrich August Johannes Loeffler was a German physician, bacteriologist, and hygienist, and a student of Robert Koch in Berlin. He described along with Paul Frosch (1860–1928) the causative agent of foot-and-mouth disease as a particulate agent smaller than a bacterium.

Frederick William Twort: Frederick William Twort, FRS (1877–1950) was an English bacteriologist and was the original discoverer in 1915 of bacteriophages (viruses that infect bacteria).

Ross Granville Harrison: Ross Granville Harrison (January 13, 1870–September 30, 1959) was an American biologist and anatomist credited as the first to work successfully with artificial tissue culture. He successfully cultured frog neuroblasts in a lymph medium and thereby took the first step toward current research on precursor and stem cells. He was considered for a Nobel prize for his work on nerve cell outgrowth, which helped form the modern functional understanding of the nervous system, and he contributed to the surgical tissue transplantation technique.

Baruch Blumberg: Baruch Samuel Blumberg (July 28, 1925–April 5, 2011) was an American doctor and corecipient of the 1976 Nobel Prize in Physiology or Medicine (with Daniel Carleton Gajdusek) for work on kuru, the first human prion disease demonstrated to be infectious, and the President of the American Philosophical Society from 2005 until his death. Blumberg received the Nobel Prize for discoveries concerning new mechanisms for the origin and dissemination of infectious diseases. Blumberg identified the hepatitis B virus, and later developed its diagnostic test and vaccine.

Ernst Ruska and Max Knoll: Max Knoll was born in Wiesbaden and studied in Munich and at the Technical University of Berlin, where he obtained his doctorate at the Institute for High Voltage Technology. In 1927, he became the leader of the electron research group there, where he and his coworker, Ernst Ruska, invented the electron microscope in 1931. In April 1932, Knoll joined Telefunken in Berlin to do developmental work in the field of television design. He was also a private lecturer in Berlin.

Wendell Meredith Stanley: Wendell Meredith Stanley (August 16, 1904–June 15, 1971) was an American biochemist, virologist, and Nobel laureate. Stanley's work contributed to lepracidal compounds, diphenyl stereochemistry, and the chemistry of the sterols. His research on the virus causing the mosaic disease in tobacco plants led to the isolation of a nucleoprotein, which displayed tobacco mosaic virus activity. Stanley was awarded the Nobel Prize in Chemistry in 1946.

Rosalind Elsie Franklin: Rosalind Elsie Franklin (July 25, 1920–April 16, 1958) was a British biophysicist and x-ray crystallographer who made critical contributions to the understanding of the fine molecular structures of DNA, RNA, viruses, coal, and graphite. Her DNA work achieved the most fame because DNA plays an essential role in cell metabolism and genetics, and the discovery of its structure helped her coworkers understand how genetic information is passed from parents to children. Franklin is best known for her work on the x-ray diffraction images of DNA, which led to the discovery of the DNA double helix. Her data, according to Francis Crick, were the data they actually used to formulate the Crick and Watson's 1953 hypothesis regarding the structure of DNA.

4.13 Knowledge builder

Scanning electron microscope: A scanning electron microscope (SEM) is a type of electron microscope that produces images of a sample by scanning it with a focused beam of electrons. The electrons interact with the atoms in the sample, producing various signals that can be detected and that contain information about the sample's surface topography and composition. The electron beam is generally scanned in a raster scan pattern, and the beam's position combines with the detected signal to produce an image. SEM can achieve resolution better than 1 nm. Specimens can be observed in high vacuum and low vacuum, and in environmental SEM, specimens can be observed in wet conditions.

Transmission electron microscope: Transmission electron microscopy (TEM) is a microscopy technique whereby a beam of electrons is transmitted through an ultrathin specimen, interacting with the specimen as it passes through. An image is formed from the interaction of the electrons transmitted through the specimen; the image is magnified and focused onto an imaging device, such as a fluorescent screen, on a layer of photographic film, or to be detected by a sensor such as a CCD camera. The first TEM was built by Max Knoll and Ernst Ruska in 1931, with this group developing the first TEM with resolution greater than that of light in 1933 and the first commercial TEM in 1939.

Enterobacteria phage T4: Enterobacteria phage T4 is a bacteriophage that infects *Escherichia coli* bacteria. The T4 phage is a member of the T-even phages, a group including enterobacteriophages T2 and T6. T4 is capable of undergoing only a lytic life cycle and not the lysogenic life cycle.

H1N1: Influenza A (H1N1) virus is the subtype of influenza A virus that was the most common cause of human influenza (flu) in 2009. Some strains of H1N1 are endemic in humans and cause a small fraction of all influenza-like illness and a small fraction of all seasonal influenza. H1N1 strains caused a small percentage of all human flu infections in 2004–2005. Other strains of H1N1 are endemic in pigs (swine influenza) and in birds (avian influenza).

Real-time RT-PCR: In molecular biology, a real-time polymerase chain reaction, also called quantitative real-time polymerase chain reaction (qPCR) or kinetic polymerase chain reaction, is a laboratory technique based on the polymerase chain reaction, which is used to amplify and simultaneously quantify a targeted DNA molecule. For one or more specific sequences in a DNA sample, real-time-PCR enables both detection and quantification. The quantity can be either an absolute number of copies or a relative amount when normalized to DNA input or additional normalizing genes.

Rapid influenza diagnostic tests: A rapid influenza diagnostic test (RIDT) is a type of antigen detection test that detects influenza viral nucleoprotein antigen. Commercially available RIDTs can provide results within 30 min or less.

RT-PCR technique: Reverse transcription polymerase chain reaction (RT-PCR) is one of many variants of polymerase chain reaction (PCR). This technique is commonly used in molecular biology to detect RNA expression levels. RT-PCR is often confused with real-time polymerase chain reaction (qPCR) by students and scientists alike. However, they are separate and distinct techniques. While RT-PCR is used to qualitatively detect gene expression through the creation of complementary DNA (CDNA) transcripts from RNA, qPCR is used to quantitatively measure the amplification of DNA using fluorescent probes. qPCR is also referred to as quantitative PCR, quantitative real-time PCR, and real-time quantitative PCR.

Metabolic pathways: In biochemistry, metabolic pathways are a series of chemical reactions occurring within a cell. In each pathway, a principal chemical is modified by a series of chemical reactions. Enzymes catalyze these reactions, and often require dietary minerals, vitamins, and other cofactors in order to function properly. Because of the many chemicals (a.k.a. "metabolites") that may be involved, metabolic pathways can be quite elaborate. In addition, numerous distinct pathways coexist within a cell. This collection of pathways is called the metabolic network. Pathways are important to the maintenance of homeostasis within an organism.

Anti-idiotypic antibodies: Anti-idiotypic vaccines comprise antibodies that have three-dimensional immunogenic regions, designated idiotopes that consist of protein sequences that bind to cell receptors. Idiotopes are aggregated into idiotypes specific of their target antigen. An example of anti-idiotype antibody is Racotumomab.

CD4: In molecular biology, CD4 (cluster of differentiation 4) is a glycoprotein found on the surface of immune cells such as T helper cells, monocytes, macrophages, and dendritic cells. It was discovered in the late 1970s and was originally known as leu-3 and T4 (after the OKT4 monoclonal antibody that reacted with it) before being named CD4 in 1984.

CCR5: C-C chemokine receptor type 5, also known as CCR5 or CD195, is a protein on the surface of white blood cells that is involved in the immune system as it acts as a receptor for chemokines. This is the process by which T cells are attracted to specific tissue and organ targets. Many forms of HIV, the virus that causes AIDS, initially use CCR5 to enter and infect host cells.

Acyclovir: Acyclovir, chemical name acycloguanosine, is a guanosine analog antiviral drug, marketed under trade names such as Cyclovir, Herpex, Acivir, Acivirax, Zovirax, Zoral, and Xovir. One of the most commonly used antiviral drugs, it is primarily used for the treatment of herpes simplex virus infections, as well as in the treatment of varicella zoster (chickenpox) and herpes zoster (shingles).

Antisense-antiviral drug: A drug made of short segments of DNA or RNA that can bind to and alter or suppress the function of viral DNA or RNA. Antisense-antivirals prevent viruses from replicating.

Protease inhibitors: Protease inhibitors are a class of antiviral drugs that are widely used to treat HIV/AIDS and hepatitis caused by hepatitis C virus. The protease inhibitors prevent viral replication by selectively binding to viral proteases (e.g., HIV-1 protease) and blocking proteolytic cleavage of protein precursors that are necessary for the production of infectious viral particles.

Rabies: Rabies is an acute and deadly disease caused by a viral infection of the central nervous system. The rabies virus is most often spread by a bite and saliva from an infected (rabid) animal (e.g., bats, raccoons, skunks, foxes, ferrets, cats, or dogs). In the United States, rabies are most often associated with bat exposures. However, there have been rare cases in which laboratory workers and explorers in caves inhabited by millions of bats were infected by rabies virus in the air.

Rabies vaccine: Rabies vaccine is a vaccine used to control rabies. Rabies can be prevented by vaccination, both in humans and in other animals.

Toxoid: A toxoid is a bacterial toxin (usually an exotoxin) whose toxicity has been inactivated or suppressed by either chemical (formalin) or heat treatment, while other properties, typically immunogenicity, are maintained. Thus, when used during vaccination, an immune response is mounted and immunological memory is formed against the molecular markers of the toxoid without resulting in toxin-induced illness.

DTP: DTP (also DPT) refers to a class of combination vaccines against three infectious diseases in humans: diphtheria, pertussis (whooping cough), and tetanus.

Further reading

Akay S and Karasu Z 2008. Hepatitis B immune globulin and HBV-related liver transplantation. *Expert Opin Biol Ther* 8 (11): 1815–1822. doi:10.1517/14712598.8.11.1815. PMID 18847315.

Almela MJ, González ME, and Carrasco L 1991. Inhibitors of poliovirus uncoating efficiently block the early membrane permeabilization induced by virus particles. *J Virol* 65 (5): 2572–2577. PMID 1850030. PMC 240614. http://jvi.asm.org/cgi/pmidlookup?view=long&pmid=1850030.

Bae K, Choi J, Jang Y, Ahn S, and Hur B 2009. Innovative vaccine production technologies: The evolution and value of vaccine production technologies. *Arch Pharm Res* 32 (4): 465–480. doi:10.1007/s12272-009-1400-1. PMID 19407962.

Bai J, Rossi J, and Akkina R 2001. Multivalent anti-CCR ribozymes for stem cell-based HIV type 1 gene therapy. *AIDS Res Hum Retroviruses* 17 (5): 385–399. doi:10.1089/088922201750102427. PMID 11282007.

Bigham M and Copes R 2005. Thiomersal in vaccines: Balancing the risk of adverse effects with the risk of vaccine-preventable disease. *Drug Saf* 28 (2): 89–101. doi:10.2165/00002018-200528020-00001. PMID 15691220.

Bishop NE 1998. Examination of potential inhibitors of hepatitis A virus uncoating. *Intervirology* 41 (6): 261–271. doi:10.1159/000024948. PMID 10325536. http://content.karger.com/produktedb/produkte.asp?typ=fulltext&file=int41261.

Bonhoeffer J and Heininger U 2007. Adverse events following immunization: Perception and evidence. *Curr Opin Infect Dis* 20 (3): 237–246. doi:10.1097/QCO.0b013e32811ebfb0. PMID 17471032.

Carlson B 2008. Adults now drive growth of vaccine market. *Genet Eng Biotechnol News* 28 (11): 22–23. http://www.genengnews.com/articles/chitem.aspx?aid=2490.

Deas TS, Binduga-Gajewska I, Tilgner M et al. April 2005. Inhibition of flavivirus infections by antisense oligomers specifically suppressing viral translation and RNA replication. *J Virol* 79 (8): 4599–4609. doi:10.1128/JVI.79.8.4599-4609.2005. PMID 15795246. PMC 1069577. http://jvi.asm.org/cgi/pmidlookup?view=long&pmid=15795246.

Demicheli V, Jefferson T, Rivetti A, and Price D 2005. Vaccines for measles, mumps and rubella in children. *Cochrane Database Syst Rev* 19: 4. doi:10.1002/14651858.CD004407.pub2. PMID 16235361. Lay summary—Cochrane press release (PDF) (2005-10-19).

Dudgeon JA 1963. Development of smallpox vaccine in England in the eighteenth and nineteenth centuries. *BMJ* (5342): 1367–1372. doi:10.1136/bmj.1.5342.1367.

Dunn PM January 1996. Dr Edward Jenner (1749–1823) of Berkeley, and vaccination against smallpox. *Arch Dis Child Fetal Neonatal Ed* 74 (1): F77–8. doi:10.1136/fn.74.1.F77. PMID 8653442. PMC 2528332. http://fn.bmjjournals.com/content/74/1/F77.full.pdf.

Flint OP, Noor MA, Hruz PW et al. 2009. The role of protease inhibitors in the pathogenesis of HIV-associated lipodystrophy: Cellular mechanisms and clinical implications. *Toxicol Pathol* 37 (1): 65–77. doi:10.1177/0192623308327119. PMID 19171928.

Giudice EL and Campbell JD 2006. Needle-free vaccine delivery. *Adv Drug Deliv Rev* 58 (1): 68–89. doi:10.1016/j.addr.2005.12.003. PMID 16564111.

Grammatikos AP, Mantadakis E, and Falagas ME 2009. Meta-analyses on pediatric infections and vaccines. *Infect Dis Clin North Am* 23 (2): 431–457. PMID 19393917.

Hardman Reis T 2006. The role of intellectual property in the global challenge for immunization. *J World Intellect Prop* 9 (4): 413–425. doi:10.1111/j.1422-2213.2006.00284.x.

Kanesa-thasan N, Sun W, Kim-Ahn G et al. 2001. Safety and immunogenicity of attenuated dengue virus vaccines (Aventis Pasteur) in human volunteers. *Vaccine* 19 (23–24): 3179–3188. doi:10.1016/S0264-410X(01)00020-2. PMID 11312014.

Kim W and Liau LM 2010. Dendritic cell vaccines for brain tumors. *Neurosurg Clin N Am* 21 (1): 139–157. doi:10.1016/j.nec.2009.09.005. PMID 19944973.

Kinney RM, Huang CY, Rose BC et al. April 2005. Inhibition of dengue virus serotypes 1 to 4 in vero cell cultures with morpholino oligomers. *J Virol* 79 (8): 5116–5128. doi:10.1128/JVI.79.8.5116-5128.2005. PMID 15795296. PMC 1069583. http://jvi.asm.org/cgi/pmidlookup?view=long&pmid=15795296.

Klein SL, Jedlicka A, and Pekosz A May 2010. The Xs and Y of immune responses to viral vaccines. *Lancet Infect Dis* 10 (5): 338–349. doi:10.1016/S1473-3099(10)70049-9. PMID 20417416.

McCaffrey AP, Meuse L, Karimi M, Contag CH, and Kay MA August 2003. A potent and specific morpholino antisense inhibitor of hepatitis C translation in mice. *Hepatology* 38 (2): 503–508. doi:10.1053/jhep.2003.50330. PMID 12883495.

Morein B, Hu KF, and Abusugra I 2004. Current status and potential application of ISCOMs in veterinary medicine. *Adv Drug Deliv Rev* 56 (10): 1367–1382. doi:10.1016/j.addr.2004.02.004. PMID 15191787.

Muzumdar JM and Cline RR 2009. Vaccine supply, demand, and policy: A primer. *J Am Pharm Assoc* 49 (4): e87–99. doi:10.1331/JAPhA.2009.09007. PMID 19589753.

Neuman BW, Stein DA, Kroeker AD et al. 2004. Antisense morpholino-oligomers directed against the 5′ end of the genome inhibit coronavirus proliferation and growth. *J Virol* 78 (11): 5891–5899. doi:10.1128/JVI.78.11.5891-5899.2004. PMID 15140987. PMC 415795. http://jvi.asm.org/cgi/pmidlookup?view=long&pmid=15140987.

Nokes JD and Cane PA 2008. New strategies for control of respiratory syncytial virus infection. *Curr Opin Infect Dis* 21 (6): 639–643. doi:10.1097/QCO.0b013e3283184245. PMID 18978532.

Odani S, Tominaga K, and Kondou S 1999. The inhibitory properties and primary structure of a novel serine proteinase inhibitor from the fruiting body of the basidiomycete, *Lentinus edodes*. *Eur J Biochem* 262 (3): 915–923. doi:10.1046/j.1432-1327.1999.00463.x. PMID 10411656.

Offit PA 2007. Thimerosal and vaccines a cautionary tale. *N Engl J Med* 357 (13): 1278–1279. doi:10.1056/NEJMp078187. PMID 17898096. http://content.nejm.org/cgi/content/full/357/13/1278.

Olesen OF, Lonnroth A, and Mulligan B 2009. Human vaccine research in the European Union. *Vaccine* 27 (5): 640–645. doi:10.1016/j.vaccine.2008.11.064. PMID 19059446.

Orenstein WA, Papania MJ, and Wharton ME 2004. Measles elimination in the United States. *J Infect Dis* 189 (Suppl 1): S1–3. doi:10.1086/377693. PMID 15106120. http://www.journals.uchicago.edu/doi/full/10.1086/377693.

Patel JR and Heldens JG 2009. Immunoprophylaxis against important virus disease of horses, farm animals and birds. *Vaccine* 27 (12): 1797–1810. Review. PMID: 19402200.

Plotkin SA 2005. Vaccines: Past, present and future. *Nat Med* 11 (4 Suppl): S5–11. doi:10.1038/nm1209. PMID 15812490.

Poland GA, Jacobson RM, and Ovsyannikova IG 2009. Trends affecting the future of vaccine development and delivery: The role of demographics, regulatory science, the anti-vaccine movement, and vaccinomics. *Vaccine* 27 (25–26): 3240–3244. doi:10.1016/j.vaccine.2009.01.069. PMID 19200833.

Ryu KJ and Lee SW 2003. Identification of the most accessible sites to ribozymes on the hepatitis C virus internal ribosome entry site. *J Biochem Mol Biol* 36 (6): 538–544. PMID 14659071. http://www.jbmb.or.kr/fulltext/jbmb/view.php?vol=36&page=538.

Samuel CE 2001. Antiviral actions of interferons. *Clin Microbiol Rev* 14 (4): 778–809. doi:10.1128/CMR.14.4.778-809.2001. PMID 11585785.

Samuelsson O and Herlitz H 2008. Vaccination against high blood pressure: A new strategy. *Lancet* 371 (9615): 788–789. doi:10.1016/S0140-6736(08)60355-4. PMID 18328909.

Sinal SH, Cabinum-Foeller E, and Socolar R 2008. Religion and medical neglect. *South Med J* 101 (7): 703–706. doi:10.1097/SMJ.0b013e31817997c9 (inactive 2008-10-26). PMID 18580731.

Sodeik B, Griffiths G, Ericsson M, Moss B, and Doms RW February 1994. Assembly of vaccinia virus: Effects of rifampin on the intracellular distribution of viral protein p65. *J Virol* 68 (2): 1103–1114. PMID 8289340. PMC 236549. http://jvi.asm.org/cgi/pmidlookup?view=long&pmid=8289340.

Soundararajan V, Tharakaraman K, Raman R, Raguram S, Shriver Z, Sasisekharan V, and Sasisekharan R 2009. Extrapolating from sequence the 2009 H1N1 'swine' influenza virus. *Nat Biotechnol* 27 (6): 510. doi:10.1038/nbt0609-510. PMID 19513050. http://www.nature.com/nbt/journal/v27/n6/full/nbt0609-510.html.

Spohn G and Bachmann MF 2008. Exploiting viral properties for the rational design of modern vaccines. *Expert Rev Vaccines* 7 (1): 43–54. doi:10.1586/14760584.7.1.43. PMID 18251693.

Stein DA, Skilling DE, Iversen PL, and Smith AW October 2001. Inhibition of Vesivirus infections in mammalian tissue culture with antisense morpholino oligomers. *Antisense Nucleic Acid Drug Dev* 11 (5): 317–325. doi:10.1089/108729001753231696. PMID 11763348.

Stern AM and Markel H 2005. The history of vaccines and immunization: Familiar patterns, new challenges. *Health Aff* 24 (3): 611–621. doi:10.1377/hlthaff.24.3.611. PMID 15886151. http://content.healthaffairs.org/cgi/content/full/24/3/611.

Suzuki H, Okubo A, Yamazaki S, Suzuki K, Mitsuya H, and Toda S April 1989. Inhibition of the infectivity and cytopathic effect of human immunodeficiency virus by water-soluble lignin in an extract of the culture medium of *Lentinus edodes* mycelia (LEM). *Biochem Biophys Res Commun* 160 (1): 367–373. doi:10.1016/0006-291X(89)91665-3. PMID 2469420.

Van Sant JE 2008. The vaccinators: Smallpox, medical knowledge, and the opening of Japan. *J Hist Med Allied Sci* 63 (2): 276–279. doi:10.1093/jhmas/jrn014.

Wang S 2010. Lancet retracts study tying vaccine to autism. *Wall Street J*. http://online.wsj.com/article/SB10001424052748704022804575041212437364420.html?mod=WSJ_hp_mostpop_emailed. Retrieved February 2, 2010.

Wolfe R and Sharp L 2002. Anti-vaccinationists past and present. *BMJ* 325 (7361): 430–432. doi:10.1136/bmj.325.7361.430. PMID 12193361. http://bmj.bmjjournals.com/cgi/content/full/325/7361/430.

chapter five

Immunological disorders and immunotherapy

5.1 Introduction

The human immune system is a defense organization within the body that protects against diseases. The immune system basically consists of several cells that identify and kill the invading pathogens and tumor cells. The immune system detects a wide variety of agents such as bacteria, viruses, and parasitic worms. The term "immunity" was first used during 430 BC and later on, in the eighteenth century, research experiments were conducted with scorpion venom that showed that certain dogs and mice are immune to scorpion venom. Various theories have been hypothesized to show that the human body has an intrinsic defense against disease and not until 1891 was it revealed that microorganisms are responsible for various infectious diseases. Besides bacteria, viruses were also established as human pathogens in 1901, with the discovery of the yellow fever virus. One of the major tasks of the immune system is to defend the body from any kind of harmful infections. It has been shown that disease detection is complicated, as pathogens can evolve rapidly and with time can produce a completely new organism to avoid the immune defense system, which allows pathogens to successfully infect hosts. It has been reported that many organisms (bacteria and viruses) have evolved that cause severe health problems around the world.

5.2 Immune system

It has been reported that all higher orders of vertebrates, including animals and humans, have more advanced defense mechanisms to fight against infection. Moreover, the human defense system consists of many types of proteins, cells, organs, and tissues that interact in an intricate and dynamic way to defend the human body against diseases and infections.

5.3 Classification of immune system

The primary function of an immune system is protecting the body from any infection. The immune system is basically creating a physical barrier to prevent pathogens such as bacteria and viruses from entering the organism. The immune system can be broadly classified into two major types: the innate immune system and adaptive immune system.

5.3.1 Innate immune system

The innate immune system contains cells and mechanisms that defend or fight against infection by other microorganisms in a generalized manner, which suggests that the cells of the innate system identify and respond to pathogens in a common way, and it does not

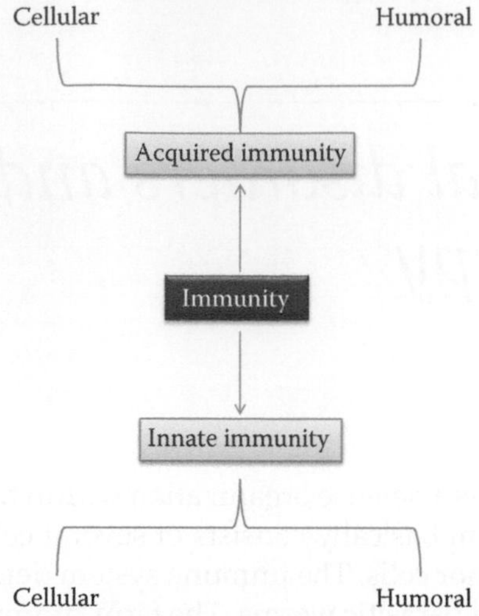

Figure 5.1 Classification of immunity.

convene long-lasting or protective immunity to the host (Figure 5.1). It has been reported that innate immune systems offer immediate defense against infection and are found in all plants and animals. It has been found that the innate immune system generally consists of three components—membrane barrier, inflammation, and complement system—to protect the cells from infections. In case a pathogen breaks these barriers, the innate immune system provides an immediate response to control pathogen entry. In case pathogens can successfully evade the innate response, a host body possesses another layer of protection called the adaptive immune system, which can be activated by the innate response. At this point, the immune system familiarizes its response during an infection to increase its recognition of the pathogen. This enhanced response against pathogens is then remembered in the form of an immunological memory after the pathogen has been removed, and allows the adaptive immune system to withstand faster and stronger attacks each time this pathogen is detected (Figures 5.2 and 5.3).

5.3.1.1 *Physical barrier*

In innate immune systems, the epithelial surfaces of a cell form a physical barrier that is highly resistant to most infectious agents and acts as the first line of defense against invading pathogenic organisms. Bacteria and other infectious agents can be removed from the skin epithelium by the process of desquamation, while bacteria and other infectious agents present in the gastrointestinal and respiratory tracts can be removed by peristalsis movement. It has been reported that the gut pathogenic bacteria can be prevented by secreting toxic substances by healthy bacteria or by competing with pathogenic bacteria for nutrients. Interestingly, the flushing act of tears and saliva helps prevent the infection of the eyes and mouth regions.

It has been reported that inflammation is one of the first responses of the immune system due to bacterial or viral infection. Inflammation is generally stimulated by chemical factors released by damaged cells and helps to establish a physical barrier against infections. Also, immune systems promote the healing of damaged tissues or cells following the removal of pathogens. During inflammation, the immune system releases various kinds of chemical factors that include histamine, bradykinin, and serotonin. Later on,

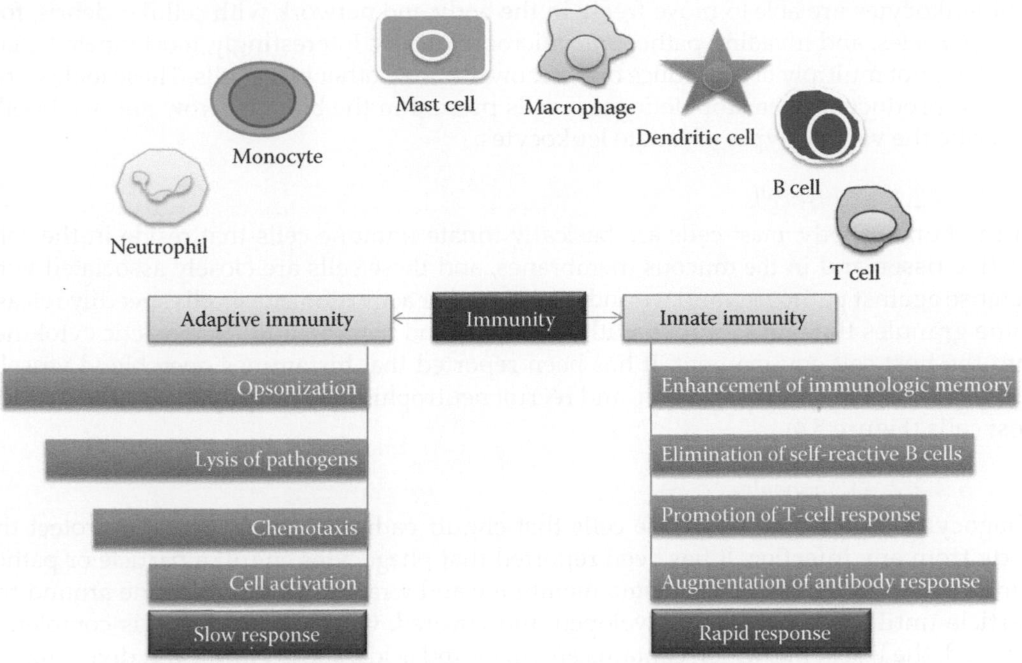

Figure 5.2 Difference between innate and adaptive (acquired) immunity.

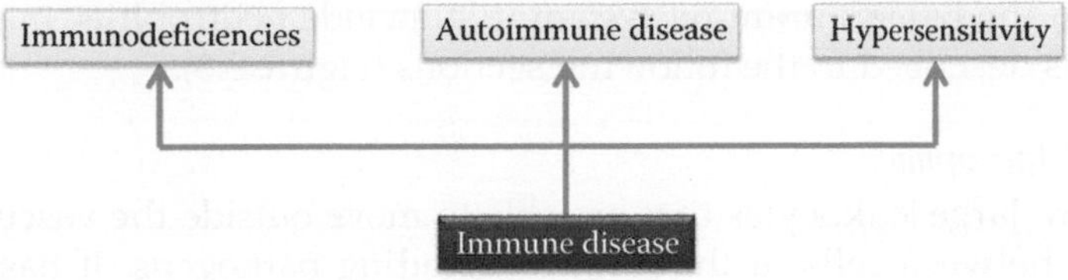

Figure 5.3 Types of immune diseases.

prostaglandins also sensitize pain receptors that cause a vasodilation of blood vessels at the location and employ phagocytes, especially neutrophils. These neutrophils then trigger other parts of the immune system to attack the pathogenic infections. Inflammation leads to the development of various symptoms that include redness of the skin, heat, swelling of the organ, pain in the body or parts of the body, and possible dysfunction of the organs or tissues involved. In addition to this, the complement system is a biochemical cascade of the immune system that helps to clear pathogens in the body. The cascade is basically composed of plasma proteins that are synthesized in the liver, mainly by hepatocytes. These proteins work together to trigger the recruitment of inflammatory cells of the immune system to upset the plasma membrane of an infected cell, resulting in the death of the pathogens.

5.3.2 *Cellular network of innate immune system*

The white blood cells (WBCs), identified as leukocytes, are different from other cells of the body because they are normally associated with a particular organ. It has been reported that leukocytes are able to move freely in the body and network with cellular debris, foreign particles, and invading pathogenic microorganisms. Interestingly, most innate leukocytes cannot multiply or reproduce on their own, unlike other body cells. These leukocytes are the products of hematopoietic stem cells present in the bone marrow and we briefly describe the various types of innate leukocytes.

5.3.2.1 *Mast cells*

In the human body, mast cells are basically innate immune cells that reside in the connective tissue and in the mucous membranes, and these cells are closely associated with defense against pathogens and wound healing. After activation, mast cells speedily release some granules that are equipped with histamine and heparin and chemotactic cytokines into the host cell environment. It has been reported that histamines open blood vessels, causing irritation or inflammation, and recruit neutrophils and macrophages to defend the host cells (Figure 5.4).

5.3.2.2 *Phagocytes*

Phagocytes are basically immune cells that engulf pathogens or particles to protect the body from any infection. It has been reported that phagocytes engulf a particle or pathogen by extending parts of its plasma membrane and wrapping the membrane around the particle until it is completely enveloped and covered. Once the pathogen is completely covered, the lysosome, which contains enzymes and acids, starts killing and digesting the foreign particle or organism. It has been described that phagocytes generally patrol the human body searching for pathogens, and are also able to respond to molecular signals produced by other cells, which are called cytokines. There are various types of phagocytic cells reported in the human immune system that include neutrophils, macrophages, and dendritic cells as described in the following sections (Figure 5.5).

5.3.2.3 *Macrophages*

Macrophages are large leukocytes that are able to move outside the vascular system and enter the areas between cells in the hunt of invading pathogens. It has been reported

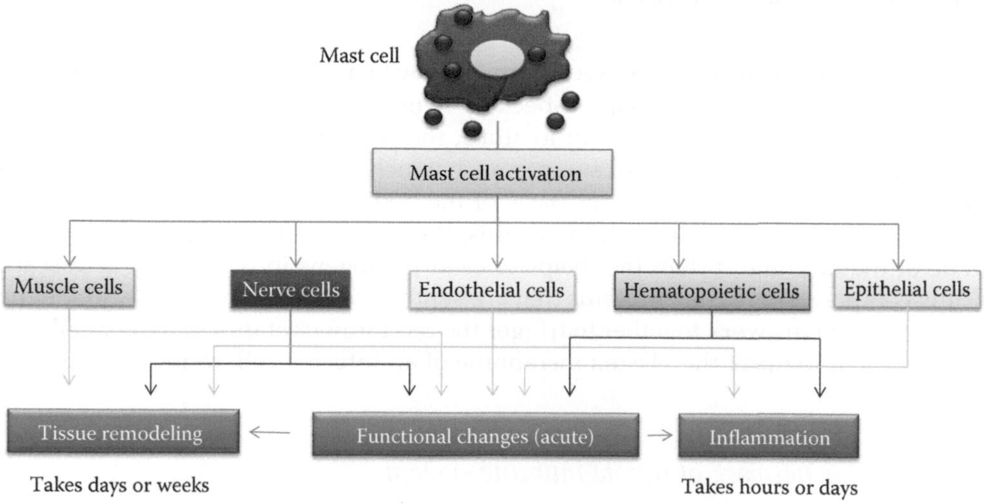

Figure 5.4 Mast cells and their role in innate and acquired immunity.

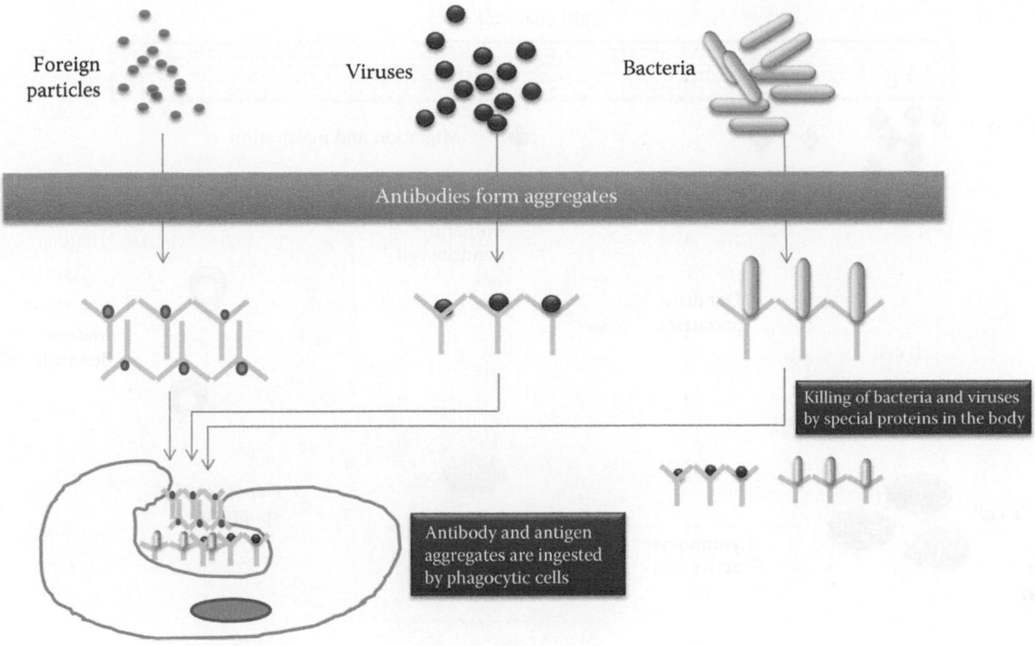

Figure 5.5 Role of phagocytic cells in immune protection.

that these macrophages are the most efficient phagocytes, and can kill large numbers of bacteria or other cells or microorganisms. The attachment of anti-bacterial molecules to receptors of a macrophage terminates the bacterial population through respiratory spurt, causing the release of reactive oxygen species. It has been reported that pathogens can also stimulate the macrophage to produce chemokines, which command other cells to the site of infection.

5.3.2.4 *Neutrophils*

Because of the presence of granules in their cytoplasm, neutrophils, eosinophils, and basophils are known as granulocytes. Neutrophils are also known as polymorphonuclear cells (PMNs) due to their typical lobed nuclei. It has been reported that neutrophil granules contain a variety of toxic elements that destroy or inhibit the growth of bacteria and fungi. Like macrophages, neutrophils attack pathogens by activating a respiratory spurt that contains oxidizing agents, including free oxygen radicals, hydrogen peroxide, and hypochlorite. It has been reported that neutrophils are the most plentiful type of phagocyte, normally representing 50–60% of the total mobile leukocytes, and they are usually the first type of cells to reach the site of an infection. It has been estimated that the bone marrow of a healthy adult human being produces more than 100 billion neutrophils per day, and produces more than 10 times more neutrophils during acute inflammation or infection.

5.3.2.5 *Dendritic cells*

Dendritic cells are phagocytic cells present in human tissues that are in contact with the external atmosphere, primarily the skin, where they are referred to as Langerhans cells, and the inner mucosal lining of the nose, stomach, intestines, and lungs. The structure of dendrite cells closely resembles neuronal dendrites; that is why they are called dendritic cells. They have no association with neuronal cells. It has been suggested that dendritic

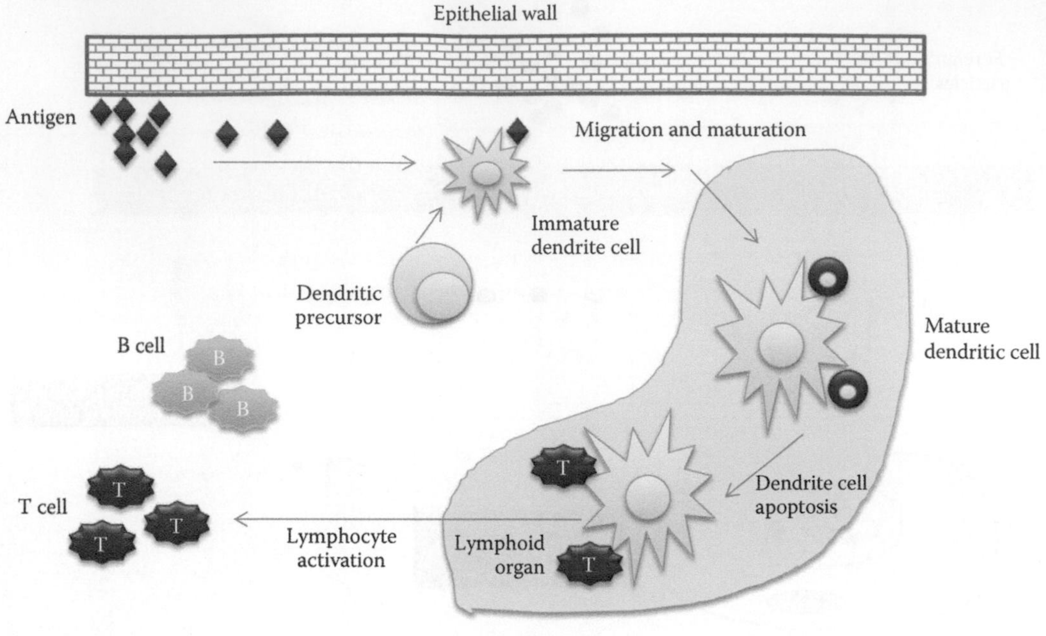

Figure 5.6 Dendritic cells and their biological actions.

cells are very vital in antigen performance and assist as a link between the innate and adaptive immune defense system (Figure 5.6).

5.3.2.6 *Basophils and eosinophils*

Basophils and eosinophils are known to relate to the neutrophils. Moreover, the basophils release histamine upon parasite entry, which are critical in the defense against parasites, and are also involved in allergic reactions. These basophils during activation secrete a highly toxic protein and free radicals that instantly kill bacteria and parasites; however, they are also known to cause cell and tissue damage during allergic-related reactions.

5.3.2.7 *Natural killer cells*

Natural killer (NK) cells are an important member of the innate immune defense system that does not attack invading pathogens or microbes. In contrast to phagocytes, NK cells can terminate compromised host cells, such as cancerous cells or virus-infected cells. They are called NK cells because of an initial idea that these NK cells do not require activation to kill cells (Figures 5.7 and 5.8).

5.3.3 *Adaptive immune system*

The adaptive immune system is basically a defense system in the human body that remembers the entry and action of each and every pathogen. Moreover, adaptive immune response is antigen specific and needs the recognition of specific antigens during antigen presentation. Antigen specificity can allow the generation of responses that are tailored to specific pathogens or pathogen-infected cells in the body. The special adaptive capability of immune cells is maintained in the body by memory cells.

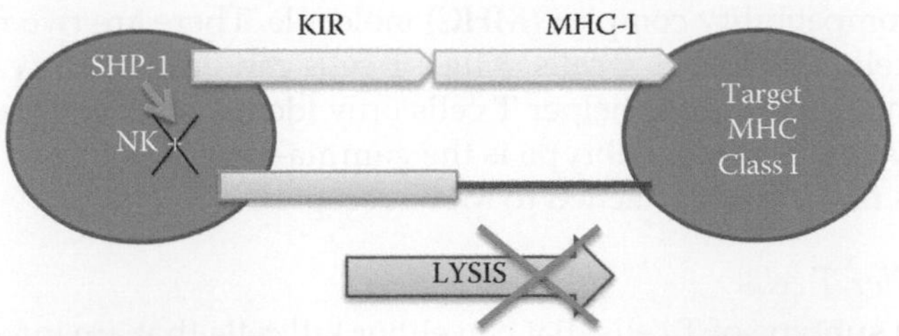

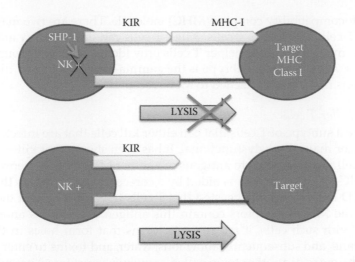

Figure 5.7 NK cell: The major histocompatibility (MHC) Class-I (MHC-I) molecules are normally expressed on the surface of virtually all cells of the body. Most pathogens do not display the MHC-I marker, and as a result, are easily identified by a killer cell.

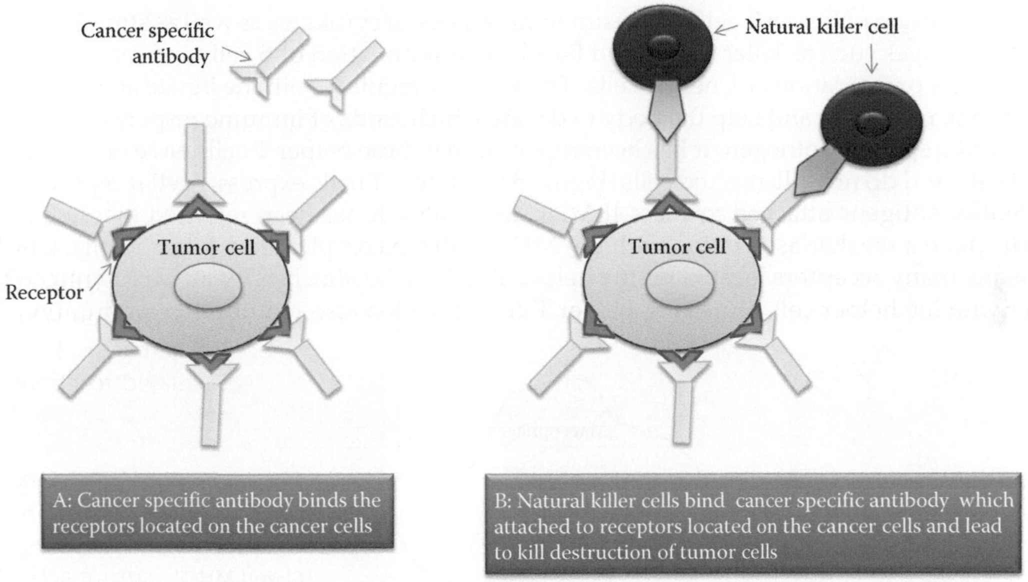

Figure 5.8 NK cell destroying cancerous cells.

5.3.3.1 *Lymphocytes*

The lymphocytes belong to the adaptive immune system. There are two different types of lymphocytes, B cells and T cells. These cells are generally derived from hematopoietic stem cells in the bone marrow. Moreover, B cells take part in the humoral immune response, while T cells are mainly involved in cell-mediated immune response. Both B and T cells contain receptor molecules that distinguish specific targets. For example, T cells recognize a pathogen only after antigens are processed and presented in combination with major histocompatibility complex (MHC) molecule. There are two major subtypes of T cells—killer T cells and helper T cells. Killer T cells can only identify antigens coupled to Class-I MHC molecules, while helper T cells only identify antigens coupled to Class-II MHC molecules. A third, minor subtype is the gamma–delta T cells that distinguish integral host antigens that are not attached to MHC receptors.

5.3.3.2 Killer T cells

Killer T cells are a subtype of T cells that can either kill cells that are infected with viruses and pathogens, or make them dysfunctional. It has been shown that killer T cells are activated when T cell receptor binds to antigens of another MHC cell. Moreover, the recognition of this MHC–antigen complex is aided by a coreceptor localized on the T cell, which is also called CD-8. It has been suggested that T cells travel throughout the body in hunt of cells where the MHC-I receptors contain this antigen. As soon as an activated T cell makes contact with such cells, it releases cytotoxins that form holes in the target cell's plasma membrane, and subsequently allow ions, water, and toxins to enter inside the cell. Furthermore, the entry of another toxin called *granulysin* (a protease) persuades the target cell to undergo apoptosis. More significantly, destroying host cells by T cells is particularly important in preventing the replication of viruses.

5.3.3.3 Helper T cells

The activation of helper T cells can result in the release of cytokines as well as stimulation of macrophages such as killer T cells and B cells. The stimulation of B cells and macrophages induces a proliferation of T helper cells. These T cells regulate both the innate and adaptive immune responses and help the body to decide which kinds of immune responses to make toward a specific pathogen. It has been reported that these helper T cells have no cytotoxic activity and do not kill infected cells (Figure 5.9). Helper T cells express T cell receptors that identify antigens attached to Class-II MHC molecules. It has been reported that helper T cells have a weaker association with the MHC–antigen complex than killer T cells, which means many receptors located on the helper T cell can be attached by an MHC antigen to activate the helper cell. Moreover, helper T cell activation also requires longer duration of

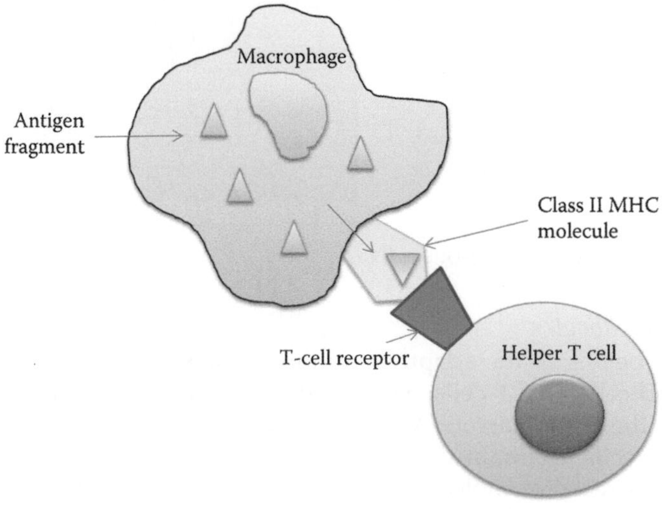

Figure 5.9 Function of T helper cells.

assurance with an antigen-presenting cell. In addition, helper T cell activation results in upregulation of molecules expressed on the T cell surface, which provide extra stimulatory signals normally required to activate antibody-producing B cells.

5.3.3.4 B lymphocytes and antibodies

The B lymphocytes and antibody cells detect pathogens when the antibodies on their surface attach to a specific foreign antigen. It has been described that this antigen–antibody complex is taken up by the B cell and processed by proteolysis into peptides. Later on, the B cells display these antigenic peptides on their surface of MHC Class-II molecules. As soon as B cells are activated, they begin to multiply, and their offspring discharges millions of copies of the antibody that recognizes this antigen. Furthermore, these antibodies can circulate in blood and stick to pathogens expressing the antigen, destroying these pathogens with phagocytes.

5.3.3.5 Immunological memory

When B cells and T cells are activated and begin to reproduce, some of their offspring can become long-lived memory cells. This process is called immunological memory. It has been suggested that in all organisms, these memory cells can remember each and every specific pathogen encountered and can enhance a strong response if the pathogen is detected or enters again. This kind of immunological response is basically adaptive in nature, because it occurs during the lifetime of an individual. It has been reported that immunological memory can be classified as passive short-term memory or active long-term memory.

5.3.3.6 Passive memory

It has been reported that newborn infants have no prior exposure to pathogens and are particularly vulnerable to infections. During this critical period of child development, the mother provides immunity against any kind of infection by producing a particular type of antibody known as immunoglobulin-G, which is transported into the baby directly across the placenta. These antibodies help the infant to fight against any infection. Furthermore, mother's breast milk contains antibodies that are transferred to the infant and protect against bacterial infections until the newborn body can produce its own antibodies. This type of development of immunity between the mother and child is called passive immunity because the fetus does not make any antibodies on its own, it only borrows them from the mother. It has been reported that passive immunity is only for a short duration of time, up to several months. Interestingly, now, it is possible to induce protective passive immunity in the infant by artificial ways.

5.3.3.7 Active memory and immunization

It has been suggested that long-term active memory is acquired following infection by activating B cells and T cells. Active immunity can be produced by vaccination. The main principle behind vaccination is called immunization where a patient is injected with an antigen developed from a nonactive or killed form of pathogens to inspire the body to develop specific immunity against that particular pathogen.

5.4 Immune diseases

The human immune system is remarkable in protecting the body from illness; however, under disease conditions, the immune system may fail to defend the body against various infections. This is called an immune-compromised immune system. This condition makes the body vulnerable to various viral, bacterial, or fungal infections. The immune-related diseases can be classified into three broad categories such as immunodeficiency, autoimmunity, and hypersensitivities.

5.4.1 Immunodeficiency

Immunodeficiency is a physiological condition where the immune system's capacity to fight infectious disease has become dysfunctional or entirely absent. In most cases, immunodeficiencies are acquired diseases, but some people are born with defects in the immune system, which is known as a primary immunodeficiency. It has been reported that a person who has an immunodeficiency of any kind is considered to be immune-compromised and such a person may be particularly vulnerable to opportunistic infections, in addition to normal infections that could affect everyone.

5.4.1.1 Primary immunodeficiency

A number of rare diseases have been reported susceptible to infections from childhood onward and many of these diseases are hereditary and autosomal recessive or X-linked in nature. There are more than 80 primary immunodeficiency syndromes reported in humans and they are generally grouped by their malfunctioning of lymphocytes or granulocyte cells. The treatment of primary immunodeficiencies depends on the nature of the defect, and may involve antibody infusions, long-term antibiotics, and stem cell transplantation.

5.4.1.2 Acquired immunodeficiency

An immune deficiency that is caused due to external processes is called secondary or acquired immunodeficiency. The common causes for secondary immunodeficiency are malnutrition, aging, and particular medications such as chemotherapy, disease-modifying antirheumatic drugs, and glucocorticoids, which are immunosuppressive drugs after organ transplants. It has been reported that there are many specific diseases that directly or indirectly impair the immune system and these include many types of cancer, predominantly those of the bone marrow and blood cells, such as lymphoma, leukemia, multiple myeloma, and certain chronic infections. Immunodeficiency is also the hallmark of AIDS, caused by HIV.

5.5 Autoimmunity

In a healthy person, immunity generally protects the person from all infectious diseases, but in some individuals, it works against itself and destroys the person's immune system. This condition is generally known as an autoimmune disease. It has been suggested that any disease fallouts from such an abnormal immune response are called an autoimmune disease. Autoimmunity is frequently caused by a deficiency of germ cell development that results in the development of a condition where body cells work against their own cells and tissues. There are several examples of autoimmunity disease such as celiac disease, Churg–Strauss syndrome, Hashimoto's thyroiditis, Graves' disease, idiopathic thrombocytopenic purpura, diabetes mellitus type 1, systemic lupus erythematosus, Sjögren's syndrome, and rheumatoid arthritis (RA).

Table 5.1 Name of Syndromes That Affect Various Body Organs

Name of syndrome	Affected organ/tissue
Diabetes mellitus type 1	Pancreas
Celiac disease, pernicious anemia	Intestine
Pemphigus vulgaris, vitiligo	Skin
Autoimmune hemolytic anemia, idiopathic thrombocytopenic purpura	Blood
Myasthenia gravis	Brain

5.5.1 Classifications of autoimmune diseases

Autoimmune diseases can be classified into systemic autoimmune disease and localized autoimmune disorders, depending on the clinical and pathological features of each disease. The examples of systemic autoimmune diseases are Sjögren's syndrome, scleroderma, RA, systemic lupus erythematosus, and dermatomyositis. It has been proposed that these disease conditions incline to be associated with autoantibodies to antigens, which are not tissue specific. The names of affected organs/tissues with autoimmune disease are listed in Table 5.1.

5.6 Diagnosis of immune diseases

After learning about the various types and causes of immune diseases, the next step would be to diagnose the various diseases to enable a physician to prescribe the appropriate treatments to the patient. The diagnosis of autoimmune disorders is largely based on a precise history and physical examination of the patient, and other pathological conditions such as an elevated C-reactive protein. It has been shown that in several systemic disorders, serological assays can be employed to detect specific autoantibodies and moreover, localized disorders are best diagnosed by immunofluorescence of biopsy tissues. The levels of autoantibodies are considered to know the level of the pathological condition of a patient.

5.6.1 Autoantibody test

Autoantibody tests are used to investigate the presence of chronic progressive arthritis-type symptoms or unexplained fevers, fatigue, muscle weakness, and rashes. The antinuclear antibody (ANA) is a marker of the autoimmune process. It is positive with a variety of different kinds of autoimmune diseases, but not very specific. Consequently, if an ANA test is positive, it is often followed up with other tests associated with arthritis and inflammation, such as a rheumatoid factor, an erythrocyte sedimentation rate, a C-reactive protein, or complements protein or complement levels. It has been shown that a single autoantibody test is not analytical, but may give signs as to whether a particular disorder is likely or unlikely to exist in patients. It has been recommended that each and every autoantibody result should be considered individually and as part of the group. However, some disorders such as systemic lupus erythematosus (SLE) may be more likely if several autoantibodies are present; others such as mixed connective tissue disease may be more likely if a single autoantibody such as a ribonucleic protein is the only one present. It has been suggested that those patients who have more than one autoimmune disorder may have several detectable autoantibodies. Whether a particular autoantibody will be present is both very individual and a matter of biostatistics. Each antibody will be present in a certain percentage of people who have a particular autoimmune disorder. For example, up to 80% of those with SLE will have a positive double-strand anti-DNA autoantibody test, but only about 25–30% will have positive ribonucleoproteins (RNPs). It has been suggested that some individuals who do have an autoimmune disorder will have negative autoantibody test results, but at a later date, as the disorder progresses, the autoantibodies can be developed.

5.7 Treatments of immune diseases

It has been suggested that most of the autoimmune diseases cannot be treated directly, but can be treated as per the symptoms associated with the disease. In general conditions, medical practitioners prescribe corticosteroid drugs, nonsteroidal anti-inflammatory drugs (NSAIDs), or more powerful immunosuppressant drugs (methotrexate, azathioprine, and cyclophosphamide) that suppress the immune response and stop the progression of the disease. Moreover, radiation of the lymph nodes and plasmapheresis, a procedure that eliminates the unhealthy cells and harmful molecules from the blood circulation, are other ways of treating an autoimmune disease.

5.7.1 Diabetes mellitus type 1

Diabetes mellitus type 1 is a disease that results from autoimmune destruction of insulin-producing β-cells of the pancreas that finally causes decreased level of blood and urine glucose. It has been reported that type 1 diabetes is lethal unless treated with insulin injection or pancreatic transplantation. It has also been reported that diet may play a role in the development of type 1 diabetes. Moreover, type 1 diabetes can be distinguished from type 2 diabetes through a C-peptide assay, which measures endogenous insulin production. It has been recommended that type 1 treatment must be continued for life in all cases; however, lifelong treatment is difficult for many people as complications may be associated with both low blood sugar and high blood sugar, as low blood sugar may lead to seizures or episodes of unconsciousness and requires emergency treatment, while high blood sugar may lead to increased exhaustion and can also result in long-term damage to body organs.

5.7.1.1 Causes

There are various causes for the development of type 1 diabetes and one of the factors is both genetic and environmental. It has been suggested that for identical twins, when one twin can have type 1 diabetes, the other twin will only have type 1 diabetes 30–50% of the time. Even with having exactly the same genome, one twin will have the disease, whereas the other twin does not; this suggests that environmental factors, in addition to genetic factors, can influence disease prevalence. It has been further shown that type 1 diabetes is a polygenic disease, meaning many different genes contribute to its expression and depending on the locus or the combination of loci on the chromosome, it can be dominant, recessive, or somewhere in between. Moreover, the strongest gene, IDDM1 is situated in the MHC Class-II region on chromosome 6, at the staining region 6p21.

5.7.1.2 Pathophysiology

Type 1 diabetes is not fully understood. In type 1 diabetes, the pancreatic β-cells produce insulin hormones in the islet of Langerhans. Type 1 diabetes (Figure 5.10) was previously

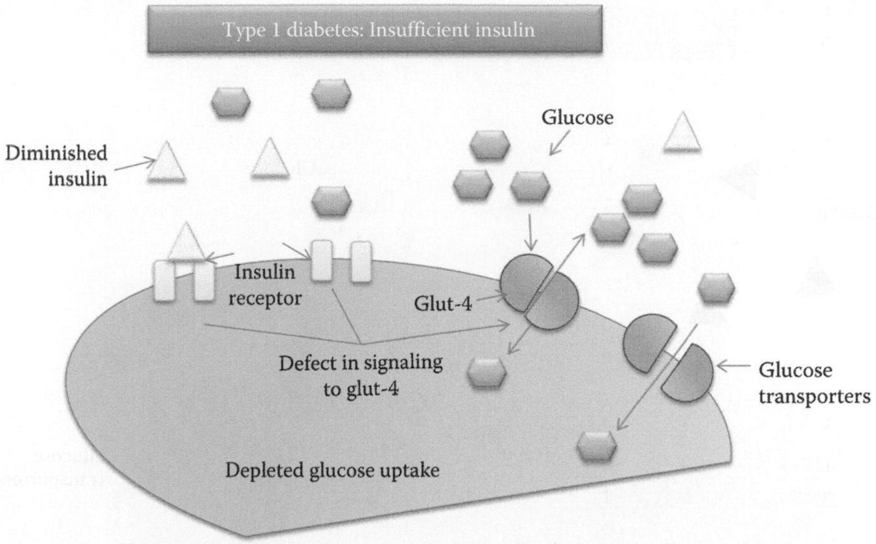

Figure 5.10 Type 1 diabetes is caused by a loss or malfunction of the insulin-producing cells, called pancreatic β-cells. Damage to β-cells results in an absence or insufficient production of insulin by the body. Most cases of type 1 diabetes have an autoimmune basis, and the immune system mistakenly attacks and destroys β-cells. Since insulin is necessary to sustain life, the missing insulin has to be replaced. The replacement insulin is administered by injection using a syringe or an insulin pump, which delivers the insulin under the skin.

known as juvenile diabetes because it is one of the most frequent chronic diseases in children; however, the majority of new-onset type 1 diabetes is observed in adults. It has been suggested that the use of antibody testing (such as glutamic acid decarboxylase antibodies, islet cell antibodies, and insulinoma-associated autoantibodies) are used to distinguish between type 1 and type 2 diabetes (Figure 5.11).

5.7.1.3 Diagnosis

One of the best approaches toward treating type 1 diabetes is first to confirm the nature of the disease by diagnostic tools. Type 1 diabetes is checked by analyzing the plasma glucose level and is diagnosed by fasting plasma glucose level at or above 126 mg/dL (considered as prediabetic conditions) and plasma glucose at or above 200 mg/dL (considered as diabetic condition). It has been suggested that the diagnosis of other types of diabetes is made in other ways that include ordinary health checkups, investigation of hyperglycemia during other medical investigations, and secondary symptoms such as vision changes or unexplainable fatigue. Diabetes is often detected when a person suffers a problem that is frequently caused by diabetes, such as a heart attack, stroke, neuropathy, poor wound healing, certain eye problems, certain fungal infections, foot ulcers, or delivering a baby with hypoglycemia.

To confirm type 1 diabetes, most physicians prefer to measure a fasting glucose level and according to the current definition, two fasting glucose measurements above 126 mg/dL are considered diagnostic for diabetes mellitus. Moreover, patients with fasting glucose levels from 100 to 125 mg/dL are considered to have impaired fasting glucose. Furthermore, patients with plasma glucose at or above 140 mg/dL but not over

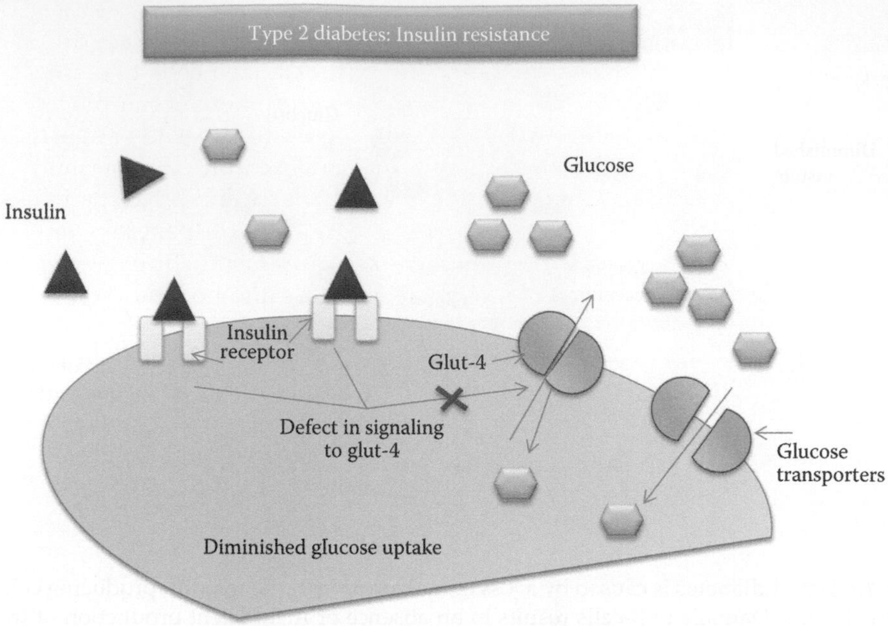

Figure 5.11 With type 2 diabetes, the pancreas still produces at least some insulin. But the cells are ignoring insulin's request for glucose transporters. For a time, the β-cells respond to this cellular insubordination by pumping out more and more insulin. But eventually, the β-cells get fed up with the overtime and quit overproducing insulin.

200 mg/dL, 2 h after a 75 g oral glucose load are considered to have impaired glucose tolerance. Interestingly, among these two prediabetic states, the latter in particular is a major risk factor for progression to full-blown diabetes mellitus as well as cardiovascular disease.

5.7.1.4 Management

One of the best practices to treat diabetic patients is control the blood insulin and glucose level all the time. There are various treatment procedures available to manage diabetes. Patients with type 1 diabetes are normally treated with insulin replacement therapy either via subcutaneous injection or insulin pump, along with dietary management such as carbohydrate tracking, and careful monitoring of blood glucose levels using glucose meters. Today, the most common insulin is the biosynthetically designed insulin that is synthesized by using recombinant DNA technology. There are major global manufacturers of insulin such as Eli Lilly and Company, Novo Nordisk, and Sanofi-Aventis, who make and sell insulin injections worldwide.

5.7.1.5 Pancreas transplantation

In some cases where drug therapy fails to improve the patient's conditions, pancreas transplants are generally performed together with, or sometime after, a kidney transplant. It has been suggested that introducing a new kidney requires taking the immunosuppressive drug treatment for a host body to accept a foreign organ. Nevertheless, pancreas transplants alone can be sensible in patients with extremely labile type 1 diabetes mellitus (Figure 5.12).

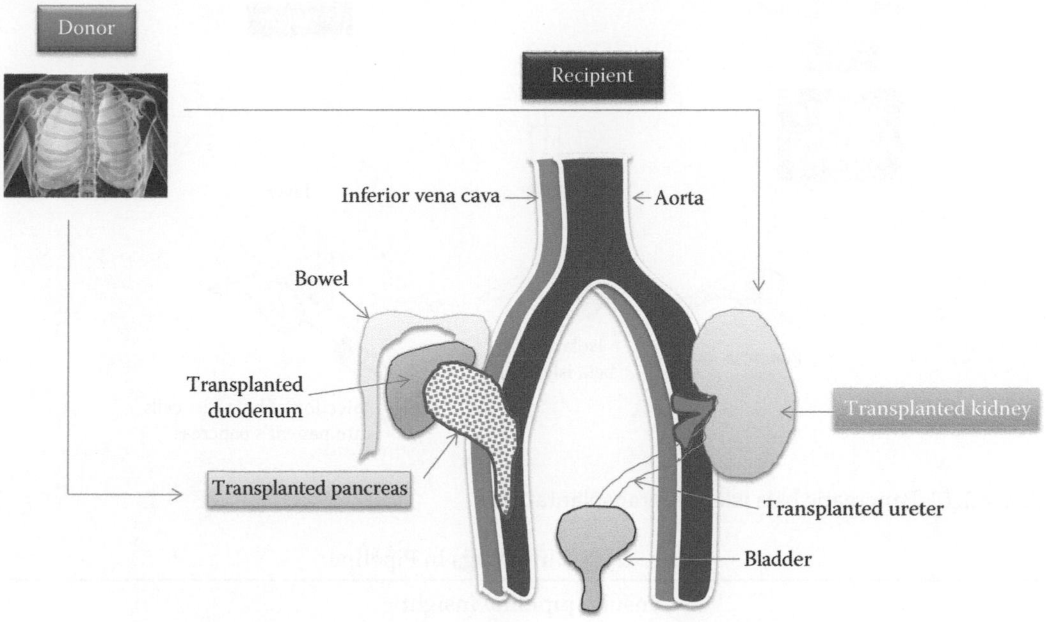

Figure 5.12 Kidney and pancreas transplantation.

5.7.1.6 Islet cell transplantation

Another approach to treat type 1 diabetes is to transplant islet cells, which are currently the most commonly used approach in humans. In one procedure, islet cells are injected into the patient's liver, where they take up host cells and begin to produce insulin. It has been suggested that the liver is expected to be the most reasonable choice because it is more accessible than the pancreas, and β islet cells appear to produce insulin well in that atmosphere. The patient's body, however, will treat the new cells as foreign cells that can be avoided by using immunosuppressor drugs. Consequently, now, patients also need to undergo treatment involving immunosuppressants, which reduce the immune system activity (Figure 5.13).

5.7.1.7 Issues with insulin injections

It has been suggested that the global diabetic population would touch near to 380 million by 2025 and nearly one-third of the total diabetes patients will be from India and China. It has been shown that 60% of the insulin available in the market today is available in the injectable form such as syringes, pens, and pumps. Interestingly, insulin is the only gold standard treatment for type 1 diabetes, and is also progressively recommended for the treatment of type 2 diabetes. However, the use of insulin has several characteristic disadvantages that include itching, allergy, local pain, and insulin lipodystrophy around the injection site.

5.7.1.8 Research trends

To minimize the side effects of current insulin injections, tremendous efforts by biotechnology or biopharmaceutical companies have been made to design a new class of insulin drugs, as depicted in Table 5.2.

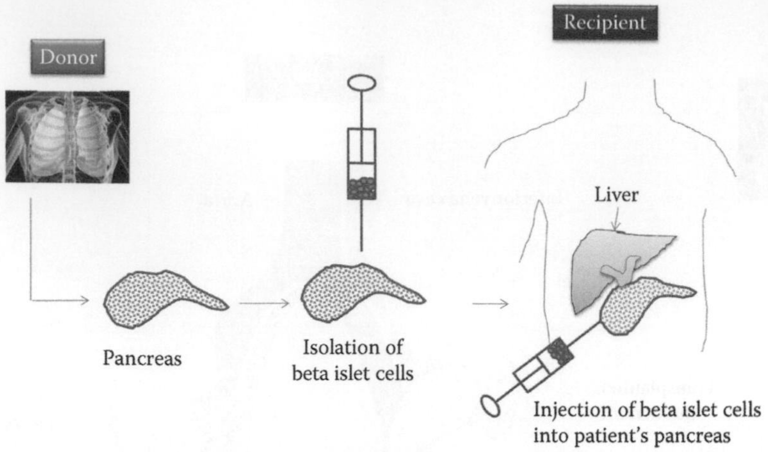

Figure 5.13 Pancreatic beta islet cell transplantation.

Table 5.2 Insulin Drugs in Pipeline

Insulin pipeline insight				
Candidate	Trial phase	Formulation	Technology	Company
Alveair	Phase I–II	Inhaler formulation	Polymer/ bioadhesive drug-delivery platform	Coremed Inc.
Oral-lyn	Phase III and commercially launched in some countries	Buccal spray	RapidMist delivery technology	Generex Biotechnology
IN-105	Phase I–II	Capsule formulation	Conjugated insulin molecule	Biocon Ltd.
Undisclosed	Preclinical phase—animal trials	Capsule formulation	Biodegradable novel polymeric nanoparticles	Transgene Biotek Ltd.
Technosphere	Phase III	Inhaler formulation and inhalant microparticle formulation	CPE-215 permeation enhancement technology	MannKind Corp.
U-Strip	Preclinical phase—animal trials	Insulin patch	U-Strip patch technology	Encapsulation Systems Inc.
Nasulin	Phase II	Intranasal insulin spray		Bentley Pharmaceuticals

5.7.2 *Myasthenia gravis*

Myasthenia gravis (MG) is an autoimmune neuromuscular disease leading to fluctuating muscle weakness. This condition is developed by blocking acetylcholine receptors at the postsynaptic neuromuscular junction that can inhibit the stimulative effect of the neurotransmitter acetylcholine. It has been reported that myasthenia can be medically treated

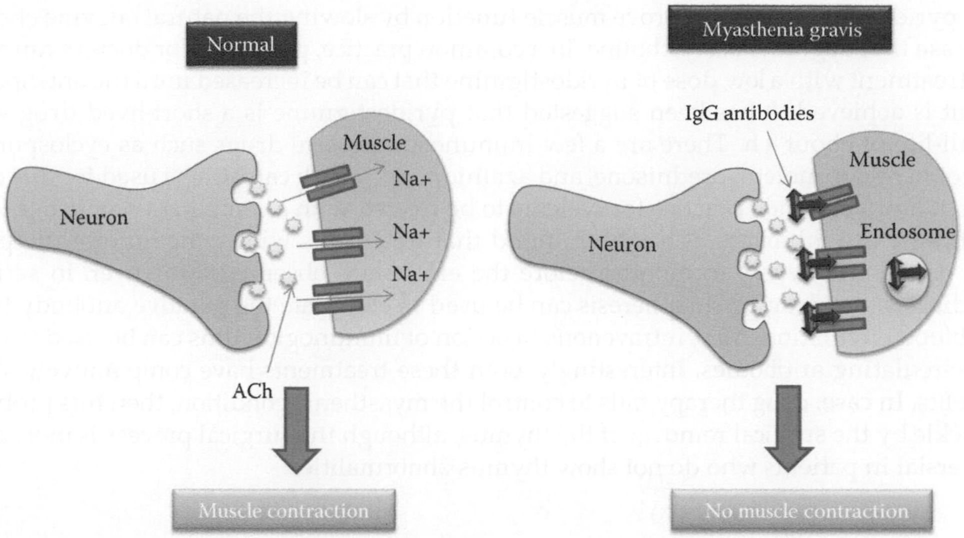

Figure 5.14 This disease is caused by the production of IgG antibodies (antiacetylcholine receptor antibodies) that attack the acetylcholine receptors of skeletal muscles. These antibodies cause a decrease in the amount of acetylcholine receptors and ultimately decrease the action potential achieved with stimulation.

with cholinesterase inhibitors or immunosuppressant drugs, and, in some selected cases, thymectomy (*surgical removal of the thymus gland*) is also considered. It has also been found that the disease can be prevalent in about 3 or 30 cases per million. Furthermore, MG needs to be distinguished from congenital myasthenia syndromes that have similar symptoms (Figure 5.14).

5.7.2.1 *Symptoms*

One of the main symptoms of MG is that muscles become gradually weaker during periods of activity and can improve after periods of rest. It has been shown that the muscles that control the eyes and face are especially vulnerable to this disease. The muscles that control the breathing function and neck and limb movements can also be affected. Interestingly, the beginning of the disorder can be unexpected and symptoms are sporadic. The diagnosis of MG may be delayed if the symptoms are variable. In most cases, the first visible symptom is weakness of the eye muscles; in others, difficulty in swallowing and inaudible speech or sound may be the first clinical signs. The amount of muscle weakness involved in MG varies among patients; extending from the eye muscles to the muscles that control breathing are affected. There are various pathological symptoms that include double vision due to weakness of the muscles, an unstable or toddling gait, and weakness on the hands. Also, in MG disease, a paralysis of the respiratory muscles can occur that requires immediate medical intervention in the form of ventilation to sustain life.

5.7.2.2 *Treatment*

Myasthenia can be treated either by medication or by surgery. It has been reported that the medication for myasthenia consists of cholinesterase inhibitors, as these drugs can improve muscle function. The use of immunosuppressant drugs can also reduce the autoimmune process. The drugs, namely, neostigmine and acetyl cholinesterase inhibitors: neostigmine and pyridostigmine, can improve muscle function by slowing the natural enzyme cholinesterase that degrades acetylcholine. In a common practice, physicians or doctors can start the treatment with a low dose of pyridostigmine that can be increased until the anticipated result is achieved. It has been suggested that pyridostigmine is a short-lived drug with a half-life of about 4 h. There are a few immunosuppressive drugs such as cyclosporine, mycophenolate mofetil, prednisone, and azathioprine, which can also be used for this condition. It is a common practice for patients to be treated with a combination of drugs with cholinesterase inhibitors. It has been found that treatments with some immunosuppressive drugs take weeks to months before the effects are observed. Moreover, in serious conditions, the drug plasmapheresis can be used to eliminate the putative antibody from the blood circulation. Also, intravenous injection of immunoglobulins can be used to bind the circulating antibodies. Interestingly, both these treatments have comparatively short benefits. In case, drug therapy fails to control the myasthenia condition, then this problem is tackle by the surgical removal of the thymus, although the surgical process is more controversial in patients who do not show thymus abnormalities.

5.8 Summary

The human immune system is a defense system against diseases and infections. The immune system basically consists of several cells that identify and kill the invading pathogens and tumor cells. The immune system detects a wide variety of agents such as bacteria, viruses, and parasitic worms. One of the major functions of the immune system is to defend the human body from any kind of harmful infections and provide immunity. There are various treatments of immunological disorders, such as antibiotics and vaccines. Monoclonal antibodies are also being used on a regular basis to treat autoimmune conditions (multiple sclerosis) where body cells actually attack and kill their own cells. In multiple sclerosis, the immune system becomes dysfunctional and starts killing the body's own healthy cells. In this chapter, we have discussed the immune system, its components, immunological disorders, and its treatment strategies.

5.9 Knowledge builder

Desquamation: Desquamation (from Latin *desquamare*, meaning "to scrape the scales off a fish"), also called skin peeling, is the shedding of the outermost membrane or layer of a tissue, such as the skin.

Lysosome: Lysosomes are cellular organelles that contain acid hydrolase enzymes that break down waste materials and cellular debris. They can be described as the stomach of the cell. They are found in animal cells, while their existence in yeasts and plants is disputed. Some biologists say the same roles are performed by lytic vacuoles, while others suggest that there is strong evidence that lysosomes are indeed found in some plant cells.

Histocompatibility complex: The MHC is a cell surface molecule encoded by a large gene family in all vertebrates. MHC molecules mediate interactions of leukocytes, also called WBCs, which are immune cells, with other leukocytes or body cells. MHC determines the compatibility of donors for organ transplant as well as one's susceptibility to an autoimmune disease via cross-reacting immunization. In humans, the MHC is also called human leukocyte antigen (HLA).

Cytotoxins: Any substance that is poisonous to living cells.

Immune-compromised: A person who has an immunodeficiency of any kind is said to be immune-compromised. An immune-compromised person may be particularly vulnerable to opportunistic infections, in addition to normal infections that could affect everyone.

Immunodeficiency syndromes: Primary immunodeficiencies are disorders in which part of the body's immune system is missing or does not function properly. To be considered a primary immunodeficiency, the cause of the immune deficiency must not be secondary in nature (i.e., caused by another disease, drug treatment, or environmental exposure to toxins). Most primary immunodeficiencies are genetic disorders; the majority is diagnosed in children under the age of 1, although milder forms may not be recognized until adulthood. About 1 in 500 people is born with a primary immunodeficiency.

Celiac disease: Celiac disease is an autoimmune disorder of the small intestine that occurs in genetically predisposed people of all ages from middle infancy onward. Symptoms include pain and discomfort in the digestive tract, chronic constipation and diarrhea, failure to thrive (in children), and fatigue. But these may be absent and symptoms in other organ systems have been described. Vitamin deficiencies are often noted in people with celiac disease owing to the reduced ability of the small intestine to properly absorb nutrients from food.

Churg–Strauss syndrome: Churg–Strauss syndrome is an autoimmune disease characterized by medium- and small-vessel vasculitis in persons with a history of asthma and allergy. Eventually leading to necrosis, it mainly involves the blood vessels of the lungs, gastrointestinal system, and peripheral nerves, but also affects the heart, skin, and kidneys. It is a rare disease that is noninheritable and nontransmissible.

Hashimoto's thyroiditis: Hashimoto's thyroiditis or chronic lymphocytic thyroiditis is an autoimmune disease in which the thyroid gland is attacked by a variety of cell- and antibody-mediated immune processes. It was the first disease to be recognized as an autoimmune disease. It was first described by the Japanese specialist Hakaru Hashimoto in Germany in 1912.

Graves' disease: Graves' disease is an autoimmune disease. It most commonly affects the thyroid, frequently causing it to enlarge to twice its size or more (goiter), and become overactive. It has related hyperthyroid symptoms such as increased heartbeat, muscle weakness, disturbed sleep, and irritability. It can also affect the eyes, causing bulging eyes (exophthalmos). It affects other systems of the body, including the skin, heart, circulation, and nervous system.

Idiopathic thrombocytopenic purpura: Idiopathic thrombocytopenic purpura, also known as primary immune thrombocytopenic purpura and autoimmune thrombocytopenic purpura, is defined as an isolated low platelet count (thrombocytopenia) with normal bone marrow and the absence of other causes of thrombocytopenia. It causes a characteristic purpuric rash and an increased tendency to bleed. Two distinct clinical syndromes manifest as an acute condition in children and a chronic condition in adults. The acute form often follows an infection and has a spontaneous resolution within 2 months. Chronic idiopathic thrombocytopenic purpura persists longer than 6 months without a specific cause.

Diabetes mellitus type 1: Diabetes mellitus type 1 (also known as type 1 diabetes), also known as insulin-dependent diabetes or juvenile diabetes, is a form of diabetes mellitus that results from autoimmune destruction of insulin-producing β-cells of the pancreas. The subsequent lack of insulin leads to increased blood and urine glucose.

Systemic lupus erythematosus: Systemic lupus erythematosus is a systemic autoimmune disease that can affect any part of the body. As it occurs in other autoimmune diseases, the immune system attacks the body's cells and tissue, resulting in inflammation and tissue damage. It is a type III hypersensitivity reaction in which antibody–immune complexes precipitate and cause a further immune response.

Sjögren's syndrome: Sjögren's syndrome is a systemic autoimmune disease in which immune cells attack and destroy the exocrine glands that produce tears and saliva. It is named after the Swedish ophthalmologist Henrik Sjögren (1899–1986), who first described it.

Rheumatoid arthritis: RA is an autoimmune disease that results in a chronic, systemic inflammatory disorder that affects many tissues and organs, but principally attacks flexible (synovial) joints. It can be a disabling and painful condition, which can lead to a substantial loss of function and mobility if not adequately treated.

C-reactive protein: C-reactive protein is a protein found in the blood, the levels of which rise in response to inflammation. Its physiological role is to bind to phosphocholine expressed on the surface of dead or dying cells (and some types of bacteria) to activate the complement system via the C1Q complex.

IDDM1: Insulin-dependent diabetes mellitus 1.

Insulin lipodystrophy: Lipodystrophy or lipoatrophy is a recognized complication of insulin injections due to loss of the adipose tissue layer at the sites of injection (prevalence of 3.6%).

Further reading

Baets MH and Oosterhuis HJGH 1993. *Myasthenia Gravis*. United Kingdom: DRD Press, pp. 158. ISBN 3805547366.

Baulcombe D 2004. RNA silencing in plants. *Nature* 431 (7006): 356–363. doi:10.1038/nature02874. PMID 15372043.

Bedlack RS and Sanders DB 2000. How to handle myasthenic crisis. Essential steps in patient care. *Postgrad Med* 107 (4): 211–214, 220–222. PMID 10778421.

Bruce A, Johnson A, Lewis J, Raff M, Roberts K, and Walters P 2002. *Molecular Biology of the Cell* (4th ed.) New York and London: Garland Science. ISBN 0-8153-3218-1. http://www.ncbi.nlm.nih.gov/books/bv.fcgi?call=bv.View..ShowTOC&rid=mboc4.TOC&depth=2.

Calhoun RF, Ritter JH, Guthrie TJ et al. 1999. Results of transcervical thymectomy for myasthenia gravis in 100 consecutive patients. *Ann Surg* 230 (4): 555–561. doi:10.1097/00000658-199910000-00011. PMID 10522725.

Carroccio A, Brusca I, Iacono G et al. 2007. IgA anti-actin antibodies ELISA in coeliac disease: A multicentre study. *Dig Liver Dis* 39: 814. doi:10.1016/j.dld.2007.06.004. PMID 17652043.

Conti-Fine BM, Milani M, and Kaminski HJ 2006. Myasthenia gravis: Past, present, and future. *J Clin Invest* 116 (11): 2843–2854. doi:10.1172/JCI29894. PMID 17080188.

de Kraker M, Kluin J, Renken N, Maat AP, and Bogers AJ 2005. CT and myasthenia gravis: Correlation between mediastinal imaging and histopathological findings. *Interact Cardiovasc Thorac Surg* 4 (3): 267–271. doi:10.1510/icvts.2004.097246. PMID 17670406.

Dittrich AM, Erbacher A, Specht S et al. 2008. Helminth infection with *Litomosoides sigmodontis* induces regulatory T cells and inhibits allergic sensitization, airway inflammation, and hyperreactivity in a murine asthma model. *J Immunol* 180 (3): 1792–1799. PMID 18209076.

Dunne DW and Cooke A 2005. A worm's eye view of the immune system: Consequences for evolution of human autoimmune disease. *Nat Rev Immunol* 5 (5): 420–426. doi:10.1038/nri1601. PMID 15864275.

Edwards JC and Cambridge G 2006. B-cell targeting in rheumatoid arthritis and other autoimmune diseases. *Nat Rev Immunol* 6 (5): 394–403. doi:10.1038/nri1838. PMID 16622478.

Edwards JC, Cambridge G, and Abrahams VM 1999. Do self perpetuating B lymphocytes drive human autoimmune disease? *Immunology* 97: 1868–1876.

Finlay B and Falkow S 1997. Common themes in microbial pathogenicity revisited. *Microbiol Mol Biol Rev* 61 (2): 136–169. PMID 9184008. PMC 232605. http://mmbr.asm.org/cgi/reprint/61/2/136.pdf.

Finlay B and McFadden G 2006. Anti-immunology: Evasion of the host immune system by bacterial and viral pathogens. *Cell* 124 (4): 767–782. doi:10.1016/j.cell.2006.01.034. PMID 16497587.

Itoh S, Ichida T, Yoshida T et al. 1998. Autoantibodies against a 210 kDa glycoprotein of the nuclear pore complex as a prognostic marker in patients with primary biliary cirrhosis. *J Gastroenterol Hepatol* 13 (3): 257–265. PMID 9570238.

Jaretzki A, Barohn RJ, Ernstoff RM et al. 2000. Myasthenia gravis: Recommendations for clinical research standards. Task Force of the Medical Scientific Advisory Board of the Myasthenia Gravis Foundation of America. *Neurology* 55 (1): 16–23. PMID 10891897. http://www.neurology.org/cgi/content/full/55/1/16.

Jerne N 1974. Towards a network theory of the immune system. *Ann Immunol (Paris)* 125C (1–2): 373–389. PMID 4142565.

Juel VC 2004. Myasthenia gravis: Management of myasthenic crisis and perioperative care. *Semin Neurol* 24 (1): 75–81. doi:10.1055/s-2004-829595. PMID 15229794.

Kerkar N, Ma Y, Davies ET, Cheeseman P, Mieli-Vergani G, and Vergani D 2002. Detection of liver kidney microsomal type 1 antibody using molecularly based immunoassays. *J Clin Pathol* 55 (12): 906–909. PMID 12461054. http://jcp.bmj.com/cgi/pmidlookup?view=long&pmid=12461054.

Kobayashi H 2005. Airway biofilms: Implications for pathogenesis and therapy of respiratory tract infections. *Treat Respir Med* 4 (4): 241–253. doi:10.2165/00151829-200504040-00003. PMID 16086598.

Kubach J, Becker C, Schmitt E, Steinbrink K, Huter E, Tuettenberg A, and Jonuleit H 2005. Dendritic cells: Sentinels of immunity and tolerance. *Int J Hematol* 81 (3): 197–203. doi:10.1532/IJH97.04165. PMID 15814330.

Leite MI, Jacob S, Viegas S et al. 2008. IgG1 antibodies to acetylcholine receptors in "seronegative" myasthenia gravis. *Brain* 131 (Part 7): 1940–1952. doi:10.1093/brain/awn092. PMID 18515870. PMC 2442426. http://brain.oxfordjournals.org/cgi/pmidlookup?view=long&pmid=18515870.

Losen M, Martínez-Martínez P, Phernambucq M, Schuurman J, Parren PW, and De Baets MH 2008. Treatment of myasthenia gravis by preventing acetylcholine receptor modulation. *Ann N Y Acad Sci* 1132: 174–179. doi:10.1196/annals.1405.034. PMID 18567867.

Losen M, Stassen MH, Martínez-Martínez P et al. 2005. Increased expression of rapsyn in muscles prevents acetylcholine receptor loss in experimental autoimmune myasthenia gravis. *Brain* 128 (Part 10): 2327–2337. doi:10.1093/brain/awh612. PMID 16150851.

McGrogan A, Sneddon S, and de Vries CS 2010. The incidence of myasthenia gravis: A systematic literature review. *Neuroepidemiology* 34 (3): 171–183. doi:10.1159/000279334.

Oertelt S, Rieger R, Selmi C, Invernizzi P, Ansari A, Coppel R, Podda M, Leung P, and Gershwin M 2007. A sensitive bead assay for antimitochondrial antibodies: Chipping away at AMA-negative primary biliary cirrhosis. *Hepatology* 45 (3): 659–665. doi:10.1002/hep.21583. PMID 17326160.

Pedreira S, Sugai E, Moreno ML et al. 2005. Significance of smooth muscle/anti-actin autoantibodies in celiac disease. *Acta Gastroenterol Latinoam* 35 (2): 83–93. PMID 16127984.

Quinnell RJ, Bethony J, and Pritchard DI 2004. The immunoepidemiology of human hookworm infection. *Parasite Immunol* 26 (11–12): 443–454. doi:10.1111/j.0141-9838.2004.00727.x. PMID 15771680.

Rojo E, Martín R, Carter C, Zouhar J et al. 2004. VPEgamma exhibits a caspase-like activity that contributes to defense against pathogens. *Curr Biol* 14 (21): 1897–1906. doi:10.1016/j.cub.2004.09.056. PMID 15530390.

Rosen FS, Cooper MD, and Wedgwood RJ 1995. The primary immunodeficiencies. *N Engl J Med* 333 (7): 431–440. doi:10.1056/NEJM199508173330707. PMID 7616993.

Sato KJ 2000. The HLA system. Second of two parts. *N Engl J Med* 343 (11): 782–786. doi:10.1056/NEJM200009143431106. PMID 10984567.

Saunders K, Raine T, Cooke A, and Lawrence C 2007. Inhibition of autoimmune type 1 diabetes by gastrointestinal helminth infection. *Infect Immun* 75 (1): 397–407. doi:10.1128/IAI.00664-06. PMID 17043101.

Scherer K, Bedlack RS, and Simel DL 2005. Does this patient have myasthenia gravis? *JAMA* 293 (15): 1906–1914. doi:10.1001/jama.293.15.1906. PMID 15840866.

Seybold ME 1986. The office tensilon test for ocular myasthenia gravis. *Arch Neurol* 43 (8): 842–843. PMID 3729766.

Szostecki C, Guldner HH, Netter HJ, and Will H 1990. Isolation and characterization of cDNA encoding a human nuclear antigen predominantly recognized by autoantibodies from patients with primary biliary cirrhosis. *J Immunol* 145 (12): 4338–4347. PMID 2258622.

Téllez-Zenteno JF, Hernández-Ronquillo L, Salinas V, Estanol B, and da Silva O 2004. Myasthenia gravis and pregnancy: Clinical implications and neonatal outcome. *BMC Musculoskelet Disord* 5: 42. doi:10.1186/1471-2474-5-42. PMID 15546494. PMC 534111. http://www.biomedcentral.com/1471-2474/5/42. (Retrieved 2008-07-10).

Thieben MJ, Blacker DJ, Liu PY, Harper CM Jr, and Wijdicks EF 2005. Pulmonary function tests and blood gases in worsening myasthenia gravis. *Muscle Nerve* 32 (5): 664–667. doi:10.1002/mus.20403. PMID 16025526.

Uz E, Loubiere LS, Gadi VK et al. 2008. Skewed X-chromosome inactivation in scleroderma. *Clin Rev Allergy Immunol* 34 (3): 352–355. doi:10.1007/s12016-007-8044-z. PMID 18157513.

Wållberg M and Harris R 2005. Co-infection with *Trypanosoma brucei* prevents experimental autoimmune encephalomyelitis in DBA/1 mice through induction of suppressor APCs. *Int Immunol* 17 (6): 721–728. doi:10.1093/intimm/dxh253. PMID 15899926. http://intimm.oxfordjournals.org/cgi/content/full/17/6/721.

Wesierska-Gadek J, Hohenuer H, Hitchman E, and Penner E 1996. Autoantibodies against nucleoporin p62 constitute a novel marker of primary biliary cirrhosis. *Gastroenterology* 110 (3): 840–847. doi:10.1053/gast.1996.v110.pm8608894. PMID 8608894.

Wohlleben G, Trujillo C, Müller J et al. 2004. Helminth infection modulates the development of allergen-induced airway inflammation. *Int Immunol* 16 (4): 585–596. doi:10.1093/intimm/dxh062. PMID 15039389.

Zaccone P, Fehervari Z, Phillips JM, Dunne DW, and Cooke A 2006. Parasitic worms and inflammatory diseases. *Parasite Immunol* 28 (10): 515–523. doi:10.1111/j.1365-3024.2006.00879.x. PMID 16965287.

chapter six

Recombinant DNA technology and therapeutic proteins

6.1 Introduction

In the previous chapters, we learned the basic constitution of DNA and its significance, and now with the advancement of molecular tools and techniques, it is also possible to manipulate DNA in order to make desirable therapeutic products. One of the interesting aspects of DNA is that the DNA of one organism (bacteria) can be mixed with the DNA of another organism (animal) to make a unique combination; such combinations are called recombinant DNA (r-DNA) and the technology used to create such combinations is called recombinant DNA technology. r-DNA is also sometimes referred to as "chimera." By combining two or more different strands of DNA, scientists are able to create a new strand of DNA. The most commonly employed recombinant processes generally involve combining the DNA of two different organisms such as human and microorganism. r-DNA technology basically differs from traditional genetic recombination where genetic recombination occurs through natural processes within the cell. r-DNA technology was made possible by the discovery, isolation, and application of restriction endonucleases in the late 1970s. These specific enzyme restriction endonucleases have really revolutionized the r-DNA technology. Scientists Werner Arber, Daniel Nathans, and Hamilton Smith, who discovered enzyme restriction endonucleases, received the 1978 Nobel Prize in Medicine.

6.2 Recombinant DNA technology

The process of r-DNA technology begins with the isolation of a gene of interest, which is then inserted into a vector; these vectors are further cloned into multiple copies. A vector is basically a piece of DNA that is capable of independent growth; bacterial plasmids and viral phages are the commonly used vectors. When the gene of interest (foreign DNA) is integrated into the plasmid or phage, this process is generally referred to as r-DNA (Figure 6.1). The next step in r-DNA technology is to introduce the vector containing the foreign DNA into host cells so that the cells can express the desirable proteins. In order to get sufficient amounts of protein, the vectors must be cloned to produce large quantities of the DNA. Once the vector is isolated in large quantities, it can be introduced into the desired host cells, which include mammalian, yeast, or special bacterial cells. Finally, the host cells can synthesize the foreign protein from the r-DNA. When the cells are grown in vast quantities in the bioreactor or fermenter, the recombinant protein can be isolated in large amounts and the entire process is commonly referred as r-DNA technology. There are three different methods available through which r-DNA products are being developed: (1) transformation, (2) phage introduction, and (3) nonbacterial transformation (Figure 6.2).

6.2.1 Steps of constructing a recombinant DNA

The making of r-DNA has been briefly described below in a stepwise manner.

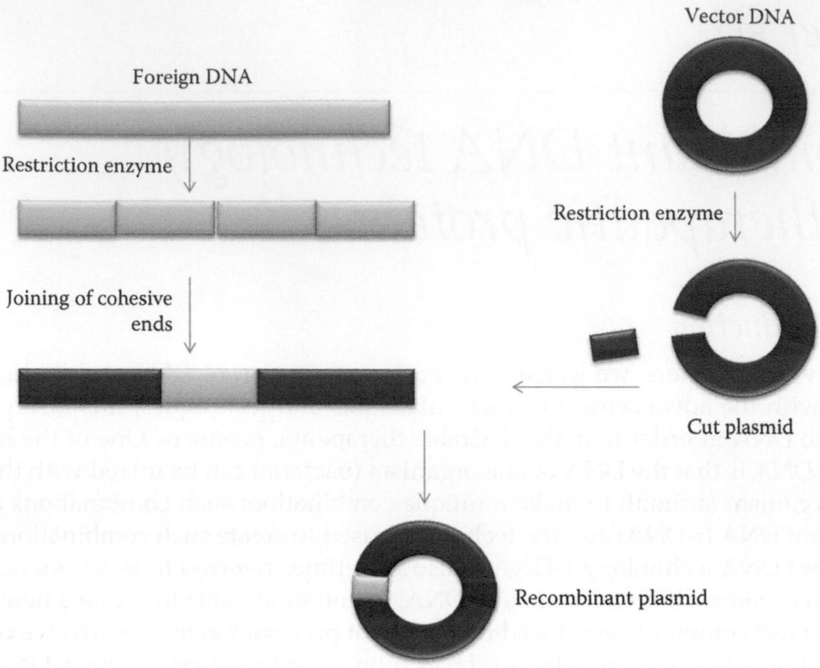

Figure 6.1 Making of recombinant DNA.

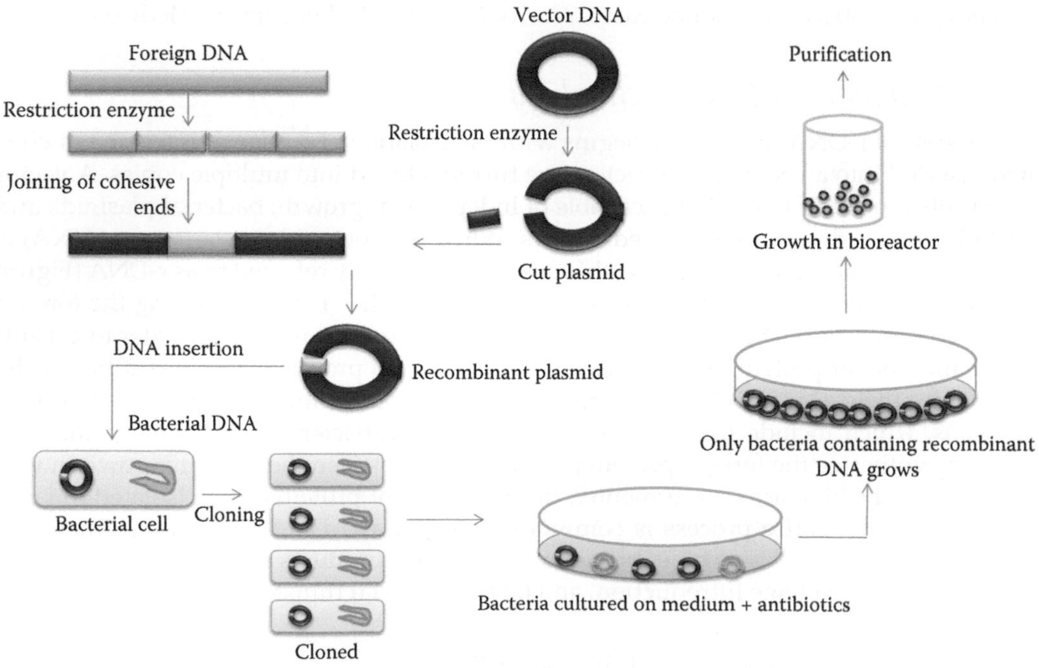

Figure 6.2 Making of recombinant DNA product.

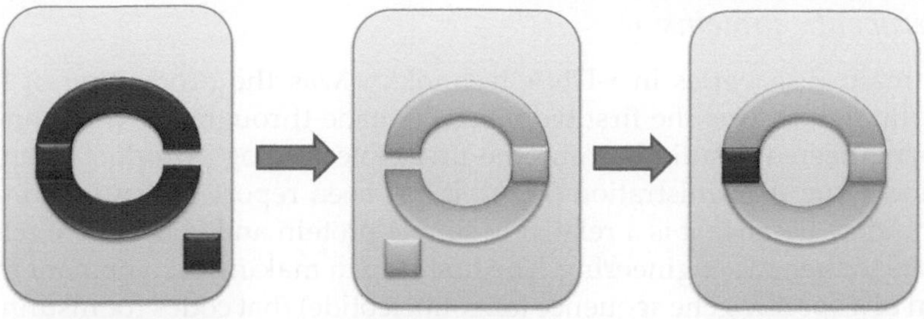

Figure 6.3 Basic concept of genetic transformation.

6.2.1.1 *Transformation*

The first step in constructing an r-DNA is to transform a select piece of DNA into a vector. The next step is to cut that piece of DNA with a restriction enzyme known as endonucleases and then ligate the DNA insert into the vector using DNA ligase. After that, the DNA insert can be visualized by a selectable marker, which permits the identification of r-DNA molecules. It has been reported that an antibiotic marker is often used to tag host cells without affecting the vector. The process of inserting a vector into a host cell is called transformation. During the making of an r-DNA product, *Escherichia coli* is found be the most widely used host organism and it has been reported that *E. coli* can easily take foreign DNA. It has been suggested that different vectors have different characteristics to make them suitable to different applications (Figure 6.3).

6.2.1.2 *Nonbacterial transformation*

This is a process very similar to transformation. The only difference between the two is that in nonbacterial transformation, there is no need for bacteria such as *E. coli* for the host cells. There are various ways through which DNA nonbacterial transformation can be achieved, which include DNA microinjection. In this process, the DNA is inserted straight into the nucleus of the cell, which is being transformed. In another method called biolistic transformation, the host cells are bombarded with a high velocity of gold or tungsten particles that are coated with DNA.

6.2.1.3 *Phage introduction*

Phage introduction is the process of DNA transfection, which is equivalent to the transformation method. The only difference is that instead of bacteria, phage is used. It has been reported that during phage introduction, various types of phages such as lambda or MI3 phages have been used to produce phage plaques that contain recombinants. The recombinants that are produced by phage introduction can be easily identified by differences in the recombinant and nonrecombinant DNA using various selection approaches.

6.3 *Applications of r-DNA technology*

r-DNA technology is not only an important tool in scientific research but also a useful tool in the diagnosis and treatment of various diseases and genetic disorders. We have discussed its various applications especially in the medical field.

6.3.1 Therapeutic proteins

One of the main discoveries in r-DNA technology was the production of biosynthetic human insulin, which was the first biomolecule made through r-DNA technology. Later on, this bioengineered insulin became the first biotechnology product approved by the U.S. Food and Drug Administration (FDA). It has been reported that insulin is basically an ideal candidate because it is a relatively simple protein and is therefore relatively easy to manipulate for genetic engineering. The first step in making recombinant insulin is the introduction of a specific gene sequence (oligonucleotide) that codes for insulin production in humans into the bacteria *E. coli*; it has been reported that only 0.94% of bacteria can pick up the sequence. Nevertheless, because the life cycle of *E. coli* is only about 30 min, there is no problem in generating a million copies of *E. coli* in a short period of time to be used for inducing insulin production.

Among all applications of r-DNA technology, therapeutic proteins have been extensively used. Therapeutic proteins are those proteins that are either removed from human cells or engineered in the laboratory for pharmaceutical use. In addition to human insulin, other human proteins such as follicle-stimulating hormone, plasminogen, erythropoietin, and growth hormones have been created by using r-DNA technology (Figure 6.4).

There are many proteins essential to for the normal function of the human body and unfortunately some people fail to produce sufficient amounts of these proteins in their body, which may lead to the development of functional deformities and genetic defects. These essential proteins include various blood-clotting factors causing hemophilia, insulin, growth hormone, and other proteins. Patients who do not produce sufficient amounts

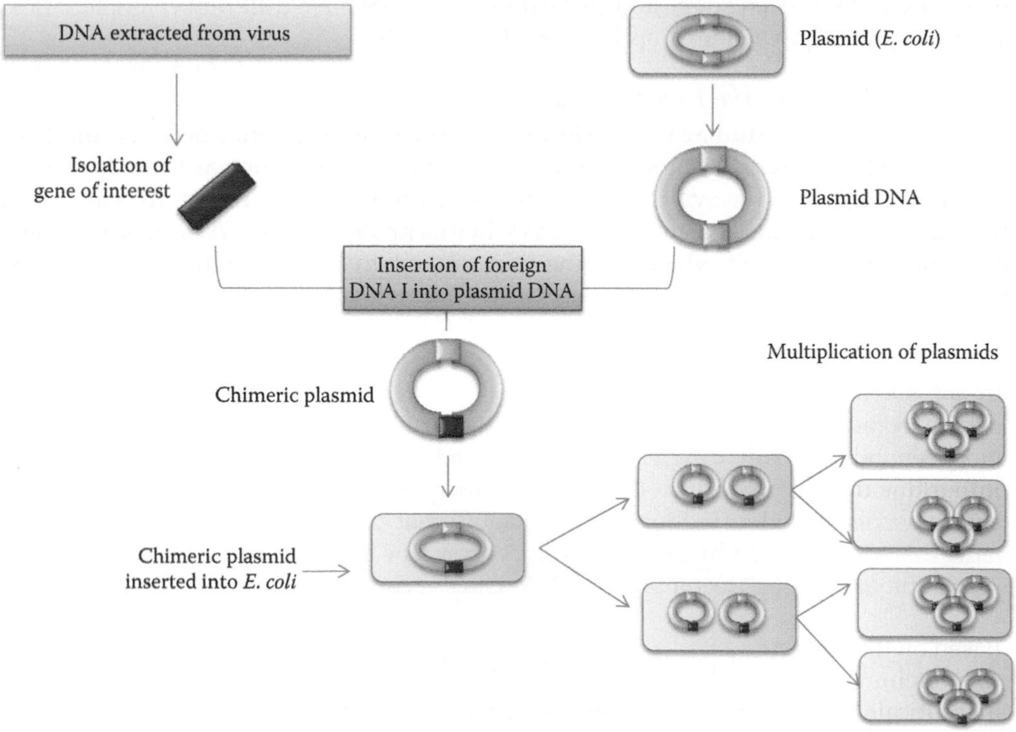

Figure 6.4 Making of chimeric proteins.

of these proteins need to take these proteins externally either in the form of a medicine or an injection. These proteins can be synthesized outside of the human body by using recombinant technology. It has been reported that the majority of therapeutic proteins are recombinant human proteins manufactured using nonhuman mammalian cell lines that are engineered to express certain human genetic sequences to produce precise proteins of human use. Over the past decade, recombinant proteins are extensively used to replace deficiencies and to strengthen the immune system to fight cancer and infectious disease.

6.3.1.1 *Recombinant human insulin*

Recombinant insulin is known to completely replace insulin in the insulin-dependent diabetic patients. This recombinant insulin is prepared from both animal and human sources. There are different kinds of recombinant insulin preparations available in the market for clinical use.

6.3.1.2 *Recombinant human growth hormone*

Human growth hormone (HGH) is administered to patients whose pituitary glands generate insufficient quantities of natural growth hormones to support normal growth and development. Before recombinant HGH became available to the patients, HGH was reported to be obtained from pituitary glands of cadavers. This unsafe practice of isolating growth hormones from cadavers led to some patients developing Creutzfeldt–Jakob disease. The development of recombinant HGH eliminated this problem, and it is now used extensively around the world. There are reports that suggest that recombinant human growth hormones have been misused as a performance-enhancing drug by athletes and sports personalities.

6.3.1.3 *Recombinant blood clotting factor VIII*

The recombinant factor VIII is a blood-clotting protein that is administered to patients with forms of the bleeding disorder hemophilia, as these patients are generally unable to produce factor VIII in sufficient quantities to support normal blood coagulation. It has been reported that before the synthesis of the recombinant blood clotting factor, the protein was obtained by processing large quantities of human blood from multiple donors. The process of recombinant factor VIII is reported to carry a high risk of the transmission of blood-borne infectious diseases such as HIV and hepatitis B.

6.3.1.4 *Recombinant hepatitis B vaccine*

There are reports that suggest that hepatitis B infection can be prevented or controlled by the use of recombinant hepatitis B vaccine. The hepatitis B vaccine basically contains a form of the hepatitis B virus surface antigen that is normally produced in yeast cells. It has been recommended that the development of the recombinant subunit vaccine is an important and necessary development because the hepatitis B virus, unlike other viruses such as poliovirus, cannot be grown in *in vitro* conditions.

6.3.2 *Current market for therapeutic proteins*

Based on the current status, it has been reported that there are about 75 approved therapeutic proteins listed by the FDA and these therapeutic proteins are also known as biopharmaceuticals, with more than 500 additional proteins under various development stages in various pharmaceutical companies. There are reports that indicate that global sales of therapeutic proteins were approximately $53 billion in 2005, and reached to $150 billion in

2012. Among all therapeutic proteins, the most widely sold proteins are erythropoietin and insulin. It has been postulated that many of the therapeutic proteins currently used in the market will lose their patent protections over the next few years. Over the past few years, we have seen surges of pharmaceutical companies that make the therapeutic proteins and many marketed proteins are facing increased competition from other therapeutic proteins approved for the same disease indications. One of the limitations of the therapeutic proteins is that these proteins are usually broken down in the gastrointestinal system and do not reach target sites; therefore, all the therapeutic proteins must be administered through injection. Upon injecting into the human body, these therapeutic proteins are broken down by enzymes and can be transported to the target sits.

6.4 Major r-DNA products

After learning the various beneficial attributes of recombinant proteins, let us also learn the benefits of some major recombinant proteins in greater detail.

6.4.1 Recombinant insulin

Among all recombinant proteins, recombinant insulin is the first and most widely used medicine for the treatment of the diabetic condition. Before learning about recombinant insulin, we can first learn about the general anatomy and function of human insulin. Human insulin is a hormone that is known to regulate the function of fat and steroid metabolism. It has been reported that insulin is responsible for liver, muscle, and fat tissue to take up glucose from the blood, and also for storing it as glycogen in the liver and muscle cells. Under pathological conditions, when the human body stops making the required amount of insulin, blood glucose is not taken up by body cells and finally leads to the development of diabetes. Insulin deficiency is known to several other anabolic effects throughout the body (Figure 6.5). In patients, when insulin levels fail regularly, this may cause the development of diabetes mellitus. Patients with diabetic condition can be treated by giving them the required amount outside or external insulin. This external insulin can be prepared by using r-DNA technology. Patients with Type 1 diabetes mellitus depend on externally created insulin for their survival because the recombinant insulin is no longer produced internally. However, patients with Type 2 diabetes mellitus are known to develop insulin resistance, and because of such resistance, they may suffer from a relative insulin shortage. In addition, some patients with Type 2 diabetes may ultimately require insulin treatment if other medications fail to control blood glucose levels sufficiently, though this is somewhat unusual. Insulin also affects other body functions, which include vascular network and cognition. As soon as insulin enters the human brain, it enhances learning and memory and, in particular, benefits verbal memory.

There are several conditions in which insulin disturbance causes diseases in human, including diabetes mellitus, autoimmune disease, Type 2 diabetes, and multifactorial syndrome. There are combined influences of genetic susceptibility and the influence of environmental factors on the human body, which may also cause insulin resistance in cells requiring insulin for glucose absorption. This form of diabetes is reported to be an inherited disease known as insulinoma, a metabolic syndrome. The basic underlying cause may be the insulin resistance of Type 2 diabetes, which is a diminished insulin response in some tissue to respond to insulin treatment. There are some common types of morbidity that are associated with hypertension, obesity, Type 2 diabetes, and cardiovascular disease.

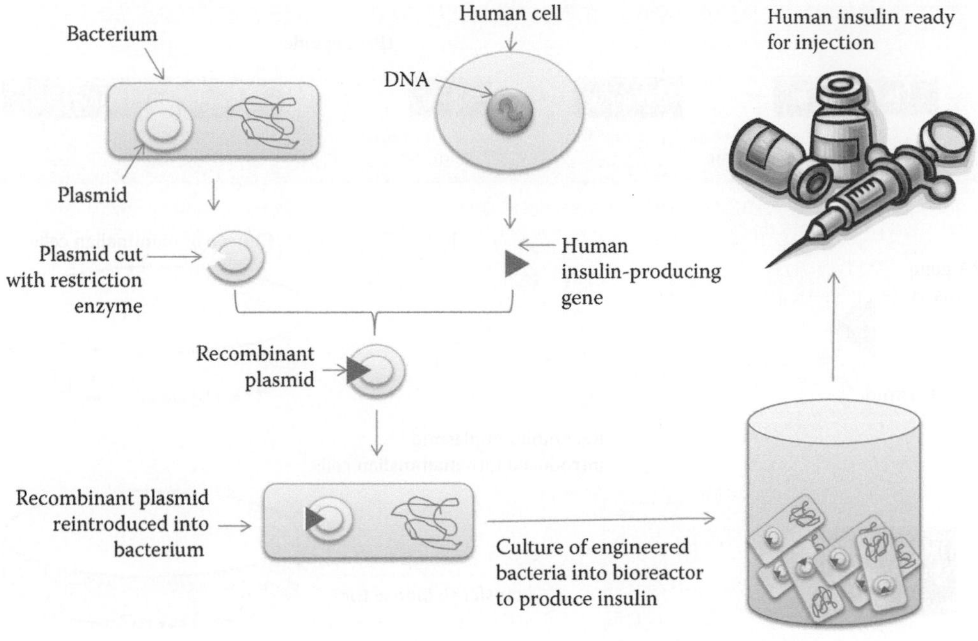

Figure 6.5 Making of human insulin by recombinant DNA technology.

6.4.2 *Recombinant tissue plasminogen activator*

Tissue plasminogen activator (tPA) is another kind of serine protease protein that is involved in the breakdown of blood clots in humans (Figure 6.6). In the human body, tissue plasminogen is found on endothelial cells, the cells that line the blood vessels. As an enzyme, tPA catalyzes the conversion of plasminogen to plasmin, the major enzyme responsible for clot breakdown. It has been reported that tPA is used as clinical medicine to treat only embolic or thrombotic stroke. Patients who have a problem related to blood clotting need a medicine to clot the blood immediately to avoid further releases of the blood from the body and tPA is considered to be an important medicine to promote blood clot. The tPA can be manufactured by using r-DNA technology and the production of tPA created this way is referred to as recombinant tissue plasminogen activator (rtPA). The basic principle behind blood clotting is that tPA catalyzes the conversion of plasminogen into plasmin, which is done by cleaving the single-chain plasminogen into two chains. These two chains are connected by a disulfide bond and the resulting molecule is called plasmin. In the patients, an increased enzymatic activity can cause hyper fibrinolysis, which demonstrates as an excessive bleeding.

tPA is used in various diseases such as pulmonary embolism, myocardial infarction, stroke, and thrombolysis. The first step in any kind of blood-clot-related disease is to stop the outflow of the blood, so the first thing any physician will do is to immediately inject tPA within the first 3 h of the event or within 6 h to be able to clot the blood. As per the guidelines used in Canada, hospitals for ischemic strokes suggest that tPA must be given within 4.5 h of the onset of symptoms, and because of this, only about 3% of patients were able to qualify for this treatment, as most patients do not seek medical assistance quickly enough. With regard to the situation in the United States, the window of the administration of tPA is 3 h from the onset of symptoms.

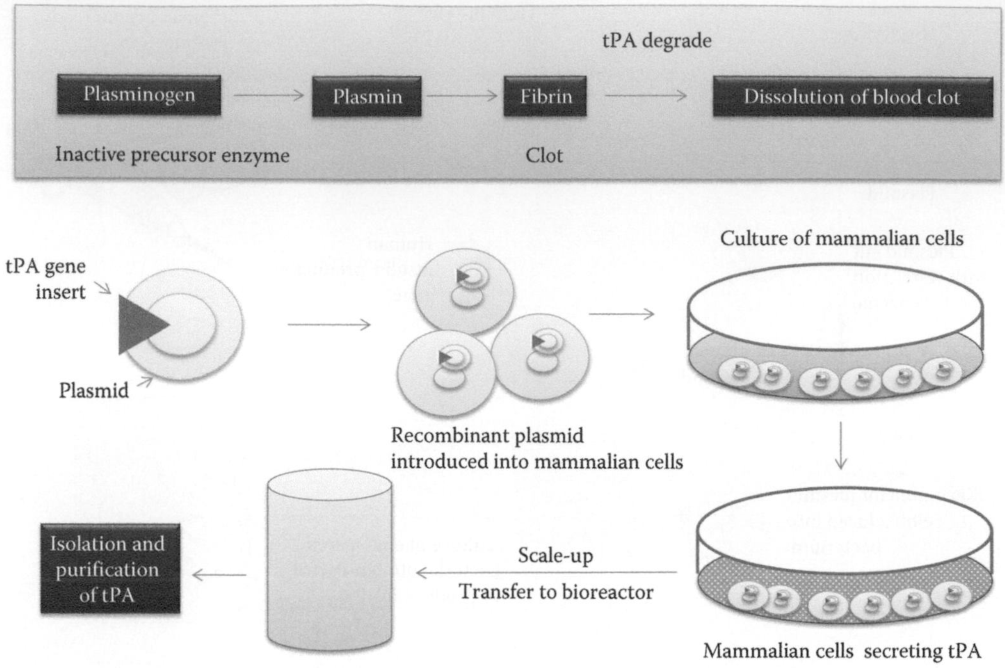

Figure 6.6 Making of recombinant tissue plasminogen activator.

There are various commercially available rtPAs in the market, which include Alteplase, Reteplase, and Tenecteplase. It has been reported that Alteplase is an FDA-approved drug for the treatment of myocardial infarction, acute ischemic stroke, and acute massive pulmonary embolism. Reteplase is also an FDA-approved drug for the treatment of acute myocardial infarction and it has more convenient administration and faster thrombolysis than Alteplase. Consequently, Tenecteplase is also specified in acute myocardial infarction, and it showed fewer bleeding complications. There are other types of tPAs are under trial phases, including Desmoteplase. One of the major concerns with regard to tPA treatment is that tPA quickly dissolves blood clots, which might lead to a risk of hemorrhage in some patients. Considering the fact that the use of tPA may cause hemorrhage, there are alternative medicines available in the market that do not cause any hemorrhage. One example is streptokinase, which is a cheaper alternative that can be used as a thrombolytic in acute treatment.

6.4.3 *Recombinant erythropoietin*

Like insulin, erythropoietin (EPO) is a glycoprotein hormone that controls red blood cell production in the body (Figure 6.7). EPO, also called hemopoietin, is known to be located as precursors in the bone marrow. It is produced by the peritubular capillary endothelial cells in the kidney and liver. Besides its role in red blood cell production, EPO also plays an important role in neuronal injury and in the wound healing process. It has been reported that EPO has its primary effect on red blood cells by protecting the blood cells from going to the apoptosis pathway. It also conjoins with various factors involved in the growth of precursor red cells. EPO has a range of actions in hypertension, stimulating angiogenesis,

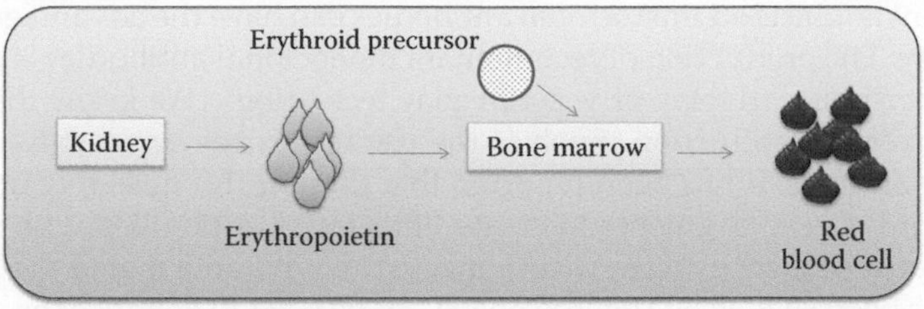

Figure 6.7 Normal synthesis of red blood cells.

Table 6.1 List of Erythropoietin Produced by r-DNA Technology

Trade name of erythropoietin	Name of manufacturer
Epogen	Amgen
Espogen	LG Life Sciences
Epotin	Gulf Pharmaceutical Industry (Julphar)
Betapoietin	CinnaGen and Zahravi
Erykine	Intas Biopharmaceutical Pvt. Ltd.
Shanpoietin	Shantha Biotechnics Ltd.
Zyrop	Cadila Healthcare Ltd.

and inducing proliferation of smooth muscle fibers. It has also been shown that EPO can upsurge iron absorption by quashing the hormone hepcidin.

6.4.3.1 *Applications of erythropoietin*

There are various applications of EPO. EPO can be used as a therapeutic agent to treat various disease conditions. It can be used in the treatment of anemia resulting from chronic kidney disease and myelodysplasia, and in the treatment of cancer. There are various types of EPO produced for patients who are suffering from anemia. These are epoetin, darbepoetin, epoetin delta, PD poetin, and methoxy polyethylene glycol-epoetin beta. The list of erythropoietin produced by using r-DNA technology is given in Table 6.1.

6.4.4 *Recombinant monoclonal antibodies*

Monoclonal antibodies have been used to treat various types of cancers. One of the problems with monoclonal antibodies is that they are produced from animal sources that might produce adverse drug reactions. Over the last few years, efforts have been made to find out an alternative approach to circumvent this problem by creating either chimeric or humanized monoclonal antibodies. These monoclonal antibodies are now produced by using r-DNA technology. It has been reported that both types of recombinant-engineered monoclonal antibodies contain human sequences. In chimeric antibodies, the human body that contains variable heavy- and light-chain domains are replaced with animal antibody, which holds the anticipated antigen specificity. It has been reported that humanized antibodies contain a minimum of rodent sequences. The most suitable cells for expression of the r-DNA monoclonal antibody genes are mammalian cell lines. These cell lines are immunoglobulin, nonproducing myeloma cells that are capable of elevated expressions of exogenous heavy- and light-chain genes and glycosylation. There are reports that suggest that recombinant engineered monoclonal antibodies can have the advantages of decreased immunogenicity. The production of recombinant monoclonal antibodies is also called repertoire cloning or phage display or yeast display technology. We know that recombinant antibody engineering production involves the use of viruses or yeast to create antibodies, rather than animals. It has been reported that these techniques rely on rapid cloning of immunoglobulin gene segments to create libraries of antibodies with somewhat dissimilar amino acid sequences from which antibodies with anticipated specificities can be produced. It has been suggested that the phage can be used to enhance the specificity with which monoclonal antibodies distinguish antigens in the human body, their stability in various environmental conditions, their therapeutic efficacy, and as well as their detectability in diagnostic applications. The large-scale production of recombinant monoclonal antibodies can be achieved by fermentation technology.

6.4.5 *Recombinant interferon*

The human body is intrinsically equipped with defense mechanisms to protect it from any kind of infection. Among these defense mechanisms, interferons (IFNs) are found to be a major player in protecting the body from any kind of infection. IFNs are basically proteins made by human host cells in the response invasion of pathogens such as viruses, bacteria, parasites, or tumor cells. In general conditions, these IFNs help the body cells to prepare to fight back against any infection and malfunction caused by pathogens or tumors. It has been reported that IFNs belong to the major class of glycoproteins known as cytokines. Interestingly, IFNs are named after their capability to interfere with viral replication within human host cells. Besides, IFNs have other functions in the human body such as they act as natural killer (NK) cells and macrophages. They are also known to increase the recognition of infection by upregulating antigen presentation to T lymphocytes. In addition, IFNs increase the ability of healthy host cells to resist new infections. During the action of IFNs, patients report certain changes in their body, which include aching muscles and fever. There are various kinds of IFNs classified in humans and they are typically divided among three major classes, which are Type I IFN, Type II IFN, and Type III IFN.

IFNs have been clinically used in several diseases and among the different types of IFNs that have been tested in humans, Imiquimod has been known to be widely used in the marketplace. Another IFN that has imidazoquinoline as the main ingredient is sold in the market as Aldara (Imiquimod) cream. This drug is approved in the United States by the FDA for treating actinic keratosis disease, superficial basal-cell carcinoma, papilloma, and external genital warts. Over the last few years, efforts have been made to develop synthetically designed IFNs and many different types have been introduced in the market. These IFNs are administered as antiviral, antiseptic, and anticarcinogenic drugs, and to treat some autoimmune diseases. Additionally, IFN beta-1a and IFN beta-1b can be clinically used to treat and control multiple sclerosis, which is an autoimmune disorder. This IFN is effective in slowing down the progression of multiple sclerosis and also reduces secondary progressive multiple sclerosis attacks in patients. Consequently, IFN therapy is used in combination with chemotherapy, and this treatment is most effective in hematological malignancy, leukemia and lymphomas, chronic myeloid leukemia, nodular lymphoma, and cutaneous T-cell lymphoma. It has been reported that patients with recurrent problem of melanomas can receive recombinant IFN-α2b as the treatment.

In addition to the treatment of cancer, IFNs have also been used in treating both hepatitis B and hepatitis C. Patients are treated with IFN-α, frequently in combination with other antiviral drugs. It has been found that some patients who are treated with IFN have a constant viral response and can eliminate the hepatitis virus. The most harmful strain of hepatitis C, genotype I virus, can only be treated with IFN-α or ribavirin. After the treatment of IFNs, biopsies of the liver showed reductions in liver damage and cirrhosis. Interestingly, some evidence shows that giving IFN immediately following infection can prevent chronic hepatitis C. With regard to the use of IFNs in various countries around the globe, it has been reported that IFN is extensively used in parts of east Europe and Russia as a method to prevent and treat viral respiratory diseases. Nevertheless, the mechanisms of such action of IFN are not well understood and it is thought that doses must be larger to have any effect on virus elimination. In contrast, most of the scientists in the Western countries are not sure about the efficacy of IFNs.

Recent findings suggest that IFN applied to mucosa may act as an adjuvant against influenza virus, and help to boost immune system response against viral infection. A flu vaccine equipped with IFN as an adjuvant is currently under clinical trials in the United States. When used in general therapy, IFNs can be administered through various routes such as intramuscular and intravenous, which are considered to be easy and well tolerable. The most frequent adverse effects are found to be flu-like symptoms, fever, tiredness, headache, muscle discomfort, seizure, dizziness, hair weakening, and depressed conditions. We have briefly described the classification of various subtypes of IFNs.

6.4.5.1 *Interferon alpha*

The interferon alpha (IFN-α) is basically proteins that are produced by human cells such as leukocytes. They are mainly involved in creating innate immune response against viral infection. Thirteen different subtypes of IFN-α have been reported: (1) IFNA1, (2) IFNA2, (3) IFNA4, (4) IFNA5, (5) IFNA6, (6) IFNA7, (7) IFNA8, (8) IFNA10, (9) IFNA13, (10) IFNA14, (11) IFNA16, (12) IFNA17, and (13) IFNA21. It has been reported that genes for the IFN-α molecule are found together in a cluster on human chromosome 9.

6.4.5.2 *Interferon beta-1a*

IFN beta-1a is an IFN family subtype that is known to treat multiple sclerosis. It has been reported that IFN beta-1a can be produced by mammalian cells, whereas IFN beta-1b can be produced by modifying *E. coli*. It has been reported that the clinical use of IFNs can reduce the rate of multiple sclerosis deteriorations by 18–38%, and can also slow down the progression of disability in multiple sclerosis patients. Although the use of IFN beta-1a does not guarantee complete cure, patients who start taking IFNs may get the beneficial effects. IFN beta-1a-based drugs are sold in the market under the brand names of mAvonex (Biogen Idec), mRebif (Merck Serono), and CinnoVex (CinnaGen).

6.4.5.3 *Interferon gamma*

Interferon-gamma (IFN-γ) is a soluble cytokine that is the only member of the IFN family type II class. IFN-γ is also called macrophage-activating factor. In humans, the IFN-γ protein is encoded by the IFNG gene and it has been reported that IFN-γ is critical for innate and adaptive immunity against viral and intracellular bacterial infections. The expression of IFN-γ in human cells is generally associated with a number of autoinflammatory and autoimmune diseases. The prominence of IFN-γ in the human immune system stems from its ability to prevent viral replication directly by its immunostimulatory and immunomodulatory effects. It has been reported that IFN-γ is produced predominantly by NK and NK T cells as part of the innate immune response, and by CD-4 and CD-8 cytotoxic T lymphocyte effector T cells once antigen-specific immunity develops.

6.4.6 Recombinant antibiotics

The importance of antibiotics has been well documented in the literature and each and every one of us has experienced the benefits of antibiotics. Many bacterial infections can be treated with various kinds of antibacterial drugs; however, the current methods of developing antibiotics are not sufficient for highly specific-target-oriented antibiotics. Over the last few years, extensive research has been done to develop highly specific antibiotics by using r-DNA technology. Modern tools based on induction and repression of genes involved in antibiotic synthesis provide a means of increasing antibiotic activity. r-DNA technology and protoplast fusion approaches are used to alter the genetics of antibiotic producers for the development of novel hybrid antibiotics. It has been reported that directed mutation and selection, and protoplast fusion are examples of alternative procedures for manipulating the biosynthetic pathways of microorganisms for strain improvement and for developing new hybrid antibiotic products. In brief, the recombinant antibiotics can be developed by using bacteria DNA, which contains an antibiotic resistance gene. These bacteria are then put on an antibiotic-containing plate. After culture, bacteria that contain vector will survive, because only they contain the antibiotic-resistant gene. After this step, these bacterial colonies that contain recombinant vector in their genome are isolated and cloned.

6.5 Problems associated with recombinant DNA technology

In the previous section, we learned the various beneficial attributes of r-DNA technology. However, r-DNA technology does raise some concerns with regard to its clinical applications and we will discuss some of the major issues related with r-DNA technology.

6.5.1 Recombinant DNA organisms

One of the major concerns associated with r-DNA technology is the manipulation of genetic information from one organism to another. If one were to enhance or elicit a characteristic of an organism by conventional mutation or selection techniques, the safety assessment of the new organism would rely heavily on the knowledge of its parent organism, as well as on an analysis of how the new organism appears to differ from the parent. In the same way, any safety assessment of organisms altered by r-DNA techniques designed for use in an industrial, agricultural, or environmental application describes initially the relevant properties of the organism. r-DNA organisms are typically constructed by introducing a small segment of DNA from a donor organism into a recipient organism. The genome of the resulting organism derived by r-DNA technique from these two parents is therefore similar to that of the recipient organism. Since all but a small fraction of the genetic information in the modified organism is that of the recipient organism, a description of the recipient's properties provides initial information useful in assessing the properties of the organism derived by r-DNA techniques. Information describing the difference between the properties of the modified organism and of the recipient organism defines the framework for safety assessment. If, as a result of risk assessment, it is concluded that the modified organism must be physically contained, this is feasible in the case of industrial use but not for agricultural or environmental applications. This distinction is even more fundamental than whether the modified organism has been derived by genetic manipulation or not.

6.5.2 Donor and recipient organisms

It has been reported that for a successful recombination, the characteristics of the recipient organism should be taken into account include genetic, pathogenic, physiological, and ecological information. While these kinds of information are generally developed during laboratory, field testing, and pilot plant stages, there may be cases where additional testing is necessary. When chemically synthesized nucleic acids are used for the construction of organisms, consideration may need to be given to the structure and function of those sequences. The essence of the assessment is the extent to which the recipient's properties are altered by the introduced DNA. A first consideration should be the degree of expression of the introduced genetic material. A second would be the extent to which relevant properties of the recipient have been modified as a result of the genetic manipulation, including significant new or unexpected effects. The close similarity between the recipient and modified organism is useful in identifying the properties of the modified organism.

r-DNA techniques can be used to modify the genome of an organism, for example, to delete a portion of a recipient genome. Compared to other kinds of manipulations, the use of a deletion technique would ordinarily suggest lesser concern about safety since a deletion typically makes smaller and more precisely defined changes, while also typically enfeebling the organism, and no new genetic information has been added to the parental organism. Deletions are also likely to mimic mutations that occur in organisms naturally. However, appropriate consideration should be given to the possibility of the expression of unanticipated functions, particularly in the case of other types of modifications.

6.5.3 Health hazards and biosafety

When r-DNA technology was first introduced, there was a natural concern as to their potential hazards, but after more than a decade of experimentation under controlled conditions, these hazards have remained hypothetical and not based on the incident. Initial uncertainty about the safety of these techniques has been ameliorated by three compelling lines of evidence. First, experimental risk assessment studies specifically designed to test the hypothesis that host organisms can acquire unexpected hazardous properties from DNA donor cells have failed to demonstrate the existence of such conjectured hazards. Second, more rigorous evaluation of existing information regarding basic immunology, pathogenicity, and infectious disease processes has resulted in the relaxation of containment specifications recommended by national authorities. Third, the experimentation conducted in recent years has elicited no observable novel hazard. The above evidence suggests that the level of safety of microorganisms derived by r-DNA techniques may be evaluated reliably by examining the known properties of the components used in the r-DNA process. For example, when DNA coding for highly potential toxins is to be cloned, special attention is warranted.

It has been reported that there is nothing intrinsically more hazardous about r-DNA organisms or their products when industrial-scale work is planned. It is primarily the scale of operation and hence the possible volume, concentration, and the duration of exposure that have increased. In addition, only under controlled fermentation conditions in a well-defined process will the biomass and the level of product per unit volume be maximized. This has to be balanced against the fact that most of the worries related to the organism at the laboratory research stage have been eliminated prior to scale-up. Furthermore, disabled laboratory host strains can be used for fermentation production, provided that the organism is efficient under the process conditions determined within the fermenter. It should also be emphasized that there is an inherent incentive for the industry to use organisms that pose a low risk. Not only does this minimize any national regulatory constraints, but it also involves lower costs by, for example, minimizing the need for expensive plant containment and associated high containment safety procedures.

6.6 Research trends in recombinant DNA technology

The field of r-DNA technology keeps expanding with the advent of new tools and knowledge. We have seen tremendous growth in recombinant-DNA-based product development. In the future, r-DNA technologies will be used in preventing genetic diseases, producing targeted medicines, customized medicine or pharmacogenomics, and providing patients with less toxic pharmaceuticals. r-DNA technology would also be in use in animal cloning, creating transgenic animals and plants, and plant tissue culture.

6.7 Summary

The cracking of the genetic code of DNA with molecular tools has made it possible to manipulate the genetic information of organisms. r-DNA is a type of bioengineered DNA that is produced by combining two or more sequences that would not normally occur together. In terms of genetic modification, it is created through the introduction of human DNA into an existing organismal DNA (bacteria) to produce human-like proteins or hormones. It differs from genetic recombination as that does not occur through natural processes within the cell, but is engineered. One of the important applications of r-DNA technology is to produce therapeutic proteins for patients who are suffering from various diseases. A protein that is produced by using r-DNA technology is known as recombinant protein. The majority of therapeutic proteins are recombinant human proteins, manufactured using nonhuman mammalian cell lines that are engineered to express certain human genetic sequences to produce specific proteins. Recombinant proteins are an important class of therapeutics used to substitute deficiencies in critical blood-borne growth factors and to strengthen the immune system to fight cancer and infectious diseases. Therapeutic proteins such as monoclonal antibodies and IFNs are also used to relieve patients' suffering from cancers. Diseases such as heart attacks, strokes, cystic fibrosis, and Gaucher's disease are treated by synthetically made enzymes and blood factors; diabetes by insulin; anemia by erythropoietin; and hemophilia by blood-clotting factors. In this chapter, we have discussed the significance of r-DNA technology and explained how this novel technology has revolutionized modern treatment modalities.

6.8 Knowledge builder

Chimera: A chimera is a single organism (usually an animal) that is composed of two or more different populations of genetically distinct cells that originated from different zygotes involved in sexual reproduction. If the different cells have emerged from the same zygote, the organism is called a mosaic. Chimeras are formed from at least four parent cells (two fertilized eggs or early embryos fused together). Each population of cells keeps its own character and the resulting organism is a mixture of tissues. The first chimeric mouse was made by Beatrice Mintz in the 1960s through the aggregation of eight-cell-stage embryos. Embryonic stem cells are also a useful tool in chimeras because genes can be mutated in them through the use of homologous recombination, thus allowing gene targeting. In the same way, the DNA of one organism (bacterial) can be integrated with the DNA of another organism (human) to make a recombinant product.

Genetic recombination: Genetic recombination is the production of new combinations of alleles, encoding a novel set of genetic information, such as by the pairing of homologous chromosomes in meiosis, or by the breaking and rejoining of DNA strands, which forms new molecules of DNA. This last type of recombination can occur between similar molecules of DNA, as in the homologous recombination of chromosomal crossover, or dissimilar molecules, as in nonhomologous end joining. Recombination is a common method of DNA repair in both bacteria and eukaryotes.

Restriction endonucleases: These are enzymes that cut a nucleic acid at specific restriction sites and produce restriction fragments, and they are obtained from bacteria (where they cripple viral invaders) and are used in recombinant DNA technology.

Escherichia coli: E. coli is a Gram-negative, anaerobic, rod-shaped bacterium that is commonly found in the lower intestine of warm-blooded organisms (endotherms). Most *E. coli* strains are harmless, but some serotypes can cause serious food poisoning in humans. The bacterium can also be grown easily and inexpensively in a laboratory setting and has been intensively investigated for many years. *E. coli* is the most widely studied prokaryotic model organism, and is an important species in the fields of biotechnology and microbiology, where it has served as the host organism for the majority of work with recombinant DNA.

Phage: Bacteriophage, also called phage, is a virus that infects and replicates within bacteria; these bacteriophages are composed of proteins that encapsulate a DNA or RNA genome, and may have relatively simple or elaborate structures. Their genomes may encode as few as four genes, and as many as hundreds of genes.

Bioengineered insulin: Recombinant insulin is a form of insulin made from recombinant DNA technology using microbial DNA and human DNA recombination and this is also called bioengineered insulin.

Follicle-stimulating hormone: Follicle-stimulating hormone (FSH) is a hormone found in humans and other animals. It is synthesized and secreted by gonadotrophs of the anterior pituitary gland. FSH regulates the development, growth, pubertal maturation, and reproductive processes of the body. FSH and luteinizing hormone (LH) act synergistically in reproduction.

Plasminogen: Plasmin is an important enzyme (EC 3.4.21.7) present in blood that degrades many blood plasma proteins, most notably, fibrin clots. The degradation of fibrin is termed fibrinolysis. Plasmin is released as a zymogen called plasminogen (PLG) from the liver into the systemic circulation. Two major glycoforms of plasminogen are present in humans—type I plasminogen contains two glycosylation moieties (N-linked to N289 and O-linked to T346), whereas type II plasminogen contains only a single O-linked sugar (O-linked to T346). Type II plasminogen is preferentially recruited to the cell surface over the type I glycoform. Conversely, type I plasminogen appears more readily recruited to blood clots.

Erythropoietin: Erythropoietin (EPO) is a glycoprotein hormone that controls erythropoiesis, or red blood cell production. It is a cytokine for erythrocyte (red blood cell) precursors in the bone marrow.

Growth hormone: Growth hormone (GH), also known as somatotropin or somatropin, is a peptide hormone that stimulates growth, cell reproduction, and regeneration in humans and other animals. It is a type of mitogen that is specific only to certain kinds of cells. Growth hormone is a 191-amino-acid, single-chain polypeptide that is synthesized, stored, and secreted by the somatotropic cells within the lateral wings of the anterior pituitary gland.

Creutzfeldt–Jakob disease: Creutzfeldt–Jakob disease is a neurodegenerative disorder that is incurable and invariably fatal. This disorder is also called the human form of mad cow disease. In this disease, the brain tissue develops holes and takes in a sponge-like texture. This is due to a type of infectious protein called prion. Prions are misfolded proteins that replicate by converting their properly folded counterparts.

Autoimmune disease: Autoimmune diseases arise from an incorrect immune response of the body against substances and tissues normally present in the body (autoimmunity). In such cases, the body immune system instead of defending the body cells starts attacking the body cells, causing damage to the body's immune system. This may be restricted to certain organs or involve a particular tissue in different places. The treatment of autoimmune diseases is typically with immunosuppression medication that decreases the immune response. A large number of autoimmune diseases are recognized.

Myocardial infarction: Myocardial infarction or acute myocardial infarction, commonly known as a heart attack, results from the partial interruption of blood supply to a part of the heart muscle, causing the heart cells to be damaged or die. This is most commonly due to the blockage of a coronary artery following the rupture of a vulnerable atherosclerotic plaque, which is an unstable collection of cholesterol, fatty acids, and white blood cells in the wall of an artery. The resulting ischemia (restriction in blood supply) and ensuing oxygen shortage, if left untreated for a sufficient period of time, can cause damage or death (infarction) of the heart muscle tissue (myocardium).

Acute ischemic stroke: Strokes can be either ischemic or hemorrhagic. In an ischemic stroke, the blood supply to a part of the brain is cut off because atherosclerosis or a blood clot has blocked a blood vessel. Blood clots can travel to the brain from another artery (artery-to-artery embolization) or they can come from the heart. In hemorrhagic condition, brain blood vessels get ruptured and can bleed into the surrounding brain.

Acute massive pulmonary embolism: Pulmonary embolism is a blockage of the main artery of the lung or one of its branches by a substance that has travelled from elsewhere in the body through the bloodstream (embolism). A small proportion of cases are due to the embolization of air, fat, talc in drugs of intravenous drug abusers, or amniotic fluid. The obstruction of the blood flow through the lungs and the resultant pressure on the right ventricle of the heart lead to the symptoms and signs of embolism.

Monoclonal antibodies: Monoclonal antibodies are mono-specific antibodies that are the same because they are made by identical immune cells that are all clones of a unique parent cell, in contrast to polyclonal antibodies, which are made from several different immune cells. Monoclonal antibodies have monovalent affinity, in that they bind to the same epitope.

Chimeric antibodies: Early on, a major problem for the therapeutic use of monoclonal antibodies in medicine was that initial methods used to produce them yielded mouse, not human antibodies. While structurally similar, differences between the two were sufficient to invoke an immune response when murine monoclonal antibodies were injected into humans, resulting in their rapid removal from the blood, as well as systemic inflammatory effects. In an effort to overcome this obstacle, approaches using recombinant DNA have been explored since the late 1980s. In one approach, mouse DNA encoding the binding portion of a monoclonal antibody was merged with human antibody-producing DNA in living cells. The expression of this chimeric DNA through cell culture yielded partially mouse, partially human monoclonal antibodies. For this product, the descriptive terms "chimeric" and "humanized" monoclonal antibody have been used to reflect the combination of mouse and human DNA sources used in the recombinant process.

Immunogenicity: Immunogenicity is the ability of a particular substance, such as an antigen or epitope, to provoke an immune response in the body of a human or animal.

Fermentation technology: Fermentation technology makes it possible to grow a number of fungi in large tanks and, in a matter of days, a large quantity of biotherapeutically products can be produced in large volume from few 100 letters to few million letters.

Actinic keratosis disease: Actinic keratosis is a premalignant condition of thick, scaly, or crusty patches of skin. It is more common in fair-skinned people and it is associated with those who are frequently exposed to the sun, as it is usually accompanied by solar damage. They are considered as potentially precancerous, since some of them progress to squamous cell carcinoma, so treatment is recommended.

Superficial basal-cell carcinoma: Basal-cell carcinoma, a skin cancer, is the most common cancer. It rarely metastasizes or kills. However, because it can cause significant destruction and disfigurement by invading surrounding tissues, it is still considered malignant. Statistically, in the United States, approximately 3 out of 10 Caucasians may develop a basal-cell cancer within their lifetime. In 80% of all cases, basal-cell cancers are found on the head and neck. There appears to be an increase in the incidence of basal-cell cancer of the trunk in recent years.

Papilloma: Papilloma refers to a benign epithelial tumor growing outwardly, projecting in finger-like fronds. In this context, papilla refers to the projection created by the tumor, not a tumor on an already-existing papilla. When used without context, it frequently refers to infections caused by human papillomavirus, such as warts. There are, however, a number of other conditions that cause papilloma, as well as many cases in which there is no known cause.

External genital warts: Genital warts are symptoms of a highly contagious sexually transmitted disease caused by some subtypes of human papillomavirus.

Leukemia: Leukemia is a type of cancer of the blood or bone marrow characterized by an abnormal increase of immature white blood cells called blasts. Leukemia is a broad term covering a spectrum of diseases. In turn, it is part of the even broader group of diseases affecting the blood, bone marrow, and lymphoid system, which are all known as hematological neoplasms.

Lymphomas: Lymphoma is a type of blood cancer that occurs when B or T lymphocytes, the white blood cells that form a part of the immune system and help protect the body from infection and disease, divide faster than normal cells or live longer than they are supposed to. Lymphoma may develop in the lymph nodes, spleen, bone marrow, blood, or other organs, and eventually they form a tumor.

Chronic myeloid leukemia: Chronic myeloid leukemia, also known as chronic granulocytic leukemia, is a cancer of the white blood cells. It is a form of leukemia characterized by the increased and unregulated growth of predominantly myeloid cells in the bone marrow and the accumulation of these cells in the blood. Chronic myeloid leukemia is a clonal bone marrow stem cell disorder in which a proliferation of matures granulocytes (neutrophils, eosinophils, and basophils) and their precursors is found.

Nodular lymphoma: Follicular lymphoma is the most common of the indolent non-Hodgkin's lymphomas, and the second-most common form of non-Hodgkin's lymphomas overall. It is defined as a lymphoma of follicle center B cells, which has at least a partial follicular pattern.

Cutaneous T-cell lymphoma: Cutaneous T-cell lymphoma is a class of non-Hodgkin's lymphoma, which is a type of cancer of the immune system. Unlike most non-Hodgkin's lymphomas, cutaneous T-cell lymphoma is caused by a mutation of T cells. The malignant T cells in the body initially migrate to the skin, causing various lesions to appear. These lesions change shape as the disease progresses, typically beginning as what appears to be a rash that can be very itchy and eventually forming plaques and tumors before metastasizing to other parts of the body.

Hepatitis C: Hepatitis C is an infectious disease primarily affecting the liver, caused by the hepatitis C virus. The infection is often asymptomatic, but chronic infection can lead to scarring of the liver and ultimately to cirrhosis, which is generally apparent after many years. In some cases, those with cirrhosis will go on to develop liver failure, liver cancer or life-threatening esophageal and gastric varices.

Autoinflammatory: Autoinflammatory diseases are a relatively new category of diseases that are different from autoimmune diseases. However, autoimmune and autoinflammatory diseases share common characteristics in that both groups of disorders result from the immune system attacking the body's own tissues, and also result in increased inflammation. This overview contains general information on the immune system, and provides brief descriptions of some of the more common autoinflammatory diseases.

Cystic fibrosis: Cystic fibrosis is an autosomal recessive genetic disorder that affects most critically the lungs, and also the pancreas, liver, and intestine. It is characterized by an abnormal transport of chloride and sodium across an epithelium, leading to thick, viscous secretions.

Gaucher's disease: Gaucher's disease is a genetic disease in which a fatty substance (lipid) accumulates in cells and certain organs. Gaucher's disease is the most common of the lysosomal storage diseases. The disorder is characterized by bruising, fatigue, anemia, low blood platelets, and enlargement of the liver and spleen.

Further reading

Aher SM and Ohlsson A 2006. Early versus late erythropoietin for preventing red blood cell transfusion in preterm and/or low birth weight infants. *Cochrane Database Syst Rev* 3: CD004865. doi:10.1002/14651858.CD004865.pub2. PMID 16856063.

Angles-Cano E and Rojas G 2003. Apolipoprotein(a): Structure-function relationship at the lysine-binding site and plasminogen activator cleavage site. *Biol Chem* 383 (1): 93–99. doi:10.1515/BC.2002.009. PMID 11928826.

Ashby DR, Gale DP, Busbridge M et al. March 2010. Erythropoietin administration in humans causes a marked and prolonged reduction in circulating hepcidin. *Haematologica* 95 (3): 505–508. doi:10.3324/haematol.2009.013136. PMID 19833632.

Bhatti Z and Berenson CS 2007. Adult systemic cat scratch disease associated with therapy for hepatitis C. *BMC Infect Dis* 7: 8. doi:10.1186/1471-2334-7-8. PMC 1810538. PMID 17319959. http://www.pubmedcentral.nih.gov/articlerender.fcgi?tool=pmcentrez&artid=1810538.

Bode W and Renatus M 1998. Tissue-type plasminogen activator: Variants and crystal/solution structures demarcate structural determinants of function. *Curr Opin Struct Biol* 7 (6): 865–872. doi:10.1016/S0959-440X(97)80159-5. PMID 9434908.

Brondyk WH 2009. Selecting an appropriate method for expressing a recombinant protein. *Methods Enzymol* 463: 131–147. doi:10.1016/S0076-6879(09)63011-1. PMID 19892171.

Brown T 2006. *Gene Cloning and DNA Analysis: An Introduction*. Cambridge, MA: Blackwell Pub. ISBN 1-4051-1121-6.

Bruen KJ, Ballard JR, Morris SE, Cochran A, Edelman LS, and Saffle JR 2007. Reduction of the incidence of amputation in frostbite injury with thrombolytic therapy. *Arch Surg* 142 (6): 546–551; discussion 551–553. doi:10.1001/archsurg.142.6.546. PMID 17576891.

Cohen SN, Chang AC, Boyer HW, and Helling RB 1973. Construction of biologically functional bacterial plasmids *in vitro*. *PNAS* 70 (11): 3240–3244. doi:10.1073/pnas.70.11.3240. PMID 4594039.

Collen D, Billiau A, Edy J, and De Somer P 1977. Identification of the human plasma protein which inhibits fibrinolysis associated with malignant cells. *Biochim Biophys Acta* 499(2): 194–220.

Colowick SP and Kapian ON 1980. *Methods in Enzymology—Volume 68; Recombinant DNA*. Waltham, MA: Academic Press. ISBN 012181968X.

Cooksley WG March 2004. The role of interferon therapy in hepatitis B. *MedGenMed* 6 (1): 16. PMC 1140699. PMID 15208528. http://www.pubmedcentral.nih.gov/articlerender.fcgi?tool=pmcentrez&artid=1140699.

Corwin HL, Gettinger A, Fabian TC et al. 2007. Efficacy and safety of epoetin alfa in critically ill patients. *N Engl J Med* 357 (10): 965–976. doi:10.1056/NEJMoa071533. PMID 17804841.

Drüeke TB, Locatelli F, Clyne N, Eckardt KU, Macdougall IC, Tsakiris D, Burger HU, and Scherhag A 2006. Normalization of hemoglobin level in patients with chronic kidney disease and anemia. *N Engl J Med* 355 (20): 2071–2084. doi:10.1056/NEJMoa062276. PMID 17108342.

Ehrenreich H, Degner D, Meller J et al. 2004. Erythropoietin: A candidate compound for neuroprotection in schizophrenia (PDF). *Mol Psychiatr* 9 (1): 42–54. doi:10.1038/sj.mp.4001442. PMID 14581931. http://physiologie.univ-lyon1.fr/enseignement/coursLB/Ehrenreich2004.pdf.

Eschbach JW, Egrie JC, Downing MR, Browne JK, and Adamson JW 1987. Correction of the anemia of end-stage renal disease with recombinant human erythropoietin. Results of a combined phase I and II clinical trial. *N Engl J Med* 316 (2): 73–78. doi:10.1056/NEJM198701083160203. PMID 3537801.

Fernandez M and Hosey R 2009. Performance-enhancing drugs snare nonathletes, too. *J Fam Practice* 58 (1): 16–23. PMID 19141266.

Fisher JW, Koury S, Ducey T, and Mendel S 1996. Erythropoietin production by interstitial cells of hypoxic monkey kidneys. *Brit J Haematol* 95 (1): 27–32. doi:10.1046/j.1365-2141.1996.d01-1864.x. PMID 8857934.

Funke T, Han H, Healy-Fried M, Fischer M, and Schönbrunn E 2006. Molecular basis for the herbicide resistance of Roundup Ready crops. *Proc Natl Acad Sci* 103 (35): 13010–13015. doi:10.1073/pnas.0603638103. PMC 1559744. PMID 16916934. http://www.pubmedcentral.nih.gov/articlerender.fcgi?tool=pmcentrez&artid=1559744.

Ge D, Fellay J, Thompson AJ et al. 2009. Genetic variation in IL28B predicts hepatitis C treatment-induced viral clearance. *Nature* 461 (7262): 399–401. doi:10.1038/nature08309. PMID 19684573.

Goldstein D and Laszlo J 1988. The role of interferon in cancer therapy: A current perspective. *Cancer J Clin* 38 (5): 258–277. doi:10.3322/canjclin.38.5.258. ISSN 0007-9235. PMID 2458171. http://caonline.amcancersoc.org/cgi/pmidlookup?view=long&pmid=2458171.

Gualandi-Signorini A and Giorgi G 2001. Insulin formulations—A review. *Eur Rev Med Pharmacol Sci* 5 (3): 73–83. PMID 12004916.

Hannig G and Makrides S 1998. Strategies for optimizing heterologous protein expression in *Escherichia coli*. *Trends Biotechnol* 16 (2): 54–60. PMID 9487731.

Haroon ZA, Amin K, Jiang X, and Arcasoy MO 2003. A novel role for erythropoietin during fibrin-induced wound-healing response. *Am J Pathol* 163 (3): 993–1000. PMID 12937140. PMC 1868246. http://ajp.amjpathol.org/cgi/content/abstract/163/3/993.

Hauschild A, Gogas H, Tarhini A, Middleton M, Testori A, Dreno B, and Kirkwood J 2008. Practical guidelines for the management of interferon-alpha-2b side effects in patients receiving adjuvant treatment for melanoma: Expert opinion. *Cancer* 112 (5): 982–994. doi:10.1002/cncr.23251. ISSN 0008-543X. PMID 18236459.

Ichinose A, Takio K, and Fujikawa K 1986. Localization of the binding site of tissue-type plasminogen activator to fibrin. *J Clin Invest* 78 (1): 163–169. doi:10.1172/JCI112546. ISSN 0021-9738. PMID 3088041.

Ishikawa T 2008. Secondary prevention of recurrence by interferon therapy after ablation therapy for hepatocellular carcinoma in chronic hepatitis C patients. *World J Gastroenterol* 14 (40): 6140–6144. doi:10.3748/wjg.14.6140. ISSN 1007-9327. PMC 2761574. PMID 18985803. http://www.wjgnet.com/1007-9327/14/6140.asp.

Jacobson LO, Goldwasser E, Fried W, and Plzak L 1957. Role of the kidney in erythropoiesis. *Nature* 179 (4560): 633–634. doi:10.1038/179633a0. PMID 13418752.

Jamall IS, Yusuf S, Azhar M, and Jamall S 2008. Is pegylated interferon superior to interferon, with ribavarin, in chronic hepatitis C genotypes 2/3? *World J Gastroenterol* 14 (43): 6627–6631. doi:10.3748/wjg.14.6627. PMC 2773302. PMID 19034963. http://www.pubmedcentral.nih.gov/articlerender.fcgi?tool=pmcentrez&artid=2773302.

Jelkmann W 2007. Erythropoietin after a century of research: Younger than ever. *Eur J Haematol* 78 (3): 183–205. doi:10.1111/j.1600-0609.2007.00818.x. PMID 17253966.

Kohler M, Ayotte C, Desharnais P, Flenker U, Lüdke S, Thevis M, Völker-Schänzer E, and Schänzer W 2008. Discrimination of recombinant and endogenous urinary erythropoietin by calculating relative mobility values from SDS gels. *Int J Sports Med* 29 (1): 1–6. doi:10.1055/s-2007-989369. PMID 18050057.

Koller BH and Smithies O 1992. Altering genes in animals by gene targeting. *Annu Rev Immunol* 10: 705–730. doi:10.1146/annurev.iy.10.040192.003421. PMID 1591000.

Lasne F, Martin L, Crepin N, and de Ceaurriz J 2002. Detection of isoelectric profiles of erythropoietin in urine: Differentiation of natural and administered recombinant hormones. *Anal Biochem* 311 (2): 119–126. doi:10.1016/S0003-2697(02)00407-4. PMID 12470670.

Lin FK, Suggs S, Lin CH, Browne JK, Smalling R, Egrie JC, Chen KK, Fox GM, Martin F, and Stabinsky Z 1985. Cloning and expression of the human erythropoietin gene. *Proc Natl Acad Sci USA* 82 (22): 7580–7584. doi:10.1073/pnas.82.22.7580. PMID 3865178. PMC 391376. http://www.pnas.org/content/82/22/7580.abstract.

Livnah O, Johnson DL, Stura EA et al. 1998. An antagonist peptide-EPO receptor complex suggests that receptor dimerization is not sufficient for activation. *Nat Struct Biol* 5 (11): 993–1004. doi:10.1038/2965. ISSN 1072-8368. PMID 9808045.

Macdougall IC, Tucker B, Thompson J, Tomson CR, Baker LR, and Raine AE 1996. A randomized controlled study of iron supplementation in patients treated with erythropoietin. *Kidney Int* 50 (5): 1694–1699. doi:10.1038/ki.1996.487. PMID 8914038.

Manco-Johnson MJ. 2010. Advances in the care and treatment of children with hemophilia. *Adv Pediatr* 57 (1): 287–294. doi:10.1016/j.yapd.2010.08.007. PMID 21056743.

Middleton, SA, Barbone, FP, Johnson, DL et al. 1999. Shared and unique determinants of the erythropoietin (EPO) receptor are important for binding EPO and EPO mimetic peptide. *J Biol Chem* 274 (20): 14163–14169. doi:10.1074/jbc.274.20.14163. ISSN 0021-9258. PMID 10318834.

Miyake T, Kung CK, and Goldwasser E 1997. Purification of human erythropoietin. *J Biol Chem* 252 (15): 5558–5564. PMID 18467. http://www.jbc.org/content/252/15/5558.long.

Mossman K 2011. *Viruses and Interferon: Current Research.* Caister Academic Press, Norfolk, England. ISBN 978-1-904455 -81-3.

Nathan PK, Nathan P, and Colowick RW 1980. *Recombinant DNA, Volume 68: Volume 68: Recombinant DNA Part F (Methods in Enzymology).* Academic Press, Massachussetts, USA. ISBN 0-1218-1968-X.

Ny T, Wahlberg P, and Brandstrom IJ 2003. Matrix remodeling in the ovary: Regulation and functional role of the plasminogen activator and matrix metalloproteinase systems. *Mol Cell Endocrinol* 187 (1–2): 29–38. doi:10.1016/S0303-7207(01)00711-0. PMID 11988309.

Ohlsson A and Aher SM 2006. Early erythropoietin for preventing red blood cell transfusion in preterm and/or low birth weight infants. *Cochrane Database Syst Rev* 3: CD004863. doi:10.1002/14651858.CD004863.pub2. PMID 16856062.

Orth K, Madison EL, Gething MJ, Sambrook JF, and Herz J 1992. Complexes of tissue-type plasminogen activator and its serpin inhibitor plasminogen-activator inhibitor type 1 are internalized by means of the low density lipoprotein receptor-related protein/alpha 2-macroglobulin receptor. *Proc Natl Acad Sci USA* 89 (16): 7422–7426. doi:10.1073/pnas.89.16.7422. ISSN 0027-8424. PMID 1502153.

Paine JA, Shipton CA, Chaggar S et al. 2005. Improving the nutritional value of Golden Rice through increased pro-vitamin a content. *Nat Biotechnol* 23 (4): 482–487. doi:10.1038/nbt1082. PMID 15793573.

Pang PT and Lu B 2005. Regulation of late-phase LTP and long-term memory in normal and aging hippocampus: Role of secreted proteins tPA and BDNF. *Ageing Res Rev* 3 (4): 407–430. doi:10.1016/j.arr.2004.07.002. PMID 15541709.

Paolicelli D, Direnzo V, and Trojano M 2009. Review of interferon beta-1b in the treatment of early and relapsing multiple sclerosis. *Biol Target Ther* 3: 369–376. ISSN 1177-5475. PMC 2726074. PMID 19707422. http://www.pubmedcentral.nih.gov/articlerender.fcgi?tool=pmcentrez&artid=2726074.

Parmar PK, Coates LC, Pearson JF, Hill RM, and Birch NP 2002. Neuroserpin regulates neurite outgrowth in nerve growth factor-treated PC12 cells. *J Neurochem* 82 (6): 1406–1415. doi:10.1046/j.1471-4159.2002.01100.x. ISSN 0022-3042. PMID 12354288.

Russell DW and Sambrook J 2001. *Molecular Cloning: A Laboratory Manual.* Cold Spring Harbor, NY: Cold Spring Harbor Laboratory. ISBN 0-87969-576-5.

Schwaber J and Cohen EP 1973. Human x mouse somatic cell hybrid clone secreting immunoglobulins of both parental types. *Nature* 244 (5416): 444–447. doi:10.1038/244444a0. PMID 4200460.

Sharieff KA, Duncan D, and Younossi Z 2002. Advances in treatment of chronic hepatitis C: "pegylated" interferons. *Cleve Clin J Med* 69 (2): 155–159. doi:10.3949/ccjm.69.2.155. PMID 11990646.

Sheehan JJ and Tsirka SE 2005. Fibrin-modifying serine proteases thrombin, tPA, and plasmin in ischemic stroke: A review. *Glia* 50 (4): 340–350. doi:10.1002/glia.20150. PMID 15846799.

Shepherd J, Waugh N, and Hewitson P 2000. Combination therapy (interferon alfa and ribavirin) in the treatment of chronic hepatitis C: A rapid and systematic review. *Health Technol Assess* 4 (33): 1–67. ISSN 1366-5278. PMID 11134916. http://www.hta.ac.uk/execsumm/summ433.htm.

Sirén AL, Fratelli M, Brines M et al. 2001. Erythropoietin prevents neuronal apoptosis after cerebral ischemia and metabolic stress. *Proc Natl Acad Sci USA* 98 (7): 4044–4049. doi:10.1073/pnas.051606598. PMID 11259643.

Teesalu T, Kulla A, Asser T et al. 2002. Tissue plasminogen activator as a key effector in neurobiology and neuropathology. *Biochem Soc Trans* 30 (2): 183–189. doi:10.1042/BST0300183. PMID 12023848.

Tsurupa G and Medved L January 2001. Identification and characterization of novel tPA- and plasminogen-binding sites within fibrin(ogen) alpha C-domains. *Biochemistry* 40 (3): 801–808. doi:10.1021/bi001789t. ISSN 0006-2960. PMID 11170397.

Watson JD 2007. *Recombinant DNA: Genes and Genomes: A Short Course.* San Francisco: W.H. Freeman. ISBN 0-7167-2866-4.

Ye X, Al-Babili S, Klöti A, Zhang J, Lucca P, Beyer P, and Potrykus I 2000. Engineering the provitamin A (beta-carotene) biosynthetic pathway into (carotenoid-free) rice endosperm. *Science* 287 (5451): 303–305. PMID 10634784.

Zagon IS, Donahue RN, Rogosnitzky M, and McLaughlin PJ 2008. Imiquimod upregulates the opioid growth factor receptor to inhibit cell proliferation independent of immune function. *Exp Biol Med* 233 (8): 968–979. doi:10.3181/0802-RM-58. PMID 18480416.

Zhuo M, Holtzman DM, Li Y, Osaka H, DeMaro J, Jacquin M, and Bu G 2000. Role of tissue plasminogen activator receptor LRP in hippocampal long-term potentiation. *J Neurosci* 20 (2): 542–549. PMID 10632583.

chapter seven

Stem cell technology

7.1 Introduction

Stem cells are extremely specialized cells of the human body that are present in all mammalian species. These cells have two distinct features: their ability to renew through mitotic cell division and their ability to differentiate into all types of body cells (Figure 7.1). In humans, stem cells are broadly classified into two types: embryonic stem cells (ESCs) that are isolated from the inner cell mass of blastocysts of a developing human embryo, and adult stem cells that are usually found in adult tissues as a reservoir. During human development, stem cells that are located in the inner cell mass can differentiate into all the specialized embryonic tissues. In adult organisms, stem cells and their progenitor cells act as a repair system for the body, but also maintain the normal reservoir of regenerative organs that include blood, skin, or intestinal tissues. It has been reported that stem cells can now be grown and transformed into specialized cells with characteristics of various tissues such as muscles or nerves. It has been shown that the adult stem cells can be isolated from a variety of sources, including umbilical cord blood and bone marrow, which are routinely used in medical therapies; it can also be isolated from dental gum, eye, and brain.

7.2 Significance of stem cells

Stem cells have the remarkable potential to develop into different cell types in the body during early life and growth (Figure 7.2). The main function of stem cells is to serve as an internal repair system, and to provide new cells to damaged organs as long as the person or animal is alive. When a stem cell multiplies, each new cell has the potential to either continue as a stem cell (reservoir) or become another type of cell of the body, such as neural cell, red blood cell, and muscle cell. Interestingly, stem cells are different from other cell types in two ways: first, stem cells are unspecialized cells that are capable of renewing themselves through cell division, and second, under special physiological or experimental conditions, they can be differentiated to become tissue or specific type of cells with special functions, such as cardiomyocytes and neurons. Furthermore, in some organs, such as the gut and bone marrow, stem cells regularly divide to repair and replace damaged tissues in the body, whereas in other organs such as the pancreas and the heart, stem cells only divide under special conditions or requirements. In principle, there are two types of stem cells in the human body; they are ESCs and nonembryonic or somatic or adult stem cells.

In 1981, ESCs were isolated from early mouse embryos, which later led to the development of a method to derive stem cells from human embryos, which can grow in the laboratory. Stem cells that are isolated from the human embryo are called human ESCs. Furthermore, human embryos used in these studies are created for reproduction by using *in vitro* fertilization procedures. When these embryos are no longer needed by the patients, they can be donated for research with the informed consent of the donor. Moreover, stem

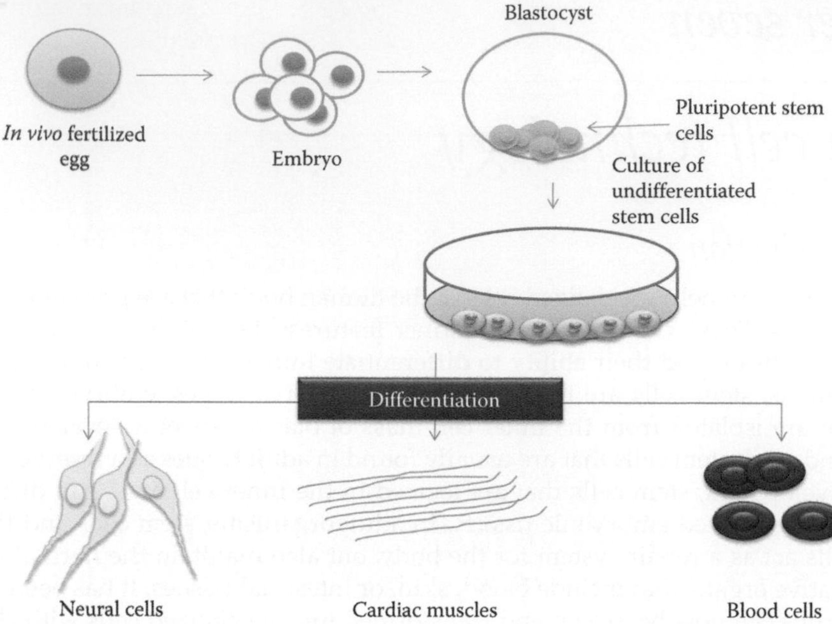

Figure 7.1 Development pathway of stem cells.

cells are important to living organisms for many reasons. The 3- to 5-day-old embryo that is called a blastocyst contains cells normally referred to as the inner cells. The inner cell mass contains stem cells that give rise to the entire body of the organism, including many specialized cell types and organs such as the skin, sperm, eggs, heart, lung, and other tissues. Stem cells are unique in many aspects as explained in Figure 7.3 as well as in Table 7.1.

Interestingly, all stem cells, regardless of their source, normally have three general properties: (i) they are capable of multiplying and renewing themselves for long periods of

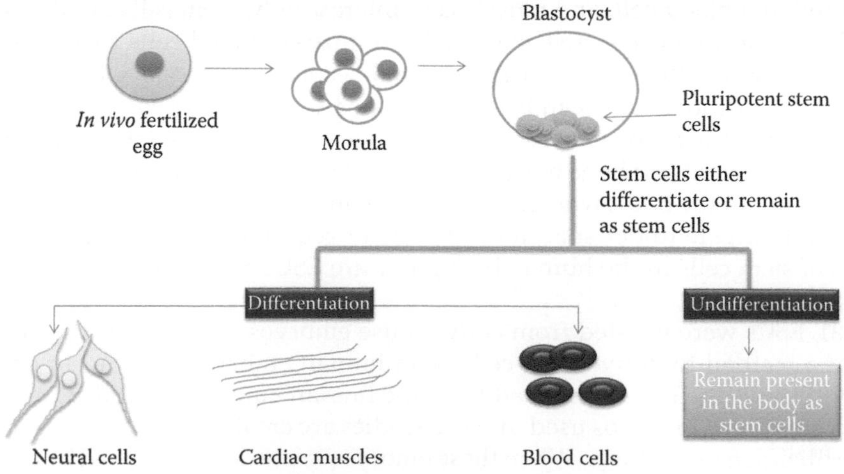

Figure 7.2 Fate of stem cells in the human body.

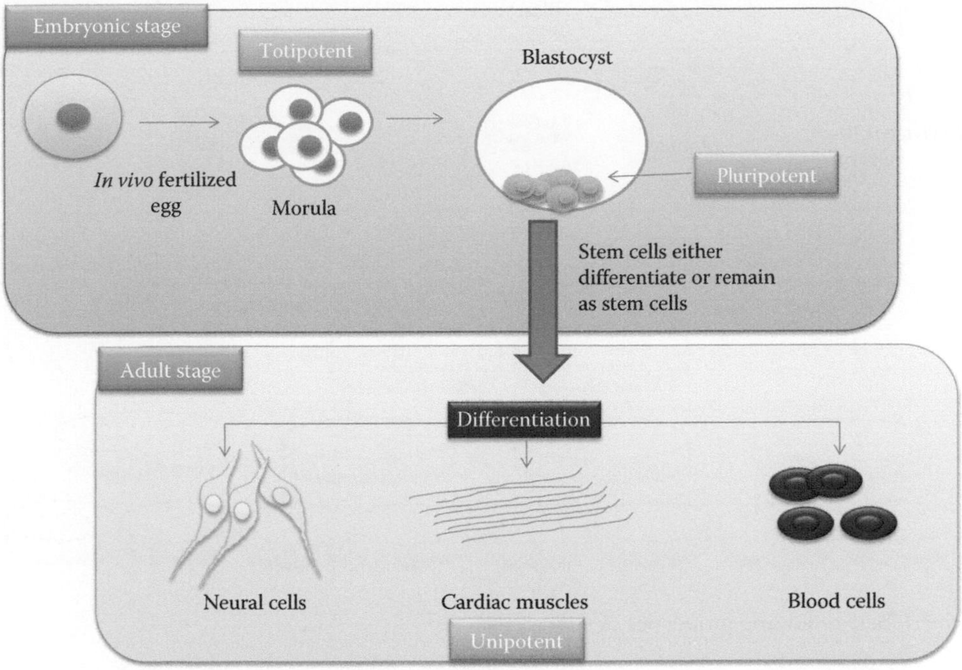

Figure 7.3 Characteristics of stem cells.

time, (ii) they are unspecialized, and (iii) they can give rise to specialized cell types upon differentiation (Figure 7.4). Furthermore, stem cells are unspecialized cells and one of the fundamental properties of stem cells is that it does not have any tissue-specific structures or morphology that allows it to perform specialized functions. For instance, a stem cell cannot work like adult or somatic cells to pump blood through the body, and stem cells cannot carry oxygen molecules through the bloodstream. Nevertheless, these unspecialized stem

Table 7.1 Properties of Stem Cells

Type of stem cells	Properties
Self-renewal	The ability to go through numerous cycles of cell division while maintaining the undifferentiated state.
Totipotent stem cells	These stem cells can differentiate into embryonic and extraembryonic cell types. Such cells can construct a complete, viable, organism. These cells are produced from the fusion of an egg and sperm cell. The cells produced by the first few divisions of the fertilized egg are also totipotent.
Pluripotent stem cells	They are the descendants of totipotent cells and can differentiate into nearly all cells, that is, cells derived from any of the three germ layers.
Multipotent stem cells	They can differentiate into a number of cells, but only those of a closely related family of cells.
Oligopotent stem cells	They can differentiate into only a few cells, such as lymphoid or myeloid stem cells.
Unipotent stem cells	They can produce only one cell type, their own, but have the property of self-renewal that distinguishes them from nonstem cells (e.g., muscle stem cells).

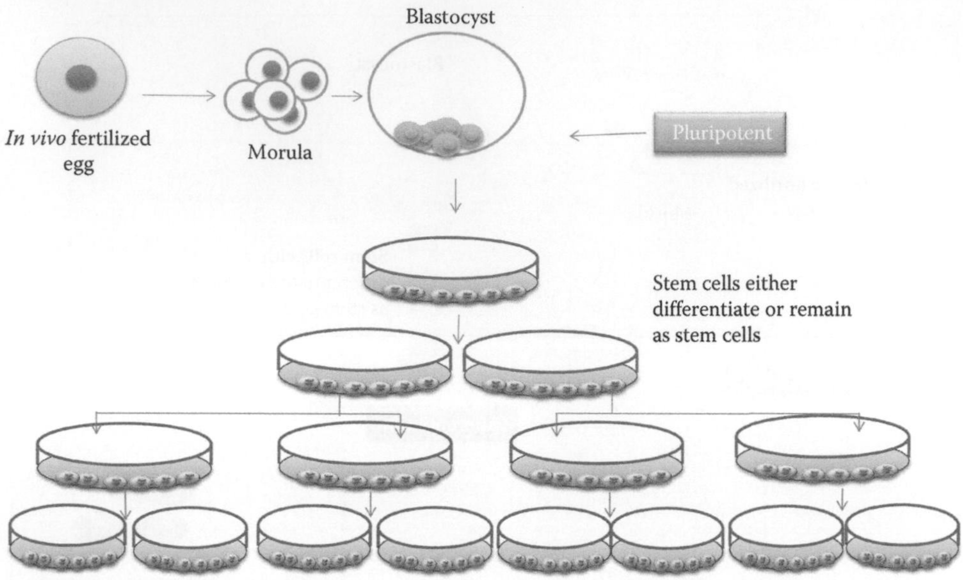

Figure 7.4 Self-renewing properties of stem cells.

cells can give rise to specialized cells through a process called differentiation. During this process, stem cells usually become specialized somatic cells in several stages.

7.3 Classification of stem cells

Stem cells are classified into two major types: ESCs that are isolated from the developing embryo known as blastocysts, and adult stem cells that are found in adult tissues or organs.

7.3.1 Embryonic stem cells

In humans, ESCs are pluripotent stem cells derived from the inner cell mass of the blastocyst (an early-stage embryo) (Figure 7.5). Moreover, human embryos reach the blastocyst stage 4–5 days postfertilization. At that time, they consist of 50–150 cells; these cells are called ESCs. ESCs are pluripotent stem cells (Figure 7.6) and they have the capability to differentiate into all three primary germ layers such as ectoderm, endoderm, and mesoderm. These three germ layers later on give rise to more than 220 different cell types in the adult body. There is a difference between ESCs and adult stem cells as far as pluripotency is concerned, as ESCs can generate all cell types in the body, whereas adult stem cells are multipotent and can only produce an inadequate number of cell types. Furthermore, under well-defined conditions, ESCs are capable of propagating themselves for long periods of time without losing their pluripotency. In view of these unique properties, ESCs can be employed as useful models both for conducting research and as regenerative medicine because ESCs can produce unlimited numbers of cells and can be transplanted into patients. With the help of ESCs, it is possible to treat various diseases such as genetic disorders, diabetes, Parkinson's disease, blindness, cancers, and spinal cord injuries.

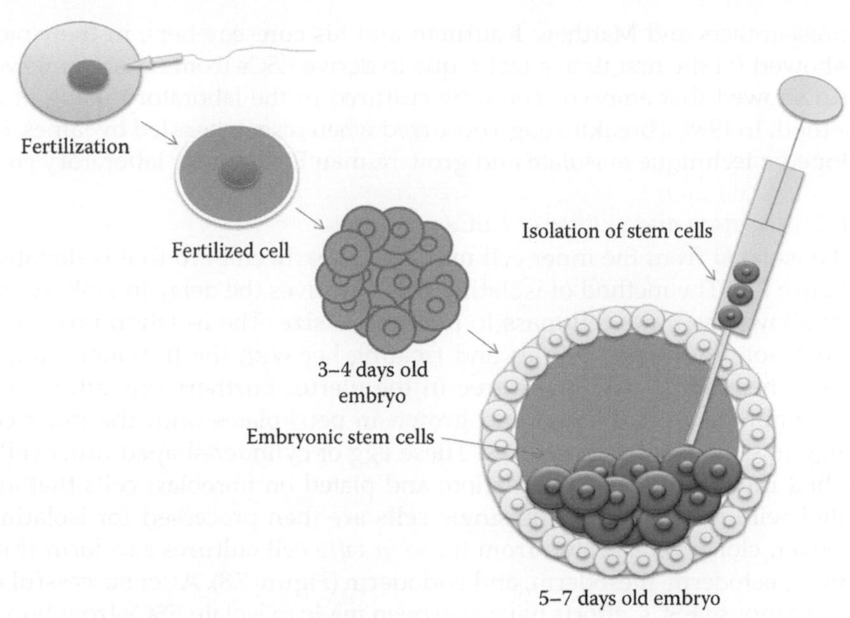

Figure 7.5 Development of human embryonic stem cells.

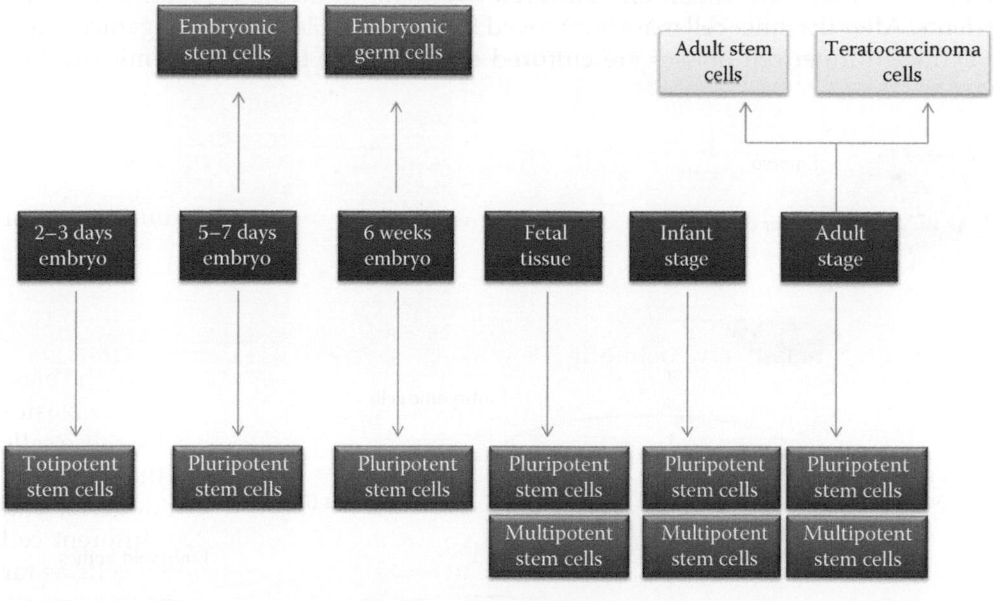

Figure 7.6 Isolation of stem cells in different stages of human life.

7.3.1.1 *Historical perspective of ES cells*

It all started in 1964 with the research work carried out to isolate a single type of cell from a teratocarcinoma, a tumor now known to be derived from a germ cell. These specialized cells were isolated from the teratocarcinoma, replicated, and grown in cell culture media; these specialized cells were later named embryonic carcinoma (EC) cells. In 1981, ESCs were derived for the first time from mouse embryos by two research groups. Martin Evans and his coresearchers and Matthew Kaufman and his coresearchers, in their pioneering research, showed for the first time a technique to derive ESCs from mouse embryos. Also, G.R. Martin showed that embryos could be cultured in the laboratory using *in vitro* cell culture method. In 1998, a breakthrough occurred when researchers led by James Thomson first developed a technique to isolate and grow human ESCs under laboratory conditions.

7.3.1.2 Isolation and culture of ESCs

ESCs can be isolated from the inner cell mass of the early embryo that is donated by the mother (Figure 7.7). The method of isolating ESCs involves the delay in embryo implantation, which allows the inner cell mass to increase in size. The isolation process includes removing the donor mother's ovaries and treating her with the hormone progesterone, which causes the embryos to remain free in the uterus. Furthermore, after 4–6 days of culture, the embryos are harvested and grown in petri-plates until the inner cell mass forms an egg or cylinder-like structures. These egg or cylinder-shaped inner cell mass is then detached into a single cell population, and plated on fibroblast cells that are previously treated with mitomycin-c. The single cells are then processed for isolating clonal cells. Moreover, clonal cells grown from these *in vitro* cell cultures can form three germ layers, namely, ectoderm, mesoderm, and endoderm (Figure 7.8). After successful isolation and culture of mouse ESCs, efforts have also been made to isolate ESCs from humans. For that purpose, a method to derive human ESCs and cultured embryonic stem (ES) cells was established. In the first step, the embryos are removed from the donor mother at approximately 76 h after fertilization and cultured overnight in media containing serum and nutrients. After the inner cell mass is removed from the late blastocyst using microsurgery, the extracted inner cell masses are cultured on fibroblasts treated with mitomycin-c in

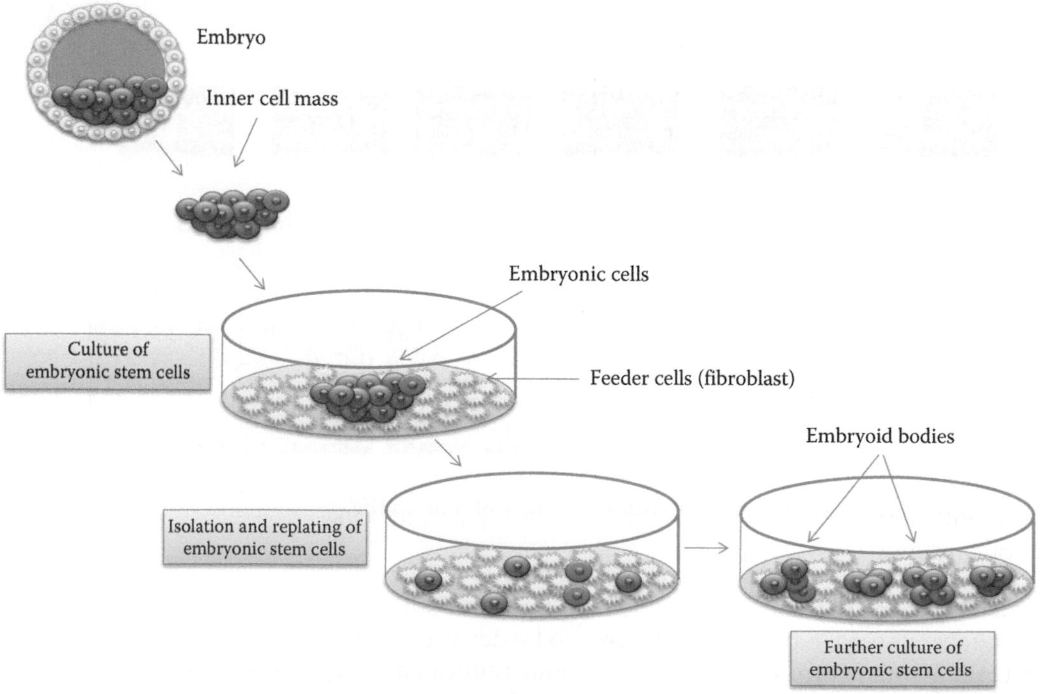

Figure 7.7 Isolation and culture of embryonic stem cells.

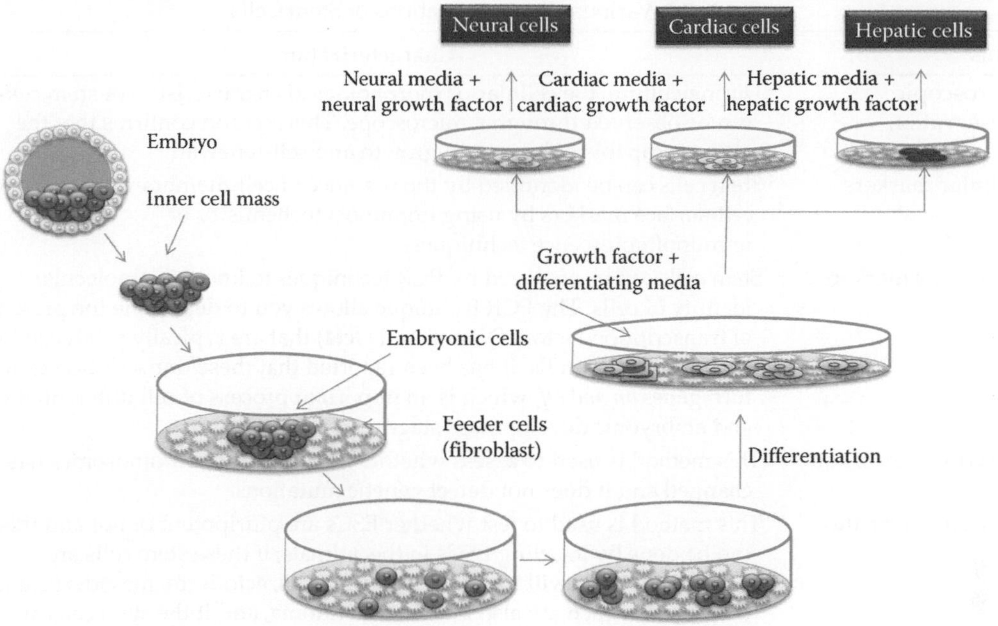

Figure 7.8 Differentiation of embryonic stem cells.

the media that contains serum. One week later, colonies of cells grow out and these cells demonstrate pluripotent characteristics. The colonies of cells have the ability to form three germ layers, differentiate *in vitro*, and form embryoid bodies. These embryoid bodies are commonly known as ESCs. Additionally, to maintain the pluripotency of stem cells, the culture media is delivered with a leukemic inhibitory factor (LIF) and bone morphogenetic proteins (BMPs) that are necessary to prevent ES cells from differentiating. Moreover, these factors are extremely important for the efficiency of deriving ES cells.

7.3.1.3 *Identification of ESCs*

While isolating and deriving ESCs, it is very important to know the identity of stem cells and their cellular, molecular, and functional characteristics. The various characteristics of ESCs are given in Table 7.2.

7.3.1.4 *Differentiation of ESCs*

One of the main characteristics of ESCs is to give rise to many cell types, which have been demonstrated in a number of experiments conducted using *in vitro* cell method. Under specific culture conditions and balanced nutrients presence, these ESCs can be differentiated to form various body cells types such as heart, skin, kidney, nerve, and many other cell types. Over the last few years, efforts have been made to develop basic methods to differentiate ESCs into some specific cell types. These differentiated cells such as neural cells or cardiomyocytes can be used to treat Parkinson's disease and heart infarction.

7.3.2 *Adult stem cells*

Unlike ESCs, adult stem cells can be found in an adult living body. The primary role of adult stem cells in an individual is to maintain and repair the body cells or tissue in which they are found. The adult stem cells are also called somatic stem cells. ESCs are defined by

Table 7.2 Various Characterizations of Stem Cells

Tools	Characterization
Microscopic observation	During culture, the cellular or morphological characteristics of stem cells can be observed through a microscope. This method confirms that the cells are capable of long-term growth and self-renewal.
Cellular markers	Stem cells can be identified by the presence of cell-membrane markers or cell-surface markers by using immunocytochemistry or immunofluorescence techniques.
Molecular markers	Stem cells can be analyzed by PCR techniques to know the molecular identity of cells. The PCR technique allows you to determine the presence of transcription factors (Nanog and Oct4) that are typically produced by undifferentiated cells. It has been reported that these transcription factors turn genes *on and off*, which is an important process of cell differentiation and embryonic development stages.
Karyotype technique	This method is used to assess whether the number of chromosomes has changed and it does not detect genetic mutations.
Teratoma formation	This method is used to test whether ESCs are pluripotent or not and this can be done by injecting ESCs in the animals; if these stem cells are pluripotent, they will form three germ layers, ectoderm, mesoderm, and endoderm, which are also known as teratoma, and if the stem cells are not pluripotent stem cells, they will not form three germ layers.
Animal studies	To check the functionality of stem cells, stem cells are injected in the animal model of diseases.

their origin, and the origin of adult stem cells is generally based on its location, for example, the neural stem cells are known to be present in the brain, whereas skin stem cells are present in the skin. Moreover, adult stem cells are located in many more tissues than once thought possible. Adult stem cells have many applications, and one of the most important applications is its use in the treatment of degenerative diseases such as Parkinson's and Alzheimer's disease (Figure 7.9).

The significance of adult stem cells has generated tremendous interest among scientists to explore its various benefits, and in 1950, researchers revealed that the bone marrow contains two types of stem cells. They are hematopoietic stem cells (HSCs), which form all types

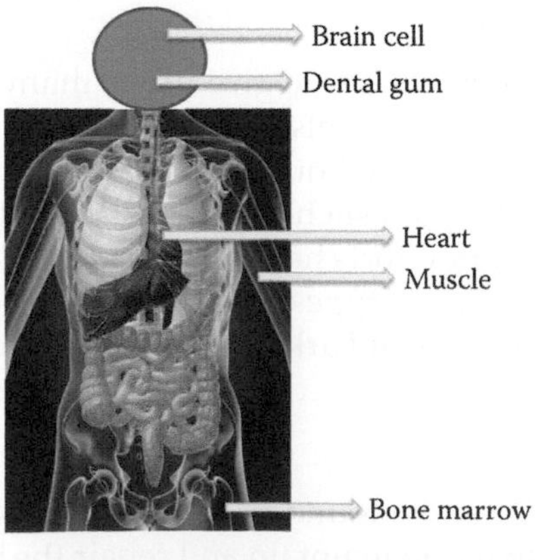

Figure 7.9 Localization of stem sells in the adult human.

of blood cells in the body, and bone marrow stromal stem cells, also known as mesenchymal stem cells or skeletal stem cells by some researchers. In an adult body, non-HSCs contain a small amount of stromal cell population located in the bone marrow that can generate cartilage, fat, and bone cells. These cells can also support the formation of blood and fiber connective tissues. Furthermore, it has been found that two areas of the brain contain dividing cells and these cells finally become nerve cells, but most researchers believed that the adult brain could not generate new nerve cells. But then, again in the 1990s, scientists accepted that the adult brain does embrace stem cells that are able to produce the brain's cells.

7.3.2.1 *Localization of adult stem cells*

Adult stem cells are known to reside in many body organs and tissues, which include brain, blood vessels, skeletal muscle, skin, teeth, heart, gut, liver, ovarian epithelium, bone marrow, peripheral blood, and testis. Furthermore, stem cells are located in a precise area of each tissue or organ, which is called a *stem cell niche*. In many tissues, it has been suggested that some types of adult stem cells are pericytes, which means cells that comprise the outermost layer of small blood vessels. In the body, these adult stem cells may remain in a nondividing state for long periods of time until they are activated by disease or tissue injury. Interestingly, the population of adult stem cells is found to be small in number in each tissue, and once isolated from the body, these adult stem cells do not divide easily and only small amounts of cells can be generated. Over the last few years, efforts have been made to find better ways to cultivate large numbers of adult stem cells in laboratory setups and to differentiate them to get specific cell types so that these cells can be used to treat injury or disease.

7.3.2.2 *Identification of adult stem cells*

Like ESCs, adult stem cells do undergo testing for cellular, molecular, and functional characterization. The markers specifically for the adult stem cells are being used to identify and confirm the nature of adult stem cells.

7.3.2.3 *Differentiation of adult stem cells*

Like other ESCs, the adult stem cells can also differentiate into tissue-specific cell lineage in the body such as nerve cells, cardiomyocytes, or hepatocytes. The process of differentiation is generally initiated based on the body's demand in the event of injury or cell dysfunction and most of the differentiation occurs in the tissue in which they reside. Moreover, HSCs can form all types of blood cells such as T lymphocytes, red blood cells, B lymphocytes, basophils, eosinophils, natural killer cells, neutrophils, monocytes, and macrophages. Moreover, mesenchymal stem cells can form a variety of cell types that include bone cells (osteocytes), fat cells (adipocytes), cartilage cells (chondrocytes), and other types of connective tissue cells such as tendon muscles. In the case of brain stem cells, three kinds of neural cells can be obtained from neural stem cells: neurons and two nonneuronal cell types, astrocytes and oligodendrocytes (Figure 7.10). Additionally, epithelial stem cells located in the lining of the digestive tract give rise to several cell types such as absorptive cells, goblet cells, and enteroendocrine cells, whereas skin stem cells occur in the basal layer of the epidermis giving rise to hair follicles.

7.3.2.4 *Transdifferentiation capabilities of adult stem cells*

Interestingly, certain adult stem cell types can be transdifferentiated into other cell types; for example, brain stem cells can be differentiated into blood cells, or blood-forming cells can be differentiated into cardiac muscle cells. The process of differentiation of neural cells into pancreatic cells is called transdifferentiation. Moreover, only a small number of cells undergo

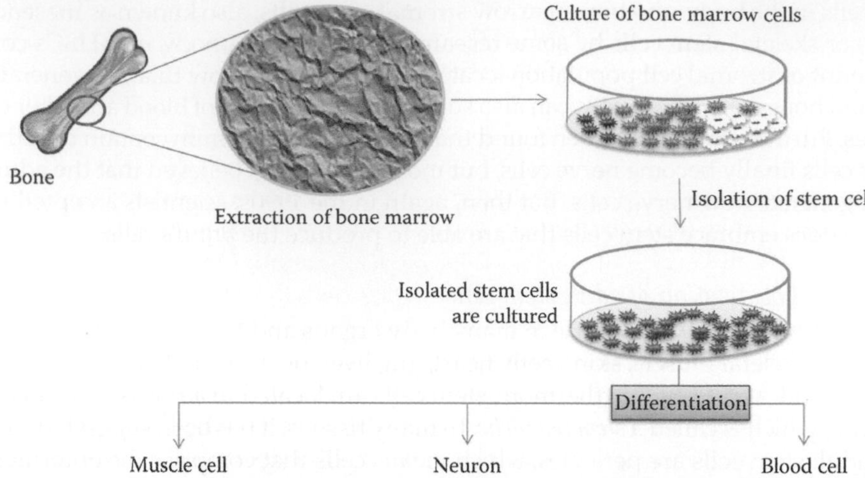

Figure 7.10 Differentiation of adult stem cells into neural cells, muscle cells, and blood cells.

transdifferentiation. The process of transdifferentiation has been observed in some vertebrate species, including humans. In humans, it has been shown that adult corneal stem cells can be differentiated into neural cells. This has led scientists to explore adult stem cells to know more about the transdifferential capabilities and a variety of experiments have been performed. It was recently established that certain adult cell types can be differentiated into other cell types *in vivo* using the genetic modification method. Furthermore, this strategy can offer a system to reprogram the available adult or somatic cells into other cell types that have become dysfunctional or damaged due to a certain disease or injury. One recent report showed that pancreatic ß-cells can be reprogrammed to make insulin-producing cells. These reprogrammed pancreatic cells did produce and secrete insulin-expressed genes specific of ß-cells, and were able to partially restore blood sugar level in animal testing.

7.3.3 Embryonic and adult stem cells: Similarities and differences

Although both adult and embryonic stem cells have plenty of applications, both have advantages and disadvantages over each other. Moreover, one major difference between adult and embryonic stem cells is pluripotency; as ESCs are pluripotent, they can form all cell types of the body, whereas if adult stem cells are multipotent, they can only form the organ- or tissue-specific cell in which they reside. Furthermore, ESCs can be grown relatively easily and in large quantities in *in vitro* culture condition, whereas adult stem cells cannot be grown in large quantities as they are difficult to grow in *in vitro* culture conditions (Figure 7.11). It has been further suggested that cells differentiated from adult stem cell source can be easily transplanted in autologous patients, whereas cells differentiated from ESCs cannot be transplanted in unrelated patients because of the likelihood of cells being rejected after transplantation.

7.4 Induced pluripotent stem cells

With a view to isolate pluripotent stem cells from adult cells, tremendous efforts have made over the last few years, and researchers were able to develop new types of pluripotent stem cells from an adult source by genetic manipulation. These types of genetically modified

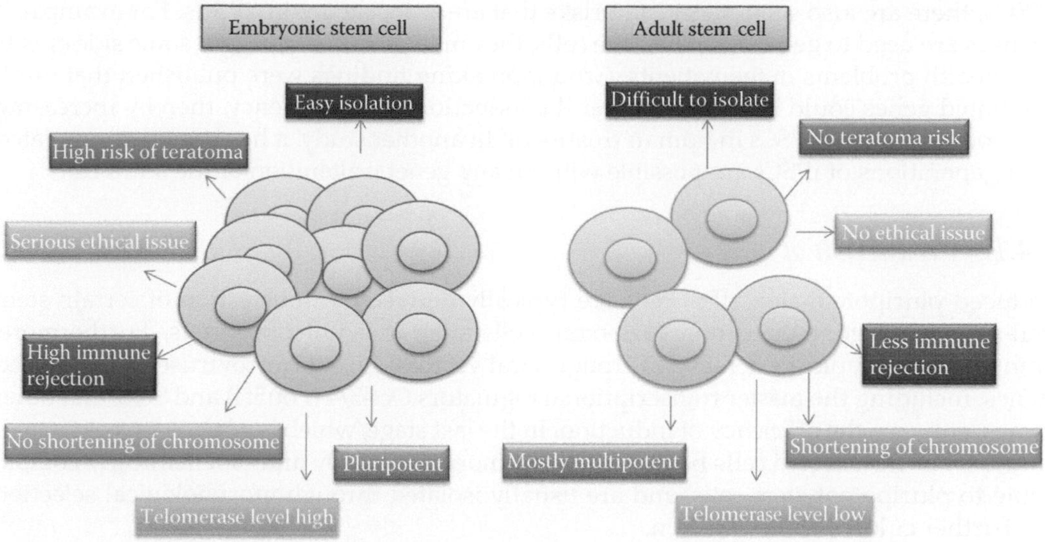

Figure 7.11 Difference between embryonic and adult stem cells.

pluripotent stem cells are known as induced pluripotent stem cells (iPSCs). Although these iPSCs meet the basic criteria of pluripotent stem cells, it is not known whether iPSCs are different from ESCs in their functionality. The first report of iPSCs was published in 2006, where mouse iPSCs demonstrated pluripotency, and data were supported by cellular and molecular analysis and functional analysis. The development of iPSCs is considered a significant development in stem cell research, as it may allow both the researcher and the clinician to use it for cell-based therapy (Figure 7.12). In addition to any benefits of having

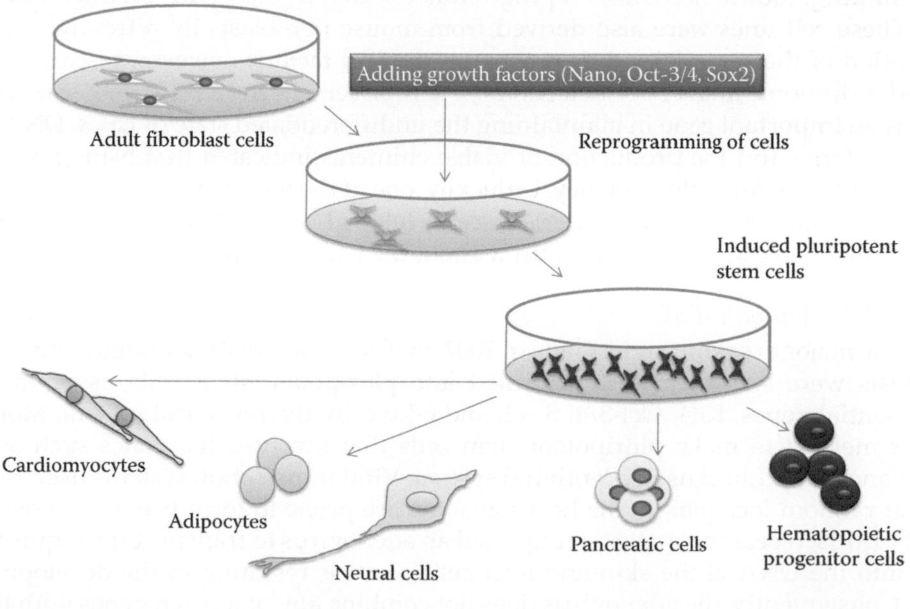

Figure 7.12 Induced pluripotent stem cells.

iPSCs, there are also some significant risks that are associated with iPSCs. For example, if viruses are used to genetically alter the cells, they may potentially trigger some side effects and health problems in the patients. Groundbreaking findings were published that viral-mediated genes could be removed after the induction of pluripotency, thereby increasing the potential use of iPSCs in human treatment. In another study, it has been demonstrated that generations of iPSCs are possible without any genetic alteration of the adult cells.

7.4.1 Production of iPSCs

Induced pluripotent stem (iPS) cells are typically derived by transfection of certain stem cell-associated genes into nonpluripotent cells such as adult fibroblasts. Furthermore, transfection is typically achieved through viral vectors, such as retroviruses. Transfected genes, including the master transcriptional regulators Oct-3/4 (Pou5f1) and Sox2 and other genes, enhance the efficiency of induction. In the last stage, which is after 3–4 weeks, small numbers of transfected cells begin to become morphologically and biochemically comparable to pluripotent stem cells, and are usually isolated through morphological selection for further culture and expansion.

7.4.1.1 First generation

iPSCs were first generated by Shinya Yamanaka's team at Kyoto University, Japan in 2006. They used genes that had been identified as particularly important in ESC development and used retroviruses to transfect mouse fibroblasts. After cell culture, pluripotency genes (Oct-3/4, Sox2, c-Myc, and Klf4) that are essential for the production of pluripotent stem cells were isolated and pluripotent stem cells were isolated by antibiotic selection of Fbx15+ cells. However, these iPSCs showed structural problem in DNA methylation and failed to produce viable chimeras upon injecting iPSCs into developing embryos.

7.4.1.2 Second generation

In one finding, mouse fibroblasts reprogrammed into iPS cells could produce viable chimera. These cell lines were also derived from mouse fibroblasts by retroviral-mediated reactivation of the same four endogenous pluripotent factors; however, researchers now selected a different marker for detection. As a replacement for Fbx15, they used Nanog, which is an important gene in maintaining the undifferentiated state of ESCs. DNA methylation patterns and the production of viable chimeras indicated that Nanog is a major determinant of cellular pluripotency. Unluckily, one of the four genes used, such as c-Myc, is oncogenic, and 20% of the chimeric mice developed cancer. Furthermore, it has been reported that one can create iPSCs even without the use of c-Myc.

7.4.1.3 Human iPSCs

One of the major breakthroughs made in 2007 on iPSCs was creating human cells. Human fibroblasts were successfully transformed into pluripotent stem cells using the same four essential genes, Klf4, Oct-3/4, Sox2, and c-Myc, by the retroviral system. Moreover, another method to make pluripotent stem cells that involved the genes such as Oct4, Sox2, Nanog, and Lin28 used a lentiviral system. Viral transfection systems used to insert genes at random locations in the host's genome are prone to form tumors. To overcome these hazards, researchers successfully used an adenovirus to transport the requisite four genes into the DNA of the skin and liver cells of mice, resulting in the development of iPSCs. Consequently, the adenovirus does not combine any of its own genes with the targeted host and the danger of creating tumors is eliminated, although this method has not yet been tested on human cells. Other methods have also been tested to generate iPSCs by using plasmid without any virus transfection system at all, but with very low success rates.

7.4.2 Identification of iPSCs

Interestingly, iPSCs that expressed cell surface antigenic markers are only known to express in ESCs. These surface markers are SSEA-3, SSEA-4, TRA-1-60, TRA-1-81, TRA-2-49/6E, and Nanog. Moreover, iPSCs are expressed in SSEA-1 but not in SSEA-3 nor SSEA-4. Interestingly, iPSC genes expressed in undifferentiated ESCs include Oct-3/4, Sox2, Nanog, GDF3, ESG1, DPPA2, DPPA4, REX1, FGF4, and hTERT.

7.4.3 Differentiation into ectoderm, mesoderm, and endoderm lineages

iPSCs can be successfully differentiated into neuronal lineages under specific culture conditions. The presence of dopamine-like immunreactivity in the differentiated cells suggests that iPSCs, such as ESCs, can also be differentiated into dopaminergic neurons. Furthermore, iPSCs can also be differentiated into cardiomyocytes that unexpectedly began beating. Another critical test for iPSCs is to disclose their ability to form three germ layers. It has been found that iPSCs injected into immunodeficient mice formed teratoma (three germ layers, ectoderm, mesoderm, and endoderm) after 9 weeks. Teratoma formation is a ground-breaking test for pluripotency.

7.5 Applications of stem cells

There are many applications of human stem cells both in research and the clinic and we have discussed some of the major applications of stem cells (Figure 7.13). Stroke and traumatic brain injury can lead to cell death, which are normally categorized by a loss of neurons and oligodendrocytes within the brain. Stem cells can be used to treat neurodegenerative diseases such as Parkinson's and Alzheimer's disease. Using traditional procedures, brain

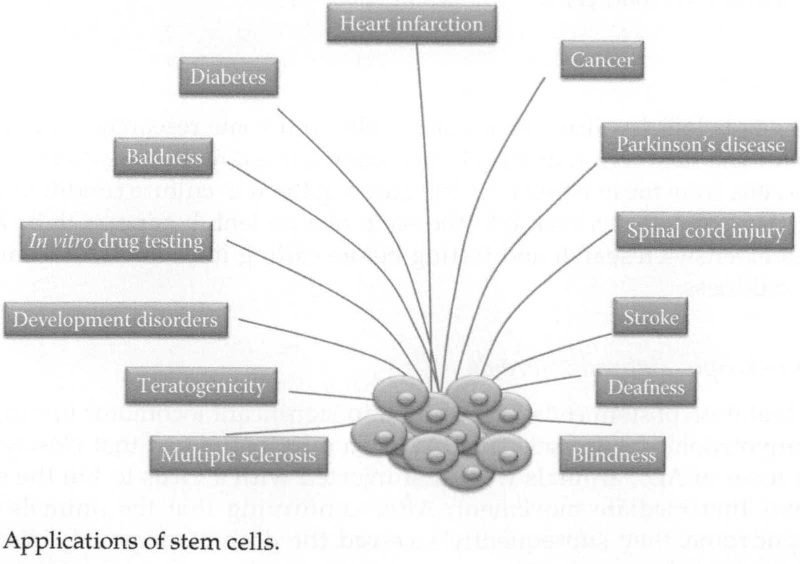

Figure 7.13 Applications of stem cells.

cancer is difficult to treat because it spreads very rapidly. Human neural stem cells were transplanted into the brain of rodents induced with intracranial tumors. After a few days, the animals were sacrificed and it was found that stem cells could migrate into the cancerous area and produced an enzyme "cytosine deaminase" that converts a nontoxic prodrug into a chemotherapeutic agent. Consequently, the injected substance was able to reduce the tumor size drastically. Moreover, these transplanted stem cells were neither differentiated nor did they turned tumorigenic.

A patient who was not able to stand for approximately 19 years due to spinal cord injury, is recovered with transplantation of stem cells derived from umbilical cord blood. Furthermore, scientists have transplanted human fetal-derived neural stem cells into paralyzed mice; the transplantation caused an improvement in locomotor functions. Additionally, the functional or behavioral recovery was due to the successful differentiation of transplanted cells into new neurons and oligodendrocytes. In addition, researchers were able to differentiate human blastocyst stem cells into neural stem cells and finally into spinal motor neurons.

7.5.1 *Heart damage*

Adult stem cell therapy is harmless, effective, and efficient in treating old and recent heart infarcts. Furthermore, adult stem cell can be used for treating heart disease with high success rate and without having ethical issues. It is now possible to differentiate bone marrow cells into heart muscle cells.

7.5.2 *Blood cell formation*

With a view to fulfill the ever-growing demand of blood requirements for patients worldwide, efforts have been made to make blood from stem cells. Now, it is possible to produce fully mature human red blood by HSCs, which are predecessors of red blood cells. In the process of generating blood, HSCs are cultured along with stromal cells by producing an environment that mimics that of the bone marrow (the site of red blood cell growth). Erythropoietin, a growth factor, is generally added to complete the terminal differentiation of HSCs into red blood cells.

7.5.3 *Baldness*

Interestingly, hair follicles also contain stem cells, and some researchers predict that the isolation of follicle stem cells may help treat baldness one day. This treatment can work by taking stem cells from the existing follicles, growing them in culture condition, and finally implanting the new follicles back into the scalp of a patient. It appears to be a nice idea, but requires extensive research and testing before calling it a successful stem cell-based therapy for baldness.

7.5.4 *Amyotrophic lateral sclerosis*

The transplantation of stem cells has resulted in significant locomotor improvements in rats with amyotrophic lateral sclerosis (ALS). In a rodent model that closely resembles the human form of ALS, animals were first injected with a virus to kill the spinal cord motor nerves that mediate movement. After confirming that the animals developed ALS-like syndrome, they subsequently received the dose of stem cells injected in the spinal cord. It has been found that transplanted stem cells migrated to the sites of injury, caused regeneration of the damages or nonfunctional nerve cells, and restored locomotor function.

7.5.5 Orthopedics

The transplantation of mesenchymal stem cells has increased cartilage and meniscus volume in individual human subjects; however, the results of clinical trials are yet to be established. In contrast, safety studies conducted in a group of 227 patients over a 3- to 4-year period showed minimal complications associated with mesenchymal cell transplantation.

7.5.6 Infertility

Human ESCs can be differentiated into precursor cells of oocytes and spermatozoa as evidenced by gene expression analysis. Although an attempt has been made to make human ESCs into spermatozoon-like cells, a normal and functional spermatozoa could not be made.

7.6 Stem cell transplantation

One of the most significant applications of stem cells is to treat various degenerative diseases in humans, which include cancer, Parkinson's disease, Huntington's disease, celiac disease, cardiac failure, Type 1 diabetes mellitus, muscle damage, neurological disorders, and many others.

7.6.1 Hematopoietic stem cell transplantation

Hematopoietic stem cell transplantation (HSCT) is the most widely used stem cell transplantation in patients who are suffering from diseases of the blood or bone marrow, or certain types of cancer. The HSCs are collected from the peripheral blood such as cord blood or placenta, instead of the bone marrow. Moreover, the collection of peripheral blood stem cells provides a bigger graft and does not require that the donor undergo anesthesia to collect the graft. The HSCT can be used in a variety of disease conditions such as multiple myeloma or leukemia, severe combined immunodeficiency, or congenital neutropenia. Additionally, there are other conditions that can be treated with stem cell transplants, including neuroblastoma, lymphoma, Ewing's sarcoma, sickle-cell disease, myelodysplastic syndrome, desmoplastic small round cell tumor, and Hodgkin's disease.

7.6.1.1 Autologous transplantation

Autologous HSCT requires the extraction of stem cells directly from the same patient or by retrieving from a stem cell bank. The patient is then treated with high-dose chemotherapy with or without radiotherapy with the intention of eradicating the patient's malignant cell population by partially or completely ablating the bone marrow population. Once the patient's own stem cells are isolated, they are stored either in the patient or in the stem cell bank. Furthermore, autologous transplants have the advantage of a lower risk of infection during the immune-compromised portion of the treatment since the recovery of immune function is rapid. Additionally, the incidence of patients experiencing rejection is very rare due to the donor and recipient being the same individual. Consequently, these advantages have established autologous HSC transplantation as one of the standard second-line treatments for diseases such as lymphoma. On the other hand, for other diseases such as acute myeloid leukemia, allogeneic HSC transplantation is not a favorable therapy and maybe autologous transplantation could be preferred for these conditions.

7.6.1.2 *Allogeneic transplantation*

Allogeneic HSC transplantation involves two people, such as the donor and the patient, who is basically the recipient. It has been recommended that the allogeneic HSC donors must have a tissue HLA type that matches the recipient. Moreover, matching is performed on the basis of inconsistency at three or more loci of the HLA gene, and a perfect match at these loci is desired. In case HLA does not match completely, the recipient requires immunosuppressive medications to diminish graft-versus-host disease (GVHD). In a broad sense, by transplanting healthy stem cells into the recipient's immune system, allogeneic HCSTs appear to improve chances for cure or at least enhance long-term survival of transplants. It has been further suggested that a mismatch of an HLA Type II gene such as HLA-DR or HLA-DQB1 can increase the risk of GVHD. In addition, race and ethnicity are known to play a major role in donor recruitment efforts, as members of the same racial individual are more likely to have matching genes, including the genes for HLA.

7.6.1.3 *Posttransplantation problems associated with HSCT*

There are problems associated with HSCT and a 10% or higher mortality rate in the recipients has been reported. It has been suggested that bone marrow transplantation usually requires that the recipient's own bone marrow needs to be destroyed to make an effective therapy. Prior to engraftment, patients generally undergo treatment for several weeks without appreciable numbers of white blood cells to help fight the infection. However, this puts a patient at a high risk of infections despite using prophylactic antibiotics, which causes a large share of treatment-related mortality. Furthermore, the use of immunosuppressive agents employed in allogeneic transplants for the prevention or treatment of GVHD further increases the risk of opportunistic infection. Immunosuppressive drugs are given for a minimum of 6 month time period after transplantation. In addition to the above-mentioned problems, there are other pathological problems that arise, which include severe liver injury that is termed as hepatic veno-occlusive disease (VOD), higher levels of bilirubin, and fluid retention. These are the clinical hallmarks of this condition. Moreover, GVHD is an inflammatory disease that is unique to allogeneic transplantation and new bone marrow immune cells can act against the recipient's tissues. This can occur even if the donor and recipient are HLA-identical because the immune system can still recognize other differences between their tissues.

7.6.2 *ESC transplantation*

The clinical trial using oligodendrocytes derived from human ES cells into spinal cord-injured individuals was initiated in 2009 and received approval from the United States. It has been reported that the U.S. FDA approved the world's first human ES cell human clinical trial. This clinical trial was mainly conducted to test the safety of cell transplantation in patients, but the trial was suspended in August 2009 due to the discovery of a small number of microscopic cysts found in several treated rat models. Suspension was lifted in July 30, 2010, and subsequently, in October 2010, researchers registered and administered ES transplantations to the first patient at Shepherd Center in Atlanta, Georgia, the USA.

7.7 Stem cell-based therapy: Global perspective

Although stem cell therapy is still under development stage around the world, in China, stem cell-based treatment is currently being practiced in many hospitals and clinics. The Ministry of Health of China has also legalized stem cell-based therapy for various degenerative diseases. In eastern China, hospitals provide numerous cell therapies to patients who are suffering from neurodegenerative and cardiovascular disorders. Although there is a demand for stem cell-based therapy in China, the regulatory policy on stem cell therapy is still unclear, and thus, in the absence of a valid clinical trial protocol, it may pose a health risk to many patients. Besides China, stem cell research has also been developed in different parts of the world, including the United Kingdom, Germany, India, Mexico, and South Korea.

7.8 Application of stem cells in drug testing

The main application of human stem cells is to generate millions of cells to be used in the treatment of various degenerative diseases. Besides being used as a cell-based therapy, human stem cells can also be used to test new drug molecules; for instance, new drug molecules can be used to test the safety of cells generated from human pluripotent cell lines. There are different kinds of cell lines that are commercially available to be used for testing new drug molecules. It has been reported that cancer cell lines are used to screen potential antitumor drugs. The availability of pluripotent stem cells will allow drug testing in a wider range of cell types, such as liver, heart, or neural cells. However, to screen drugs effectively, the conditions must be identical when comparing different drugs; subsequently, scientists need to make a precise differentiation of stem cells into the precise cell type on which drugs are to be tried.

7.8.1 Significance of testing using human cells

Drug development is an amazingly expensive and lingering process. Typically, it costs around $1 billion to bring a new drug to the market and the whole process usually takes about 10–15 years. Before new drugs can go forward for clinical trials, it is necessary for the biochemical compounds that make up a drug to undergo extensive testing before beginning trials on animals. Moreover, it is really important for the pharmaceutical industry to have proper test systems work on these kinds of things. Stem cell-based drug testing is already being promoted in the United Kingdom by the public/private initiatives.

7.8.2 ESCs and drug testing

ESCs also hold promise on the front end of drug discovery. Disease genes are inserted into ESCs, which are then persuaded to differentiate into human disease tissues that can be used to screen for drugs. The kinds of *in vitro* models of the human tissue based on ESCs are as diverse as the cell types they generate, although many stem cell researchers in both academia and industry see the primary promise of stem cells as direct therapeutics. Furthermore, the most successful development of stem cells as *in vitro* models for toxicology testing is in the human cardiac tissue. Many drugs have been removed from the market as a consequence of cardiac toxicity. An infamous example is terfenadine, an antihistamine that caused close to 100 deaths as a consequence of adverse cardiac events when it was released in the market. ESCs have since been differentiated into cardiac tissue, which shows potential as a toxicological model of the disease, and many companies involved in using ESCs have research programs in this area. Developing stem cell models of the liver, the other major organ that animal models fail to emulate, has been more difficult but is nevertheless a main focus of many researchers and companies working in this area. Where the promise of stem cells falls short is in their modeling of systemic toxicity. Sometimes, one organ alters a drug in some way, but this subsequent metabolite is toxic only to a different organ. Since stem cells in a dish reflect only a single organ's response to a drug, there would be no way to check the impact of subsequent metabolites on the whole organism.

7.9 Stem cell banks

Over the last two decades, enormous interest has been generated to collect stem cells from different sources, and both private and governmental agencies have established stem cell banks in various parts of the world. The main objective of the creation of such stem cell bank facilities is to provide the access of stem cells to physicians for patients suffering from diseases. One of the highly successful and rewarding stem cell banks is umbilical cord stem cells, also known as cord blood stem cell banks.

7.9.1 Cord blood bank

The cord blood bank is a facility that normally stores umbilical cord blood for future use. The cord blood comprises HSCs, which are basically progenitor cells that form red blood cells, white blood cells, and platelets. It has been reported that both private and public cord blood banks have been established in the mid-1990s in response to the potential demand for cord blood. Unlike private cord blood banking, public cord blood banking is supported/sponsored by federal or state government agencies. It has been recommended that an expectant mother who is interested in cord blood donation must contact the bank before the 34th week of pregnancy. In the United States, the National Marrow Donor Program has listed public cord blood banks on their website and once the cord blood is donated, it loses all identifying information after a short period of initial testing, whereas families are not able to recover their own blood after it has been donated. In the case of private banks, the family can recover it later if it is needed. It has been suggested that the parents have custody of the cord blood until the child is an adult. It has been reported that private banks charge a fee of around 1000–$2000 to preserve the harvested cord blood for family biological insurance. In the United States, the FDA regulates cord blood under the group of human cells, tissues, and cellular- and tissue-based products category. It is found in the Code of Federal Regulations under which the U.S. FDA regulates public and private cord blood banking. It has been suggested that both public and private cord blood banks are eligible for voluntary certification with either the American Association of Blood Banks or the Foundation for the Accreditation of Cellular Therapy.

7.9.1.1 Banking umbilical cord tissue

Expectant parents can collect and preserve stem cells from the donated umbilical cord, also known as Wharton's jelly. This cord blood is known to be a rich source of HSCs that upon differentiation form blood cells. Additionally, this cord tissue is also a rich source of mesenchymal stem cells. Mesenchymal stem cells differentiate to form bone, cartilage, and connective tissues, and are effective in facilitating the body's inflammatory response to damaged or injured cells. Furthermore, the umbilical cord can produce between 21 and 500 million mesenchymal stem cells.

7.9.1.2 Collection and preservation of umbilical cord stem cells

The cord blood collection can take place after the umbilical cord has been surgically cut and is removed from the fetal end of the cord. It is typically done within 10–15 min of giving birth. Moreover, additional stem cells may be collected from the placenta through placenta cord banking. Once the health-care provider draws the cord blood from the end of the placenta umbilical cord, the placenta is then dispatched to the cell culture laboratory, where stem cells are isolated. An adequate cord blood collection requires a minimum of 75 mL to ensure that there are enough cells to be used for transplantation in the patients. Before the blood is stored in the freezer, the blood is processed for viral testing such as for HIV and hepatitis B and C, and tissue typing to determine the HLA type. After the completion of collection and testing phases, the cord blood unit is shipped to the laboratory and then cryopreserved in liquid nitrogen tank. Moreover, there are many procedures to process a cord blood unit as some method allows the separation of the red blood cells and others keep the red blood cells. Upon processing blood units, a cryopreservant is added to the cord blood to allow the cells to live in the cryogenic condition for a long period of time. Once the unit is slowly cooled to minus 90°C, cells can be kept in a liquid nitrogen tank that will keep the cord blood cells frozen at minus 196°C. The slow-freezing process is important to keep the cells alive. Furthermore, the protocols used for the cryopreservation of stem cells are similar to the bone marrow hematopoietic stem or progenitor cells. There is no consensus yet on optimal procedures for the cryopreservation of these cord blood cells, although many cryopreservation strategies suggest that dimethyl sulfoxide (DMSO) generally is a good cryopreservant for stem cells.

7.9.1.3 Therapeutics use of umbilical cord stem cells

Cord blood stem cells can be used in treating brain injury and Type 1 diabetes, stroke, and hearing loss. It has been estimated that approximately one in three Americans could benefit from stem cells, and children whose cord blood stem cells are stored in the bank can also benefit in the future. Moreover, there is no risk of the immune rejection of the cells for autologous transplantation. A clinical trial is being conducted to examine how transplantation of autologous cord blood stem cells into children with Type 1 diabetes will affect the metabolic control over time, compared to standard insulin treatments. Interestingly, preliminary results establish that transplantation of cord blood stem cells is a safe procedure and therapeutically effective in slowing down the loss of insulin production in children with Type 1 diabetes. Additionally, umbilical cord blood stem cells carry great promise in cardiovascular repairs as investigators are finding several positive results in animal studies.

7.10 Hurdles in ESC research

To make ESCs an effective and realistic therapy, several key issues need to be addressed. It has been reported that the use of human ESCs need a lifelong use of drugs to prevent rejection of the tissue. A more serious disadvantage of using ESCs is that they can produce unwanted tumors when injected into adult patients. Another disadvantage is the use of animal-contaminated ESCs, where ESCs are grown on mouse fibroblast that can cause the animal diseases upon transplantation. If any of this research is to turn into treatments, it will need endorsement from the U.S. FDA, which requires special safeguards to prevent the transmission of animal diseases to people. It is uncertain how many of these cell lines were developed with the safety measure in place. This may cause a host of problems related to transgenic issues. A fourth disadvantage reported that mice cloned from ESC were genetically defective. If human ESC is also genetically unstable, it could cause serious health problems.

7.11 Summary

Stem cells are highly specialized cells of the human body that are present in all mammalian species. These specialized stem cells have two distinct features: their ability to renew through mitotic cell division and their ability to differentiate into all types of body cells. Broadly speaking, there are two types of mammalian stem cells: adult stem cells and ESCs. The ESCs are isolated from the inner cell mass of blastocysts, whereas adult stem cells are those that are found in adult tissues. One of the interesting characteristics of stem cells is that they can now be grown and differentiated into specialized cells with characteristics of various tissues such as muscle, kidney, or brain cells. There are many applications of stem cells and it has been suggested that stem cell therapy has the potential to change the treatment of human disease, especially Parkinson's disease and Alzheimer's disease. Interestingly, a number of stem cell therapies have been in use in clinics, predominantly bone marrow transplants from adult stem cells that are used to treat leukemia. In the near future, ESCs could be used to treat a variety of diseases, including cancer, spinal cord injuries, ALS, multiple sclerosis, muscle damage, and other degenerative diseases. Nevertheless, there still exists a great deal of technical issues to be resolved to make stem cell-based therapy a success. One apprehension of treatment is the possible risk that transplanted ESCs isolated from the embryo could form tumors and have the likelihood of becoming malignant if cell division continues nonstop.

7.12 Scholar's achievements

Martin Evans: Sir Martin John Evans, FRS, is a British scientist who, with Matthew Kaufman, was the first to culture mice ESCs and cultivate them in the laboratory in 1981. He is also known, along with Mario Capecchi and Oliver Smithies, for his work in the development of the knockout mouse and the related technology of gene targeting, a method of using ESCs to create specific gene modifications in mice. In 2007, the three shared the Nobel Prize in Physiology or Medicine in recognition of their discovery and contribution to the development of new treatments for illnesses in humans.

Matthew Kaufman: Matthew H. Kaufman is a professor emeritus at the University of Edinburgh having been the professor of anatomy there from 1985 to 2007. He has taught anatomy and embryology for more than 30 years, initially at the University of Cambridge, when he was a Fellow of King's College, and more recently (from 1985 to 1997) in Edinburgh. In 1981, Kaufman and Martin Evans at the University of Cambridge in England and Gail R. Martin in America were the first to derive ES cells from mouse embryos.

G.R. Martin: Professor Gail R. Martin is in charge of the developmental biology program at the University of California, San Francisco. She is a member of the American Academy of Arts and Sciences, a member of the National Academy of Sciences (cellular and developmental biology), and is the president of the Society for Developmental Biology. In 1981, Martin, working at the University of California, San Francisco, and Martin Evans and Matthew Kaufman, working at the University of Cambridge, England, separately and simultaneously discovered techniques for extracting stem cells from mouse embryos. Martin is attributed with coining the term "embryonic stem cell."

James Thomson: James Alexander Thomson (born December 20, 1958) is an American developmental biologist best known for deriving the first human embryonic stem cell (SC) line in 1998 and for deriving human iPS cells in 2007. He serves as the director of regenerative biology at the Morgridge Institute for Research in Madison, Wisconsin, as a professor in the Department of Cell and Regenerative Biology at the University of Wisconsin

School of Medicine and Public Health, and as a professor in the Molecular, Cellular, and Developmental Biology Department at the University of California, Santa Barbara. He is also a founder and chief scientific officer for Cellular Dynamics International, a Madison-based company producing derivatives of human iPSCs for drug discovery and toxicity testing.

7.13 Knowledge builder

Embryonic stem cells: ES cells are pluripotent stem cells derived from the inner cell mass of a blastocyst, an early-stage embryo. Human embryos reach the blastocyst stage 4–5 days postfertilization, at which time they consist of 50–150 cells. Isolating the embryo blast or inner cell mass (ICM) results in the destruction of the fertilized human embryo, which raises ethical issues. Human embryonic stem cells have the potential to differentiate into various cell types in the body, and are considered to be useful for cell-based therapy or tissue engineering.

Adult stem cells: Adult stem cells are undifferentiated cells, found throughout the body after development, which multiply by cell division to replenish dying cells and regenerate damaged tissues. Also known as somatic stem cells, they can be found in juvenile as well as adult animals and human bodies. Scientific interest in adult stem cells is centered on their ability to divide or self-renew indefinitely, and generate all the cell types of the organ from which they originate, potentially regenerating the entire organ from a few cells. Unlike ESCs, the use of adult stem cells in research and therapy is not considered to be controversial, as they are derived from adult tissue samples rather than destroyed human embryos. They have mainly been studied in humans and model organisms such as mice and rats.

In vitro fertilization: In vitro fertilization (abbreviated as IVF) is a process by which an egg is fertilized by a sperm outside the body: *in vitro.* IVF is a major treatment for infertility when other methods of assisted reproductive technology have failed. The process involves monitoring a woman's ovulatory process, removing egg or eggs from the woman's ovaries, and letting the sperm fertilize them in a fluid medium in a laboratory. When a woman's natural cycle is monitored to collect a naturally selected egg for fertilization, it is known as natural cycle IVF. The fertilized egg, also known as a zygote, is then transferred to the patient's uterus with the intention of establishing a successful pregnancy. The first successful birth of a "test tube baby," Louise Brown, occurred in 1978. Louise Brown was born as a result of the natural cycle IVF. Robert G. Edwards, the physiologist who developed the treatment, was awarded the Nobel Prize in Physiology or Medicine in 2010 for his discovery.

Inner cell mass: In early embryogenesis of most mammals, the inner cell mass (abbreviated as ICM and also known as the embryoblast or pluriblast, the latter term being applicable to all mammals) is the mass of cells inside the primordial embryo that will eventually give rise to the definitive structures of the fetus. This structure forms in the earliest stages of development, before implantation into the endometrium of the uterus has occurred.

Extraembryonic cell: Extraembryonic is external to the embryo.

Pluripotent stem cells: Pluripotent stem cells are often termed "true" stem cells because they have the potential to differentiate into almost any cell in the body. This means that under the right circumstances, a stem cell that is isolated from an embryo can produce almost all the cells in the body. Yet, after this embryonic developmental stage is over, stem cells no longer have this unlimited potential to develop into all cell types. Their pluripotency is thus lost and they can only become certain types of cells.

Teratocarcinoma: Teratocarcinoma, a malignant neoplasm, consisting of elements of the teratoma with those of the embryonal carcinoma or choriocarcinoma, or both, occurrs most often in the testis.

Mitomycin-c: The mitomycins are a family of aziridine-containing natural products isolated from *Streptomyces caespitosus* or *Streptomyces lavendulae*. One of these compounds, mitomycin-c, finds use as a chemotherapeutic agent by virtue of its antitumor antibiotic activity. It is given intravenously to treat upper gastrointestinal (e.g., esophageal carcinoma), anal cancers, and breast cancers, as well as by bladder instillation for superficial bladder tumors.

Self-renewal: It is the ability to go through numerous cycles of cell division while maintaining the undifferentiated state.

Hematopoietic stem cells: HSCs are the blood cells that give rise to all the other blood cells. They give rise to the myeloid (monocytes and macrophages, neutrophils, basophils, eosinophils, erythrocytes, megakaryocytes/platelets, and dendritic cells), and lymphoid lineages (T cells, B cells, and NK cells). The definition of HSCs has changed in the last two decades. The hematopoietic tissue contains cells with long-term and short-term regeneration capacities and committed multipotent, oligopotent, and unipotent progenitors. HSCs constitute 1:10.000 of cells in the myeloid tissue.

Mesenchymal stem cells: Mesenchymal stem cells, or MSCs, are multipotent stromal cells that can differentiate into a variety of cell types, including osteoblasts (bone cells), chondrocytes (cartilage cells), and adipocytes (fat cells). This phenomenon has been documented in specific cells and tissues in living animals and their counterparts growing in tissue culture.

Induced pluripotent stem cells: Induced pluripotent stem cells, commonly abbreviated as iPS cells or iPSCs, are a type of pluripotent stem cell, artificially derived from a nonpluripotent cell—typically an adult somatic cell—by inducing a "forced" expression of specific genes. iPSCs are similar to natural pluripotent stem cells, such as ES cells, in many aspects, such as the expression of certain stem cell genes and proteins, chromatin methylation patterns, doubling time, embryoid body formation, teratoma formation, viable chimera formation, and potency and differentiability, but the full extent of their relation to natural pluripotent stem cells is still being assessed. iPSCs have been made from adult stomach, liver, skin cells, and blood cells. iPSCs were first produced in 2006 from mouse cells and in 2007 from human cells in a series of experiments by Shinya Yamanaka's team at Kyoto University, Japan, and by James Thomson's team at the University of Wisconsin-Madison.

Pluripotency: The ability of a cell to differentiate into different cell types is called pluripotency. The more cell types a stem cell can differentiate into, the greater its potency. Potency is also described as the gene activation potential within a cell, which like a continuum begins with totipotency to designate a cell with the most differentiation potential, pluripotency, multipotency, oligopotency, and finally unipotency.

Transfection: Transfection is the process of deliberately introducing nucleic acids into cells. The term is notably used for nonviral methods in eukaryotic cells. It may also refer to other methods and cell types, although other terms are preferred: "transformation" is more often used to describe nonviral DNA transfer in bacteria, nonanimal eukaryotic cells, and plant cells—a distinctive sense of transformation refers to spontaneous genetic modifications (mutations to cancerous cells (carcinogenesis), or under stress (UV irradiation). Transduction is often used to describe virus-mediated DNA transfer. The word "transfection" is a blend of trans and infection.

DNA methylation: DNA methylation is a biochemical process, involving the addition of a methyl group to the cytosine or adenine DNA nucleotides. DNA methylation stably alters the expression of genes in cells as cells divide and differentiate from ESCs into specific tissues. The resulting change is normally permanent and unidirectional, preventing one organism from reverting to a stem cell or converting into another type of tissue.

Plasmid: A plasmid is a small DNA molecule that is physically separate from, and can replicate independently of, the chromosomal DNA within a cell. Most commonly found as small circular, double-stranded DNA molecules in bacteria, plasmids are sometimes present in archaea and eukaryotic organisms. In nature, plasmids carry genes that may benefit the survival of the organism (e.g., antibiotic resistance), and can frequently be transmitted from one bacterium to another (even of another species) via horizontal gene transfer.

Parkinson's disease: Parkinson's disease is a degenerative disorder of the central nervous system. The motor symptoms of Parkinson's disease result from the death of dopamine-generating cells in the substantia nigra, a region of the midbrain; the cause of this cell death is unknown. Early in the course of the disease, the most obvious symptoms are movement related; these include shaking, rigidity, slowness of movement, and difficulty with walking and gait. Later, thinking and behavioral problems may arise, with dementia commonly occurring in the advanced stages of the disease, whereas depression is the most common psychiatric symptom. Other symptoms include sensory, sleep, and emotional problems. Parkinson's disease is more common in the elderly, with most cases occurring after the age of 50.

Alzheimer's disease: Alzheimer's disease (AD), also known in the medical literature as Alzheimer disease, is the most common form of dementia. There is no cure for the disease, which worsens as it progresses, and eventually leads to death. It was first described by a German psychiatrist and neuropathologist Alois Alzheimer in 1906 and was named after him. Most often, AD is diagnosed in people over 65 years of age, although the less-prevalent early-onset Alzheimer's can occur much earlier. In 2006, there were 26.6 million sufferers worldwide. Alzheimer's is predicted to affect 1 in 85 people globally by 2050.

Neurons: A neuron is an electrically excitable cell that processes and transmits information through electrical and chemical signals. A chemical signal occurs via a synapse, a specialized connection with other cells. Neurons connect to each other to form neural networks. Neurons are the core components of the nervous system, which includes the brain, spinal cord, and peripheral ganglia. A number of specialized types of neurons exist: sensory neurons respond to touch, sound, light, and numerous other stimuli affecting cells of the sensory organs that then send signals to the spinal cord and brain. Motor neurons receive signals from the brain and spinal cord, cause muscle contractions, and affect glands. Interneurons connect neurons to other neurons within the same region of the brain or spinal cord.

Oligodendrocytes: Oligodendrocytes are a type of brain cell. They are a variety of neuroglia. Their main functions are to provide support and to insulate the axons (the long projection of nerve cells) in the central nervous system (the brain and spinal cord) of some vertebrates. Oligodendrocytes do this by creating the myelin sheath, which is 80% lipid and 20% protein. A single oligodendrocyte can extend its processes to 50 axons, wrapping approximately 1 μm of myelin sheath around each axon; Schwann cells, on the other hand, can wrap around only one axon. Each oligodendrocyte forms one segment of myelin for several adjacent axons.

Neuroblastoma: Neuroblastoma (NB) is the most common extracranial solid cancer in childhood and the most common cancer in infancy, with an annual incidence of about 650 cases per year in the United States and a hundred cases per year in the United Kingdom. Nearly half of the neuroblastoma cases occur in children younger than 2 years. It is a neuroendocrine tumor, arising from any neural crest element of the sympathetic nervous system.

Lymphoma: Lymphoma is a type of blood cancer that occurs when B or T lymphocytes, the white blood cells that form a part of the immune system and help protect the body from infection and disease, divide faster than normal cells or live longer than they are supposed to. Lymphoma may develop in the lymph nodes, spleen, bone marrow, blood, or other organs, and eventually, they form a tumor.

Ewing's sarcoma: Ewing's sarcoma is a malignant small, round, blue cell tumor. It is a rare disease in which cancer cells are found in the bone or in the soft tissue. The most common areas in which it occurs are the pelvis, the femur, the humerus, the ribs, and the clavicle (collar bone).

Sickle-cell disease: Sickle-cell disease, or sickle-cell anemia or drepanocytosis, is a hereditary blood disorder, characterized by red blood cells that assume an abnormal, rigid, sickle shape. Sickling decreases the cells' flexibility and results in a risk of various complications. The sickling occurs because of a mutation in the hemoglobin gene. Individuals with one copy of the defunct gene display both normal and abnormal hemoglobin.

Myelodysplastic syndrome: The myelodysplastic syndromes, formerly known as preleukemia are a diverse collection of hematological (blood-related) medical conditions that involve ineffective production (or dysplasia) of the myeloid class of blood cells.

Desmoplastic small round cell tumor: Desmoplastic small round cell tumor is classified as a soft-tissue sarcoma. It is an aggressive and rare tumor that primarily occurs as masses in the abdomen. Other areas affected may include the lymph nodes, the lining of the abdomen, diaphragm, spleen, liver, chest wall, skull, spinal cord, large intestine, small intestine, bladder, brain, lungs, testicles, ovaries, and the pelvis. Reported sites of metastatic spread include the liver, lungs, lymph nodes, brain, skull, and bones.

Hodgkin's disease: Hodgkin's lymphoma, also known as Hodgkin lymphoma and previously known as Hodgkin's disease, is a type of lymphoma, which is a cancer originating from white blood cells called lymphocytes. It was named after Thomas Hodgkin, who first described abnormalities in the lymph system in 1832.

Immunosuppressive agents: Immunosuppressive drugs or immunosuppressive agents are drugs that inhibit or prevent the activity of the immune system. They are used in immunosuppressive therapy to prevent the rejection of transplanted organs and tissues (e.g., bone marrow, heart, kidney, and liver).

Further reading

Allison C, McLaughlin L, Sledge B, Waters-Pick S, and Kurtzberg J 2010. Differences in quality between privately and publicly banked umbilical cord blood units: A pilot study of autologous cord blood infusion in children with acquired neurological disorders. *Transfusion* 50 (9): 1980–1987. doi:10.1111/j.1537-2995.2010.02720.x. PMID 20546200.

Assmus B, Schächinger V, Teupe C et al. 2002. Transplantation of progenitor cells and regeneration enhancement in acute myocardial infarction (TOPCARE-AMI). *Circulation* 106 (24): 3009–3017.

Awad HA, Butler DL, Boivin GP et al. 1999. Autologous mesenchymal stem cell-mediated repair of tendon. *Tissue Eng* 5 (3): 267–277. doi:10.1089/ten.1999.5.267. PMID 10434073.

Black LL, Gaynor J, Adams C et al. 2008. Effect of intraarticular injection of autologous adipose-derived mesenchymal stem and regenerative cells on clinical signs of chronic osteoarthritis of the elbow joint in dogs. *Vet Ther* 9 (3): 192–200. PMID 19003780.

Bruder SP, Kraus KH, Goldberg VM, and Kadiyala S 1998. The effect of implants loaded with autologous mesenchymal stem cells on the healing of canine segmental bone defects. *J Bone Joint Surg Am* 80 (7): 985–996. PMID 9698003. http://www.ejbjs.org/cgi/pmidlookup?view=long&pmid=9698003.

Centeno CJ, Busse D, Kisiday J, Keohan C, Freeman M, and Karli D 2008a. Increased knee cartilage volume in degenerative joint disease using percutaneously implanted, autologous mesenchymal stem cells. *Pain Physician* 11 (3): 343–353. PMID 18523506. http://www.painphysicianjournal.com/linkout_vw.php?issn=1533-3159&vol=11&page=343.

Centeno CJ, Busse D, Kisiday J, Keohan C, Freeman M, and Karli D 2008b. Regeneration of meniscus cartilage in a knee treated with percutaneously implanted autologous mesenchymal stem cells. *Med Hypotheses* 71 (6): 900–908. doi:10.1016/j.mehy.2008.06.042. PMID 18786777.

Centeno CJ, Schultz JR, Cheever M, Robinson B, Freeman M, and Marasco W 2010. Safety and complications reporting on the re-implantation of culture-expanded mesenchymal stem cells using autologous platelet lysate technique. *Curr Stem Cell Res Ther* 5 (1): 81–93. doi:10.2174/157488810790442796. PMID 19951252.

Chen J, Li Y, Wang L et al. 2001. Therapeutic benefit of intravenous administration of bone marrow stromal cells after cerebral ischemia in rats. *Stroke* 32 (4): 1005–1011. PMID 11283404. http://stroke.ahajournals.org/cgi/pmidlookup?view=long&pmid=11283404.

Csaki C, Matis U, Mobasheri A, Ye H, and Shakibaei M 2007. Chondrogenesis, osteogenesis and adipogenesis of canine mesenchymal stem cells: A biochemical, morphological and ultrastructural study. *Histochem Cell Biol* 128 (6): 507–520. doi:10.1007/s00418-007-0337-z. PMID 17922135.

Fraser JK, Wulur I, Alfonso Z, and Hedrick MH 2006. Fat tissue: An underappreciated source of stem cells for biotechnology. *Trends Biotechnol* 24 (4): 150–154. doi:10.1016/j.tibtech.2006.01.010. PMID 16488036. http://linkinghub.elsevier.com/retrieve/pii/S0167-7799(06)00028-X.

Fu YS, Cheng YC, Lin MY et al. 2006. Conversion of human umbilical cord mesenchymal stem cells in Wharton's jelly to dopaminergic neurons *in vitro*: Potential therapeutic application for Parkinsonism. *Stem Cells* 24 (1): 115–124. PMID 16099997.

Giarratana MC, Kobari L, Lapillonne H et al. 2005. *Ex vivo* generation of fully mature human red blood cells from hematopoietic stem cells. *Nat Biotechnol* 23 (1): 69–74. doi:10.1038/nbt1047. PMID 15619619.

Gluckman E, Rocha V, Boyer-Chammard A et al. 1997. Outcome of cord blood transplantation from related and unrelated donors. *N Engl J Med* 337 (6): 373–381. doi:10.1056/NEJM199708073370602. PMID 9241126.

Gurtner GC, Callaghan MJ, and Longaker MT 2007. Progress and potential for regenerative medicine. *Annu Rev Med* 58: 299–312.

Kang KS, Kim SW, Oh YH et al. 2005. A 37-year-old spinal cord-injured female patient, transplanted of multipotent stem cells from human UC blood, with improved sensory perception and mobility, both functionally and morphologically: A case study. *Cytotherapy* 7 (4): 368–373. doi:10.1080/14653240500238160. PMID 16162459.

Keirstead HS, Nistor G, Bernal G et al. 2005. Human embryonic stem cell-derived oligodendrocyte progenitor cell transplants remyelinate and restore locomotion after spinal cord injury. *J Neurosci* 25 (19): 4694–4705. doi:10.1523/JNEUROSCI.0311-05.2005. PMID 15888645.

Klimanskaya I, Chung Y, Becker S, Lu SJ, and Lanza R 2006. Human embryonic stem cell lines derived from single blastomeres. *Nature* 444 (7118): 481–485. doi:10.1038/nature05142. PMID 16929302.

Klimanskaya I, Chung Y, Meisner L, Johnson J, West MD, and Lanza R 2005. Human embryonic stem cells derived without feeder cells. *Lancet* 365 (9471): 1636–1641. doi:10.1016/S0140-6736(05)66473-2. PMID 15885296.

Koch TG and Betts DH 2007. Stem cell therapy for joint problems using the horse as a clinically relevant animal model. *Expert Opin Biol Ther* 7 (11): 1621–1626. doi:10.1517/14712598.7.11.1621. PMID 17961087. http://informahealthcare.com/doi/abs/10.1517/14712598.7.11.1621%20.

Kraus KH and Kirker-Head C 2006. Mesenchymal stem cells and bone regeneration. *Vet Surg* 35 (3): 232–242. doi:10.1111/j.1532-950X.2006.00142.x. PMID 16635002. http://www3.interscience.wiley.com/resolve/openurl?genre=article&sid=nlm:pubmed&issn=0161-3499&date=2006&volume=35&issue=3&spage=232.

La Rocca G, Anzalone R, Corrao S et al. 2009. Isolation and characterization of Oct-4+/HLA-G+ mesenchymal stem cells from human umbilical cord matrix: Differentiation potential and detection of new markers. *Histochem Cell Biol* 2009 Feb;131(2): 267–282. doi: 10.1007/s00418-008-0519-3. Epub 2008 Oct 3.

Ledermann B and Burki K 1991. Establishment of a germ-line competent C57BL/6 embryonic stem cell line. *Exp Cell Res* 197 (2): 254–258. doi:10.1016/0014-4827(91)90430-3. PMID 1959560.

Liu Y, Mu R, Wang S et al. 2010. Therapeutic potential of human umbilical cord mesenchymal stem cells in the treatment of rheumatoid arthritis. *Arthritis Res Therapy* 12: R210. doi:10.1186/ar3187. PMID 21080925.

Martin MJ, Muotri A, Gage F, and Varki A 2005. Human embryonic stem cells express an immunogenic nonhuman sialic acid. *Nat Med* 11 (2): 228–232. doi:10.1038/nm1181. PMID 15685172.

Murphy JM, Fink DJ, Hunziker EB, and Barry FP 2003. Stem cell therapy in a caprine model of osteoarthritis. *Arthritis Rheum* 48 (12): 3464–3474. doi:10.1002/art.11365. PMID 14673997.

Nathan S, Das De S, Thambyah A, Fen C, Goh J, and Lee EH 2003. Cell-based therapy in the repair of osteochondral defects: A novel use for adipose tissue. *Tissue Eng* 9 (4): 733–744. doi:10.1089/107632703768247412. PMID 13678450.

Nixon AJ, Dahlgren LA, Haupt JL, Yeager AE, and Ward DL 2008. Effect of adipose-derived nucleated cell fractions on tendon repair in horses with collagenase-induced tendinitis. *Am J Vet Res* 69 (7): 928–937. doi:10.2460/ajvr.69.7.928. PMID 18593247.

Revoltella RP, Papini S, Rosellini A et al. 2008. Cochlear repair by transplantation of human cord blood CD133+ cells to nod-scid mice made deaf with kanamycin and noise. *Cell Transplant* 17 (6): 665–678. doi:10.3727/096368908786092685. PMID 18819255.

Richards M, Fong CY, and Bongso A 2008. Comparative evaluation of different *in vitro* systems that stimulate germ cell differentiation in human embryonic stem cells. *Fertil Steril* 93 (3): 986–994. doi:10.1016/j.fertnstert.2008.10.030. PMID 19064262.

Richardson LE, Dudhia J, Clegg PD, and Smith R 2007. Stem cells in veterinary medicine attempts at regenerating equine tendon after injury. *Trends Biotechnol* 25 (9): 409–416. doi:10.1016/j.tibtech.2007.07.009. PMID 17692415. http://linkinghub.elsevier.com/retrieve/pii/S0167-7799(07)00188-6.

Sampaolesi M, Blot S, D'Antona G et al. 2006. Mesoangioblast stem cells ameliorate muscle function in dystrophic dogs. *Nature* 444 (7119): 574–579. doi:10.1038/nature05282. PMID 17108972.

Singec I, Jandial R, Crain A, Nikkhah G, and Snyder EY 2007. The leading edge of stem cell therapeutics. *Annu Rev Med* 58:313–328. doi:10.1146/annurev.med.58.070605.115252. PMID 17100553. http://arjournals.annualreviews.org/doi/abs/10.1146/annurev.med.58.070605.115252?url_ver=Z39.88-2003&rfr_id=ori:rid:crossref.org&rfr_dat=cr_pub%3dncbi.nlm.nih.gov.

Smith RKW 2008. Principles of stem cell therapy in the horse—The science behind the technology. *Pferdeheilkunde* 24 (4): 508.

Strauer BE, Schannwell CM, and Brehm M 2009. Therapeutic potentials of stem cells in cardiac diseases. *Minerva Cardioangiol* 57 (2): 249–267. PMID 19274033.

Taguchi A, Toshihiro S, Hidekazu T et al. 2004. Administration of CD34+ cells after stroke enhances neurogenesis via angiogenesis in a mouse model. *J Clin Invest* 114 (3): 330–338. doi:10.1172/JCI20622. PMC 484977. PMID 15286799. http://www.pubmedcentral.nih.gov/articlerender.fcgi?tool=pmcentrez&artid=484977.

Takahashi K, Tanabe K, Ohnuki M, Narita M, Ichisaka T, Tomoda K, and Yamanaka S 2007. Induction of pluripotent stem cells from adult human fibroblasts by defined factors. *Cell* 131 (5): 861–872. doi:10.1016/j.cell.2007.11.019. PMID 18035408.

Takahashi K and Yamanaka S 2006. Induction of pluripotent stem cells from mouse embryonic and adult fibroblast cultures by defined factors. *Cell* 126: 663–676. PMID 16904174.

Taylor SE, Smith RK, and Clegg PD 2007. Mesenchymal stem cell therapy in equine musculoskeletal disease: Scientific fact or clinical fiction? *Equine Vet J* 39 (2): 172–180. doi:10.2746/042516407X180868. PMID 17378447.

Tecirlioglu RT and Trounson AO 2007. Embryonic stem cells in companion animals (horses, dogs and cats): Present status and future prospects. *Reprod Fertil Dev* 19 (6): 740–747. doi:10.1071/RD07039. PMID 17714628. http://www.publish.csiro.au/journals/abstractHTML.cfm?J=RD&V=19&I=6&F=RD07039abs.XML.

Tran I, Seshareddy K, Weiss ML, and Detamore MS 2009. A comparison of human bone marrow-derived mesenchymal stem cells and human umbilical cord-derived mesenchymal stromal cells for cartilage tissue engineering. *Tissue Eng Part A* 15 (8): 2259–2266. doi:10.1089/ten.tea.2008.0393.

Vastag B 2001. Stem cells step closer to the clinic: Paralysis partially reversed in rats with ALS-like disease. *JAMA* 285 (13): 1691–1693. doi:10.1001/jama.285.13.1691. PMID 11277806. http://jama.ama-assn.org/cgi/pmidlookup?view=long&pmid=11277806.

Vergano D 2010. Embryonic stem cells used on patient for first time. *USA Today*. http://www.usatoday.com/tech/science/2010-10-12-stemcells12_ST_N.htm (retrieved 2010-10-12).

Wakitani S, Nawata M, Tensho K, Okabe T, Machida H, and Ohgushi H 2007. Repair of articular cartilage defects in the patello-femoral joint with autologous bone marrow mesenchymal cell transplantation: Three case reports involving nine defects in five knees. *J Tissue Eng Regen Med* 1 (1): 74–79. doi:10.1002/term.8. PMID 18038395.

Weissman IL 2000. Stem cells: Units of development, units of regeneration, and units in evolution. *Cell* 100 (1): 157–168. doi:10.1016/S0092-8674(00)81692-X. PMID 10647940.

Yamada Y, Ueda M, Naiki T, Takahashi M, Hata K, and Nagasaka T 2004. Autogenous injectable bone for regeneration with mesenchymal stem cells and platelet-rich plasma: Tissue-engineered bone regeneration. *Tissue Eng* 10 (5–6): 955–964. doi:10.1089/1076327041348284. PMID 15265313.

Yen AH and Sharpe PT 2008. Stem cells and tooth tissue engineering. *Cell Tissue Res* 331 (1): 359–372. doi:10.1007/s00441-007-0467-6. PMID 17938970.

Young RG, Butler DL, Weber W, Caplan AI, Gordon SL, and Fink DJ 1998. Use of mesenchymal stem cells in a collagen matrix for Achilles tendon repair. *J Orthop Res* 16 (4): 406–413. doi:10.1002/jor.1100160403. PMID 9747780.

chapter eight

Cell and tissue engineering

8.1 Introduction

A commonly applied definition of tissue engineering, as stated by Langer and Vacanti is an interdisciplinary field that applies the principles of engineering and life sciences toward the development of biological substitutes to restore, maintain, or improve tissue function or a whole organ. Over the past decade, the field of cell and tissue engineering has emerged as a multidisciplinary field concerning biology, medicine, and engineering. The field of tissue engineering is likely to revolutionize the ways we improve the health and quality of life for millions of patients worldwide by restoring, maintaining, or enhancing tissue and organ function. In addition to having a therapeutic application such as cell-based therapy or tissue reconstruction, where the cells or tissues are grown in the controlled conditions in the laboratory, they can be used for transplantation studies. Tissue engineering can also be used in diagnostic purposes where the cells and tissues can be used for testing new drug molecules. Over the last few years, the bioengineered cells or tissues have been used extensively in both treating the degenerative diseases and in the diagnostic field (Figure 8.1).

8.2 Animal cell culture

The beginning of animal tissue culture can be traced back to 1880 when scientist Arnold showed that leukocytes can divide outside the body. In 1903, the behavior of animal tissue explants immersed in serum, lymph, or ascites fluid was reported. Later on, in 1907, it was shown that frog tadpole spinal cord cells can be successfully cultured and was considered to be an important breakthrough in cell and tissue culture. In 1913, another complicated methodology was developed for maintaining cultures free from microorganism contamination and subsequently, a suitable culture media was developed and the cell and tissue techniques of cell culture developed as well.

8.3 Organ culture

Efforts have also been made to construct bioengineered organs outside the human body, which in fact is the biggest challenge. Culture methods have been tested and developed to make anatomical and functional human body organs which can give rise to organs consisting of multiple tissues such as parenchyma and stoma and can be easily cultured together to make a single organ. We will briefly describe various types of organ culture techniques (Figure 8.2).

8.3.1 Organ culture technique

The first attempt to develop an organ culture method was attempted in 1897, which employed an adult rabbit liver, kidney, and thyroid on small plasma clots and observed

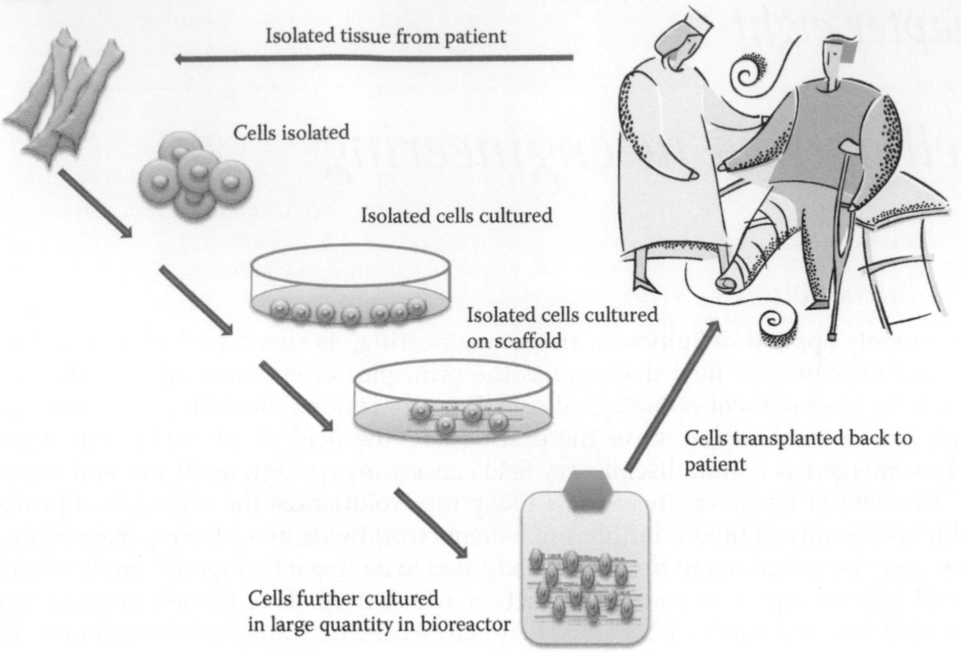

Figure 8.1 Cell and tissue engineering.

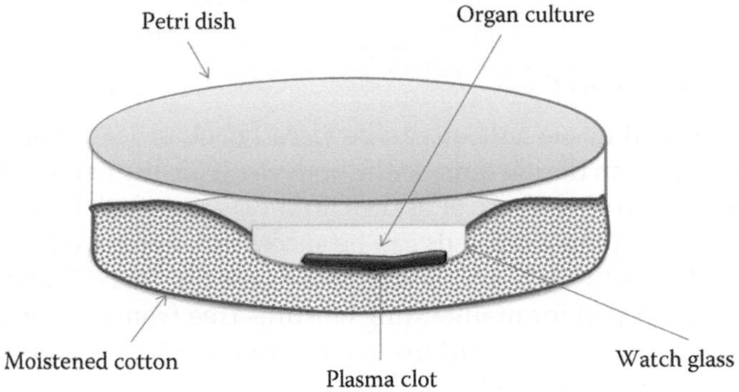

Figure 8.2 Classical example of organ culture.

that these bioengineered organs retained their normal histological features for 3 days. Later in 1919 it was reported that the culture tube can be filled with oxygen to prevent necrosis of the cells. The various organ culture methods are briefly described.

8.3.1.1 Plasma clot

Plasma clot is a culture technique where explant is cultured on the surface of a clot consisting of chick plasma and chick embryo extract. This technique has been in use for studying morphogenesis in embryonic organ rudiments. It has also been adapted to study the action of hormones, vitamins, and cancer-causing agents on adult mammalian tissues. A widely used watch glass approach is as follows. The cell explant is placed on a suitably prepared clot which is kept in a watch glass. One or two such watch glasses are kept in a Petri dish lined with a moist filter paper or cotton wool to minimize evaporation of the clot. The Petri dish is generally incubated at 37.5°C temperature. In order to maintain the culture, fresh clots can be added every 2–3 days derived from avian tissues and every 3–4 days for mammalian tissues.

The technique has been little modified by keeping organ rudiments or pieces on plasma clots kept on a coverslip, which is then inverted onto the cavity in a microconcavity microscopic slide; the coverslip is sealed with paraffin wax. The plasma clot is prepared by mixing three drops of chicken plasma with one drop of chick embryo extract (50%) onto the coverslip. The plasma clot can be replaced by fresh clots by lifting the coverslip. This method is inexpensive, permits light microscopic observations during culture and is suitable for studies such as hair growth, fetal mouse skin differentiation, and so on. One of the chief disadvantages of all plasma clot methods is that the clot liquefies in the vicinity of explants so that they become partly or fully immersed in the medium. The duration of culture is rather short and biochemical analysis is not possible due to the complexity of the medium.

8.3.1.2 Raft methods

In this method, the cell or tissue explant is placed on a raft which is made of rayon acetate. The chemical (rayon acetate) rafts are basically made to float on the serum with silicone. Correspondingly, floatability of lens paper is boosted by treating it with silicone. On each raft, four or more cells or tissue explants are usually positioned. In an amalgamation of the raft and clot techniques, the explants are first placed on a suitable raft, which is then kept on a plasma clot and this modification makes media changes easy, and prevents the sinking of explants into plasma (Figure 8.3).

8.3.1.3 Agar gel

In this methodology, the medium consisting of a suitable serum, sodium chloride solution, chick embryo extract, or a mixture of certain amino acids and vitamins is crystallized with agar (1%). This agar-based method avoids immersion of explants into the medium and permits the use of defined media. Generally, explants need to be subcultured on fresh agar gels every 5–7 days. The agar mixed with gel is generally kept in watch glasses and wrapped with paraffin wax. The explants can be examined using a stereoscopic microscope. This method has been used to study many developmental aspects of normal organs as well as of tumors.

8.3.1.4 Grid method

This method was initially used in 1954. It utilizes 25 mm × 25 mm pieces of a suitable wire mesh or perforated stainless-steel sheets whose edges are bent to form four legs of about 4 mm height. The culture tissue derived from skeletal muscle are generally placed directly

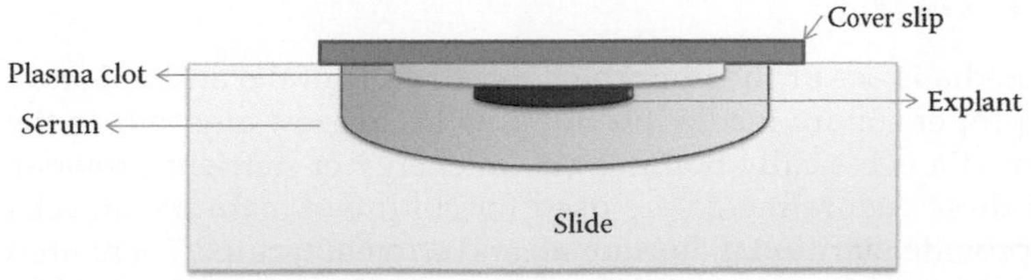

Figure 8.3 Raft method of organ culture.

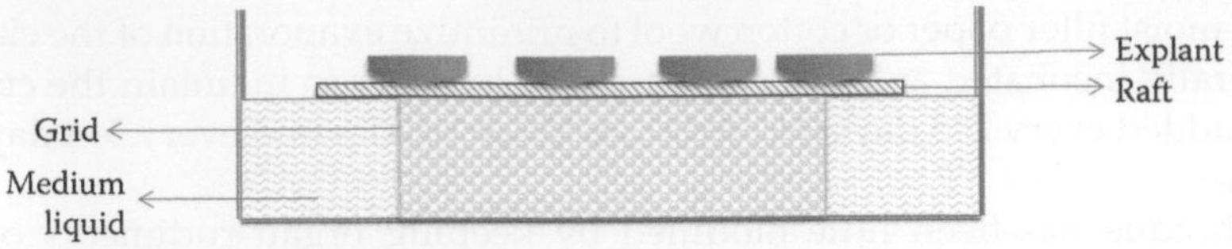

Figure 8.4 Grid method of organ culture.

on the grid, but softer tissues like glands can be first placed on rafts, which are then kept on the grids. The grids are placed in a culture chamber packed with culture medium and the chamber is supplied with a mixture of oxygen and carbon dioxide to meet the high oxygen requirements of adult mammalian organs. A modification of the original grid method is widely used to study the growth and differentiation of adult and embryonic cell and tissues (Figure 8.4).

8.3.1.5 Cyclic exposure to medium and gas phase

This technique has been successful in the long term (up to 4–5 months) culture of human adult tissues such as esophagus, mammary epithelium, uterine endocervix, and so on. The explants are intermittently exposed to the fluid medium and the gas phase. The number of explants per dish varies from 2 to 18 depending on the organ cultured. Moreover, the explants are normally attached to the bottom of a plastic culture dish and are covered with fluid medium. The dishes are enclosed in a chamber containing a suitable gas mixture and mounted on a rocker platform. The chamber is rocked at several cycles/min to ensure cyclic exposure of the organ explants to the medium and the gas phases.

8.3.2 Advantages of organ culture

There are various advantages of organ culture which suggest that explants remain comparable to the *in vivo* organs both in structure and function aspects, which makes them more suitable than cell cultures for physiological and functional studies. The *in vitro* development of fetal organ culture is equivalent to that *in vivo* method. Another advantage of organ culture is that organs such as endocrine organs generally secretes the specific hormones which can be easily studied and analyzed. Consequently, *in vitro* organ culture method also provides information on the patterns of cell growth, cell differentiation, and tissue development. In a few cases, organ cultures can also be replaced with whole animals in experimentation to avoid ethical approvals. Finally, the results obtained with organ cultures usually give an idea of the *in vivo* events that happened in the body; this so often reduces significantly the number of experiments necessary with whole animals to investigate.

8.4 Culture media

The culture media is one of the important constituents of the any cell and tissue culture and without proper culture media it is not possible to grow any cells in the laboratories. The culture media is basically nothing but an energy or nutrient provider to the growing cells and these culture media are used for culture of mammalian cells. The culture media must provide nutritional, hormonal, and stromal factors. There are various types of culture media used for cell and tissue culture and can be assembled into two broad categories: natural media and artificial media. The choice of medium depends mainly on the type of cells to be cultured, for example, culture media for normal cells will be different than immortalized cell or transformed cells. The culture media generally provides support for the growth, survival, and differentiation processes. The normal cells and primary cell cultures from healthy tissues contain defined quantities of proteins, growth factors, and hormones in addition to the basic culture media. It has been shown that immortalized cells produce most of the growth factors, but may still need some of the growth factors present in the serum. In contrast, transformed cells synthesize their own growth factors and sometime the addition of growth factors leads to harmful effects. There are various types of culture media commercially available in the market and are described below.

8.4.1 Natural media

These media mainly consist of naturally occurring biological fluids which include cagula or plasma clots, biological fluids, and tissue extracts. The natural media are generally used for organ culture, whereas artificial media with or without serum are used in the cell culture method. While culturing the organ, the culture media must contain the plasma clots which in fact improve the quality of the organ culture. These plasma clots are now commercially available either in liquid or lyophilized form. In case plasma clots are not commercially available, the same can be also be prepared in the laboratory. This is done by taking blood of a male fowl; blood clotting must be avoided during the preparation. Among all biological fluids used as a culture medium, serum is found to be the most widely used. The serum can be obtained from adult human blood, placental cord blood, and also from animals such as horse blood or calf blood. Among all animals, serum from a fetal calf is the most commonly used.

8.4.2 Artificial media

Artificial media contain either partly or fully defined components. The artificial media can be used for various conditions such as immediate survival of cells, prolonged survival of cells or tissues, and indefinite growth of cells. The various artificial media developed for cell cultures may be grouped into the following four classes: serum-containing media, serum-free media, chemically defined media, and protein-free media.

8.4.2.1 Functions of serum in the culture medium

One of the main functions of the serum is to provide the basic nutrients to growing cells. The nutrients are present in the serum and also contain several hormones such as insulin, which is essential for growth of nearly all cells in culture, progesterone, cortisone, somatostatin, testosterone, and prostaglandin. The serum also contains several growth factors which include platelet-derived growth factor, transforming growth factor β, and epidermal growth factor. Moreover, both hormones and growth factors are involved in cell growth promotion and cell maturation. Not all the growth factors have similar effects on the growing cells, but varied effects as one type of hormone or growth factor may stimulate growth of one cell type, may have no effects on another and may even be inhibitory to some others. For instance, platelet-derived growth factors induce proliferation in fibroblasts, but then induces differentiation of some types of epithelial cells. Additionally, proliferation of a single cell type may be induced by more than one growth factor. For example, fibroblasts are known to respond to platelet-derived growth factor, epidermal growth factor, and fibroblast growth factor, respectively. Another important function of serum is to supply proteins such as fibronectin or fibrinogen, which are known to promote attachment of cells to the substrate. The serum also provides spreading factors that help the cells to spread out in the culture flask before they can begin to divide. It is true that growing cells produce these factors but with little amount and, therefore, it is very important to provide growing cells with additional serum as it contains several binding proteins such albumin and transferrin which are very important for cell adhesion and growth. Furthermore, transferrin usually increases the viscosity of medium and, thus, protects growing cells from mechanical damages like shear forces during agitation of suspension cultures.

8.4.2.1.1 Disadvantages of serum in the culture medium. There are also some disadvantages of using serum in the culture as it has been reported that serum can inhibit growth of some cell types, for example, epidermal keratinocytes. It has also been found that serum contains some potentially cytotoxic constituents which can be harmful to the growing cells. For example, fetal calf serum which is the most extensively used in culture is known to contain the enzyme polyamine oxidase, which converts polyamines into cytotoxic poly-amino aldehyde. Another problem with commercially available serums is the large variation in serum quality from one batch to another; this needs expensive and time-consuming testing process.

8.4.2.1.2 Serum-free media. In view of the various disadvantages of use of serum in the culture, researchers have done an extensive research to develop serum-free preparations of culture media. The technology to make serum-free media has resulted in several elaborate media formulations in which serum is basically replaced with the mixture of amino acids, vitamins, several other organic compounds, hormones, growth factors, and other protein supplements when required. Even though serum has some disadvantages, the use of it in the culture is very essential and at least 5–20% of serum even in these media is essential for optimal cell growth.

8.4.2.2 Advantages of serum-free media

It is easy to culture live cells in the serum-free media, which is one of its advantages to improve reproducibility of results. You can also avoid the toxic effects of serum. The culture may also face interference due to the presence of serum proteins. In addition to this, there is no danger of degrading serum proteases that are present in the serum. Serum-free media permit selective culture of differentiated and producing cell types from the heterogeneous cultures.

8.4.2.3 Disadvantages of serum-free media

It has been reported that most of serum-free media are specific to one cell type. Therefore, it has been recommended that different media may be required for different cell lines. Additionally, it has been noticed that reliable serum-free preparations for most of the media formulations are not available commercially, and to prepare the serum-free media is a laborious and time-consuming process. During cell culture, great care is required to control pH and temperature while using serum-free media. There are reports which suggest the use of serum-free media can curtail the cell growth rate and the cell density compared to serum-containing media. There are also reports that suggest the use of serum-free media makes the cells fragile during prolonged agitated cultures unless biopolymers or synthetic polymers are added.

8.4.2.4 *Chemically defined media*

The media which contain the defined quantity of organic chemicals, growth factors, vitamins are called chemically defined media. The culture media also contain protein and hormones such as insulin and epidermal growth factors.

8.4.2.5 *Protein-free media*

As the name indicates, protein-free media do not contain any protein; they only contain nonprotein constituents necessary for the culture of the cells. The formulations MEM, DME, RPM-1640 are protein-free media generally in supplementation of required proteins.

8.5 *Culture wares*

In addition to having the required culture media to support the growth of cells, it is also equally important to have vessels or containers on which the cells can grow. These vessels or containers are normally known as Petri dishes or flasks made of either glass or plastics.

8.5.1 *Roux bottle*

The Roux bottle is commonly used in the laboratory, and is kept stationary so that only a part of its internal surface is available for cell docking. Each bottle has a capacity up to 175–200 cm^2 surface area for cell attachment and occupies 750–1000 cm^3 space.

8.5.2 *Roller bottle*

This vessel permits a limited scale up as it is rocked or, preferably, rolled so that its entire internal surface is available in anchorage. It has been reported that several modifications of roller bottle can further enhance the available surface such as a spiral polystyrene cartridge, glass tube (roller bottle packed with a parallel cluster of small glass tubes separated by silicone spacer rings), and an extended surface area roller bottle (the bottle surface is corrugated enhancing the surface by a factor of 2).

8.5.3 *Multi-tray unit*

The cells can also be cultured in multi-tray units. A standard unit has 10 chambers stacked on each other, which have interconnecting channels; this enables the various operations to be carried out in one go for all the chambers. Each chamber has a surface area of 600 cm^2 and this polystyrene unit is basically disposable and gives good results, similar to plastic flasks.

8.5.4 *Synthetic hollow fiber cartridge*

The cells can also be cultured in the synthetic hollow fiber cartridge. The fibers enclosed in a sealed cartridge provide a large surface area for cell attachment on the outside surface of the fibers. The capillary fibers made up of acrylic polymer are 350 μm in diameter with 75 μm thick walls. The medium is pumped in through the fiber, goes through the fiber walls and becomes available to the cells. The available surface area is found to be very high. This synthetic hollow fiber cartridge system is mainly used for suspension cells, but is also suitable for cell docking.

8.5.5 Opticell culture system

In this type of a cell culture system, a cylindrical ceramic cartridge in which two channels run through the length of the unit provides for successful cell growth. This system gives about 40 cm^2 surface area per mL of medium to be used for the cell culture. Interestingly, this type of the cell culture method is suitable for virus culture, cell surface antigen, and monoclonal antibody production, and also for both suspension and monolayer cell cultures.

8.5.6 Plastic film

Teflon which is basically fluoro-ethylene-propylene copolymer is biologically inert and highly permeable to gas. Teflon bags (dimension 5 × 30 cm) filled with cells and medium (dimension 2–10 mm deep) serve as good culture vessels and it has been found that cells can attach to the inside surface of the bags. On the other contrary, Teflon tubes are enfolded around a whirl with a bar and the medium is pumped through the tube; cells can grow on the inside surface of the tube.

8.5.7 Heli cell vessels

This is another useful method where cells are cultured using Heli cell vessels; these vessels are packed with polystyrene ribbons (dimension 3 mm × 5–10 mm × 100 μm) that are twisted in a helical shape. The culture medium is pumped through the vessel. It has been reported that the helical shape of ribbons ensures good circulation of the culture media so that growing cells could get sufficient nutrients. One of the interesting aspects of the vessels culture method is the scale-up method for many folds using multiple units.

8.6 Classifications of cell transplantation

In cell transplantation, the cells or tissues can be classified based on their utilization in different parts of the body. We have given a few examples where cell-based transplantation is effectively used in clinical research.

8.6.1 Autologous cells

The autologous cell transplantation is basically a transplantation in which cells obtained from patients can be transplanted into the same patient. One significance of the autologous transplantation is that there is a high rate of success as the transplanted cells easily can be accepted by the patient's body and there are few problems associated with ejection and pathogen transmission. There are however, a few shortcomings in the autologous cell transplantation as the availability of required cells to be transplanted are found in very low in numbers and also genetic disease-suitable autologous cells are not available. Another disadvantage of autologous cell transplantation is that older patients do not have sufficient numbers of autologous cells to be used for cell transplantation. The old patients need to undergo a surgical operation in order to isolate the cells which might lead to donor site infection or chronic pain. Autologous cells also must be cultured from samples before they can be used and these are lengthy procedures, so autologous cell transplantation might take a long time. In recent times there has been a trend toward the use of human mesenchymal stem cells (MSCs) isolated from bone marrow and fat cells. These MSCs can be differentiated into a variety of tissue types including bone, cartilage, fat, and nerve cells. A large number of cells can be easily and quickly isolated from a fat source, consequently opening the potential for large numbers of cells to be quickly and easily obtained.

8.6.2 Allogeneic cells

Allogeneic cells come from the body of a donor of the same species; for example, the cells from one person (donor) can be used by another person (patient). There are some ethical restraints on the use of human cells for *in vitro* studies, however, the use of dermal fibroblasts from human foreskin has been demonstrated to be clinically safe and consequently a viable choice for tissue engineering of skin.

8.6.3 Xenogeneic cells

The cells which are isolated from two different species are called as xenogeneic cells; for example, the cells from one species (sheep) can be used in another species (human). In particular, animal cells have been widely used in experiments aimed at the construction of cardiovascular implants which later can be used in humans.

8.6.4 Syngeneic or isogenic cells

This type of cell isolates from genetically identical individuals, such as twins, clones, or extremely inbred research animal models.

8.7 Bioengineered cells

In vitro cell culture techniques have successfully cultured and constructed the human cells outside of the body. These outside body constructed cells are often referred to as bioengineered cells. There are various applications of bioengineered cells in clinical conditions.

8.7.1 Construction of scaffold

The *in vitro* culture cells are frequently embedded into an artificial structure which is capable of supporting three-dimensional tissue formation. These cell structures are typically called scaffolds and are often critical for tissue repairing and bioengineering. Interestingly, scaffolds usually serve at least one of the following purposes: (i) scaffolds allow cell attachment and migration, (ii) scaffolds deliver and retain cells and biochemical factors, (iii) scaffolds enable diffusion of vital cell nutrients, and (iv) scaffolds exert certain mechanical and biological influences to modify the behavior of the cell phase and cell growth. It has been recommended that scaffolds must meet some specific requirements to successfully make the tissue reconstruction. One requirement is that scaffolds should have a high porosity; an adequate pore size is essential to enable cell seeding and diffusion for the cell to get nutrients. Another requirement is that scaffold should have biodegradability, which is often a vital factor since scaffolds should be absorbed by the neighboring tissues. Additionally, the rate at which degradation of scaffold occurs has to concur as much as possible with the rate of cell and tissue formation, which means that while cells are fabricating their own natural material around themselves, the scaffold is able to provide structural reliability within the body.

The materials used in the medical field before the advent of tissue engineering are biodegradable sutures. These biodegradable sutures are made of collagen and some polyester. Over the past years, the new technology has developed various kinds of biomaterials that are biocompatible, nonimmunogenetics, transparent, easily accessible, and functional. The most commonly used material is synthetic which is basically polylactic acid. Polylactic acid is a polyester known to degrade in the human body to form lactic acid; lactic acid is a naturally occurring chemical which can be easily removed from the body. There are also different kinds of materials which have been tested such as poly-glycolic acid and poly-caprolactone, and it has been found that their degradation process is similar to that of polylactic acid, but they exhibit correspondingly slower rate of degradation compared to polylactic acid. In addition to the use of polylactic acid as the scaffold, these materials can also be used as extracellular matrix to support cell growth, protein materials (collagen or fibrin), and polysaccharide materials (chitosan or glycos-amino-glycans), which have all proven to be suitable for cell compatibility.

8.7.2 *Synthesis of bioengineered cells*

A number of different methods have been reported for constructing porous structures to be employed as tissue scaffolds and each of these techniques presents its own advantages and disadvantages.

8.7.2.1 *Nanofiber self-assembly*

It has been reported that nanofiber-based self-assembly is one of the few approaches for constructing biomaterials with properties similar to that of the natural *in vivo* extracellular matrix. Additionally, these hydrogel scaffolds have shown superiority in *in vivo* studies and biocompatibility compared to traditional macro-scaffolds and animal-derived materials.

8.7.2.2 *Textile materials*

The scaffold can also be prepared by using textile materials; particularly, the use of nonwoven poly-glycolide materials have been tested for tissue engineering applications. The textile fiber-based materials are fibrous and have been found to be useful in growing different types of cells. One big disadvantage of the textile-based materials is that it is very difficult to obtain high porosity and regular pore size.

8.7.2.3 *Solvent casting and particulate leaching*

There is another method which allows the preparation of porous materials with regular porosity. This method is simple as the polymer is first dissolved in a suitable organic solvent such as polylactic acid (could also be dissolved into dichloro-methane). Then the solution is cast into a mold filled with porogen particles. These porogens are usually inorganic salts such as sodium chloride, crystals of saccharose, or gelatin spheres. It has been reported that the size of the porogen particles can affect the size of the scaffold pores and, hence, the polymer–porogen ratio is directly correlated to the amount of porosity of the final structure. After this, the solution in which polymer has been cast is allowed to evaporate; then the composite structure in the mold is immersed in a liquid solution which is suitable for dissolving the porogens. When the porogen has been fully dissolved, a porous structure is obtained.

8.7.2.4 *Gas foaming*

This technique uses gas as a porogen to overcome the need to use organic solvents and solid porogens. In brief, the first step is to make a disc-shaped structure by means of compression using a heated mold and then the discs are placed in a chamber where they are exposed to high pressure of carbon dioxide for many days. It has been found that the pressure inside the chamber is gradually restored to atmospheric level. During this process, the pores are formed by the carbon dioxide molecules that abandon the polymer, resulting in a form of sponge-like structure. It has been found that there were difficulties associated with this technique which caused an excessive release of heat during the process.

8.7.2.5 Emulsification/freeze drying

This emulsification and freeze-drying techniques do not require the use of a solid bargain. The process is simple as a synthetic polymer which first is dissolved in a suitable solvent, and water is added to the polymeric solution; then the two liquids are mixed properly to obtain an emulsion. Before separation of two phases, the prepared emulsion is casted into a mold and quickly frozen by means of dipping into liquid nitrogen. Later on, the frozen emulsion is subsequently freeze dried to remove the isolated water moisture and the solvent, thus leaving behind a solidified and porous polymeric structure. It has been suggested that though emulsification and freeze drying allow for a faster preparation of emulsion structure compared to the SCPL technique, it still requires the use of many solvents. Additionally, pore size is relatively small and porosity is often found to be irregular.

8.7.2.6 Thermally induced phase separation

Similar to the emulsification or freeze-drying techniques, this thermally induced phase separation technique needs the use of a solvent with a low melting point that is easy to sublime. For instance, dioxane could be used to dissolve poly-lactic acid, then phase separation is induced through the addition of a small quantity of water which leads to the formation of a polymer-rich and a polymer-poor phase. After cooling the polymer for some time, vacuum drying is done to obtain a porous scaffold. However, this phase separation presents the same disadvantages of emulsification and freeze drying.

8.8 Significance of cell and tissue engineering

There are two alternative approaches available for tissue engineering. It may involve either injection of a growth factor required for *in situ* regeneration of lost tissue or may involve transplantation of a three-dimensional structure (bio-artificial or bio-hybrid organ) made up of scaffolds of biodegradable polymers with tissues made up of cells harvested from the patient or a donor individual. When a growth factor is injected, the patient's own cells migrate into the wound site and regenerate the desired tissue/organ. However, when a bio-hybrid organ is transplanted at the site of injury, the tissue/organ regenerates using the polymer as a scaffold and later the artificial polymer as a scaffold and later the artificial polymer component of the organ breaks down, thus leaving only a completely natural final product in the body of the patient. In US hospitals and other developed countries, artificial tissues that are already being used for medical treatment include fabricated skin, cartilage, bone, ligament, and tendon. It is also hoped that at least some of the whole organs such as liver, lung, kidney, pancreas, breast, intestine, and so on will become available off-the-shelf for treatment by the year 2018, if not earlier. Considerable research has also been done on the nature and use of biomaterials that can be used for tissue engineering. A brief account of the two different approaches mentioned above and also of the biomaterials that are used for tissue engineering, including the achievements of the art and science of tissue engineering, will be presented in this chapter.

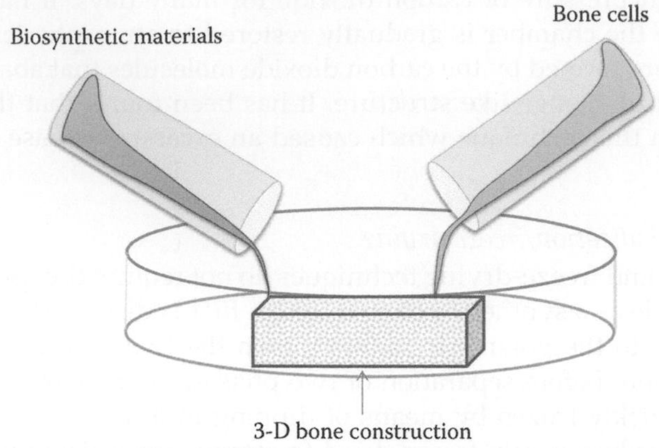

Figure 8.5 3-Dimensional construction of bone scaffolds.

8.8.1 *Biomaterials in tissue engineering*

It has been reported that a variety of biomaterials have been utilized in tissue engineering. These may range from synthetic polymers with biological characteristics to biologically derived polymers. They are used for repair of damaged or diseased tissues and to create entirely new tissues for transplantation. For example, they serve as matrices to guide tissue regeneration and to release growth factors. Biomaterials are also available that block antibody permeation in transplanted tissue, which could otherwise lead to transplant rejection. Recombinant DNA technology has also been used to generate self-assembly of biomaterials, which are designed to mimic natural tissue matrices that are potentially useful for engineering tissue for an injured bone (Figure 8.5).

8.8.2 *Synthetic polymers*

Biological recognition ability can be imparted to material surfaces by immersing a synthetic polymer in a fluid containing the cell adhesion proteins that, in turn, will form an adherent monolayer on the polymer surface. These adhesion proteins include fibronectin and vitronectin, both present in blood plasma and many other biological fluids. Cells will attach to these surfaces, spread and flatten utilizing their own cell-surface receptors, which will help in recognizing adhesion molecules adsorbed on polymer surface. In due time, a cell may secrete its own adhesion proteins and the extracellular matrix (ECM). This attachment of cells to polymer surface induces several intracellular activities, which can be exploited in engineering tissues. The most important receptor molecules recognizing adhesion proteins are integrins. The recognition sites in these adhesion proteins have been tracked to a mere three amino acid peptide, that is, arginine–glycine–aspartic acid (RGD), which is the consensus sequence in many integrins. The sequence RGD is recognized by many integrin receptors. Several other oligopeptide sequences have also been identified which bind to nonintegrin receptors.

8.8.3 *Synthetic peptides*

In view of the availability of information on cell binding domains of adhesion molecules, arginine–glycine–aspartic acid and other oligopeptide have also been incorporated (as a substitute to adhesion protein) into polymer molecules (e.g., polyurethanes) to stimulate cell adhesion through direct interaction with the cells. These peptides have been shown to support adhesion of many cell types. The density of these peptides, however, needs to be optimized, because densities that are too low may yield low strength of adhesion, while those that are too high may inhibit the ability of a cell to migrate. Further, the peptides may be so selected as to provide selectivity to biomaterials in supporting cell adhesion, that is, it may be selectively adhesive to one set of cell types but not to the others. Such biomaterials with selectivity may be useful for tissue engineering under certain conditions. For instance, in the vascular graft, growth of endothelial cells lining the blood vessels is desired, but the adhesion and spreading of blood platelets is not desired, since the latter may lead to occlusion of the graft by thrombus.

8.8.4 Amine-rich oligopeptides

There is another class of oligopeptides that are amine rich and known to support cell adhesion with low specificity. These oligopeptides bear several positive charges (e.g., arginine, lysine), uninterrupted by negative charges such as glutamic acid and aspartic acid. These sequences are known as heparin binding domains, and help in cell adhesion by binding to cell surface heparan sulfate or chondroitin sulfate proteoglycans.

8.8.5 Natural polymers as biomaterials

It has been reported that collagen (protein) can be purified from animal or human tissues and can also be obtained in the form of gels to be used as biomaterials for tissue engineering. Porosity of such a gel may differ and the pore size may influence cell behavior. This property is utilized in tissue engineering. Polysaccharides have also been used to get biopolymer gels that are useful in tissue engineering. Diluted solutions of the polymer are used as a coating on tissue surfaces to reduce damage during handling of such tissue. Hyaluronic acid is an important example and can be modified to meet the requirements of material property needed for tissue engineering. Protein polymers found in nature are also used for tissue engineering. Silk is one example, which consists of alanine–glycine (AG) repeats forming stacked antiparallel β-sheets. Length of AG repeats can be altered using recombinant DNA technology. Individual amino acids can also be introduced or substituted to alter the properties of these biomaterials.

8.8.6 Polymer matrices

Several approaches are being currently used for engineering structural tissues. One of these approaches involves transplanting cells on biodegradable polymer matrices, which offer the following advantages: (i) deliver cells to specific anatomical sites; (ii) provide space for tissue development, and (iii) guide tissue formation before being degraded. However, it requires isolation and multiplication of cells *in vitro* and many cell types show poor survivals on transplantation. In another strategy, tissue inductive proteins (e.g., bone morphogenic proteins, and platelet-derived growth factor (PDGF) are also delivered. However, decreased stability of these proteins causes a problem. To overcome this problem, delivery of plasmid DNA, encoding tissue-inductive factors has been proposed. A limited exposure of cells to the plasmid leads to low expression of the genes carried by the plasmid; therefore, incorporation of plasmid DNA into tissue engineering matrices and its subsequent sustained release *in vivo* has recently been suggested as a means to engineer tissues. This will allow the transaction of a large number of cells at a defined site to facilitate production of a therapeutic protein to enhance tissue development. A plasmid, encoding PDGF, has already been used for this purpose, and its other uses include DNA vaccines and correction of metabolic deficiencies.

8.8.7 *Resorption of biomaterials*

All the above biomaterials described in the previous section of this chapter are resorbable. The structural features that communicate resorption ability, include polyesters and copolyesters of hydroxy-acids which are widely used. Their ester bonds are labile and undergo nonenzymatic degradation in two steps; the first step lead to lowering of molecular weight and the second step involves fragmentation, when the fragments are taken up by cells or macrophages for excretion. These polyesters have been successfully used as matrices for cell transplantation and tissue generation. The process of resorption may take 6 months to 3 years depending upon the nature of the polyester. Copolymers have been formed with polyethylene glycol to reduce inflammation during degradation to improve biocompatibility (due to hydrophilicity). Cross-linking of polymers for *in situ* formation of biomaterials has also been used in tissue engineering. A copolymer of polyethylene glycol and polypropylene glycol (known as Pluronic or Poloxamer) is one such biomaterial. It is soluble in water and forms a hydrogel at 37°C (human body temperature). This feature allows in situ formation of adherent biomaterials on tissue surfaces and also allows resorption by dissolution from the hydrogel phase. These biomaterials can also be made to develop biological recognition properties with the help of amino acids.

8.8.8 *Inducing tissue regeneration*

Often tissue does not regenerate except under healthy conditions, so that the biomaterials need to be designed so that the tissue is induced not only to regenerate but also to acquire the desired architecture in healthy conditions. While designing biomaterials, the density of adsorbed proteins may be adjusted so that it supports cell spreading, receptor clustering, and cytoskeleton organization. For example, in one study it was shown that the desired level of density is 12,000 ligands/m^2 in the case of an immobilized RGD peptide based on fibronectin. To induct regeneration of single cells, sometimes islands of single cell dimensions were created on gold substrata, using alkanethiols as the adsorbed biomaterial. Similarly, complex patterns of many cells may be created using photolithography and amino-functional alkoxysilanes. These approaches have been used to fabricate arrays of direct neurons in culture. Multilayered cellular structures have also been produced, which histologically appear very similar to the dermis. These tissues can be as large as 100 cm^2 per sheets. The tissues are tested in vitro for toxicity of drugs and cosmetics, and also tested for transplantation in place of skin auto grafts.

This approach is being commercialized by the company Organogenesis in the United States. Porous degradable polymers are used as supports for cells to be cultured, so that these polymers making the support will degrade after the cultured cells are used in surgery. For example, chondrocytes are seeded and cultured within such polymers, and used to generate cartilage for surgery, ordinarily done for reconstruction of a damaged tissue. Engineering of a tissue with more than one type of cell is also possible, but poses a serious challenge. A large tissue, with vascularization and specific function, such as a functional liver, is an example. In the liver, both hepatocytes and bile duct cells are organized. Vascularization can be facilitated by the following; (i) use of tissue that is conducive to vascularization; (ii) pre-implantation of devices in the tissue to facilitate vascularization, for example, poly (I-lactic acid); and (iii) large pore size for faster vascularization. For instance, hepatocytes transplanted in the rat on poly-glycolic acid filamentous sheets were shown to vascularize rapidly. Inducing a desired functional state within cells is another important area, where hepatocytes provide a good example. Although hepatocytes rapidly dedifferentiate and lose their hepatocyte-specific function, biomaterials have been used to induce prolonged retention of hepatocyte phenotype in culture.

8.8.9 Growth factors

It has been suggested that growth factors can be introduced to the site of damage or loss of tissue through injections for regeneration of tissue. In this connection, some success has been achieved for the regeneration of bone and blood vessels. For instance, during the mid-1960s it was shown in animals that if powdered bone is implanted, new bony tissue will be formed. This also led to the identification and isolation of bone morphogenetic proteins (BMPs) and the genes coding for this protein, so that when genes for BMPs were inserted into mammalian cell lines, BMPs were produced in large quantities. Clinical trials are being conducted to find out the potential of the above approach in healing acute bone fractures and some positive results have already been obtained. Another use of growth-promoting molecules in tissue engineering involved production of new blood vessels, a phenomenon described as angiogenesis. Many angiogenesis-stimulating molecules that are produced through recombinant DNA technology are now commercially available, and have been shown to promote growth of new blood vessels that bypass blockages in arteries. Small-scale trials on human beings are also being conducted in this connection.

The pharmaceutical industry is busy in resolving some of the above issues for the therapeutic use of tissue engineering and there are some examples: (i) new injectable biodegradable polymers have been tried for bone regeneration. These polymers are moldable, so that they can fill irregular spaces in damaged bones, and harden in 10–15 min. The regenerated skeletal region would have mechanical properties similar to those of the bone they replace and the polymers degrade within weeks to months, thus filling the gaps in bones, caused due to injury. (ii) Biodegradable and injectable hydrogels containing useful molecules have been tried for dental defects involving poor bondage between teeth and the underlying bone. These hydrogels provide a scaffold, on which new bone can grow without the formation of a scar. (iii) Genes encoding growth factors may be cloned in plasmid vectors and inserted, so that the cells take up the DNA and with its help synthesize the desired growth factor for bone regeneration. Since the DNA does not get inserted in the cellular DNA and remains free floating, it eventually degrades. This DNA can also be inserted in the form of three-dimensional biodegradable polymers spiked with cloned DNA, so that the DNA will synthesize the growth factor over an extended period and the structure will serve as a scaffold for new tissue formation.

8.8.10 In situ tissue regeneration

Appropriate types of cultured living cells can also be introduced at the site of tissue damage or loss, so that these cells can help in the tissue regeneration. During the 1970s and 1980s, this approach was actually tried in patients with skin wounds and cartilage damage. A small sample of cells, that may be available in stock, can be quickly used for this purpose. In the United States, living skin cells have already been approved for this purpose and are being used for treatment of diabetic ulcers, skin cancer, and severe burns.

Cartilage is another tissue which is being produced artificially and used for orthopedic, craniofacial, and urological applications. Since cartilage has low nutrient needs, it does not require new blood vessels. In the United States, approval has been granted to a company (Genzyme Tissue Repair) to engineer tissues (derived from patients own cells) for the repair of knee-cartilage damage. Full regeneration in this case takes 12–18 months. It has also been shown that new cartilage can be grown in the shapes of an ear, nose, and other forms. The possibility of using this approach in treating urological disorders, such as incontinence, and in regenerating breasts removed due to breast cancer is being explored in the United States.

Skin is perhaps the only organ that can be artificially made from cell culture and used for grafting when skin is completely damaged due to severe burns. Of the few cell types that can be cultured, keratinocytes, which make 90% of the epidermis of skin, are the most important. They are responsible for giving rise to corneocytes making the external cornified layers of skin, and their proliferation is facilitated by the fibroblasts found in the dermis layer of the skin. Since fibroblasts are useful for culturing keratinocytes, fibroblast cells, called 3T3 cells, were used to cover the bottom of a vessel before adding epidermal cells for culturing them. Other substances added in culture medium included epidermal growth factors, cholera toxin, and a mixture of other growth factors. Only 1–10% epidermal cells proliferate, others having already started the process of differentiation. These cells form colonies, are separated again, and transferred to fresh culture to allow better growth. The process of separating cells from colonies and reculturing them is continued to discourage stratification of cell layers and to allow the cell colonies to become confluent forming a sheet of pure epithelium. Moreover, these cells of pure epithelium are linked by desmosomes and this cultured epithelium can be detached from the vessel using the enzyme dispase.

Extraneous protein attached to a backing of gauze can be brought to the hospital to be used for grafting on patients having severe burns. Meticulous reparation of wounds is required, since they are often contaminated, and complete elimination of microorganisms are essential. It is important that cultured keratinocytes used to generate epidermis must come from the unburned portion of the skin of the patient himself; otherwise these will soon be rejected. Starting from a 3 cm^2 skin of the patient, it can be expanded 5000-fold in 3–4 weeks to supply 1.7 m^2 of the skin needed for an adult human. The entire body may need 350 grafts, each of 25 cm^2 to cover only the front or back surface. Before the cultured epithelium became available, split thickness grafts were used which involved transfer of 0.3 mm thick skin (epidermis + part of dermis) from one part of body to the other. Such grafting leads to quick recovery and normalization of skin. However, in grafting of cultured skin, the samples of regenerated skin are taken over a period of five years; the different elements of normal skin return at different rates, but eventually normal skin, with all essential components, is regenerated.

A variety of diseases have also been treated using cultured keratinocytes. The following are some examples: (i) Scars on the skin can be removed using cultured skin. (ii) Cultured oral keratinocytes have been used to regenerate epithelium of the mouth. (iii) Cultured urethral keratinocytes have been used to repair congenital penile defects. (iv) For some middle ear diseases with troublesome discharge, cultured epidermal keratinocytes are used. (v) Chronic skin ulcers have also been treated with cultured grafts; even allografts (skin from another individual) are successful in these ulcers. More than 500 patients throughout the world have already received cultured keratinocytes for treatment of burns, ulcers, or other conditions. However, this is a very small number in comparison with the number of patients who need this help. In the future, other cell types may also be successfully cultured and used for the following applications: (i) use of cultured endothelial cells for lining of vascular prostheses (artificial limbs, etc.); (ii) use of cultured urothelial cells to repair urinary tracts; (iii) use of pancreatic islet cells to treat diabetes; (iv) use of cultured liver cells to provide for hepatic function; and (v) use of cultured myoblasts to treat muscle diseases.

8.8.11 Bone grafts

It has been reported that millions of orthopedic operations take place in many parts of the world every year. Often these procedures involve repair of injured bones. Autogenous bone grafts are generally used for repair of these injured bones. In these autogenous grafts, bone segments are taken from one part of the body (nonessential part of a bone, like brim of the pelvis) and transplanted to repair bones that are essential for weight bearing or other functions such as leg bones (Figure 8.6). In this procedure of auto grafts, the patient suffers the pain and potential complications due to the harvesting from one bone to repair another bone. Revolutionary alternatives to autogenous bone grafts are now becoming available.

In recent years, it is possible to engineer bone tissue in the laboratory from a combination of cells, bioactive factors, and supportive three-dimensional matrices. There were two studies published in September 2000 (*Nature Biotechnology*). In one study, the bony precursor cells were triggered to aggregate by transforming growth factor β1 (TGF- β1) This was followed by the formation of organized bone tissue *in vitro* in a manner, similar to that in vivo. In the second study, sea coral (calcium carbonate-based ceramic) was used in combination with autogenous mesenchymal stem cells (MSCs) to produce orthopedic implants that facilitated the healing of bone defects in sheep. Thus, it became the first such device (containing living human cells) to receive FDA's approval. Apligraf was shown to repair various ulcers, diabetic ulcers, skin lesions (due to leaky veins) and serious burns, efficiently. It has also been tried with patients undergoing dermatological surgery.

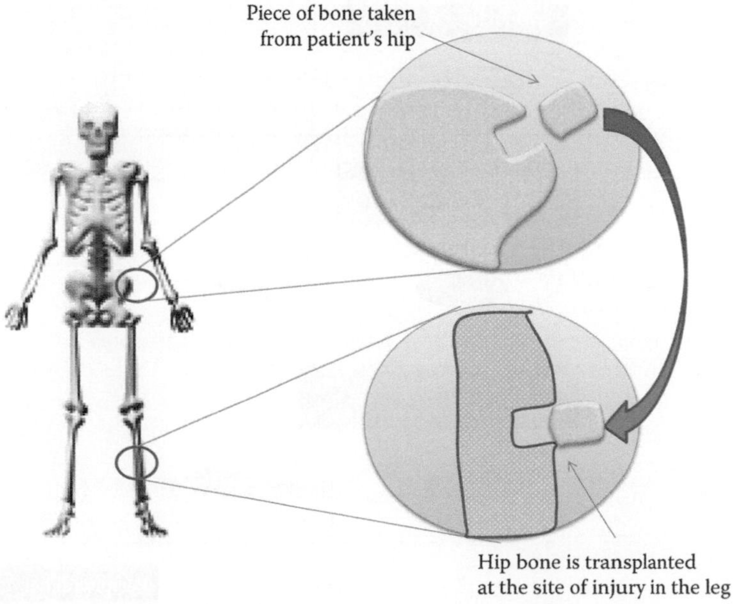

Figure 8.6 Autologous bone grafts.

Apligraf is being already marketed in the United States and Canada and is delivered fresh with a shelf life of five days at room temperature. Two skin products were also created by the company Advanced Tissue Sciences. These products are known by the trade names Transcyte and Dermagraft. Transcyte consists of functional dermis and is alive only until frozen for shipment and until taken for off-the shelf use; it does not carry any living cells when used by the patient.

8.8.12 *Artificial nerve grafts*

Nerve injuries are a class of most serious injuries in the human body, since neurons do not replicate. However, under suitable conditions, axon extensions do regenerate over gaps caused by injury, thus reconnecting with the distal stumps and reestablishing functional contacts. When a nerve is cut or crushed and nerve function is lost, the portion of the nerve distal to the injury dies and degenerates. In such cases, the proximal segment may be able to regenerate the distal part and reestablish nerve function (Figure 8.7). Although, small gaps created by injury can be repaired by axon regeneration, large gaps need the insertion of grafts that work as guides for axon regeneration. For the nerve injuries noted above, a typical graft is an autograft, which is a segment of nerve removed from another part of the body. Therefore, artificial nerve grafts, also known as a nerve guiding channels, have been used for extending the length on which nerves can successfully regenerate. These artificial nerve grafts are synthetic conduits, which bridge the gaps between nerve stumps (produced due to injury), thus directing and supporting the nerve regeneration.

8.8.12.1 *Synthetic nonresorbable nerve grafts*

It has been reported that silicon tubing was one of the first and most frequently used synthetic material for nerve grafts. These could be used for filling a gap of about 10 mm; a longer distance could be bridged by filling the graft with neuro-trophic substances.

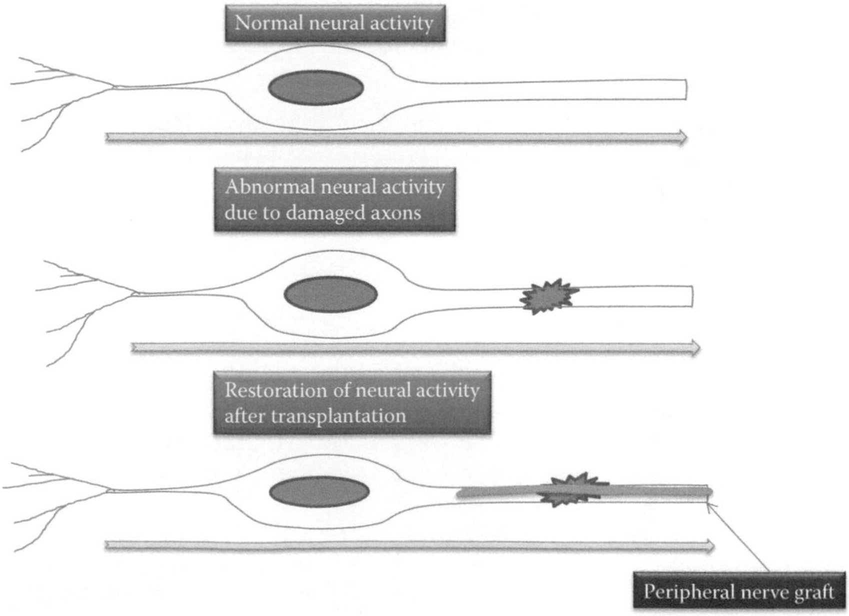

Figure 8.7 Artificial nerve transplantation.

8.8.12.2 Synthetic resorbable nerve grafts

Since silicon tubes may be toxic and may cause constriction of the nerve after regeneration, a bio-resorbable material is preferred over nonresorbable. Nonresorbable conduits may need to be removed, after nerve regeneration, by a surgical operation, while resorbable conduits eventually degrade, thus promoting long-term recovery. Polyglycolic acid and similar other polymers have been shown to be better suited for the manufacture of bio-resorbable nerve grafts.

8.8.12.3 Bio-artificial nerve grafts

Bio-artificial nerve grafts are synthetic nerve grafts seeded in their lumen with cultured Schwann cells suspended in a gel. It has been reported that Schwann cells secrete neurotrophic factors and express cell adhesion molecules that enhance nerve regeneration. These bio-artificial nerve grafts, making use of biodegradable channels seeded with Schwann cells and equipped with release of trophic factors, have shown great promise and are making their way into clinics. Since the use of Schwann cells, causes immune response, immuno-suppression is generally required while making use of bio-artificial nerve grafts. However, efforts are made to obtain universal Schwann cells, which can be frozen and thawed whenever needed for seeding conduits. These developments and future research will lead to improved methods for repair of the peripheral and central nervous systems.

8.8.13 Hemoglobin-based blood substitutes

It has been well known to all of us that hemoglobin is required for a variety of clinical applications ranging from local oxygen delivery to more complex applications in trauma and sickle cell anemia, which exploit hemoglobin effects on the circulatory system and capillary blood pressure. Hemoglobin-based blood substitutes are being developed for this purpose to be used as oxygen carriers or for maintaining blood pressure in critically ill patients. Many such hemoglobin-based blood substitutes have actually been prepared, but there are concerns about the toxicity of such cell-free hemoglobin outside the RBCs. Chemical engineering and genetic engineering are also being used to develop second-generation hemoglobin prototypes, that carry oxygen and have suppressed ability to cause vasoconstriction and oxidative inactivation. Despite the progress made toward the use of these blood substitutes, intrinsic toxicity of the hemoglobin molecule is a matter of concern. It is hoped that in the future, safer hemoglobin-based blood substitutes will become available and used as therapeutics.

8.8.14 Bio-hybrid organs

Over the last few years the use of artificial skin, bone cartilage, and blood substitutes have completely revolutionized the tissue engineering field. Though artificial skin is already being marketed, artificial bone and artificial cartilage should become available by the year 2018, if not earlier. However, the ultimate objective of tissue engineering remains to provide complete internal organs such as pancreas, liver, lung, kidney, heart, and so on. Some progress has already been achieved. For instance, in animals new liver-like tissue could be created from transplanted liver cells. Biomaterial and drugs that facilitate growth of transplanted liver cells have also been identified in some cases, but the entire function of the organ could not be replicated. Kidney cells have also been used to make neo-organs that possess the filtering capability of the kidney. In recent animal studies, intestines or urinary bladders could also be grown within the abdominal cavity and then spliced into the existing intestinal tissue or urinary bladder. Human versions of these neo-intestines when available will be a boon to patients suffering with short-bowel syndrome from birth. Efforts are also being made to grow new hearts. Although it may take 10–20 years to get an entire heart through tissue engineering, but heart valves and blood vessels of the heart may become available sooner.

8.9 Bioreactor

As you know, cells can grow on Petri dishes, but the large quantity of cells cannot grow on them. Over the last few years attempts have been made to grow cells in large volume by using a special vessel which is known as bioreactor or fermenter. Large-scale cultures are essential where cell cultures are used for producing useful product-like biochemicals such as interferon, hormones, interleukins, enzymes, and antibodies. Fermenters up to 10,000 L are used for this purpose (Figure 8.8). Large-scale cell culture is a major industry in biotechnology, with millions of dollars turn around especially in Europe, North and South America, Africa, Japan, and India. The list of some of the major commercial bioreactors are given in Table 8.1.

8.9.1 Types of bioreactor

A fermentation process is a biological process divided into two main types, with various combinations and modifications.

8.9.1.1 Batch fermentation process

In batch fermentation process, a tank is filled with the prepared mash of raw materials to be fermented. It has been reported that the temperature and pH of microbial fermentation can be properly adjusted, and occasionally nutritive supplements are added to the prepared mash. Moreover, the mash is steam sterilized in a pure culture process and,

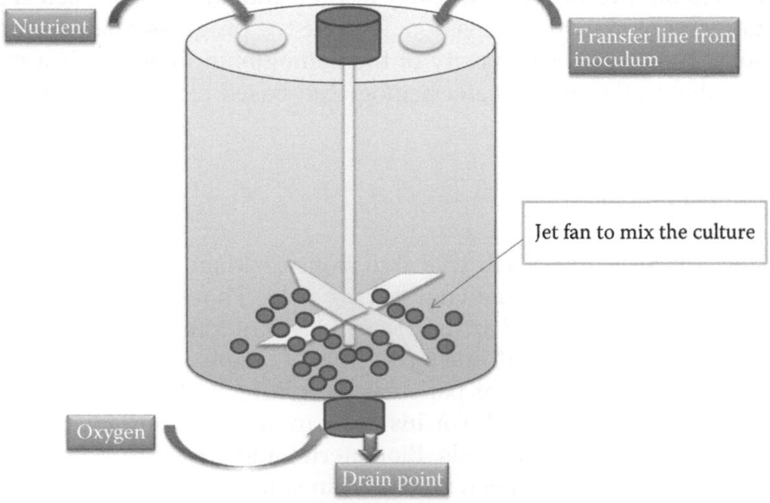

Figure 8.8 Large-scale cell production by bioreactor.

Table 8.1 Major Types of Commercial Bioreactors

Types of bioreactor	Products
Microbial cell culture	Singly cell's protein, baker's yeast, *Lactobacillus, E. coli*
Microbial enzyme culture	Catalase, amylase, protease, pectinase, glucose, isomerase, cellulose, hemicellulose, lipase, lactose, streptokinase
Microbial metabolite culture	Ethanol, citric acid, glutamic acid, lysine, vitamins, polysaccharides
Recombinant protein	Insulin, HBV, interferon, GCSF
Biotransformation	Phenyl acetyl carbinol, steroid biotransformation

afterwards, inoculum of a pure culture is added to the fermenter. The process of fermentation is started and after some time, the contents of the fermenter are taken out for further processing. The fermenter must be cleaned and the process is repeated.

8.9.1.2 *Continuous fermentation process*

In a continuous fermentation process, growth of microorganisms is monitored by a growth curve, with a lag phase followed by a logarithmic phase. The culture process is terminated by progressive decrement growth rate until the stationary phase is reached. It has been reported that in continuous fermentation, the substrate is added to the fermenter continuously at a fixed rate which maintains the organisms in the logarithmic growth phase. The fermentation products are taken out on a regular basis and it has been reported that the design and arrangements for continuous fermentation are somewhat complex.

8.9.1.3 *Aerobic fermentation*

A number of industrial processes called fermentations are carried on by microorganisms under aerobic conditions. Moreover, in older aerobic processes it was necessary to furnish a large surface area by exposing fermentation media to air, whereas in modern fermentation processes, the aerobic conditions are maintained in a closed fermenter with submerged cultures. The culture contents of the fermenter can be agitated with an impeller and aerated by forcing sterilized air.

8.9.1.4 *Anaerobic fermentation*

In principle, a fermenter is designed to operate under anaerobic conditions, generally the same as that designed to operate under aerobic conditions except that arrangements for intense agitation and aeration are unnecessary. However, other anaerobic fermentation require minor aeration for the initial growth phase, and enough agitation for mixing and maintenance of temperature.

8.9.2 *Bioreactor design*

Bioreactor design is a relatively complex engineering task, which is studied in the discipline of biochemical engineering. It has been reported that under optimum conditions, the microorganisms are able to perform their desired function with very high rate of success. The bioreactor's environmental conditions such as oxygen, nitrogen, carbon dioxide, temperature, pH and dissolved oxygen levels, and agitation speed/circulation rate need to be closely monitored and controlled. Moreover, most industrial bioreactor manufacturers use vessels, sensors, and a control system networked together. It has been reported that biological fermentation is a major source of heat; therefore, in most cases bioreactors need be refrigerated. In general, refrigeration can be done with an external jacket. In an aerobic process, optimal oxygen transfer is perhaps the most difficult task to accomplish because oxygen is poorly soluble in water and is relatively scarce in air. It has been shown that oxygen transfer is usually done by agitation, which is also needed to mix nutrients and to keep the fermentation homogeneous. In practice, bioreactors are often pressurized; this increases the solubility of oxygen in water.

8.10 Cell banking

It has been advocated that cell banking is an essential and preliminary prerequisites for a large-scale cell culture and its scaling up. For these, master cell banks (MCB) are first established. These master cell banks are then utilized to develop master working cell banks (MWCB). The development of MWCB should be sufficient to satisfy the needs of the production system. If the MWCB is not adequate, a new master cell bank has to be developed. In order to confirm cell stability MWCB is repeatedly subcultured and each generation subjected to screening to rule out any change in the cellular material. It has been reported that the scaling up of cell cultures can be done as monolayer cultures, suspension cultures, or immobilized cell systems. Production of the Master Cell Bank (MCB) is one of the first steps in therapeutic development as it will support not only the clinical development of the product but also the profitable supply phase.

8.11 Trends in tissue engineering

The biomanufacturing additive processes (BMAP) signify a new group of nonconventional fabrication techniques, which have been recently introduced in the biomedical engineering field. The main benefits of these techniques are to rapidly produce complex 3-D models in a layer-by-layer manner and their ability to use various raw materials. During diagnostic imaging, these fabrication techniques can be used to produce constructs to identify shape of the defect or injury. Interestingly, some processes can operate at room temperature, which allows cell encapsulation without significantly affected cell viability. In the tissue engineering, BMAPs are used to manufacture scaffolds with tailored external shape and predefined internal morphology, which allows better control of pore size and pore distribution. It has been reported that additive biomanufacturing processes have remarkably improved the range and diversity of scaffolds and is extensively studied in many innovative process techniques such as bio-electro-spraying, hydrogel micro-patterning, organ bio-printing, laser writing of cells, and microvasculature fabrication.

8.12 Challenges of tissue engineering

The potential of tissue engineering in overcoming human suffering is no longer a fiction; science creation of bio-hybrid organs have been shown to be possible. It has already been shown that the biotechnology companies had a market worth more than US$4 billion in 2000 and this market will grow, with the progress in this new field of biotechnology. However, there are some limitations that will have to be overcome before tissue engineering is widely used to relieve human beings from suffering caused by defects and injuries in a wide range of tissue/organs. These various limitations are described in brief.

8.12.1 Nonavailability of reliable source of cells

A reliable source of cell for tissue engineering is necessary, since animal cells are often rejected by the human immune system. The following possibilities are available and are now being explored. For example, human progenitor cells from bone marrow can be induced to form either the osteoblasts (for bones) or chondrocytes (for cartilage). However, it is still difficult to obtain bone marrow stem or progenitor cells since they are often contaminated with fibroblasts, which overgrow and replace stem cells. Similarly, progenitor cells from adult liver can be made to mature into hepatocytes (producing bile) or epithelial cells. Donor cell lines are another approach, in which proteins on the surfaces of cells are either removed or masked by other molecules, so that they lose their identity and are not rejected on transplantation. Both animal cells and unmatched human cells are being tried for this purpose.

8.12.2 Adequate quantities of cells and tissues with desired properties

It has been reported that existing methods for cell and tissue culture in bioreactors often yield too few cells, or yield sheets of tissues that are either thin or lacked uniform thickness or the desired mechanical properties. Solutions for this problem are being sought. For instance, success has been achieved in getting segments of cartilage thick enough to replace worn-out cartilage in the knee. Mechanical properties of the cultured tissue can also be manipulated, by manipulating the force exerted by the fluid in cultured cells in the bioreactor. For example, cartilage cultured in rotating vessels has been shown to be stiffer, durable, and responsive to external forces. Osteoblasts cultured in a base of stirring collagen beads make more bone material than they do on a flat surface. Methods are similarly being developed for engineering blood vessels, skeletal tissue, and cardiac muscles, which develop mechanical properties and become strong enough to be able to respond to physical stress. Tissue engineering becomes more complicated, when used for designing organs like the liver, which has six types of cells that are organized in lobules and vary not only in their behavior/function, but also in their interaction with other cells. Therefore, in order to be able to get a bio-artificial liver, we should know how to grow hepatocytes and other cells of the liver to maximize their abilities to perform their normal physiological roles. Angiogenesis will also be necessary for sustaining many tissue-engineered organs such as pancreas, livers, and kidneys, which need a large blood supply. Success in stimulating angiogenesis in bio-artificial organs has been achieved by coating the polymer scaffold with growth factors that trigger blood vessel formation. The activity of these growth factors needs to be regulated, so that blood vessels are formed only when and where they are needed. The use of specific biodegradable biomaterials to allow for remodeling of the transplanted bio-artificial organs is another active area of future research which has already been discussed earlier in this chapter.

8.12.3 Tissue engineering and reperfusion injury

One of the essential requirements of tissue engineering is that the artificial tissue is stored and preserved for long periods of time. Much of the injury to a transplanted organ occurs during reperfusion, when the organ is connected to a blood supply in the recipient patient. It is during this process that many cells of transplanted tissue die. However, molecules have been identified, which if added to the preservation solution will protect the tissue-engineered products from reperfusion injury.

8.13 Summary

With the emergence of *in vitro* cell culture methods, which means to culture living cells outside of body, it become possible to easily grow human body cells in Petri dishes in the laboratories. The definition of tissue engineering usually covers the replacement or reconstruction of the human body tissue or organs such as bone, cartilage, blood vessels, liver, bladder, skin, and so on. The main function of reconstructed cells or tissues is to perform the normal body function. The cell and tissue engineering term has been useful in performing biochemical functions through a bioengineered-created support system like an artificial pancreas or a bioengineered liver. The term regenerative medicine is frequently used synonymously with cell and tissue engineering, though in regenerative medicine, cell-based therapy is considered to be a main branch of regenerative medicine. In human tissue, bioengineering utilizes living cells as bioengineered materials which include using living fibroblasts in skin repair, whereas cartilage can be repaired with living chondrocytes.

8.14 Scholar's achievements

R.S. Langer: Robert Samuel Langer, Jr. (born August 29, 1948 in Albany, New York) is an American engineer and the David H. Koch Institute Professor at the Massachusetts Institute of Technology. He is a widely recognized and cited researcher in biotechnology, especially in the fields of drug delivery systems and tissue engineering.

J. Vacanti: Dr. Joseph Vacanti has been working in the field of tissue engineering since its beginnings in the early 1980s; a mission that stems from his long-held interest in solving the problem of organ shortages. His approach to developing tissue involves a scaffold made of an artificial, biodegradable polymer, seeding it with living cells, and bathing it in growth factors. The cells can come from living tissue or stem cells.

S.V. Arnold: S.V. Arnold is a pioneer in tissue culture.

8.15 Knowledge builder

Aerobic Fermentation: Fermentation is a metabolic process converting sugar into acids, gases, and/or alcohol using yeast or bacteria. In its strictest sense, fermentation is the absence of the electron transport chain and takes a reduced carbon source, such as glucose, to make products like lactic acid or acetate. No oxidative phosphorylation is used, only substrate level phosphorylation, which yields a much lower amount of ATP. Fermentation is also used much more broadly to refer to the bulk growth of microorganisms on a growth medium. The science of fermentation is known as zymology.

Anaerobic fermentation: Anaerobic digestion is a collection of processes by which microorganisms break down biodegradable material in the absence of oxygen. The process is used for industrial or domestic purposes to manage waste and/or to produce fuels. Much of the fermentation used industrially to produce food and drink products, as well as home fermentation, uses anaerobic digestion. Silage is produced by anaerobic digestion.

Apligraf: Apligraf is living cell-based product for chronic venous leg ulcers and diabetic foot ulcers. Apligraf is supplied as a living, bi-layered skin substitute.

Bioassays: Bioassay or biological assay, or biological standardization is a type of scientific experiment. Bioassays are typically conducted to measure the effects of a substance on a living organism and are essential in the development of new drugs and in monitoring environmental pollutants. Both are procedures by which the potency or the nature of a substance is estimated by studying its effects on living matter. Bioassay is a procedure for the determination of the concentration of a particular constitution of a mixture.

Biocompatibility: Biocompatibility is related to the behavior of biomaterials in various contexts. The term refers to the ability of a material to perform with an appropriate host response in a specific situation. The ambiguity of the term reflects the ongoing development of insights into how biomaterials interact with the human body and eventually how those interactions determine the clinical success of a medical device (such as pacemaker, hip replacement, or stent). Modern medical devices and prostheses are often made of more than one material so it might not always be sufficient to talk about the biocompatibility of a specific material.

Biodegradable polymers: Biodegradable polymers are polymers that break down and lose their initial integrity. Biodegradable polymers are used in medical devices to avoid a second operation to remove them, or to gradually release a drug.

Biopolymers: Biopolymers are polymers produced by living organisms. Since they are polymers, biopolymers contain monomeric units that are covalently bonded to form larger structures. There are three main classes of biopolymers, classified according to the monomeric units used and the structure of the biopolymer formed: polynucleotides (RNA and DNA), which are long polymers composed of 13 or more nucleotide monomers; polypeptides, which are short polymers of amino acids; and polysaccharides, which are often linear bonded polymeric carbohydrate structures.

Degenerative diseases: A degenerative disease is a disease in which the function or structure of the affected tissues or organs will increasingly deteriorate over time, whether due to normal bodily wear or lifestyle choices such as exercise or eating habits [1]. Degenerative diseases are often contrasted with infectious diseases.

DME: Dulbecco's modified Eagle's medium.

Epidermal keratinocytes: Keratinocyte is the predominant cell type in the epidermis, the outermost layer of the skin, constituting 90% of the cells found there. Those keratinocytes found in the basal layer (Stratum germinativum) of the skin are sometimes referred to as "basal cells" or "basal keratinocytes."

Immortalized cell: An immortalized cell line is a population of cells from a multicellular organism which would normally not proliferate indefinitely but, due to mutation, have evaded normal cellular senescence and instead can keep undergoing division. The cells can therefore be grown for prolonged periods in vitro. The mutations required for immortality can occur naturally or be intentionally induced for experimental purposes.

Morphogenesis: Morphogenesis is the biological process that causes an organism to develop its shape. It is one of three fundamental aspects of developmental biology along with the control of cell growth and cellular differentiation.

MEM: Minimum essential media is patterned after Eagle's media and is well suited for the growth of a broad spectrum of mammalian cells.

Organogenesis: In animal development, organogenesis is the process by which the ectoderm, endoderm, and mesoderm develop into the internal organs of the organism. The germ layers in organogenesis differ by three processes: folds, splits, and condensation. Developing early during this stage in chordate animals is the notochord, which induces the formation of the neural plate, and ultimately the neural tube. Vertebrate animals all differentiate from the gastrula the same way.

RPM-1640: RPMI-1640 medium was developed by Moore et al., at Roswell Park Memorial Institute, hence the acronym RPMI. The formulation is based on the RPMI-1630 series of media utilizing a bicarbonate buffering system and alterations in the amounts of amino acids and vitamins. RPMI-1640 medium has been used for the culture of human normal and neoplastic leukocytes. RPMI-1640 when properly supplemented, has demonstrated wide applicability for supporting growth of many types of cell cultures, including fresh human lymphocytes in the 72-h phytohemagglutinin (PHA) stimulation assay.

Schwann cells: Schwann cells, which are named after physiologist Theodor Schwann, are the principal glia of the peripheral nervous system (PNS). Glial cells function to support neurons and in the PNS, also include satellite cells, olfactory ensheathing cells, enteric glia, and glia that reside at sensory nerve endings, such as the Pacinian corpuscle. There are two types of Schwann cell, myelinating and nonmyelinating. Myelination Schwann cells wrap around axons of motor and sensory neurons to form the myelin sheath.

Stromal factors: The stromal cell-derived factor 1 (SDF-1) also known as C-X-C motif chemokine 12 (CXCL12) is a chemokine protein that in humans is encoded by the CXCL12 gene. Stromal cell-derived factors 1-alpha and 1-beta are small cytokines that belong to the intercrine family, members of which activate leukocytes and are often induced by proinflammatory stimuli such as lipopolysaccharide, TNF, or IL1.

Synthetic polymers: Polymer that is chemically manufactured from separate materials. Synthetic polymers require human intervention.

Tissue culture: Tissue culture is the growth of tissues or cells separate from the organism. This is typically facilitated via use of a liquid, semi-solid, or solid growth medium, such as broth or agar. Tissue culture commonly refers to the culture of animal cells and tissues, with the more specific term plant tissue culture being used for plants.

Tissue regeneration: Tissue regeneration are technologies that restore the function of diseased and damaged organs and tissues such as bone, cartilage, blood vessels, and pancreas.

Transformed cells: In molecular biology, transformation is genetic alteration of a cell resulting from the direct uptake, incorporation and expression of exogenous genetic material (exogenous DNA) from its surroundings and taken up through the cell membrane(s). Transformation occurs naturally in some species of bacteria, but it can also be affected by artificial means in other cells. For transformation to happen, bacteria must be in a state of competence, which might occur as a time-limited response to environmental conditions such as starvation and cell density.

Further reading

Abeyewickremea A, Kwoka A, McEwanb JR, and Jayasinghe SN 2009. Bio-electrospraying embryonic stem cells: Interrogating cellular viability and pluripotency. *Itegr Biol* 1, 260–266.

Adachi T, Osako Y, Tanaka M, Hojo M, and Hollister SJ 2006. Framework for optimal design of porous scaffold microstructure by computational simulation of bone regeneration. *Biomaterials* 27 (21): 3964–3972.

Ang TH, Sultana FS, Hutmacher DW, Wong YS, Fuh JY, Mo XM, Loh HT, Burdet E, and Teoh SH 2002. Fabrication of 3D chitosan-hydroxyapatite scaffolds using a robotic dispersing system. *Mater Sci Eng* C20, 35–42.

Barry R III, Shepherd R, Hanson J, Nuzzo R, Wiltzius P and Lewis J 2009. Direct-write assembly of 3D hydrogel scaffolds for guided cell growth. *Adv Mater* 21 (23), 2407–2410.

Bartolo PJS, Almeida H, and Laoui T 2009. Rapid prototyping and manufacturing for tissue engineering scaffolds. *Int J Comput Appl Technol* 36 (1): 1–9.

Bartolo PJ, Almeida HA, Rezende RA, Laoui T, Bidanda B, and Brtolo, P. (eds) 2007. Advanced processes to fabricate scaffolds for tissue engineering. In *Virtual Prototyping & Bio Manufacturing in Medical Applications*. Berlin: Springer Verlag, p. 299.

Bartolo PJ and Mitchell G 2003. Stereo-thermal-lithography. *Rapid Prototyping J* 9, 150–156.

Bucklen, Wettergreen W, Yuksel E, and Liebschner M 2008. Bone-derived CAD library for assembly of scaffolds in computer-aided tissue engineering. *Virtual Phys Prototyping* 3 (1), 13–23. [informaworld]

Cai S and Xi J 2008. A control approach for pore size distribution in the bone scaffold based on the hexahedral mesh refinement. *Comput-Aided Des* 40 (10–11), 1040–1050.

Chan G and Mooney DJ 2008. New materials for tissue engineering: Towards greater control over the biological response. *Trends Biotechnol* 26 (7), 382–392.

Cheah CM, Chua CK, Leong KF, Cheong CH and Naing MW 2004. Automatic algorithm for generating complex polyhedral scaffold structures for tissue engineering. *Tissue Eng* 10 (3–4), 595–610.

Chu TM, Halloran JW, Hollister SJ and Feinberg SE 2001. Hydroxyapatite implants with designed internal architecture. *J Mater Sci Mater Med* 12 (6): 471–478.

Chua CK, Leong KF, and Tan KH 2009. Specialized fabrication processes: Rapid prototyping. In: Narayan R. (ed.) *Biomedical Materials.* New York: Springer Science+Business Media.

Chua CK, Leong KF, Tan KH, Wiria FE and Cheah CM 2004. Development of tissue scaffolds using selective laser sintering of polyvinyl alcohol/hydroxyapatite biocomposite for craniofacial and joint defects. *J Mater Sci: Mater Med* 15 (10): 1113–1121.

Cooke MN, Fisher JP, Dean D, Rimnac C and Mikos AG 2002. Use of stereolithography to manufacture criticalsized 3D biodegradable scaffolds for bone ingrowth. *J Biomed Mater Res Part B: Appl Biomater* 64B, 65–69.

Crump SS 1992. Apparatus and method for creating three-dimensional objects Patent US5121329, June 9 1992.

Cui X and Boland T 2009. Human microvasculature fabrication using thermal inkjet printing technology. *Biomaterials* 30 (31): 6221–6227.

Domingos M, Dinucci D, Cometa S, Alderighi M, Bártolo PJ, and Chiellini F 2009. Polycaprolactone scaffolds fabricated via bioextrusion for tissue engineering applications. *Int J Biomater* 2009, 239643. doi: 10.1155/2009/239643.

Engel E, Michiardi A, Navarro M, Lacroix D, and Planell JA 2007. Nanotechnology in regenerative medicine: The materials side. *Trends Biotechnol* 26, 39–47.

Griffith ML and Halloran JW 1996. Free-form fabrication of ceramics via stereolithography. *J Am Ceramic Soc* 79, 2601–2608.

He J, Li D, Liu Y, Gong H, and Lu B 2008. Indirect fabrication of microstructured chitosan-gelatin scaffolds using rapid prototyping. *Virtual Phys Prototyping* 3 (3), 159–166.

Hollister SJ 2005. Porous scaffold design for tissue engineering. *Nat Mater* 4 (7), 518–524.

Jayasinghe S 2007. Bio-electrosprays: The development of a promising tool for regenerative and therapeutic medicine. *Biotechnol J* 2 (8), 934–937.

Kim SS, Utsunomiya H, Koski JA, Wu BM, Cima MJ, Sohn J, Mukai K, Griffith LG, and Vacanti JP 1998. Survival and function of hepatocytes on a novel three-dimensional synthetic biodegradable polymer scaffold with an intrinsic network of channels. *Annals Surg* 228 (1): 8–13.

Lam C, Olkowski R, Swieszkowski W, Tan K, Gibson I, and Hutmacher D. 2008 Mechanical and *in vitro* evaluations of composite PLDLLA/TCP scaffolds for bone engineering. *Virtual Phys Prototyping* 3 (4): 193–197. [informaworld]

Lam CX, Mo XM, Teoh SH, and Hutmacher DW 2002. Scaffold development using 3D printing with a starchbased polymer. *Mater Sci Eng* 20, 49–56.

Lan PX, Lee JW, Seol YJ, and Cho DW 2009. Development of 3D PPF/DEF scaffolds using micro-stereolithography and surface modification. *J Mater Sci Mater Med* 20 (1), 271–279.

Lee G and Barlow JW 1996. Selective laser sintering of bioceramic materials for implants. *96 SFF Symposium* August 12–14, Austin, TX.

Leong K, Chua C, Sudarmadji N and Yeong W 2008. Engineering functionally graded tissue engineering scaffolds. *J Mech Behav Biomed Mater* 1 (2): 140–152.

Leong KF, Cheah CM and Chua CK 2003. Solid freeform fabrication of three-dimensional scaffolds for engineering replacement tissues and organs. *Biomaterials* 24 (13): 2363–2378.

Levy RA, Chu TM, Halloran JW, Feinberg SE, and Hollister S. 1997. CT-generated porous hydroxyapatite orbital floor prosthesis as a prototype bioimplant. *AJNR Am J Neuroradiol* 18 (8): 1522–1525.

Liu VA, Jastromb WE, and Bhatia SN 2002. Engineering protein and cell adhesivity using PEO-terminated triblock polymers. *J Biomed Mater Res* 60 (1): 126–134
Matsumoto T and Mooney DJ 2006. Cell instructive polymers. *Adv Biochem Eng Biotechnol* 102: 113–137.
Melchels FPW, Feijen J, and Grijpma DW 2009. A poly(D,L-lactide) resin for the preparation of tissue engineering scaffolds by stereolithography. *Biomaterials* 30 (23–24): 3801–3809.
Mironov V, Boland T, Trusk T, Forgacs G, and Markwald RR 2003. Organ printing: Computer-aided jet-based 3D tissue engineering. *Trends Biotechnol* 21 (4): 157–161.
Mironov V, Gentile C, Brakke K, Trusk T, Jakab K, Forgacs G, Kasyanov V, Visconti R, and Markwald R 2009. Designer "blueprint" for vascular trees: Morphology evolution of vascular tissue constructs. *Virtual Phys Prototyping* 4 (2): 63–74. [informaworld]
Mironov V, Prestwich G, and Forgacs G 2007. Bioprinting living structures. *J Mater Chem* 17 (20): 2054–2060.
Mironov V, Visconti R, Kasyanov V, Forgacs G, Drake C, and Markwald R 2009. Organ printing: Tissue spheroids as building blocks. *Biomaterials* 30 (12): 2164–2174.
Mistry AS and Mikos AG 2005. Tissue engineering strategies for bone regeneration. *Adv Biochem Eng Biotechnol* 94: 1–22.
Mota C, Chiellini F, Brtolo PJ, and Chiellini E 2009. A novel approach to the fabrication of polymeric scaffolds for tissue engineering applications. *VII Convegno Nazionale Scienza e Tecnologia Dei Materiali June*, Tirrenia, Italy.
Mota C, Mateus A, Brtolo PJ, Almeida H, and Ferreira N 2009. Processo e equipamento de fabrico rapido por bioextrusao/Process and equipment for rapid fabrication through bioextrusion—Portuguese Patent Application.
Nair LS and Laurencin CT 2006. Polymers as biomaterials for tissue engineering and controlled drug delivery. *Adv Biochem Eng Biotechnol* 102: 47–90.
Ramanath HS, Chandrasekaran M, Chua CK, Leong KF, and Shah KD 2007. Modeling of extrusion behavior of biopolymer and composites in fused deposition modeling. *Key Eng Mater* 334–335: 1241–1244.
Ramanath HS, Chua CK, Leong KF, and Shah KD 2008. Melt flow behaviour of poly-epsilon-caprolactone in fused deposition modelling. *J Mater Sci Mater Med* 19 (7): 2541–2550.
Rath S, Cohn D, and Hutmacher D 2008. Comparison of chondrogenesis in static and dynamic environments using a SFF designed and fabricated PCL-PEO scaffold. *Virtual Phys Prototyping* 3 (4): 209–219. [informaworld]
Sachlos E, Reis N, Ainsley C, Derby B, and Czernuszka JT 2003. Novel collagen scaffolds with predefined internal morphology made by solid freeform fabrication. *Biomaterials* 24 (8): 1487–1497.
Sachs EM, Haggerty JS, Cima MJ, and Williams PA 1993. Three-dimensional printing techniques—Patent US5204055, April 20 1993.
Schiele N, Koppes R, Corr D, Ellison K, Thompson D, Ligon L, Lippert T, and Chrisey D 2009. Laser direct writing of combinatorial libraries of idealized cellular constructs: Biomedical applications. *Appl Surf Sci* 255 (10): 5444–5447.
Skalak R and Fox CF 1988 *Tissue Engineering*. New York: Alan R. Liss.
Tan JY, Chua CK, and Leong KF 2009. Indirect fabrication of tissue engineering scaffolds using rapid prototyping and a foaming process. *4th International Conference on Advanced Research in Virtual and Rapid Prototyping*, 6–10 October, Leiria, Portugal.
Tan KH, Chua CK, Leong KF, Cheah CM, Cheang P, Abu Bakar MS, and Cha SW 2003. Scaffold development using selective laser sintering of polyetheretherketone-hydroxyapatite biocomposite blends. *Biomaterials* 24 (18): 3115–3123.
Tan KH, Chua CK, Leong KF, Naing MW, and Cheah CM 2005. Fabrication and characterisation of hydroxyapatite biocomposite Scaffolds using Laser Sintering. *Proc Inst Mech Eng J Eng Med UK*, May 219, pp. 183–194.
Tellis BC, Szivek JA, Bliss CL, Margolis DS, Vaidyanathan RK, and Calvert P 2008. Trabecular scaffolds created using micro CT guided fused deposition modeling. *Mater Sci Eng* C 28, 171–178.
Velema J, and Kaplan D 2006. Biopolymer-based biomaterials as scaffolds for tissue engineering. *Adv Biochem Eng Biotechnol* 102, 187–238.

Wang F, Shor L, Darling A, Khalil S, Geri S, and Lau A 2004. Precision deposition and characterization of cellular polycaprolactone tissue scaffolds. *Rapid Prototyping J* 10, 42–49.

Williams JM, Adewunmi A, Schek RM, Flanagan CL, Krebsbach PH, Feinberg SE, Hollister SJ, and Das S 2005. Bone tissue engineering using polycaprolactone scaffolds fabricated via selective laser sintering. *Biomaterials* 26 (23): 4817–4827.

Wiria FE, Chua CK, Leong KF, Quah ZY, Chandrasekaran M, and Lee MW 2008. Improved biocomposite development of poly(vinyl alcohol) and hydroxyapatite for tissue engineering scaffold fabrication using selective laser sintering. *J Mater Sci Mater Med* 19 (3): 989–996.

Wiria FE, Leong KF, Chua CK, and Liu Y 2007. Poly-epsilon-caprolactone/hydroxyapatite for tissue engineering scaffold fabrication via selective laser sintering. *Acta Biomater* 3 (1): 1–12.

Woodfield TBF, Malda J, de Wijn J, Pters F, Riesle J, and van Blitterswijk CA 2004. Design of porous scaffolds for cartilage tissue engineering using a three-dimensional fiber-deposition technique. *Biomaterials* 25 (18): 4149–4161.

Yan Y, Zhang R, and Lin F 2003. Research and applications on bio-manufacturing. *1st International Conference on Advanced Research in Virtual and Rapid Prototyping Leiria*, Portugal.

Yang S, Leong K, Du Z, and Chua C 2001. The design of scaffolds for use in tissue engineering. Part I. Traditional factors. *Tissue Eng* 7 (6): 679–689.

Yang S, Leong K, Du Z, and Chua C 2002. The design of scaffolds for use in tissue engineering. Part II. Rapid prototyping techniques. *Tissue Eng* 8 (1): 1–11.

Yeong WY, Chua CK, and Leong KF 2006. Indirect fabrication of collagen scaffold based on inkjet printing technique. *Rapid Prototyping J* 12 (4): 229–237.

Yeong WY, Chua CK, Leong KF, and Chandrasekaran M 2004. Rapid prototyping in tissue engineering: Challenges and potential. *Trends Biotechnol* 22 (12): 643–652.

Yeong WY, Chua CK, Leong KF, Chandrasekaran M, and Lee MW 2007. Comparison of drying methods in the fabrication of collagen scaffold via indirect rapid prototyping. *J Biomed Mater Res B Appl Biomater* 82 (1): 260–266.

Yildirim E, Besunder R, Guceri S, Allen F, and Sun W 2008. Fabrication and plasma treatment of 3D polycaprolactane tissue scaffolds for enhanced cellular function. *Virtual Phys Prototyping* 3 (4): 199–207. [informaworld]

Yuan D, Lasagni A, Shao P, and Das S 2008. Rapid prototyping of microstructured hydrogels via laser direct-write and laser interference photopolymerisation. *Virtual Phys Prototyping* 3 (4): 221–229. [informaworld]

Zeltinger J, Sherwood JK, Graham DA, Meller R, and Griffith LG 2001. Effect of pore size and void fraction on cellular adhesion, proliferation, and matrix deposition. *Tissue Eng* 7 (5): 557–572.

Zhou J, Lu L, Byrapogu K, Wootton D, Lelkes P, and Fair R 2007. Electrowetting-based multi-microfluidics array printing of high resolution tissue construct with embedded cells and growth factors. *Virtual Phys Prototyping* 2 (4): 217–223.

Zhou WY, Lee SH, Wang M, Cheung WL, and Ip WY 2008. Selective laser sintering of porous tissue engineering scaffolds from poly (L: -lactide)/carbonated hydroxyapatite nanocomposite microspheres. *J Mater Sci Mater Med* 19 (7): 2535–2540.

chapter nine

Molecular diagnostics and forensic science

9.1 Introduction

Medical diagnosis is basically a procedure to determine the identity of a possible cause of disease or disorder. Moreover, the term "diagnostic criteria" includes the signs, symptoms, and laboratory test results that the clinician uses to make the correct diagnosis. Normally, a person with abnormal symptoms will consult a health care provider such as a physician, who will then obtain a medical history of the patient's illness and perform a physical examination for signs of disease. The health provider will formulate a hypothesis of likely diagnoses and in many cases will obtain further testing to confirm the diagnosis before providing treatment. Moreover, medical tests are commonly performed by measuring blood pressure, checking the pulse rate, urine tests, fecal tests, saliva tests, blood tests, listening to the heart with a stethoscope, medical imaging, electrocardiogram, hydrogen breath test, and occasionally biopsy. For instance, pneumonia was used as a diagnosis before the germ theory was established, and the disease was defined as complex-symptom disease consisting of cough, sputum production, fever, and chills.

9.2 History of diagnostic tests

The history of medical diagnosis goes back several centuries and the practice of diagnosis continues to be used for many centuries. It has been reported that the Arab physician Abu al-Qasim al-Zahrawi, commonly known as Abulcasis, wrote a book on hematology. His book *Al-Tasrif* written during the period 1000 AD provided the first description of hemophilia, a hereditary genetic disorder. Later on, the Persian physician Ibn Sina, commonly known as Avicenna, pioneered the idea of a syndrome/disease in the diagnosis of specific diseases. There are four components of medical diagnostics (Figure 9.1) and each one is essential for understanding body homeostasis; they are (i) anatomy to understand the structure of the human body, (ii) physiology to know how the body works, (iii) pathology to know what can go wrong with the anatomy and physiology, and (iv) psychology to know thought and behavior. As soon as the health provider knows what normal condition is and can measure the patient's current condition/status against those norms, she or he can then determine the patient's particular departure from homeostasis (normal condition) and the degree of variability, and the whole process of knowing the difference between normal condition and disease condition is called diagnosis. The minute a diagnosis has been established, the provider will be able to propose a management plan, which will include treatment as well as plans for follow-up. Moreover, the health provider educates the patient about the causes of diseases and possible treatments of his ailments, as well as providing advice for maintaining health. In contrast to this, it should be noted

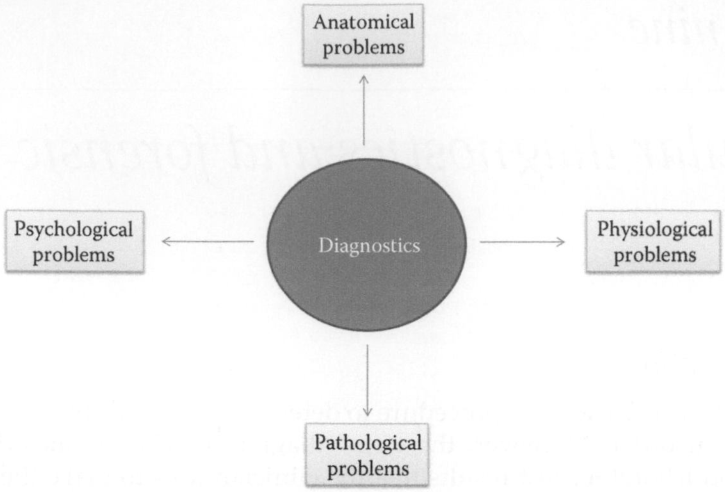

Figure 9.1 Human disease identification by diagnostic tests.

that medical diagnosis in psychology or psychiatry is difficult, and apart from the fact that there are differing theoretical views toward mental conditions, there are only few laboratory tests available for various major disorders.

9.3 Diagnostic process

In order to better understand disease progression, it is very important to know the diagnosis process followed by physicians. There are a number of techniques used by providers to obtain a correct diagnosis such as the exhaustive method (every possible question is asked and all possible data are collected), algorithmic method (the provider follows the steps of a proven strategy), pattern recognition method (the provider uses experience to recognize a pattern of clinical characteristics), and differential diagnosis (the provider uses the hypothetico-deductive method, a systematic, problem-focused method of inquiry) (Figure 9.2). The physician or clinician uses a combination of the pattern recognition and hypothetico-deductive approaches. The mere presence of some medical conditions cannot be recognized from examination or testing; therefore, diagnosis is important for establishing the cause and reason. It has been reported that the process of diagnosis begins when the patient consults the health provider and presents a set of health-related issues. If the patient is in an

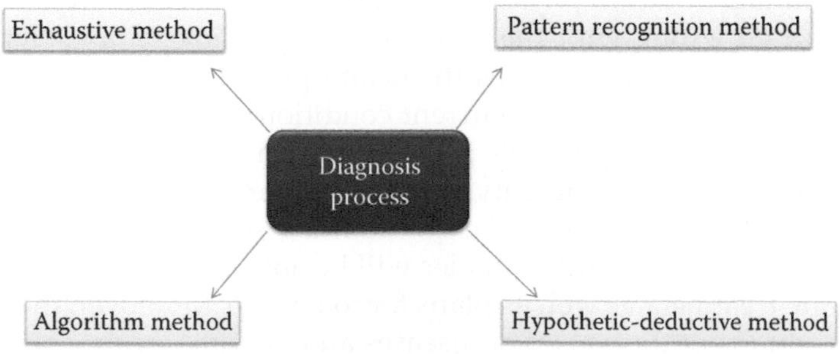

Figure 9.2 Process of diagnosis of human diseases.

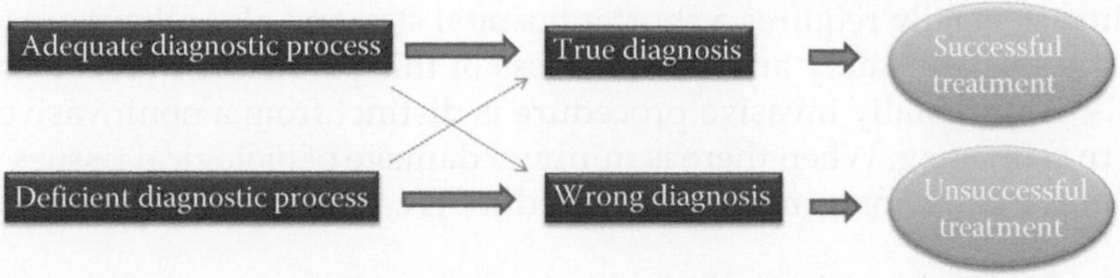

Figure 9.3 Failures and successes of diagnosis of human diseases.

unconscious state, this means that the patient is suffering from some illness and requires immediate attention. In that case, the health provider obtains further information from those who know him or her, if present, about the patient's symptoms, their previous state of health, living conditions, and so forth. Rather than consider the myriad diseases that could afflict the patient, the provider narrows down the possibilities to his/her illnesses with apparent symptoms, and the health provider then conducts a physical examination of the patient. When the list of probabilities is narrowed down to a solitary condition, this is called differential diagnosis and this provides the basis for a patient's sickness.

Until and unless the health provider is convinced of the condition present in the patient, further medical tests are performed to establish the reasons, and, moreover, consultations with other health specialists in the field can be pursued. In spite of all of these complexities, most patient consultations are relatively brief because many diseases are obvious and can be diagnosed with current tools. Once the health provider completes the diagnostic process, the prognosis is described to the patient and a treatment plan is suggested, which includes therapy and follow-up checkups or consultations. Furthermore, a laboratory diagnosis can be a substitution to the diagnosis made by the examination of the patient, for example, a proper diagnosis of infectious diseases usually requires both an examination of symptoms and laboratory test of characteristics of the pathogen involved. The success or failure of diagnostic tests depends on adequate and accurate diagnosis (Figure 9.3).

9.4 Classification of diagnostic tests

Medical tests can be classified into three categories: invasive, minimally invasive, and noninvasive.

9.4.1 Invasive test

This is an invasive procedure that penetrates the skin or enters a body cavity; examples include those that involves perforation, such as an incision, or catheterization; surgery is a typical medical invasive procedure. An open surgery means cutting skin and tissues so that the surgeon has direct access to the structures or organs involved. In this procedure, the organs and tissues can be observed and manipulated, and they are directly exposed to the air of the operating room; this is also an invasive procedure. There are several examples of open surgery, which include the removal of organs, such as the kidney and liver, or certain types of heart surgery.

9.4.2 Minimally invasive procedure

This procedure is less invasive than open surgery. Minimally invasive procedures typically involve the use of laparoscopic devices and remote-controlled handling of instruments.

This procedure generally requires a shorter hospital stay and also allows outpatient treatment. Nevertheless, the safety and effectiveness of this procedure must be confirmed by various trials. A minimally invasive procedure is distinct from a noninvasive procedure, such as external imaging. When there is minimal damage of biological tissues or organs at the point of entry of the instrument, the procedure is called minimally invasive.

9.4.2.1 Minimal incision technique

The minimal incision technique is a specialized surgical technique that has been practiced by some physicians and surgeons to remove masses (tumor) or growths with minimal scarring and less recovery time. Moreover, most surgeons usually cut only 10–15% of the total length of the mass (tumor) to access it or remove it. A smaller incision forms a much reduced scar and results in less recovery time. This technique is particularly useful for cyst identification and removal, and patients with obesity can gain great benefit from such techniques.

9.4.3 Noninvasive test

A medical procedure is strictly defined as noninvasive when no incision is made on the skin and when there is no contact with the skin or internal body. Deep palpation and thumping are noninvasive, but a rectal examination is considered an invasive procedure. Correspondingly, the examination of the ear drum or the inside of the nose or a bandage change all fall outside the strict definition of noninvasive procedures. It has been reported that for centuries physicians have been using many simple noninvasive methods based on physical parameters in order to assess body function in health and disease, such as pulse rate measuring, peripheral vascular examination, the auscultation of heart and lung sounds, oral examination, abdominal examination, external percussion and palpation, temperature examination, respiratory examination, and blood pressure measurement by using the sphygmomanometer.

9.5 Characteristics of diagnostic tests

The success of any diagnostic test is based on the precision and accuracy of the data; in other words, the precise or accurate data that help physicians to treat their patients with a high success rate. Furthermore, the accuracy of a laboratory test is its correspondence with the true value. Accuracy of data can be maximized by calibrating laboratory equipment on a regular basis. In addition, precision is a measure of test reproducibility when repeated on the same sample, whereas an imprecise test is one that yields different results of repeated measurement.

9.6 Molecular diagnostic

Molecular diagnostics assess your biological makeup at the genetic level and unlocking the DNA code can reveal variations between individuals, which may represent a predisposition to develop a disease or even treatment options that may be more effective in some people. Over the last few years, the field of molecular diagnostics is growing rapidly. With the use of molecular diagnostic tests, you can detect specific sequences in DNA or RNA that may or may not be associated with the disease, including single nucleotide polymorphism (SNP), deletions, rearrangements, insertions, and others. The clinical applications can be found in at least six general areas: infectious diseases, oncology, pharmacogenomics, genetic disease screening, human leukocyte antigen typing, and coagulation.

The main techniques of molecular assay require three basic steps: (1) the extraction and purification of nucleic acid, (2) the amplification or making copies of the nucleic acid of interest (target) or attaching multiple copies of a dye to a single target copy, and (3) the detection of the amplified target using real-time polymerase chain reaction (PCR) or end product detection, including microarrays, Luminex (similar to flow cytometry), or DNA sequencing. The Federal Drug Administration (FDA) and Clinical Laboratory Improvement Act regulate clinical molecular tests like all other clinical laboratory tests. Molecular assays may be qualitative to see if the virus exists or quantitative to see how much of the virus exists. Basic molecular assay economics suggest two other categories of assays. The first is assays that may be reported in the same patient, including recurrence of an infectious disease or cancer, and detection of minimal residual disease. The second category refers to tests that only need to be performed once in a patient's lifetime. With a view to limit the movement of pathogens and reduce the economic and socioeconomic impact of disease, there is considerable scope for more effective use of DNA-based methods of pathogen detection. DNA-based pathogen detection method offers rapid results with potentially high sensitivity and specificity, at relatively low cost. Recognition of these advantages has led to rapid adoption of available DNA-based and genetic tests, particularly in human sample for which histological procedures lack specificity and culture-based methods have not been possible. Over the last few decades, there has been a surge of information pertaining to molecular and genetic techniques for identification of human diseases, especially in those diseases that are caused due to mutated or dysfunctional genes. The identification of dysfunctional genes is the prime aim of any diagnostic approach. It has been reported that fluorescence *in situ* hybridization (FISH) and PCR techniques are the two most commonly used diagnostic methods for analysis, whereas other techniques have been proposed or are currently in development. Moreover, PCR is generally used to diagnose DNA/RNA-related disorders and FISH is used for the detection of chromosomal abnormalities, for example, aneuploidy screening or chromosomal translocations. In the recent past, various advancements happened in genetic disease testing, which have allowed for the collection of diagnostic data. Recently, a method was developed to allow fixing metaphase plates from single blastomeres. This technique in conjunction with FISH, metaphase-FISH, can produce more reliable results since analysis is done on whole metaphase plates.

9.6.1 *Fluorescence in situ hybridization*

FISH is a cytogenetic technique used to identify the presence or absence of specific DNA sequences on chromosomes. It has been reported that FISH employs fluorescent probes that bind to only those parts of the chromosome of a patient's sample with which they show a high degree of sequence similarity. Additionally, fluorescence-based microscopy can be used to find out where the fluorescent probe bound to the chromosomes. It has been reported that FISH is frequently used for finding specific topographies in DNA for use in genetic counseling, medicine, and person's identification, and can also be used to detect and localize specific mRNAs in the samples (Figure 9.4). Furthermore, molecular probes are derived from DNA that were isolated, purified, and amplified for use in the Human Genome Project. The size of the human DNA is so large that it was essential to divide the genome into fragments or small pieces. The DNA is fragmented into smaller pieces by employing sequence-specific endonucleases. To preserve the fragments with

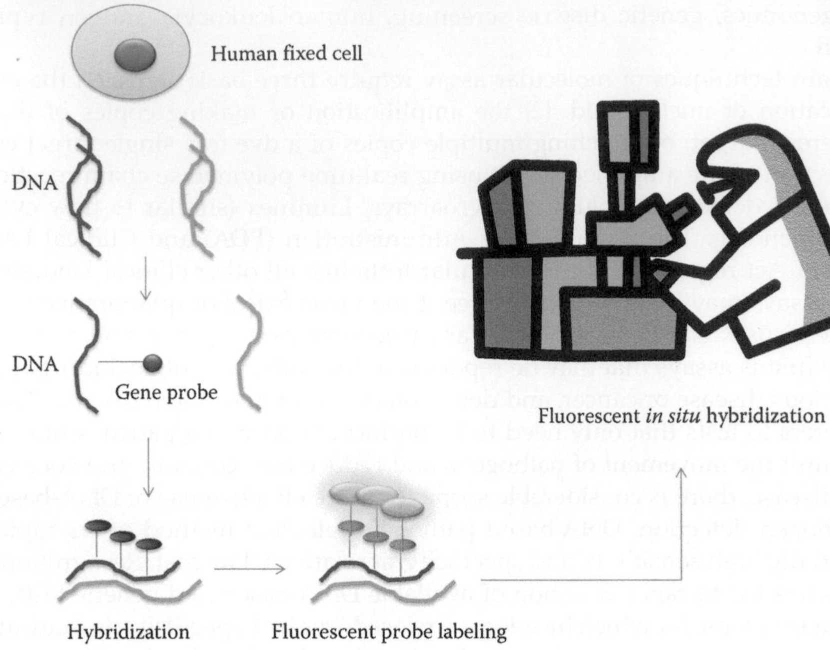

Figure 9.4 Fluorescence *in situ* hybridization technique.

their individual DNA sequences, they are added into a system of continually replicating bacteria populations. The clonal populations of bacteria that maintain a single artificial chromosome are stored in various laboratories around the world. The artificial chromosomes can be grown, extracted, and labeled, and are the foundation for most FISH probe construction.

9.6.2 Preparation, hybridization process, and types of FISH techniques

One of the main steps in FISH labeling is the preparation and hybridization of probes. The first step is the construction of a probe; the probe must be big enough to hybridize specifically to its target but must not be so large as to obstruct the hybridization process. Later on, the probe can be tagged directly with fluorophores, with targets for antibodies, or with biotin molecules. It has been reported that tagging can be used in various ways, such as nick translation, and PCR-based tagging nucleotides. After making a probe, interphase or metaphase chromosome preparation is shaped and the chromosomes are firmly attached to a substrate, usually glass. After that, a solution containing short fragments of DNA is added to the sample to block the repetitive DNA sequences. Thereafter, the probe is then applied to the chromosomal DNA and incubated for approximately 12 h in a hybridizing chamber. The solution is then washed several times to remove all unhybridized or partially hybridized probes and the results are visualized and quantified using a fluorescent microscope. It has been shown that FISH experiments are designed to detect or localize gene expression within cells and tissues and rely on the use of a reporter gene (green fluorescent protein) to provide the fluorescence signal. There are various types of FISH techniques, which are described below in brief.

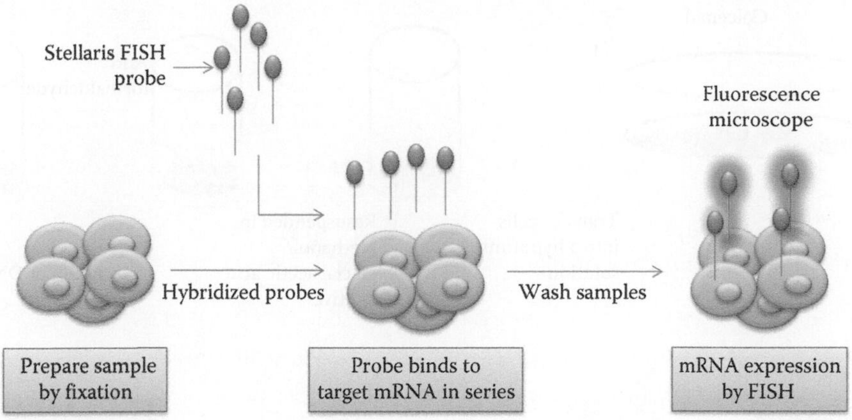

Figure 9.5 Single molecule RNA FISH.

9.6.2.1 Single molecule RNA FISH

A single molecule RNA FISH is a technique of identifying and measuring messenger RNA (mRNA) and other long RNA molecules in tissue samples derived from patients. It has been shown that target sites can be visualized through the application of multiple short single labeled oligonucleotide probes. These probes can bind to the target site precisely and when each probe binds to the single-stranded mRNA, it causes cooperative unwinding of the mRNA, which in turn causes the binding of many fluorescent labels to a single molecule of mRNA. These probe binding provides sufficient fluorescence to consistently locate each target mRNA in a wide-field fluorescent microscopy image. Moreover, those probes that are not able to bind to the intended sequence do not show any fluorescence and can be distinguished from the background. The single molecule RNA FISH has potential applications in gene expression analysis, cancer diagnosis, neuroscience, and companion diagnostics (Figure 9.5).

9.6.2.2 Q-FISH

Quantitative fluorescence *in situ* hybridization (Q-FISH) is another type of FISH technique, which is basically a cytogenetic technique-based FISH methodology. In Q-FISH, fluorescence-labeled probes (Cy3 or FITC) are used to quantify target sequences in chromosomal DNA using fluorescent microscopy and analysis software. Q-FISH is most commonly used to study the telomere length in a patient's sample (blood or tissue); it has been suggested that telomeres are necessary at chromosome ends to prevent DNA damage. Additionally, Q-FISH has also been used to quantify the telomere length distribution, which is associated with various sicknesses (Figure 9.6).

Though Q-FISH provides an accurate evidence about telomere length, its relevance can be extended by combining Q-FISH with other FISH-related techniques, such as flow-FISH, which is based on flow cytometry. In flow-FISH, flow cytometry is employed to measure fluorescence intensity in a population of cells rather than just a handful of cells in Q-FISH. Unlike Q-FISH, flow-FISH is unable to determine telomere length in a particular chromosome within an individual cell. However, it should be clear that although Q-FISH is generally considered low-throughput and not suitable for population studies, researchers have developed high-throughput protocols that use computerized machinery to perform Q-FISH. Similarly, other methods such as multiplex-FISH and multicolor

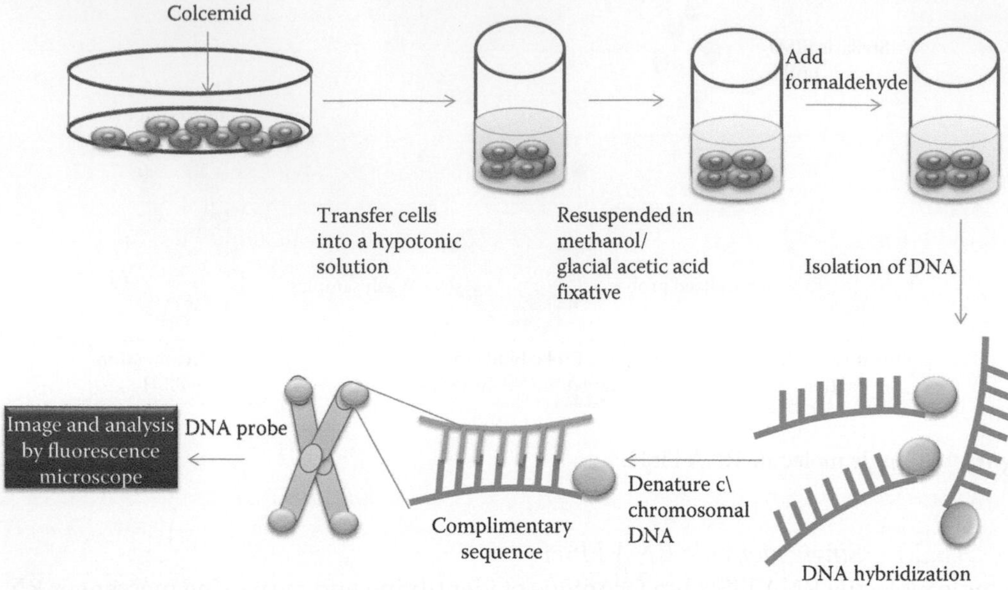

Figure 9.6 The process of Q-FISH.

FISH (cenM-FISH) have been established, which can also be used in combination with Q-FISH. It has been reported that multiplex-FISH uses a variety of probes to visualize multiple chromosomes in different color combinations and is also able to identify changes in chromosomal rearrangements. Moreover, centromere-specific multicolor FISH (cenM-FISH) uses the multicolor probes from multiplex-FISH as well as centromere-specific labeled probes to recognize and distinguish centromere regions in the chromosomes. It has been suggested that the relation between centromere abnormalities or chromosomal rearrangements and telomere length can have high clinical significance in cancer developments. In addition to the above-mentioned applications, Q-FISH can also be used in the detection of telomeric fusions, where the ends of chromosomes are fused together at the telomere, which are sometimes called interstitial chromosome telomere sequences (ITSs). Furthermore, studying telomeric fusions can infrequently show the course of evolution; for example, one human chromosome has an ITS that is hypothesized to be the equal of two chromosomes in chimpanzees that are fused together. By observing the regulation of telomere length in different species such as human and animals, it reveals important information about karyotype evolution and its relevance to human illnesses.

9.6.3 *Medical applications of FISH*

There are various applications of the FISH technique in the medical diagnostics fields, which will be described in brief, although some of the applications have already been discussed in the previous sections.

9.6.3.1 Species identification

The FISH technique is often used in clinical studies to identify pathogens. For example, if a patient is infested with a suspected pathogen, patients tissues are normally grown on agar plates to determine the identity of the kind of pathogen. It has been reported that many harmful bacteria do not grow well under laboratory conditions and the FISH technique can be used to identify the uniqueness of the pathogens on small samples of the patient's tissue. The FISH technique can also be used to compare the genomes of two different biological species, also called *zoo blot*. Furthermore, FISH is widely used in the field of microbial biology to recognize microorganisms.

9.6.3.2 Lab-on-a-chip

Although interphase FISH is a profound diagnostic tool used for the detection of chromosomal aberrations, the cost and technical complexity of FISH protocols have inhibited its widespread use. To overcome this problem, researchers have identified solutions in the form of lab-on-a-chip, which is basically microfluidic devices that incorporate networks of microchannels, reducing the operational cost. Moreover, microchannels allow sophisticated levels of fluid control and may reduce analysis times, lower reagent consumption, and also minimize human involvement. At present, the FISH technique has been done on glass microfluidic platforms that standardize much of the procedure offering results that are precise, cost-effective, and easier to obtain. Furthermore, lab-on-a-chip FISH provides a 10-fold higher throughput and a 10-fold reduction in the cost of testing compared to conventional FISH methods.

9.7 Diagnostic application of polymerase chain reaction

PCR is a molecular technique to amplify a single copy of DNA and generates millions of copies of a particular DNA sequence derived from a patient's sample (blood and tissue). This method relies on thermal cycling of repeated heating and cooling of the reaction for DNA, causing replication of the DNA. It was invented by Kary Mullis. Moreover, primers that contain sequences complementary to the target region of the DNA are key components to enable selective and frequent amplification of DNA. During PCR, the DNA produced is itself used as a template for replication, and sets into motion a chain reaction in which the DNA template is exponentially amplified. It has been shown that PCR can be extensively altered to perform a wide array of genetic manipulations and changes. Furthermore, almost all PCR applications use a heat-stable DNA polymerase, such as Taq polymerase. This DNA polymerase can build a new DNA strand from DNA building blocks, the nucleotides, by using single-stranded DNA as a template. Furthermore, DNA oligonucleotides, also called DNA primers, are required for the initiation of DNA synthesis. The vast majority of PCR methods use thermal cycling, as these are necessary to separate two DNA strands of a double helix at a high temperature; this process is called DNA melting. Thereafter, at a lower temperature, each DNA strand is used as the template in DNA synthesis (Figure 9.7).

9.7.1 Application of PCR technology

PCR technology has become an essential methodology for research and diagnostics. Moreover, the PCR technique allows scientists to take a specimen of genetic material and generate a test sample sufficient to detect the identity of a specific virus or microorganism. Medical research and clinical medicine are benefiting from PCR technology mainly in two areas: (i) detection of infectious organisms, including viruses that cause AIDS and hepatitis, and other microorganisms that affect women's health and cause tuberculosis, and (ii) detection of genetic variations, including mutations, in human genes.

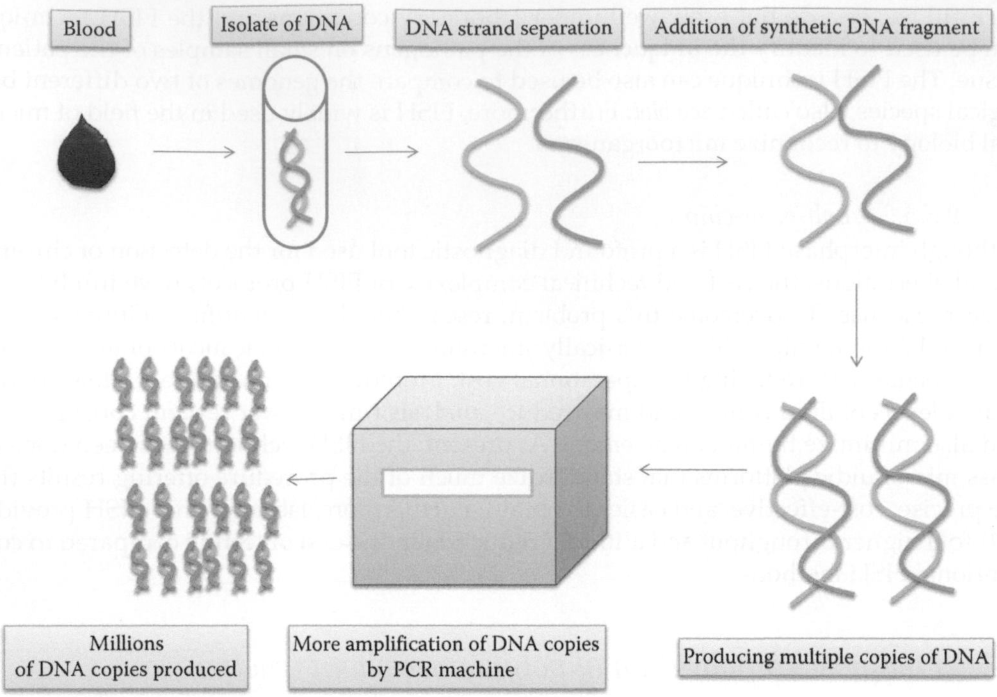

Figure 9.7 Process of polymerase chain reaction.

9.7.1.1 *Infectious disease*

The PCR technique can be used to detect the DNA or RNA of pathogenic organisms such as viruses and bacteria. These PCR-based tests have several advantages over traditional antibody-based diagnostic methods that measure the body's immune response to a pathogen. In particular, PCR-based tests are able to detect the presence of pathogenic agents earlier than serologically based methods, as patients can take weeks to develop antibodies against an infectious agent. The PCR technique is an easy and fast way to detect the disease in order to start treatment procedures. Moreover, PCR-based diagnostics tests are available for detecting and/or quantifying several pathogens.

9.7.1.2 *Blood screening*

Serological tests have been used to screen donated blood samples for the presence of infectious agents. Nevertheless, a small risk of viral transmission remains primarily due to the failure of such screening tests to identify recently infected donors during the period (the time delay postinfection in which the body develops an immune response to the infectious agent). Moreover, tests using PCR nucleic acid amplification testing (NAT) technology detect the actual virus. Experts consider that including such tests in blood screening programs could provide an additional measure of protection by detecting viral infection at an earlier stage. Highly sensitive PCR-based tests are available for detecting early markers of HIV-1, hepatitis B, and hepatitis C infection, namely, viral DNA or RNA, in blood. Furthermore, these tests can help to improve blood safety and also help patients by reducing the waiting period for blood transfusion. The PCR technique can also be used to screen for several pathogens, including hepatitis C, hepatitis B, and HIV-1.

9.7.1.3 Genetic testing

We all know that PCR technology can be used to easily distinguish among the tiny variations in DNA that make people genetically unique. In the future, PCR technology may be used in predictive test methods for finding out who is predisposed to common disorders, such as heart disease and many cancers. Roche is developing new molecular-based tests in disease predisposition, cancer screening, and cancer therapy. It has been suggested that genetic analysis can provide information as to whether an individual has the right metabolic system to metabolize a particular drug. With the use of PCR technology, it will be possible to prescribe drugs that do not have side effects. Physicians will also have a clearer understanding of which treatments will work best for patients and there will be improvements in the quality of life for patients.

9.8 Forensic science

One of the best-known applications of forensic science is to answer questions of interest to a legal system. Moreover, forensic science can be used in relation to a crime or a civil action. It has been reported that the word "forensic" is derived from the Latin word forensic, and it becomes a investigation tool to address many crime, to establish an individual's identity and to establish parenting issue (Figure 9.8).

9.8.1 Classification of forensic science

The field and scope of forensic science keeps expanding with the emergence of new technology and methodology. The forensic field can be classified into various subfields.

9.8.1.1 Forensic anthropology

The application of the science of physical anthropology and human skeleton in a legal setting, most often in criminal cases, is known as forensic anthropology, where the victim's remains (body or tissue) are in advanced stages of decomposition. Furthermore, a forensic anthropologist can also assist in the identification of cadaver individuals, whose remains are decomposed, burned, mutilated, or otherwise unrecognizable.

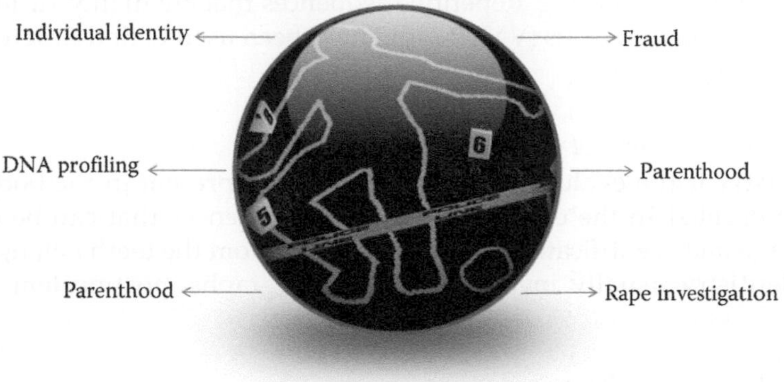

Figure 9.8 Application of forensic science.

9.8.1.2 *Forensic archaeology*

Forensic archaeology is the application of archaeological principles, techniques, and methodologies in a legal context, predominately medico-legal. Moreover, forensic archaeologists are employed by police and other agencies to help locate evidence at a crime scene typically using specialized skills to excavate the hidden treasure or gather mass grave evidence from the past.

9.8.1.3 *Forensic fingerprinting*

A fingerprint is nothing but an impression left by the friction ridges of a human finger and in a broader sense, fingerprints are impressions from the friction ridges of any part of a human hand. It has been suggested that all human being have a very unique set of ridges in their hand that are different in each individual. These unique ridges can be used to identify an individual's identity. It has been suggested that a print from the foot can also leave an impression of friction ridges. A friction ridge is basically the raised portion of the epidermis on the fingers consisting of one or more connected ridge units of friction ridge skin. These are occasionally known as epidermal ridges, which are produced by the core interface between the dermal papillae of the dermis and the interpapillary hooks of the epidermis. Furthermore, these epidermal ridges serve to amplify vibrations triggered due to touching uneven or even surfaces. These ridges can also assist in gripping rough surfaces as well as smooth wet surfaces. After touching any object, the human fingers leave impressions of prints on a surface by the natural secretions of sweat from the exocrine glands that are present in the friction ridge. It has been reported that fingerprint records normally contain impressions of fingers, though fingerprint cards also typically record portions of lower joint areas of the fingers.

9.8.1.4 *DNA profiling*

In criminal science, DNA profiling has been extensively used by forensic scientists to establish the identification of persons on the basis of their respective DNA outlines. It has been reported that DNA profiles are encoded sets of numbers that reflect a person's DNA makeup, which can also be used as the person's identity. There is a caution here that DNA profiling should not be confused with full genome sequencing. DNA profiling has been used in parental testing and rape investigation. Moreover, more than 99% of the human DNA sequences are the same in every person; there are few unique characteristics in each individual and in DNA profiling. Repetitive sequences that are highly variable are called variable number tandem repeats (VNTRs) and have been used to find differences between two individuals (Figure 9.9).

9.8.1.5 *Forensic dentistry*

Forensic dentistry is the evaluation of dental evidence present in the body or cadaver, that can be presented in the court of justice. The evidences that can be derived from teeth are the age and identification of the person to whom the teeth belong. The process of forensic dentistry usually involves dental radiographs, postmortem photographs, and DNA.

9.8.1.6 *Forensic pathology*

Forensic pathology is a branch of pathology concerned with determining the cause of death by the examination of a corpse. The autopsy is performed by the pathologist at the request of the medical examiner usually during the examination of criminal law cases and

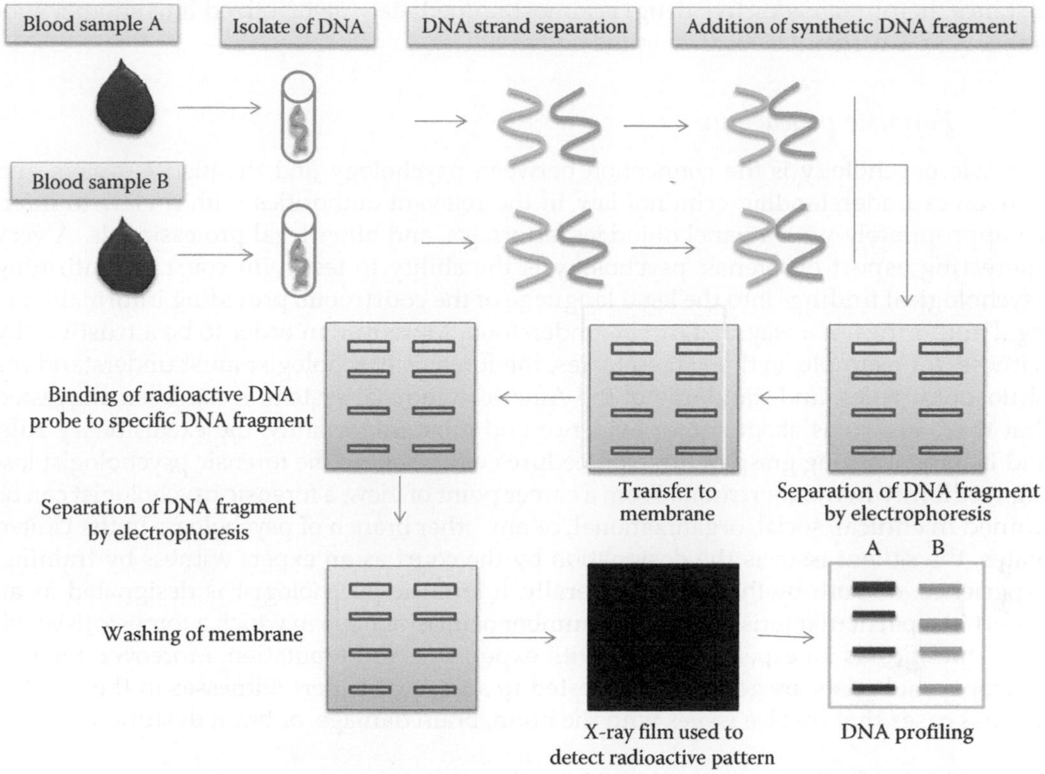

Figure 9.9 Forensic DNA fingerprinting.

civil law cases in some authorities. Furthermore, forensic pathologists are also commonly asked to confirm the identity of a corpse.

9.8.1.7 *Forensic serology*

Forensic serology is commonly used to detect, classify, and study various bodily fluids such as semen, fecal matter, blood, and their relationship to a crime scene. Furthermore, a forensic serologist can also be involved in DNA analysis and blood stain pattern analysis.

9.8.1.8 *Forensic toxicology*

Forensic toxicology is the use of toxicology and other disciplines such as analytical chemistry, biochemistry, pharmacology and clinical chemistry aid, medical or legal investigation of death, poisoning, and drug use. The primary concern for forensic toxicology is not the legal outcome of the toxicological investigation or the technology utilized, but rather the obtaining and interpreting of the results. Moreover, a toxicological analysis can be made to various kinds of samples and a forensic toxicologist must consider the background of an investigation, and collection of any evidence at a crime scene, which includes pill bottles, cigarette bud, hair, powders, shoe impressions, residue of soil in shoe base, and so on. The sample can be collected from the crime scene and handed over to the forensic toxicologist. The forensic toxicologist will determine the identity of a substance and its concentration, and will tell the likely effect of those chemicals on the person. Additionally, determining the substance (chemical) ingested is often complicated by the body's natural processes as it is rare for a chemical to remain in its original form once taken inside the body. For instance, heroin (an addictive drug) is almost immediately metabolized into another substance and is difficult to localize in the body.

9.8.2 Forensic psychology

Forensic psychology is the connection between psychology and the justice system and it involves understanding criminal law in the relevant authorities with a view to interact appropriately with a panel of judges, attorneys, and other legal professionals. A very interesting aspect of forensic psychology is the ability to testify in court, reconfirming psychological findings into the legal language of the courtroom, providing information to legal authorities in a way that can be understood. Moreover, in order to be a trustworthy witness, for example, in the United States, the forensic psychologist must understand the philosophy, rules, and standards of the American judicial system. It has been suggested that there are rules about rumor evidence and most importantly, the exclusionary rule, and lacking a strong grasp of these procedures will result in the forensic psychologist losing credibility in the courtroom. From a career point of view, a forensic psychologist can be trained in clinical, social, organizational, or any other branch of psychology. In the United States, the salient issue is the designation by the court as an expert witness by training, experience, or both by the judge. Generally, a forensic psychologist is designated as an expert in a particular jurisdiction. The number of jurisdictions in which a forensic psychologist qualifies as an expert increases with experience and reputation. Moreover, forensic neuropsychologists are generally requested to appear as expert witnesses in the court to discuss cases that involve issues with the brain, brain damage, or brain dysfunction.

9.8.2.1 Career opportunities in forensic psychology

There are numerous professional positions and employment possibilities for forensic psychologists. They can be practiced at several different employment settings.

University researcher: University forensic psychologists are normally engaged in teaching, research, training and supervision of students, and other education-related activities. Professionals usually have an advanced degree in psychology or neuroscience (most likely a PhD). While their main focus is research, it is not rare for them to take on any of the other positions of forensic psychologists. Moreover, these professionals may be employed at various locations, which include colleges and universities, research institutes, government or private agencies, and mental health agencies. Psychology researchers generally test hypotheses using empirical methods and apply the research on issues related to psychology and law. They also conduct research on neural disorder law and policy evaluation. Some famous psychologists in the field include Saul Kassin, very widely known for studying false confessions, and Elizabeth Loftus, known for her research in eyewitness memory and who has provided expert witness testimony in many cases.

Federal forensic consultant: Forensic psychologists can assist law enforcement authorities to tackle criminal cases. These experts work in collaboration with the police force or other law enforcement agencies and are frequently trained to help with crisis intervention, including posttrauma and suicide-based cases. Most importantly, these law enforcement psychologists also help to provide training in stress management, personnel management, and referral of departmental personnel as well as their families for specialized treatment and counseling.

Forensic evaluators: Forensic psychologists are responsible for evaluating parties in criminal or civil cases on mental health issues related to their case. In criminal cases, they may be called upon to evaluate issues including, but not limited to, the defendants' competency to stand trial, their mental state at the time of the offense (insanity), and their risk for future violent acts. In addition to this, they may be called upon to evaluate issues including, but not limited to, an individual's psychological state after an accident or the families of custody cases. Moreover, any assessment made by an evaluator is not considered a counseling session, and, therefore, whatever is said or done is not confidential. It is the obligation of the evaluator to inform the parties that everything in the session will be open to scrutiny in a forensic report or expert testimony. Forensic evaluators work closely with expert witnesses as many are called into court to testify to what they have come to conclude from their evaluations.

Treatment benefactor: Treatment benefactor is a forensic psychologist who administers a psychological intervention to individuals in both criminal and civil cases. In criminal proceedings of the court, treatment benefactors may be requested to provide psychological interventions to individuals who require treatment for the restoration of his/her competency, after having been determined by the courts as incompetent to stand trial. They are generally asked to provide treatment for the mental illness of those believed insane at the crime. Moreover, they may also be requested to administer treatment to minimize the likelihood of future acts of violence for individuals who are at a high risk of committing a violent crime. As for civil proceedings, treatment providers may have to treat families going through divorce and/or custody cases. They may also provide treatment to individuals who have suffered psychological injuries due to some kind of trauma. In addition, the treatment benefactor and evaluator work in the same type of settings; not surprisingly, their work may greatly overlap. The forensic psychologist may take on the role of both treatment benefactor and evaluator for the same client.

Trial consultant: Forensic psychologists are regularly involved in trial consulting. Trial consultants are social scientists who work with legal professionals such as trial attorneys to support case preparation, which includes selection of the jury, development of case strategy, and witness preparation. Moreover, trial consultants may also attend seminars directed at the improvement of jury selection and trial presentation skills. Interestingly, to become a trial consultant does not necessarily require a doctoral degree; all that is really needed is some level of training. However, trial consultants are faced with many ethical issues as they are not only social scientists; they may be entrepreneurs as well, marketing their business and keeping fixed costs. It is a challenge to their ethical responsibilities as applied researchers who need to be following the guidelines of ethical research. Trial consultants can be hired by attorneys and conflicts may arise when each party has a different viewpoint on a certain issue.

9.8.3 Forensic accounting

Forensic accounting is the practice area of accountancy that defines engagements that result from financial disputes or litigation. Forensic accountants, also referred to as forensic auditors or investigative auditors, frequently have to give expert evidence at the eventual trial. Most of the financial companies, as well as many banks and financial institutes, and police and federal government organizations, do have specialist forensic accounting departments. Furthermore, forensic accounting may be further subspecialized into insurance claims, personal injury claims, fraud, construction, or royalty audits. Forensic accounting also deals with economic damage calculations, postacquisition disputes, bankruptcy, insolvency, securities fraud, and computer forensics. Moreover, forensic auditors often assist in professional negligence claims where they assess and comment on the work of other professionals. Forensic accountants are also engaged in marital and family law of analyzing lifestyles for spousal support purposes, determining income available for child support, and equitable distribution. The activities relating to criminal matters typically arise in the aftermath of fraud. They are frequently involved with the assessment of accounting systems and account presentations, in essence, checking if the numbers reflect reality. Additionally, some forensic accountants specialize in forensic analytics, which is the procurement and analysis of electronic data to reconstruct, detect, or otherwise support a claim of financial fraud. The main steps in forensic analytics are data collection, data preparation, data analysis, and reporting. Moreover, forensic analytics may be used to review an employee's purchasing card activity to assess whether any of the purchases were diverted for personal use.

9.9 *Genetic fingerprinting*

Genetic fingerprinting, also called DNA fingerprinting, is a technique employed by forensic researchers to support the identification of persons on the basis of their respective DNA profiles. Moreover, the DNA profiling process is normally begun with a collection of a DNA sample of a person, typically called a reference sample. The most anticipated method of collecting a sample is the use of a buccal swab, as this cuts the likelihood of contamination. DNA is also obtained from blood, saliva, semen, or other appropriate fluid or tissue from personal items, or from stored samples. The samples obtained from blood relatives or biological relatives can provide an indication of an individual's profile and its identity. There are different ways in which an individual's DNA can be measured and analyzed. They are described below.

9.9.1 *Restriction fragment length polymorphism analysis*

This method for DNA profiling involves restriction enzyme digestion followed by Southern blot analysis. It has been reported that polymorphisms exist in the restriction enzyme cleavage sites, and to analyze VNTR loci, the enzymes and DNA probes are used. Nevertheless, the Southern blot technique is painstaking, and requires large amounts of undegraded sample DNA. In addition, Karl Brown's technique can be used to study minisatellite loci at the same time, increasing the observed variability, but making it hard to differentiate individual alleles and therefore it cannot be used for parental testing. These early techniques have been supplanted by PCR-based assays (Figure 9.10).

9.9.1.1 *Short tandem repeat analysis*

Short tandem repeat (STR) method uses highly polymorphic regions of DNA that have short repeated sequences. It has been observed that unrelated (not related to family) people certainly have different numbers of STR units; therefore, STR can be used to discriminate between unrelated individuals. During PCR, primers specific for STR are used to target the STR loci in the samples. Later, DNA fragments obtained through gel electrophoresis are analyzed for STR status in the sample. Each STR is polymorphic, but the number of alleles is very small and normally each STR allele can be shared by 5–20% of individuals. The STR analysis deals with mapping multiple STR loci concurrently and, thus, the pattern of alleles can identify an individual quite precisely. Therefore, STR analysis provides an excellent tool for establishing person's identity.

Moreover, different STR-based DNA-profiling systems are in use in different countries. In the North American region, STR systems that amplify the CODIS 13 core loci are almost universal, whereas in the United Kingdom, the SGM plus system that is compatible

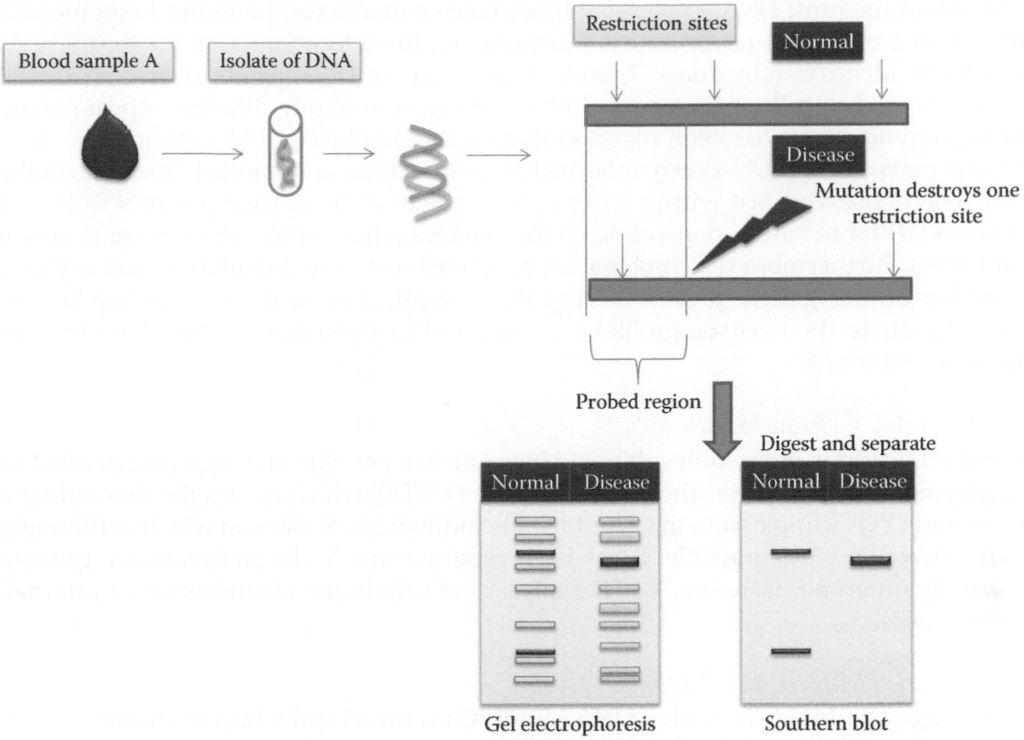

Figure 9.10 Restriction fragment length polymorphism.

with the National DNA Database is in practice. Furthermore, whichever system is used, most of the STR regions used are the most similar. We are aware that DNA-based profiling systems are generally based on multiplex reactions, where many STR regions can be examined at the same time. The main strength of STR analysis is in its statistical power of discrimination because the 13 loci that are currently used for discrimination in CODIS are independently assorted; the product rule for probabilities can be applied. This means that if some person has the DNA type of XYZ, where the three loci are independent, then we can assume that the likelihood of having that DNA type is the chance of having type X times the chance of having type Y times the probability of having type Z, respectively.

9.9.1.2 *DNA family relationship analysis*

DNA analysis is widely employed to establish genetic family relationships, which include paternity issue, maternity issue, siblingship, and other kinships. As we know a baby carries the genes from both mother's and father's sides, and during conception, the father's sperm and the mother's egg fuse to form a fertilized egg, which is called a zygote. This zygote contains a complete set of DNA structure, which is basically a unique combination of DNA from both parents (mother and father). Later on, this zygote divides and multiplies into an embryo and finally develops into a full human being. At each stage of development, all the cells contain the DNA received from the father and mother in equal proportions. In order to establish the individual's identity, testing is done by collecting the samples from buccal swabs or blood from individuals. DNA that contains information pertaining to certain functions, which is called junk DNA, can be used for human identification. At some special locations in the junk DNA, expectable inheritance patterns can be found to be useful in determining biological relationships. Furthermore, these locations contain specific DNA markers to identify individuals. Therefore, in a routine DNA paternity test, STR markers, which are basically short pieces of DNA, are used in highly different repeat patterns among individuals. It has been reported that each individual's DNA contains two copies of these markers, one DNA copy inherited from the father and another from the mother. It has been observed that within a population, the markers at each person's DNA location could differ in length, depending on the markers inherited from both parents (mother and father). Furthermore, the combination of marker sizes found in each person makes up his or her unique genetic profile. During the determination of the relationship between two individuals, their genetic profiles are compared to understand if they share the same inheritance designs.

9.9.1.3 Y chromosome analysis

Recent innovations in the molecular field have made it possible to design primers that target polymorphic regions on the Y chromosome (Y-STR), which allows the determination of a mixed DNA sample from male and female individuals or cases in which a differential DNA extraction is not possible. It has been reported that Y chromosomes are generally paternally inherited; therefore, Y-STR analysis can help in the identification of paternally related males.

9.9.1.4 Mitochondrial DNA analysis

Interestingly, for highly degraded DNA samples, it is occasionally impossible to get a complete profile of the 13 CODIS STRs and in these situations, mitochondrial DNA (mtDNA) can be used for identification. It has been shown that forensic scientists can amplify the HV1 and HV2 regions of the mtDNA, and then sequence each region and compare single nucleotide differences to a reference sample. Also, mtDNA that is maternally inherited come from the mother and can be directly linked to maternal relatives and can be used as match references to establish family relationships through the mother's side. Additionally, mtDNA analysis can be useful in determining clear family identities, such as those of misplaced or lost individuals when a maternally linked relative can be found.

9.10 Summary

The term "molecular diagnostics" refers to the measurement of DNA, RNA, proteins, or metabolites to detect genotypes, mutations, or biochemical changes in the patient's samples such as blood, cells, or tissues. Molecular diagnostics assess the patient's biological makeup at the genetic level. Decoding the DNA code can reveal variations between individuals, which may characterize a predisposition to develop a disease or to find out its treatment option. It has been reported that molecular diagnostic tests can analyze genetic content related to diseases. These tests sequence specific regions of the DNA to identify genetic alterations or quantify the levels of certain genetic materials that are expressed by a bacterium, virus, or cancer. With the molecular diagnostic information, the doctors usually alert the patients to make certain lifestyle choices in order to avoid or monitor the development of a particular disease. It has been reported that certain mutations can also affect treatment options as if the drug target contains critical mutations. Therefore, doctors use this genetic information to select the optimal therapeutic strategy for each individual and illness. Molecular techniques have also been used to confirm a person's identity and paternity issues, and is extensively used in forensic analysis. In this chapter, we discussed the significance of molecular tools in diagnosing various diseases and conditions and explained how these tools are being used in forensic and criminal laboratories.

9.11 Scholar's achievements

Abu al-Qasim al-Zahrawi: Abu al-Qasim Khalaf ibn al-Abbas Al-Zahrawi (936–1013), also known in the West as Albucasis, was an Arab Muslim physician who lived in Al-Andalus. He is considered the greatest medieval surgeon to have appeared from the Islamic world, and has been described by many as the father of modern surgery. His greatest contribution to medicine is the Kitab al-Tasrif, a 30-volume encyclopedia of medical practices. His pioneering contributions to the field of surgical procedures and instruments had an enormous impact on the East and West well into the modern period, where some of his discoveries are still applied in medicine to this day.

Ibn Sina: Abu Ali al-Husayn ibn Abd Allah ibn Sina, commonly known as Ibn Sina or by his Latinized name Avicenna, was a Persian who wrote almost 450 treatises on a wide range of subjects, of which around 240 have survived. In particular, 150 of his surviving treatises concentrate on philosophy and 40 of them concentrate on medicine. His most famous works are *The Book of Healing*, a vast philosophical and scientific encyclopedia, and *The Canon of Medicine*, which was a standard medical text at many medieval universities.

Kary Mullis: Kary Banks Mullis (born 1944) is a Nobel Prize-winning American biochemist, author, and lecturer. In recognition of his improvement of the polymerase chain reaction (PCR) technique, he shared the 1993 Nobel Prize in Chemistry with Michael Smith and earned the Japan Prize in the same year. The improvements made by Mullis allowed PCR to become a central technique in biochemistry and molecular biology, described by *The New York Times* as highly original and significant, virtually dividing biology into the two epochs of before PCR and after PCR.

9.12 Knowledge builder

Hypothetico-deductive approaches: The hypothetico-deductive model or method is a proposed description of scientific method. According to it, scientific inquiry proceeds by formulating a hypothesis in a form that could conceivably be falsified by a test on observable data. A test that could and does run contrary to predictions of the hypothesis is taken as a falsification of the hypothesis. A test that could but does not run contrary to the hypothesis corroborates the theory. It is then proposed to compare the explanatory value of competing hypotheses by testing how stringently they are corroborated by their predictions.

Differential diagnosis: A differential diagnosis is a systematic diagnostic method used to identify the presence of an entity where multiple alternatives are possible (and the process may be termed differential diagnostic procedure), and may also refer to any of the included candidate alternatives (which may also be termed candidate condition). This method is essentially a process of elimination or at least of obtaining information that shrinks the "probabilities" of candidate conditions to negligible levels.

Peripheral vascular examination: In medicine, the peripheral vascular examination is a series of maneuvers to elicit signs of peripheral vascular pathology. It is performed as part of a physical examination, or when a patient presents with leg pain suggestive of a cardiovascular pathology.

Sphygmomanometer: A sphygmomanometer or blood pressure meter is a device used to measure blood pressure. It is composed of an inflatable cuff to restrict blood flow, and a mercury or mechanical manometer to measure the pressure. It is always used in conjunction with a means to determine at what pressure blood flow is just starting, and at what pressure it is unimpeded. Manual sphygmomanometers are used in conjunction with a stethoscope.

Aneuploidy screening: Aneuploidy screening is a term used to screen a chromosome problem that is caused by an extra or missing chromosome.

Chromosomal translocations: In molecular genetics, a chromosome translocation is a chromosome abnormality caused by the rearrangement of parts between nonhomologous chromosomes. A gene fusion may be created when the translocation joins two otherwise separated genes, the occurrence of which is common in cancer. It is detected on cytogenetic or a karyotype of affected cells. There are two main types: reciprocal (also recognized as non-Robertsonian) and Robertsonian. Also, translocations can be balanced (in an even exchange of material with no genetic information extra or missing, and ideally full functionality) or unbalanced (where the exchange of chromosomal material is unequal resulting in extra or missing genes).

Metaphase-Fish: FISH provides a powerful tool for identifying the location of a cloned DNA sequence on metaphase chromosomes.

Human Genome Project: The Human Genome Project is an international scientific research project with a primary goal of determining the sequence of chemical base pairs that make up the DNA, and of identifying and mapping the approximately 20,000–25,000 genes of the human genome from both a physical and functional standpoint.

Size-exclusion chromatography: Size-exclusion chromatography (SEC) is a chromatographic method in which molecules in solution are separated by their size, and in some cases molecular weight. It is usually applied to large molecules or macromolecular complexes such as proteins and industrial polymers. Typically, when an aqueous solution is used to transport the sample through the column, the technique is known as gel-filtration chromatography, versus the name gel permeation chromatography, which is used when an organic solvent is used as a mobile phase. SEC is a widely used polymer characterization method because of its ability to provide good molar mass distribution results for polymers.

Antibodies: An antibody also known as an immunoglobulin is a large Y-shaped protein produced by B-cells that is used by the immune system to identify and neutralize foreign objects such as bacteria and viruses. The antibody recognizes a unique part of the foreign target, called an antigen.

Green fluorescent protein: The green fluorescent protein (GFP) is a protein composed of 238 amino acid residues that exhibits bright green fluorescence when exposed to light in the blue to ultraviolet range. Although many other marine organisms have similar green fluorescent proteins, GFP traditionally refers to the protein first isolated from the jellyfish *Aequorea victoria*. In cell and molecular biology, the GFP gene is frequently used as a reporter of expression. In modified forms, it has been used to make biosensors, and many animals have been created that express GFP as a proof-of-concept that a gene can be expressed throughout a given organism. The GFP gene can be introduced into organisms and maintained in their genome through breeding, injection with a viral vector, or cell transformation. To date, the GFP gene has been introduced and expressed in many bacteria, yeast and other fungi, fish (such as zebrafish), plant, fly, and mammalian cells, including human. Martin Chalfie, Osamu Shimomura, and Roger Y. Tsien were awarded the 2008 Nobel Prize in Chemistry for their discovery and development of the GFP.

Flow cytometry: Flow cytometry is a laser-based, biophysical technology employed in cell counting, cell sorting, biomarker detection, and protein engineering, by suspending cells in a stream of fluid and passing them by an electronic detection apparatus. It allows simultaneous multiparametric analysis of the physical and chemical characteristics of up to thousands of particles per second.

Telomere: A telomere is a region of repetitive nucleotide sequences at each end of a chromatid, which protects the end of the chromosome from deterioration or from fusion with neighboring chromosomes.

Karyotype: A karyotype is the number and appearance of chromosomes in the nucleus of a eukaryotic cell. The term is also used for the complete set of chromosomes in a species, or an individual organism. Karyotypes describe the number of chromosomes, and what they look like under a light microscope.

DNA polymerase: A DNA polymerase is a cellular or viral polymerase enzyme that synthesizes DNA molecules from their nucleotide building blocks. DNA polymerases are essential for DNA replication, and usually function in pairs while copying one double-stranded DNA molecule into two double-stranded DNAs in a process termed semiconservative DNA replication. DNA polymerases also play key roles in other processes within cells, including DNA repair, genetic recombination, reverse transcription, and the generation of antibody diversity via the specialized DNA polymerase, terminal deoxynucleotidyl transferase. DNA polymerases are widely used in molecular biology laboratories, notably for PCR, DNA sequencing, and molecular cloning.

Cadaver: A corpse, also called a cadaver in medical literary and legal usage or when intended for dissection, is a dead human body.

Forensic archaeologists: Forensic archaeology, a forensic science, is the application of archaeological principles, techniques, and methodologies in a legal context, predominately medico-legal. The individual who performs such action is called a forensic archaeologist. Forensic archaeologists are employed by police and other agencies to help locate evidence at a crime scene using the skills normally used on archaeological sites to uncover evidence from the past. Forensic archaeologists are employed to locate, excavate, and record buried remains; the variety of such targets is large and each case is unique in its requirements.

Further reading

Baerlocher GM, Vultro I, de Jong G, and Lansdorp, PM 2006. Flow cytometry and FISH to measure the average length of telomeres. *Nat Protoc* 1 (5): 2365–2376.

Bailey SM and Goodwin EH 2004. DNA and telomeres: Beginnings and endings. *Cytogenet Genome Res* 104: 109–115.

Canela A, Vera E, Klatt P, and Blasco MA 2007. High-throughput telomere length quantification by FISH and its application to human population studies. *Proc Natl Acad Sci* 104 (13): 5300–5305.

Carson SA, Gentry WL, Smith AL, and Buster JE 1993. Trophectoderm microbiopsy in murine blastocysts: Comparison of four methods. *J Assist Reprod Genet* 10 (6): 427–433. doi:10.1007/BF01228093. PMID 8019091.

Cheng S, Fockler C, Barnes WM, and Higuchi R 1994. Effective amplification of long targets from cloned inserts and human genomic DNA. *Proc Natl Acad Sci* 91 (12): 5695–5699. doi:10.1073/pnas.91.12.5695. PMID 8202550.

Chien A, Edgar DB, and Trela JM 1976. Deoxyribonucleic acid polymerase from the extreme thermophile *Thermus aquaticus*. *J Bacteriol* 174 (3): 1550–1557. PMID 8432.

Coutelle C, Williams C, Handyside A, Hardy K, Winston R, and Williamson R 1989. Genetic analysis of DNA from single human oocytes: A model for preimplantation diagnosis of cystic fibrosis. *BMJ* 299 (6690): 22–24. doi:10.1136/bmj.299.6690.22. PMID 2503195.

Crumbley DL, Heitger LE, and Smith GS 2005. *Forensic and Investigative Accounting*. Chicago, IL: CCH Group. ISBN 0-8080-1365-3.

David F and Turlotte E 1998. An isothermal amplification method. *CR Acad Sci Paris Life Sci* 321 (1): 909–914.

Demko Z, Rabinowitz M, and Johnson D 2010. Current methods for preimplantation genetic diagnosis. *J Clin Embryol* 13 (1): 6–12. http://www.genesecurity.net/wp-content/uploads/2010/04/Current-Methods-for-Preimplantation-Genetic-Diagnosis.pdf.

Fagagna F, Hande MP, Tong WM, Roth D, Lansdorp PM, Wang ZQ, and Jackson SP 2001. Effects of DNA nonhomologous end-joining factors on telomere length and chromosomal stability in mammalian cells. *Curr Biol* 15: 1192–1196.

Falconer E, Chavez EA, Henderson A, Poon SSS, McKinney S, Brown L, Huntsman DG, and Lansdorp PM 2010. Identification of sister chromatids by DNA template strand sequences. *Nature* 463: 93–98.

Gardner RL and Edwards RG 1968. Control of the sex ratio at full term in the rabbit by transferring sexed blastocysts. *Nature* 218 (5139): 346–349. doi:10.1038/218346a0. PMID 5649672.

Gianaroli L, Magli MC, Ferraretti AP, and Munné S 1999. Preimplantation diagnosis for aneuploidies in patients undergoing *in vitro* fertilization with a poor prognosis: Identification of the categories for which it should be proposed. *Fertil Steril* 72 (5): 837–844. doi:10.1016/S0015-0282(99)00377-5. PMID 10560987. http://linkinghub.elsevier.com/retrieve/pii/S0015-0282(99)00377-5.

Handyside AH, Lesko JG, Tarín JJ, Winston RM, and Hughes MR 1992. Birth of a normal girl after *in vitro* fertilization and preimplantation diagnostic testing for cystic fibrosis. *N Engl J Med* 327 (13): 905–909. doi:10.1056/NEJM199209243271301. PMID 1381054.

Hemann MT, Strong MA, Hao LY, and Greider CW 2001. The shortest telomere, not average telomere length, is critical for cell viability and chromosome stability. *Cell* 107: 67–77.

Herman JG, Graff JR, Myöhänen S, Nelkin BD, and Baylin SB 1996. Methylation-specific PCR: A novel PCR assay for methylation status of CpG islands. *Proc Natl Acad Sci U S A* 93 (13): 9821–9826. doi:10.1073/pnas.93.18.9821. PMID 8790415.

Holding C and Monk M 1989. Diagnosis of beta-thalassaemia by DNA amplification in single blastomeres from mouse preimplantation embryos. *Lancet* 2 (8662): 532–535. doi:10.1016/S0140-6736(89)90655-7. PMID 2570237. http://linkinghub.elsevier.com/retrieve/pii/S0140-6736(89)90655-7.

Innis MA, Myambo KB, Gelfand DH, and Brow MA 1988. DNA sequencing with *Thermus aquaticus* DNA polymerase and direct sequencing of polymerase chain reaction-amplified DNA. *Proc Natl Acad Sci U S A* 85 (24): 9436–4940. doi:10.1073/pnas.85.24.9436. PMID 3200828.

Isenbarger TA, Finney M, Ríos-Velázquez C, Handelsman J, and Ruvkun G 2008. Miniprimer PCR, a new lens for viewing the microbial world. *Appl Environ Microbiol* 74 (3): 840–849. doi:10.1128/AEM.01933-07. PMID 18083877.

Kahraman S, Bahçe M, Samli H et al. 2000. Healthy births and ongoing pregnancies obtained by preimplantation genetic diagnosis in patients with advanced maternal age and recurrent implantation failure. *Hum Reprod* 15 (9): 2003–2007. doi:10.1093/humrep/15.9.2003. PMID 10967004. http://humrep.oxfordjournals.org/cgi/pmidlookup?view=long&pmid=10967004.

Khan Z, Poetter K, and Park DJ 2008. Enhanced solid phase PCR: Mechanisms to increase priming by solid support primers. *Anal Biochem* 375 (2): 391–393. doi:10.1016/j.ab.2008.01.021. PMID 18267099.

Kleppe K, Ohtsuka E, Kleppe R, Molineux I, and Khorana HG 1971. Studies on polynucleotides. XCVI. Repair replications of short synthetic DNA's as catalyzed by DNA polymerases. *J Mol Biol* 56 (2): 341–361. doi:10.1016/0022-2836(71)90469-4. PMID 4927950.

Klitzman R, Zolovska B, Folberth W, Sauer MV, Chung W, and Appelbaum P 2009. Preimplantation genetic diagnosis on *in vitro* fertilization clinic websites: Presentations of risks, benefits and other information. *Fertil Steril* 92 (4): 1276–1283. doi:10.1016/j.fertnstert.2008.07.1772. PMID 18829009.

Lawyer FC, Stoffel S, Saiki RK, Chang SY, Landre PA, Abramson RD, and Gelfand DH 1993. High-level expression, purification, and enzymatic characterization of full-length *Thermus aquaticus* DNA polymerase and a truncated form deficient in 5′ to 3′ exonuclease activity. *PCR Methods Appl* 2 (4): 275–287. PMID 8324500.

Lewis CM, Pinêl T, Whittaker JC, and Handyside AH 2001. Controlling misdiagnosis errors in preimplantation genetic diagnosis: A comprehensive model encompassing extrinsic and intrinsic sources of error. *Hum Reprod* 16 (1): 43–50. doi:10.1093/humrep/16.1.43. PMID 11139534. http://humrep.oxfordjournals.org/cgi/pmidlookup?view=long&pmid=11139534.

Li M, DeUgarte CM, Surrey M, Danzer H, DeCherney A, and Hill DL 2005. Fluorescence *in situ* hybridization reanalysis of day-6 human blastocysts diagnosed with aneuploidy on day 3. *Fertil Steril* 84 (5): 1395–1400. doi:10.1016/j.fertnstert.2005.04.068. PMID 16275234.

Liu YG and Whittier RF 1995. Thermal asymmetric interlaced PCR: Automatable amplification and sequencing of insert end fragments from P1 and YAC clones for chromosome walking. *Genomics* 25 (3): 674–681. doi:10.1016/0888-7543(95)80010-J. PMID 7759102.

Marcondes AM, Bair S, Rabinovitch PS, Gooley T, Deeg HJ, and Risques R 2009. No telomere shortening in marrow stroma from patients with MDS. *Ann Hematol* 88: 623–628.

McArthur SJ, Leigh D, Marshall JT, de Boer KA, and Jansen RP 2005. Pregnancies and live births after trophectoderm biopsy and preimplantation genetic testing of human blastocysts. *Fertil Steril* 84 (6): 1628–1636. doi:10.1016/j.fertnstert.2005.05.063. PMID 16359956.

Montag M, van der Ven K, Dorn C, and van der Ven H. 2004. Outcome of laser-assisted polar body biopsy and aneuploidy testing. *Reprod Biomed Online* 9 (4): 425–429. doi:10.1016/S1472-6483(10)61278-3. PMID 15511343. http://openurl.ingenta.com/content/nlm?genre=article&issn=1472-6483&volume=9&issue=4&spage=425&aulast=Montag.

Mueller PR and Wold B 1988. *In vivo* foot printing of a muscle specific enhancer by ligation mediated PCR. *Science* 246 (4931): 780–786. doi:10.1126/science.2814500. PMID 2814500.

Mullis K 1990. The unusual origin of the polymerase chain reaction. *Sci Am* 262 (4): 56–61, 64–65. doi:10.1038/scientificamerican0490-56.

Mullis K 1998. *Dancing Naked in the Mind Field*. New York: Pantheon Books. ISBN 0-679-44255-3.

Munné S, Cohen J, and Sable D 2002. Preimplantation genetic diagnosis for advanced maternal age and other indications. *Fertil Steril* 78 (2): 234–236. doi:10.1016/S0015-0282(02)03239-9. PMID 12137856. http://linkinghub.elsevier.com/retrieve/pii/S0015028202032399.

Munné S, Dailey T, Sultan KM, Grifo J, and Cohen J 1995. The use of first polar bodies for preimplantation diagnosis of aneuploidy. *Hum Reprod* 10 (4): 1014–1020. PMID 7650111. http://humrep.oxfordjournals.org/cgi/pmidlookup?view=long&pmid=7650111.

Munné S, Magli C, Cohen J et al. 1999. Positive outcome after preimplantation diagnosis of aneuploidy in human embryos. *Hum Reprod* 14 (9): 2191–2199. doi:10.1093/humrep/14.9.2191. PMID 10469680. http://humrep.oxfordjournals.org/cgi/pmidlookup?view=long&pmid=10469680.

Myrick KV and Gelbart WM 2002. Universal fast walking for direct and versatile determination of flanking sequence. *Gene* 284 (1–2): 125–131. doi:10.1016/S0378-1119(02)00384-0. PMID 11891053.

Navidi W and Arnheim N 1991. Using PCR in preimplantation genetic disease diagnosis. *Hum Reprod* 6 (6): 836–849. PMID 1757524. http://humrep.oxfordjournals.org/cgi/pmidlookup?view=long&pmid=1757524.

Newton CR, Graham A, Heptinstall LE et al. 1989. Analysis of any point mutation in DNA. The amplification refractory mutation system (ARMS). *Nucl Acid Res* 17 (7): 2503–2516. doi:10.1093/nar/17.7.2503. PMID 2785681.

Nietzel A, Rocchi M, Starke H et al. 2001. A new multi-colour FISH approach for the characterization of marker chromosomes: Centromere-specific multicolor-FISH (cenM-FISH). *Hum Genet* 108: 199–204.

Nigrini M 2011. *Forensic Analytics: Methods and Techniques for Forensic Accounting Investigations*. Hoboken, NJ: John Wiley & Sons Inc. ISBN 978-0-470-89046-2.

Ochman H, Gerber AS, and Hartl DL 1988. Genetic applications of an inverse polymerase chain reaction. *Genetics* 120 (3): 621–623. PMID 2852134.

Park DJ 2004. 3′RACE LaNe: A simple and rapid fully nested PCR method to determine 3′-terminal cDNA sequence. *Biotechniques* 36 (4): 586–588, 590. PMID 15088375.

Park DJ 2005. A new 5′ terminal murine GAPDH exon identified using 5′RACE LaNe. *Mol Biotechnol* 29 (1): 39–46. doi:10.1385/MB:29:1:39. PMID 15668518.

Pavlov AR, Pavlova NV, Kozyavkin SA, Slesarev AI 2012. Cooperation between catalytic and DNA binding domains enhances thermostability and supports DNA synthesis at higher temperatures by thermostable DNA polymerases. *Biochemistry* 51 (10):2032–2043. doi: 10.1021/bi2014807. Epub 2012 Mar 1.

Pavlov AR, Pavlova NV, Kozyavkin SA, and Slesarev AI 2004. Recent developments in the optimization of thermostable DNA polymerases for efficient applications. *Trends Biotechnol* 22 (5): 253–260. doi:10.1016/j.tibtech.2004.02.011. PMID 15109812.

Pehlivan T, Rubio C, Rodrigo L et al. March 2003. Impact of preimplantation genetic diagnosis on IVF outcome in implantation failure patients. *Reprod Biomed Online* 6 (2): 232–237. doi:10.1016/S1472-6483(10)61715-4. PMID 12676006. http://openurl.ingenta.com/content/nlm?genre=article&issn=1472-6483&volume=6&issue=2&spage=232&aulast=Pehlivan.

Pernthaler A, Pernthaler J, and Rudolf A 2002. Fluorescence *in situ* hybridization and catalyzed reporter deposition for the identification of marine bacteria. *Appl Environ Microbiol* 68 (6): 3094–3101. doi: 10.1128/AEM.68.6.3094-3101.2002.

Pierce KE and Wangh LJ 2007. Linear-after-the-exponential polymerase chain reaction and allied technologies Real-time detection strategies for rapid, reliable diagnosis from single cells. *Methods Mol Med* 132: 65–85. doi:10.1007/978-1-59745-298-4_7. PMID 17876077.

Rychlik W, Spencer WJ, and Rhoads RE 1990. Optimization of the annealing temperature for DNA amplification *in vitro*. *Nucl Acid Res* 18 (21): 6409–6412. doi:10.1093/nar/18.21.6409. PMID 2243783. PMC 332522. http://www.pubmedcentral.nih.gov/articlerender.fcgi?tool=pubmed&pubmedid=2243783.

Saiki RK, Gelfand DH, Stoffel S et al. 1988. Primer-directed enzymatic amplification of DNA with a thermostable DNA polymerase. *Science* 239 (4839): 487–491. doi:10.1126/science.2448875. PMID 2448875. http://sunsite.berkeley.edu/cgi-bin/ebind2html/pcr/009.

Sambrook J and Russel DW (eds) 2001. Chapter 8: *In vitro* amplification of DNA by the polymerase chain reaction, In *Molecular Cloning: A Laboratory Manual (3rd ed.)*. Cold Spring Harbor, NY: Cold Spring Harbor Laboratory Press. ISBN 0-87969-576-5.

Sandalinas M, Sadowy S, Alikani M, Calderon G, Cohen J, and Munné S 2001. Developmental ability of chromosomally abnormal human embryos to develop to the blastocyst stage. *Hum Reprod* 16 (9): 1954–1958. doi:10.1093/humrep/16.9.1954. PMID 11527904. http://humrep.oxfordjournals.org/cgi/pmidlookup?view=long&pmid=11527904.

Sarrate Z, Vidal F, and Blanco J 2010. Role of sperm fluorescent *in situ* hybridization studies in infertile patients: Indications, study approach, and clinical relevance. *Fertil Steril* 93 (6): 1892–1902. doi:10.1016/j.fertnstert.2008.12.139. PMID 19254793.

Sharkey DJ, Scalice ER, Christy Jr. KG, Atwood SM, and Daiss JL 1994. Antibodies as thermolabile switches: High temperature triggering for the polymerase chain reaction. *Bio-Technology* 12: 506–509. doi:10.1038/nbt0594-506.

Shkumatov A, Kuznyetsov V, Cieslak J, Ilkevitch Y, and Verlinsky Y 2007. Obtaining metaphase spreads from single blastomeres for PGD of chromosomal rearrangements. *Reprod Biomed Online* 14 (4): 498–503. doi:10.1016/S1472-6483(10)60899-1. PMID 17425834. http://openurl.ingenta.com/content/nlm?genre=article&issn=1472-6483&volume=14&issue=4&spage=498&aulast=Shkumatov.

Sieben VJ, Debes Marun CS, Pilarski PM et al. 2007. FISH and chips: Chromosomal analysis on microfluidic platforms. *IET Nanobiotechnol* 1 (3): 27–35. doi:10.1049/iet-nbt:20060021. PMID 17506594. http://link.aip.org/link/?NBT/1/27/1 (Retrieved 2009-01-26).

Sieben VJ, Debes-Marun CS, Pilarski LM, and Backhouse CG 2008. An integrated microfluidic chip for chromosome enumeration using fluorescence *in situ* hybridization. *Lab Chip* 8 (12): 2151–2156. doi:10.1039/b812443d. PMID 19023479. http://www.rsc.org/publishing/journals/LC/article.asp?doi=b812443d (Retrieved 2009-03-24).

Staessen C, Platteau P, Van Assche E et al. 2004. Comparison of blastocyst transfer with or without preimplantation genetic diagnosis for aneuploidy screening in couples with advanced maternal age: A prospective randomized controlled trial. *Hum Reprod* 19 (12): 2849–2858. doi:10.1093/humrep/deh536. PMID 15471934.

Stemmer WP, Crameri A, Ha KD, Brennan TM, and Heyneker HL 1995. Single-step assembly of a gene and entire plasmid from large numbers of oligodeoxyribonucleotides. *Gene* 164 (1): 49–53. doi:10.1016/0378-1119(95)00511-4. PMID 7590320.

Stender H 2003. PNA-FISH: An intelligent stain for rapid diagnosis of infectious diseases. *Expert Rev Mol Diagn* 5: 649–655.

Summers PM, Campbell JM, and Miller MW 1988. Normal in-vivo development of marmoset monkey embryos after trophectoderm biopsy. *Hum Reprod* 3 (3): 389–393. PMID 3372701. http://humrep.oxfordjournals.org/cgi/pmidlookup?view=long&pmid=3372701.

Uhrig S, Schuffenhauer S, Fauth C et al. 1999. Multiplex-FISH for pre- and post-natal diagnostic applications. *Am J Hum Genet* 65: 448–462.

Verlinsky Y, Ginsberg N, Lifchez A, Valle J, Moise J, and Strom CM 1990. Analysis of the first polar body: Preconception genetic diagnosis. *Hum Reprod* 5 (7): 826–829. PMID 2266156. http://humrep.oxfordjournals.org/cgi/pmidlookup?view=long&pmid=2266156.

Verlinsky Y, Rechitsky S, Schoolcraft W, Strom C, and Kuliev A 2001. Preimplantation diagnosis for Fanconi anemia combined with HLA matching. *JAMA* 285 (24): 3130–3133. doi:10.1001/jama.285.24.3130. PMID 11427142. http://jama.ama-assn.org/cgi/pmidlookup?view=long&pmid=11427142.

Vincent M, Xu Y, and Kong H 2004. Helicase-dependent isothermal DNA amplification. *EMBO Rep* 5 (8): 795–800. doi:10.1038/sj.embor.7400200. PMID 15247927.

Zietkiewicz AR and Labuda D 1994. Genome fingerprinting by simple sequence repeat (SSR)-anchored polymerase chain reaction amplification. *Genomics* 20 (2): 176–183. doi:10.1006/geno.1994.1151. PMID 8020964.

chapter ten

Genetic disorders and gene therapy

10.1 Introduction

A genetic disease is the result of structural or functional modifications in the DNA and the disease in which the DNA sequence is altered is called a gene mutation. It has been reported that DNA which makes the proteins, the molecules that carry out most of the work, and perform most life functions. These proteins make up the minority of cellular structures when a gene is mutated, the gene which makes a particular protein become dysfunctional, which finally leads to the development of a disorder or disease. Furthermore, diseases can be genetically inherited from parents to children and can also result from structural or functional changes in DNA in the body cells. Some genetic diseases are called Mendelian disorders, including Huntington's disease and cystic fibrosis, which are caused by single gene mutation. Moreover, there are many types of genetic diseases related to heart disease, cancer, and diabetes that are multigene in nature and are normally caused by mutations in multiple genes.

10.2 Genetic epidemiology

The genetic epidemiology is the study of the role of genetic factors in determining health and disease in families and in populations, and the interplay of such genetic factors with environmental factors. Genetic epidemiology was defined by N.E. Morton as a science which deals with the distribution, and control of disease in groups of relatives in populations. It is closely associated to both molecular epidemiology and statistical genetics, but these overlapping fields have distinct emphases and societies. This customary method has proved highly successful in identifying monogenic disorders and locating the genes responsible. More recently, the scope of genetic epidemiology has expanded to include common diseases for which many genes make a smaller contribution. This has developed rapidly in the first decade of the twenty-first century following completion of the Human Genome Project, as advances in genotyping technology and associated reductions in cost has made it feasible to conduct large-scale genome-wide association studies in thousands of individuals. These studies have led to the discovery of many genetic polymorphisms that influence the risk of developing many genetic diseases.

10.3 Epigenetics

Epigenetics is the study of changes in gene expression caused by mechanisms other than changes in the underlying DNA sequence; henceforth, the name epigenetics was coined. Some of these changes have been shown to be genetic. It also refers to functionally relevant modifications to the genome that do not involve a change in the nucleotide sequence. Examples of such modifications are DNA methylation and histone modification, both of which serve to regulate gene expression without altering the underlying DNA sequence. Gene expression can be controlled through the action of repressor proteins that attach to silencer regions of the DNA. These variations may remain through cell divisions for the remainder of the cell's life and may also last for multiple generations. However, there is no change in the underlying DNA sequence of the organism; instead, nongenetic factors cause the organism's genes to behave (or "express themselves") differently. Interestingly, there are oppositions to the use of the term epigenetics to describe chemical modification of histone, since it remains unclear whether or not histone modifications are genetic. In eukaryotic biology the process of cellular differentiation is an example of epigenetics. During the morphogenesis process, totipotent stem cells can become pluripotent cell lines, which in turn become fully differentiated cells. In other words, in a single fertilized egg cell the zygote changes into the many cell types including neurons, muscle cells, epithelium, endothelium of blood vessels, and they continue to divide. The situation does so by activating some genes while inhibiting others. Moreover, it was investigated that the methylation of messenger RNA (mRNA) has a critical role in human energy homeostasis.

10.3.1 Mechanism of epigenetics

There are several types of epigenetic inheritance systems which play a role that has been identified as cell memory. We have described a few of them for the readers understanding.

10.3.1.1 DNA methylation

The phenotype of a cell or individual is affected by particular genes that are transcribed and have heritable transcription states that can give rise to epigenetic effects. There are numerous regulation layers of gene expression and one way is through the remodeling of chromatin. Chromatin is basically the complex of DNA and the histone proteins with which it allies. Histone proteins are little spheres in shape that DNA wraps around. In case DNA which is enveloped around the histones changes, gene expression can also change as well. Furthermore, chromatin remodeling is accomplished through two main mechanisms as briefly explained: (a) The first way is posttranslational modification of the amino acids that make up histone proteins and histone proteins consist of long chains of amino acids. If the amino acids that are in the chain are modified, the shape of the histone sphere may be changed. During replication, DNA is not completely unwound. It is possible, then, that the modified histones may be carried into each new copy of the DNA. Once there, these histones may act as templates, initiating the surrounding new histones to be shaped in a new manner. By altering the shape of the histones around it, these modified histones would ensure that a differentiated cell would stay differentiated, and not convert back into being a stem cell. (b) The second way is the addition of methyl groups to the DNA, mostly at CpG sites, to convert cytosine to 5-methylcytosine, 5-methylcytosine does much like a regular cytosine, pairing up with a guanine. Nevertheless, some areas of the genome are methylated more heavily than others, and highly methylated areas tend to be less transcriptionally active, through a mechanism not fully understood. Moreover, methylation of cytosines can also persist from the germ line of one of the parents into the zygote, marking the chromosome as being inherited from this parent.

The way that the cells stay differentiated in the case of DNA methylation is clearer to us than it is in the case of histone shape. Fundamentally, certain enzymes have a higher affinity for the methylated cytosine. If this enzyme reaches a hemimethylated portion of DNA (where methylcytosine is in only one of the two DNA strands) the enzyme will methylate the other half. Although histone modifications occur throughout the entire sequence, the unstructured N-termini of histones also called as histone tails are particularly highly modified which include acetylation, methylation, ubiquitylation, phosphorylation, and sumoylation. Interestingly, acetylation is the most exceedingly studied of these modifications. For example, acetylation of the K14 and K9 lysines of the tail of histone H3 by histone acetyltransferase enzymes is generally correlated with transcriptional competence.

One mode of thinking is that the tendency of acetylation to be associated with "active" transcription is biophysical in nature. Because it normally has a positively charged nitrogen at its end, lysine can bind the negatively charged phosphates of the DNA backbone. The acetylation event converts the positively charged amine group on the side chain into a neutral amide linkage and this gets rid of the positive charge, thus loosening the DNA from the histone. When this occurs, complexes like SWI/SNF and other transcriptional factors can bind to the DNA and allow transcription to occur and this is called as the *cis* model of epigenetic function. In other words, changes to the histone tails have a direct effect on the DNA itself.

A different model of epigenetic function is the *trans* model where changes to the histone tails act indirectly on the DNA. For example, lysine acetylation may create a binding site for chromatin-modifying enzymes (and basal transcription machinery as well). This chromatin remodeler can cause changes to the state of the chromatin. Indeed, the bromodomain, a protein segment (domain) that specifically binds acetyl–lysine, is found in many enzymes that help activate transcription, including the SWI/SNF complex (on the protein polybromo). It may be that acetylation acts in this and the previous way to aid in transcriptional activation. The idea that modifications act as docking modules for related factors is borne out by histone methylation as well. Methylation of lysine 9 of histone H3 has long been associated with constitutive transcriptionally silent chromatin (constitutive heterochromatin). It has been determined that a chromodomain (a domain that specifically binds methyl–lysine) in the transcriptionally repressive protein HP1, recruits HP1 to K9 methylated regions. One example that seems to refute this biophysical model for methylation is that trimethylation of histone H3 at lysine 4 is strongly associated with (and required for full) transcriptional activation. Trimethylation in this case would introduce a fixed positive charge on the tail.

DNA methylation frequently occurs in repeated sequences and helps to suppress the expression and mobility of transposable elements. Because 5-methylcytosine can be spontaneously deaminated (replacing nitrogen with oxygen) to thymidine, CpG sites are frequently mutated and become rare in the genome, except at CpG islands where they remain unmethylated. Epigenetic changes of this type have the potential to direct increased frequencies of permanent genetic mutation. DNA methylation patterns are known to be established and modified in response to environmental factors by a complex interplay of at least three independent DNA methyltransferases, DNMT1, DNMT3A, and DNMT3B; the loss of any of which is lethal in mice. DNMT1 is the most abundant methyltransferase in somatic cells,. It is localized to replication foci, has a 10–40-fold preference for hemimethylated DNA, and interacts with the proliferating cell nuclear antigen (PCNA).

By favorably modifying hemimethylated DNA, DNMT1 transfer patterns of methylation to a newly synthesized strand after DNA replication is often referred to as the "maintenance" methyltransferase. Moreover, DNMT1 is critical for proper embryonic development and imprinting. To emphasize the difference of this molecular mechanism of inheritance from the canonical Watson–Crick base-pairing mechanism of transmission of genetic information, the term epigenetic templating was introduced. In addition to the maintenance and transmission of methylated DNA states, the same principle could work in the maintenance and transmission of histone modifications and even cytoplasmic heritable states.

Histones H3 and H4 can also be manipulated through demethylation process using histone lysine demethylase (KDM) and it has been recently identified an enzyme which has a catalytic active site called the Jumonji domain C (JmjC). The demethylation occurs when JmjC utilizes multiple cofactors to hydroxylate the methyl group, thereby removing it. Moreover, Jumonji domain C is capable of demethylating mono-, di-, and trimethylated substrates. Chromosomal regions can adopt stable and heritable alternative states resulting in bistable gene expression without changes to the DNA sequence. Epigenetic control is often associated with alternative covalent modifications of histones. The stability and heritability of larger chromosomal regions are often thought to involve positive feedback where modified nucleosomes recruit enzymes that similarly modify nearby nucleosomes.

Because DNA methylation plays such a central role in many types of epigenic inheritance, the word epigenetics is sometimes used as a synonym for these processes. However, this can be misleading. The chromatin remodeling process is not always inherited and not all epigenetic inheritance involves chromatin remodeling. It has been suggested that the histone code could be mediated by the effect of small RNAs. The recent discovery and characterization of a vast array of small (21- to 26-nt), noncoding RNAs suggests that there is an RNA component, possibly involved in epigenetic gene regulation. Small interfering RNAs can modulate transcriptional gene expression via epigenetic modulation of targeted promoters.

10.3.1.2 RNA transcripts and their encoded proteins

At times, after being turned on a gene transcribes a product that maintains the activity of that gene. For example, Hnf4 and MyoD enhance the transcription of many liver- and muscle-specific genes, respectively through the transcription factor activity of the proteins they encode. RNA signaling includes the differential recruitment of a hierarchy of generic chromatin-modifying complexes and DNA methyltransferases to specific loci by RNAs during differentiation and development. Other epigenetic changes are mediated by the production of different splice forms of RNA, or by the formation of double-stranded RNA (RNAi). Moreover, descendants of the cell in which the gene was turned on will inherit this activity, even if the original stimulus for gene activation is no longer present. These genes are most often turned on or off by signal transduction, although in some systems where syncytia or gap junctions are important, RNA may spread directly to other cells or nuclei by diffusion. A large amount of RNA and protein is contributed to the zygote by the mother during oogenesis or via nurse cells, resulting in maternal effect phenotypes. A smaller quantity of sperm RNA is transmitted from the father, but there is recent evidence that this epigenetic information can lead to visible changes in several generations of the offspring.

10.3.1.3 MicroRNAs

MicroRNAs (miRNAs) are members of noncoding RNAs that range in size from 17 to 25 nucleotides and miRNAs regulate a large variety of biological functions in plants and animals. So far, in 2013, about 2000 miRNAs have been discovered in humans and these can be found online in an miRNA database. Each miRNA expressed in a cell may target about 100–200 messenger RNA that it downregulates. Most of the downregulation of mRNAs occurs by causing the decay of the targeted mRNA, while some downregulation occurs at the level of translation into protein. It appears that about 60% of human protein coding genes are regulated by miRNAs. Many miRNAs are epigenetically regulated. About 50% of miRNA genes are associated with CpG islands, that may be repressed by epigenetic methylation. Transcription from methylated CpG islands is strongly and heritably repressed. Other miRNAs are epigenetically regulated by either histone modifications or by combined DNA methylation and histone modification.

10.3.1.4 Small RNA

Small RNAs (sRNAs) are small (50–250 nucleotides), highly structured, noncoding RNA fragments found in bacteria. They control gene expression including virulence genes in pathogens and are viewed as new targets in the fight against drug-resistant bacteria. They play an important role in many biological processes, binding to mRNA and protein targets in prokaryotes. Their phylogenetic analyses, for example, through sRNA–mRNA target interactions or protein-binding properties, are used to build comprehensive databases. sRNA–gene maps based on their targets in microbial genomes are also constructed.

10.3.1.5 Prions

Prions are infectious forms of proteins. In normal circumstances, proteins fold into isolated units that perform distinct cellular functions, but some proteins are also capable of forming an infectious conformational state known as a prion. Although often viewed in the context of infectious disease, prions are more loosely defined by their ability to catalytically convert other native state versions of the same protein to an infectious conformational state. It is in this latter sense that they can be viewed as epigenetic agents capable of inducing a phenotypic change without a modification of the genome. Fungal prions are considered epigenetic because the infectious phenotype caused by the prion can be inherited without modification of the genome. PSI+ and URE3, discovered in yeast in 1965 and 1971, are the two best studied of this type of prion. Prions can have a phenotypic effect through the sequestration of protein in aggregates, thereby reducing that protein's activity. In PSI+ cells, the loss of the Sup35 protein (which is involved in the termination of translation) causes ribosomes to have a higher rate of read-through of stop codons, an effect that results in suppression of nonsense mutations in other genes. The ability of Sup35 to form prions may be a conserved trait. It could confer an adaptive advantage by giving cells the ability to switch into a PSI+ state and express dormant genetic features normally terminated by stop codon mutations.

10.4 Genetic disorders: Classification

The genetic disease is caused by an abnormality in an individual's genome and this abnormality can range from single gene mutation to whole chromosome abnormality. Moreover, some genetic disorders are inherited from the infected parents, while other genetic diseases are caused by mutations in a preexisting gene or cluster of genes. Furthermore, mutations occur either randomly or due to some environmental contact. We have described different types of genetic disorders briefly (Figure 10.1).

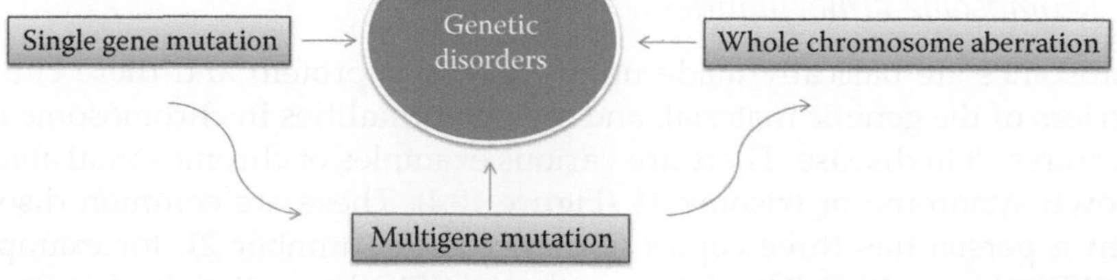

Figure 10.1 Nature of genetic disorders in humans.

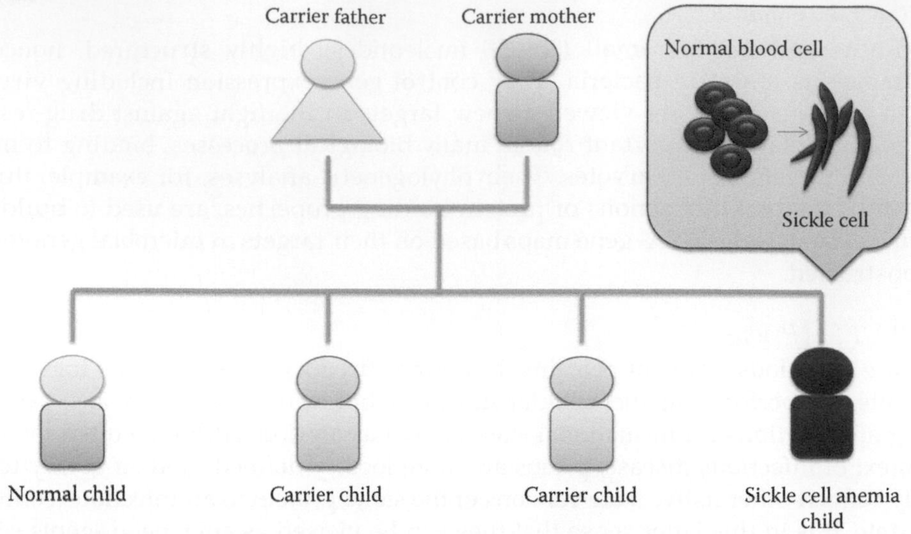

Figure 10.2 Single gene inheritance which causes sickle cell anemia.

10.4.1 *Single gene inheritance*

The single gene inheritance is called Mendelian or monogenetic inheritance. Moreover, this type of inheritance is triggered by mutations that occur in the DNA sequence of a single gene. There are more than 6000 known single gene disorders that exist in humans. These single gene disorders are called monogenetic disorder; examples include Huntington's disease, hemochromatosis, cystic fibrosis, sickle cell anemia, and Marfan syndrome (Figure 10.2). Moreover, single gene disorders can be inherited in identifiable patterns such as an autosomal dominant, autosomal recessive, and x-linked-like condition.

10.4.2 *Multifactorial inheritance*

The multifactorial inheritance is caused by a combination of environmental factors and mutations in multiple genes (Figure 10.3). For example, different genes that influence breast cancer vulnerability have been found on chromosome numbers 6, 11, 13, 14, 15, 17, and 22. The examples of multifactorial disorders are Alzheimer's disease, arthritis, diabetes, cancer, heart disease, high blood pressure, and obesity. It has been reported that multifactorial inheritance is also associated with genetic traits such as height, eye color, fingerprint patterns, and skin color.

10.4.3 *Chromosome abnormalities*

The chromosomes are basically made up of DNA and protein and these chromosomes are the carriers of the genetic material, and any abnormalities in chromosome number or structure can result in disease. There are various examples of chromosomal abnormalities such as Down syndrome or trisomy 21 (Figure 10.4). These are common disorders that occur when a person has three copies of chromosome number 21, for example, Turner syndrome (45X) (Figure 10.5), Klinefelter syndrome (47XXY), and cri du chat syndrome (46, XX, or XY). It has been reported that abnormalities in chromosomes typically occur during

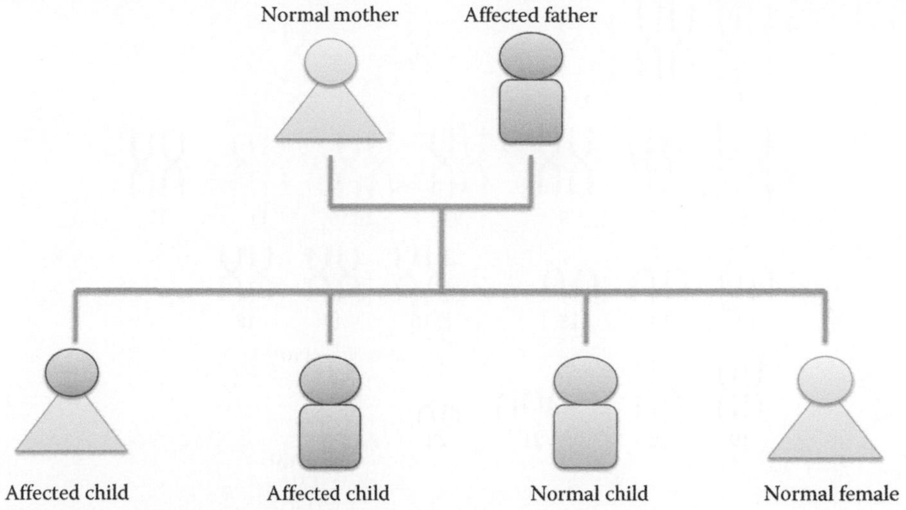

Figure 10.3 Poly gene inheritance in humans.

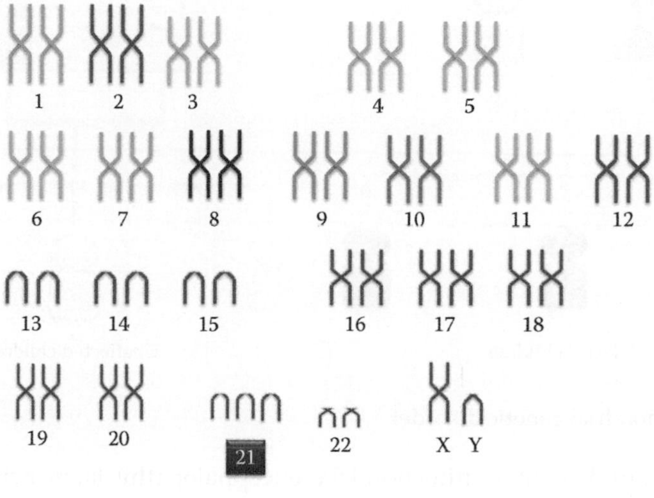

Figure 10.4 Down syndrome.

cell division process and diseases may also occur because of chromosomal translocation in which portions of two chromosomes are exchanged.

10.4.4 Mitochondrial inheritance

It has been reported that mitochondria are involved in cellular respiration and are found in the cytoplasm of plant and animal cells. Each mitochondrion may contain 5–10 circular pieces of DNA. It has been reported that female egg cells usually contain mitochondria; mitochondrial DNA is always inherited from the female parent. The structural and functional changes in mitochondria can cause several diseases which include eye disease (Leber's hereditary optic atrophy); a type of epilepsy (myoclonus epilepsy with ragged

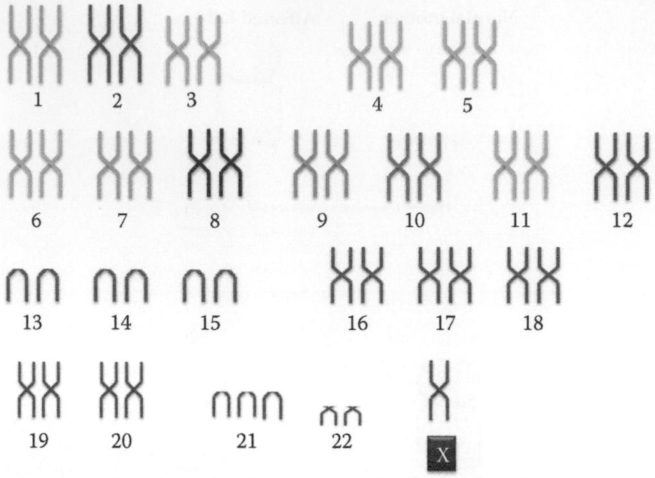

Figure 10.5 Turner syndrome (45 X).

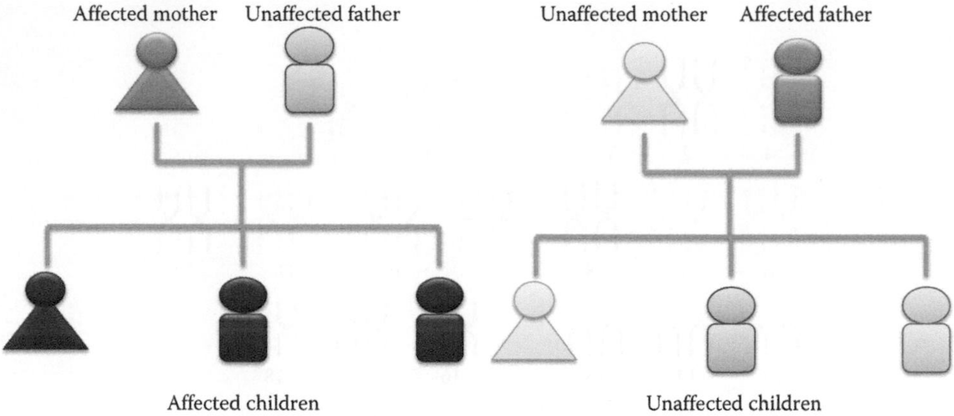

Figure 10.6 Mitochondrial genetic disorder.

red fibers); a form of dementia (mitochondrial encephalopathy, lactic acidosis) and stroke (Figure 10.6).

10.5 Causes of genetic diseases

Genetic disease can be caused by mutations in the genetic information. One abnormal gene is sufficient to cause genetic diseases. In some cases, one normal gene can avoid the development of a genetic disease. When a the potentially harmful gene is in a recessive state, then its normal counterpart will carry out all the tasks assigned to both; only if one person inherits from his/her parents two copies of the same recessive gene then it will lead to disease. In case the gene is dominant, then in that condition it can cause the disease even if its counterpart is normal. Moreover, only the children of a parent with the disease can be afflicted, and then on average only half the children will be affected. Huntington's chorea, a severe disease of the nervous system, which becomes active only in adulthood, is a model of a dominant genetic disease.

Furthermore, there are genetic diseases which are linked with the X chromosome; examples of such diseases are Duchenne muscular dystrophy and hemophilia. It has been reported that Queen Victoria was a carrier of the defective gene responsible for the development of hemophilia, and through her it was transmitted to the royal families of Spain, Russia, and Prussia. One of the major concerns of hemophilia is that patients lose blood clotting abilities caused due to lack of proteins (factors VIII and IX) involved in the clotting of blood. Not all defective genes necessarily produce harmful effects, since the environment in which the gene operates is also of importance. A typical instance of a genetic disease having a beneficial effect on survival is demonstrated by the relationship between sickle cell anemia and malaria. Individuals who have two copies of the sickle cell gene produce a defective blood protein and suffer from the disease. Furthermore, individuals with one sickle cell gene and one normal gene are unaffected and, more notably, are able to resist infection by malarial parasites.

10.6 Gene therapy and types

One of the most sought after techniques to treat genetic disorders is gene therapy. Iin this technique, the absent or faulty gene can be replaced by a working or normal gene (Figure 10.7), so that the human body can make the correct protein and consequently eliminate the root cause of the disease. This type of gene therapy generally involves somatic cells, whereas gene therapy can also use germline cells which contribute to the genetic heritage of the offspring. It has been reported that gene therapy in germline cells has the probability to affect not only the individual being treated, but also his or her children as well. The gene therapy can be classified into two major types: somatic gene therapy and germline gene therapy.

10.6.1 Somatic gene therapy

By using somatic gene therapy, somatic cells can be treated by inserting a vector loaded with the correct gene into a person's body. The somatic cells are cells that form in the body and cannot produce progenies. Gene therapy, in its present stage only treats somatic cells in humans. There are two types of somatic gene therapy, *ex vivo* and *in vivo*. In *ex vivo* gene therapy genes or cells are modified outside the body and then transplanted back into

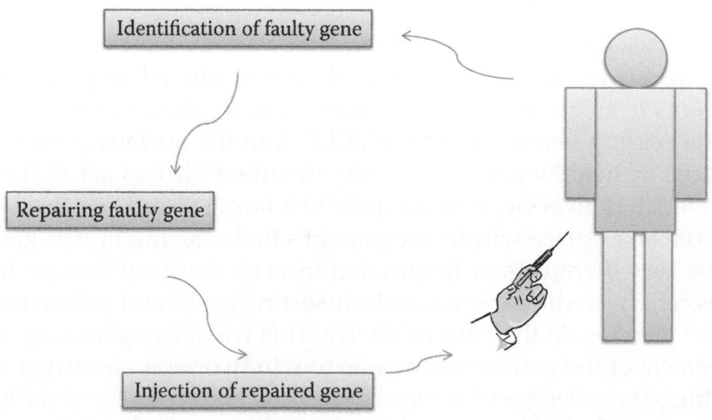

Figure 10.7 Gene therapy.

the body, whereas *in vivo* gene therapy, cells are modified or treated within the patient's body. It has been suggested that somatic gene therapy does not affect any descendants of the person being treated. It has been reported that scientists used gene therapies on genetic diseases which include hemophilia, muscular dystrophy, sickle cell anemia, and cystic fibrosis. Furthermore, the legal issues related to the use of somatic gene therapy varies from country to country. It has been found that some countries limit the use of gene therapy for certain diseases, including diseases that may not be cured with other medical methods and that may eventually cause an early death. In some other countries, the laws require that any research that takes place follow certain health regulations, which include the establishment of committees and organizations for monitoring. Moreover, many countries now require research to be approved by federal or state committees that have been established to deal with somatic gene therapy research.

In addition to legal issues related to somatic gene therapy, there are moral and ethical issues pertaining to the effectiveness of the therapy. Moreover, somatic gene therapy is not as affected by ethics when compared to the germline gene therapy, as somatic gene therapy only treats body cells, not mitotically active cells like germ cells. Nevertheless, there are some ethical concerns which have been raised in different parts of the world, and some ethical organizations have released recommendations to resolve the gene therapy issues and these recommendations include (a) establishing a national ethics body in each country to look at somatic gene therapy; (b) supporting somatic gene therapy research that follows the recommendations; (c) asking researchers, organizations, and governments to listen and respond to public concerns about gene therapy research; and (d) asking that research follows quality and safety controls.

10.6.1.1 *Ex vivo somatic gene therapy*

Ex vivo somatic gene therapy involves the introduction of vectors directly into the body of the person, most usually into the afflicted tissue. For example, if the aim was to treat skin cancer, the vectors would be introduced into the melanoma itself. Eventually, there is hope that vectors will be found that can be introduced directly into the bloodstream, however, there are difficulties with the immune system response that have slowed development in this area to date. One might recall that the body is programmed to mount an immune response if ever a foreign cell should be introduced. Thus, because *in vivo* somatic gene therapy involves the introduction of thousands of what amount to being viruses into the human body, it has been a particularly difficult field to master (Figure 10.8).

10.6.1.2 *In vivo somatic gene therapy*

The process by which the genetic makeup of cells is altered to produce a therapeutic effect that prevents or treats diseases in the patients is called *in vivo* somatic gene therapy. Defective or missing hereditary material DNA in the nucleus of the patient's cells is altered or replaced by healthy genes. Specially modified viruses act as the carriers of the new genetic material, delivering it to the patient's targeted cells or tissues. The transfer of genetic material takes place within the patient's body during *in vivo* gene therapy. The process of *in vivo* gene therapy is differentiated from *ex vivo* gene therapy in that the latter procedure takes cells from the patient's body, inserting genes and culturing the cells in the laboratory rather than inside the patient's body. This treatment generally requires extraction and replacement of the patient's bone marrow in two separate surgeries.

One of the biggest challenges of *in vivo*-based gene therapy is the insertion of genes into respective sites in the cells. The vector which carries the gene has a challenging task to complete as they have to deliver the genes to all affected cells for results and at the same time

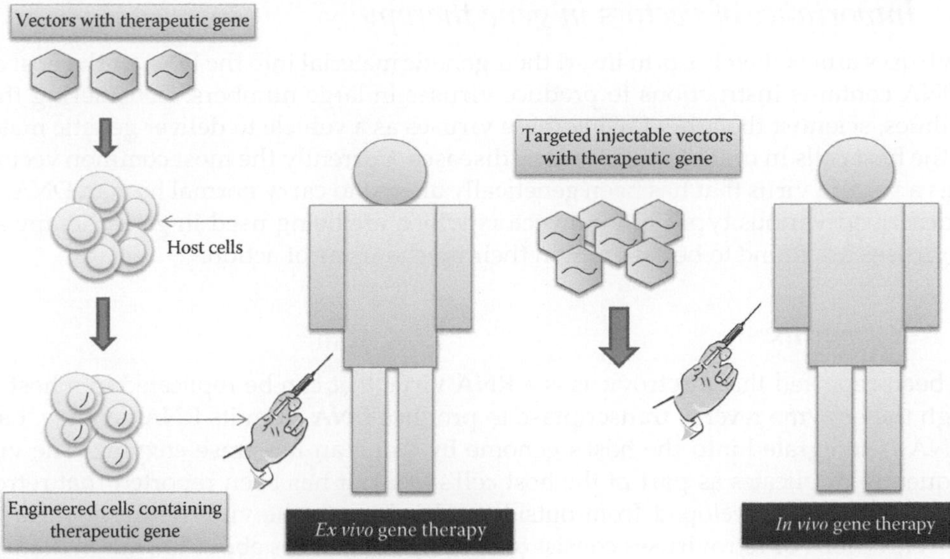

Figure 10.8 *Ex vivo* and *in vivo* gene therapy.

these vectors remain undetected by the body's immune system to avoid immune rejection. The use of virus as a vector to deliver the gene inside the cells is primarily owing to the fact that viruses are known to deliver genetic information from cell to cell, this is what viruses normally do to insert their genes into host cells so that their host cells can replicate them. It has been reported that through millions of years of evolution, viruses have developed very sophisticated ways of transforming genetic information. To make gene therapy effective, there are two classes of viruses—retroviruses and adenoviruses—found to be critical in gene delivery. Adenoviruses are medium-sized nonenveloped (without an outer lipid bilayer) viruses with an icosahedral nucleocapsid containing a double stranded DNA genome. Their name derives from their initial isolation from human adenoids in 1953. They have a broad range of vertebrate hosts; in humans, 57 distinct adenoviral serotypes have been found to cause a wide range of illnesses, from mild respiratory infections in young children to life-threatening multi-organ disease in people with a weakened immune system. Retroviruses are sRNA-based viruses, because they reproduce by integrating their RNA into the host's DNA; they carry the prospect of incorporating new genes into chromosomes (host cells) so that cells that divide will pass the genes to their progeny. It has been cautioned that using such viruses may cause health problems to the ailing patients because there is a possibility that the gene which causes infection can also be transferred to the host cells, to avoid such problems scientists remove certain harmful genes from the viral genome so that they cannot damage the host.

Moreover, a French pharmaceutical company has conducted experiments by injecting retroviruses into lung cancer patients and after the injections of vectors containing p53, a gene that suppresses tumors directly into the cancerous tissue, the tumors stopped growing. One of the major problems in all virus-based vectors is recognition by the immune system; when acquainted viruses are detected in the bloodstream, the body produces and sends antibodies to bind to those viruses and kill them. Additionally, while using retroviral and other recombination-based approaches, another problem arises in an unpredictable way, where the new DNA inserts into the chromosomes of transfected cells. For example, if the gene is inserted in an untargeted place then the cell will never translate to produce protein and could become cancerous.

10.7 *Importance of vectors in gene therapy*

Most viruses attack their hosts to insert their genetic material into the DNA of the host and this DNA contains instructions to produce viruses in large numbers. Considering these capabilities, scientist thought of using these viruses as a vehicle to deliver genetic materials to the host cells in order to treat genetic diseases. Currently the most common vector is used as a vehicle virus that has been genetically altered to carry normal human DNA. We have described various types of viral vectors which are being used in gene therapy and these viruses are found to be different in their mechanisms of action.

10.7.1 *Retroviruses*

It has been reported that a retrovirus is a RNA virus that can be replicated in a host cell through the enzyme reverse transcriptase to produce DNA from its RNA genome. Later, the DNA is integrated into the host's genome by using an integrase enzyme. The virus subsequently duplicates as part of the host cell's DNA. It has been reported that retroviruses are generally enveloped from outside and belong to the viral family *Retroviridae.* Moreover, virions of retroviruses consist of enveloped particles about 100 nm in diameter and it also contains two identical single-stranded RNA molecules. Even though virions of different retroviruses do not have the same morphology or biology, all the virion components are very comparable. Moreover, the key brain component is the envelope which is composed of a protein capsid (Figure 10.9).

Retroviruses have better capabilities to integrate efficiently into the genomic DNA of animal cells and can be replicated and transmitted to all of the progeny of these cells. Moreover, severe oncogenic retroviruses often arise as the result of attaining of sequences derived from cellular protooncogenes provided an additional stimulus. It was clear from

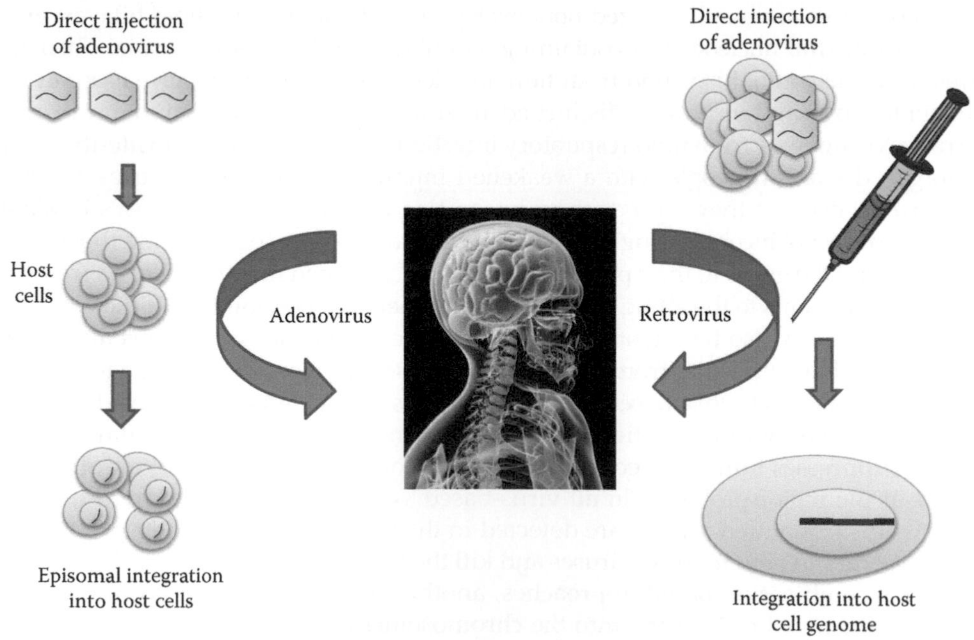

Figure 10.9 Gene therapy by using adenovirus and retrovirus vectors.

many studies that retroviral genomes could house wide changes, and even though these changes often resulted in defects in replication. Certainly, early synthetic retroviral vectors were produced by using helper virus; nevertheless, the presence of helper virus prohibited many types of trials where viral spread after infection was objectionable, especially for many genetic studies or for human gene therapy. A major development is taking place in retroviral vector design with the improvement of retroviral packaging cells that but do not allow the replication of the competent virus. Furthermore, many of the first generation of packaging cell lines are produced by a helper virus as a result of recombination events. The large range of vectors produced by packaging cell lines has also been protracted by the development of cell lines based on a variety of mammalian and avian retroviruses. More interestingly, retroviral vectors have also been improved by the elimination of all viral coding regions and by the reduction of the residual viral elements to the minimum required for high proficiency transfer. It became possible because of the early steps in the viral life cycle where retroviral entry into cells, reverse transcription of the viral genome into DNA, do not depend on viral protein synthesis. As a consequence, retroviral vectors can be used to transfer only the genes of interest.

Bioengineered vectors with surface protein of vesicular stomatitis virus (VSV) are considered to be an important advance in retroviral vector technology. This modification has prolonged the host range of retroviral vectors to include insect, fish, and amphibian cells and, because the VSV G-protein is associated more with virions than retroviral envelope proteins, it allows effective ways to produce high titer vectors. In contrast to typical vectors derived from oncoviruses, lentiviruses such as the human HIV can also infect nondividing cells. This property will be especially useful for gene therapy applications, especially those involving *in vivo* gene transfer using hematopoietic stem cells. In addition, vectors of this type are able to infect neurons in rats.

Retroviral vectors have advantages when compared to many other gene transfer systems and these include the ability to transduce a wide range of cell types from different animal species, to integrate genetic material carried by the vector into recipient cells accurately, and to be able to express the transduced genes at high levels. Additionally, retroviral vectors have been engaged in the study of viral replication and it is typically much simpler to track the replication than from unmarked viruses. Moreover, the ability to limit viral replication to a single round improves the measurement of rates of mutation and recombination.

10.7.2 Adenoviruses

Adenoviruses are viruses that contain their genetic material in the form of DNA when these viruses infect host cells and they introduce their DNA into the host cells for replications. Genetic material of the adenoviruses is not integrated into the host cells genetic material and the adenovirus DNA molecule is left free in the nucleus of the host cell,. The genetic messages in this extra DNA molecule are transcribed just like any other gene and the only difference is that these extra DNA does not get replicated when the host cell is about to undergo cell division. Therefore, the progenies of that cell will not have the extra DNA in their nucleus (Figures 10.10 and 10.11).

10.7.3 Adeno-associated viruses

Adeno-associated viruses (AAV) belong to the parvovirus family—small viruses with a genome of single-stranded DNA. There are a few disadvantages of using AAV in gene therapy as the DNA of AAV is small and it is difficult to carry and to produce DNA.

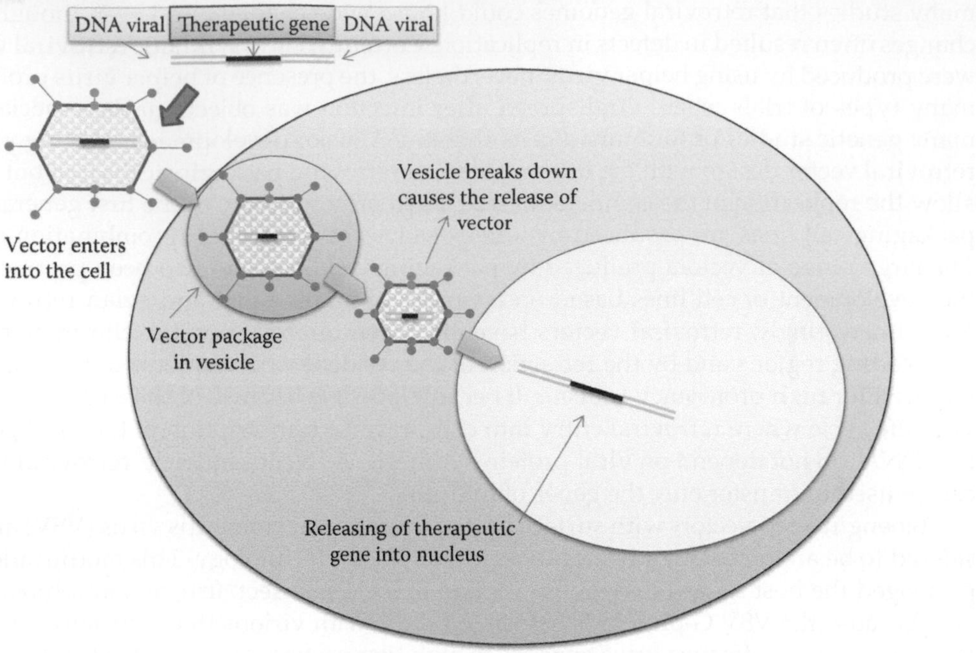

Figure 10.10 Gene therapy by using an adenovirus.

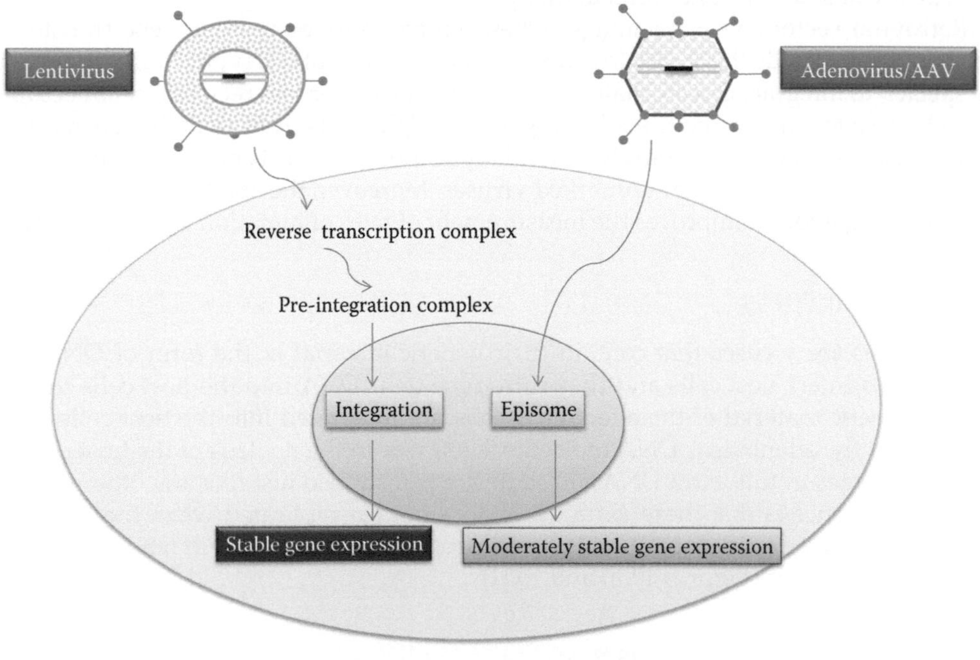

Figure 10.11 Difference of gene expression using lentivirus and adenovirus/AAV.

Nevertheless, this type of virus is being employed because it is nonpathogenic in function. Furthermore, in contrast to adenoviruses, most patients treated with AAV may not build an immune response to remove the virus. Several clinical trials with AAV are in progress, primarily trying to treat muscle and eye diseases, the two tissues where the virus seems to be particularly useful.

10.7.4 *Envelope protein viruses*

The adenoviruses are known to infect host cells most efficiently, whereas retroviruses have limited access to natural host cell ranges and do not infect the cells that efficiently. Moreover, retroviruses and AAV have a single protein coating on their membrane, while adenoviruses are coated with both an envelope protein and fibers that spread away from the surface of the virus. The envelope proteins of these viruses bind to cell surface molecules, which localize them on the surface of the host cells, as well as with the specific protein receptor that either induces entry promoting structural changes in the viral protein. However, in either case, entry into potential host cells requires a desirable interface between a protein on the surface of the virus and a protein on the surface of the host cell.

In the case of gene therapy, one might either want to limit or expand the range of cells susceptible to transduction by a gene therapy vector and, in that case, many factors have been developed in which the endogenous viral envelope proteins can be replaced by either envelope proteins from other viruses, or by chimeric proteins. It has been reported that viruses in which the envelope proteins have been replaced are referred as pseudotyped viruses. For instance, the most popular retroviral vector for use in gene therapy trials is lentivirus. Over the past few years, many attempts have been made to limit the *"tropism"* of viral vectors to one or a few host cell populations. Moreover, this advance can allow for the systemic administration of a relatively small amount of vector. Many attempts to limit tropism have been made using chimeric envelope proteins bearing antibody fragments and have great promise for the development of gene therapy.

10.7.5 *Replication competent viruses*

A replication-competent vector called ONYX-015 is used in replicating tumor cells. It was found that in the absence of the E1B-55kd viral protein, adenovirus caused very rapid apoptosis of infected, p53 positive cells, and these results dramatically reduced virus progeny and no subsequent spread. Moreover, apoptosis was primarily the consequence of the ability of EIA to inactivate p300. It has been reported that in p53 negative cells, deletion of E1B 55kd has no result in terms of apoptosis. Viral replication is likened to that of wild-type virus, resulting in the enormous killing of cells. It has been suggested that a replication defective vector deletes some essential genes. These deleted genes are essential in the body so they are changed with either a helper virus or a DNA molecule.

10.7.6 *Nonviral-mediated gene therapy*

Besides virus-mediated gene-delivery systems, there are several nonviral options for gene delivery. It has been reported that nonviral methods have certain advantages over viral methods, with a simple way to produce in large scale and low host immunogenicity. One of the major reasons why scientists were not serious about using nonviral approach of gene therapy was because of its low levels of transfection and expression of the gene, nevertheless, recent developments in vector technology have yielded molecules and techniques

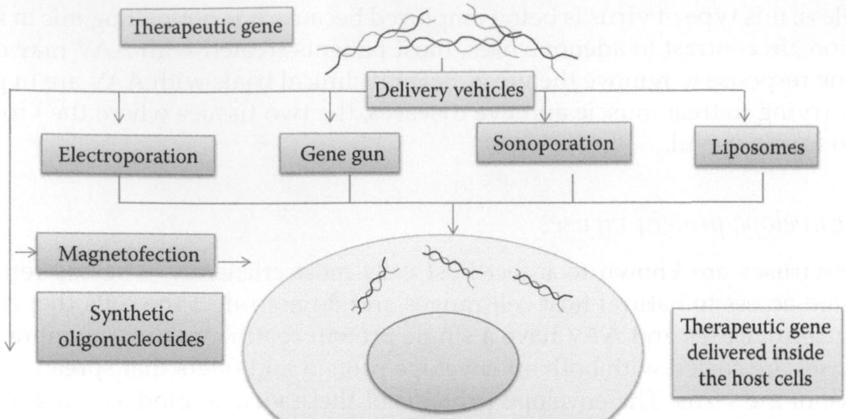

Figure 10.12 Synthetic cationic vectors such as cationic polymers, branched dendrimers, cell-penetrating (CP) peptides, and cationic liposomes can be used to deliver genes into cells.

with transfection efficiencies similar to those of viruses. The nonviral method of viral transfection is the simplest and clinical trials are carried out using intramuscular injection of a naked DNA plasmid have transpired with some success, though the gene expression was found to be very low in comparison to other methods of transaction. In addition to trial with plasmids, there have been trials with the naked PCR product, which are known to have similar or better results. Moreover, research efforts focusing on improving the efficiency of naked DNA uptake have yielded several new and novel methods, such as electroporation, sonoporation, and the use of a gene gun to shoot DNA-coated gold particles into the cell using high-pressure gas (Figure 10.12).

10.7.6.1 Electroporation

In this method, DNA molecules pass through cell membrane by using short pulses of high voltage and it has been suggested that this shock is thought to cause temporary formation of pores in the cell membrane, allowing DNA molecules to pass through. It has been suggested that electroporation is generally efficient and works across a broad range of cell types; nonetheless, a high rate of cell death following electroporation has been reported which has limited its application. Recently, scientists have developed a newer method of electroporation, which is termed electron-avalanche transfection and has been used in gene therapy experiments. By using a high-voltage plasma discharge, DNA was proficiently delivered following very short pulses.

10.7.6.2 Gene gun

The use of particle bombardment, or the gene gun, is another physical method of DNA transfection. In this technique, DNA is coated with gold particles and loaded into a device which generates a force to achieve penetration of DNA–gold into the cells.

10.7.6.3 Sonoporation

It has been reported that DNA can be delivered into cells by using ultrasonic frequencies and the process of acoustic vibration is believed to disturb the cell membrane and permit DNA to move into the cells.

10.7.6.4 Magnetofection

In this method DNA is mixed with magnetic particles, and a magnet is placed beneath the tissue culture dish to bring DNA complexes into contact with a cell monolayer.

10.7.6.5 Synthetic oligonucleotides

The synthetic oligonucleotides can be used to inactivate the genes involved in the disease development and there are several methods by which this is achieved. Moreover, antisense specific to the target gene can be used to disrupt the transcription of the faulty gene. Another way to use small molecules of RNA called siRNA is to signal the cell to cleave specific unique sequences in the m-RNA transcript of the faulty gene, disrupting translation of the defective mRNA, and consequent expression of the gene. Furthermore, in another strategy double-stranded oligo-deoxy-nucleotides have been used as a decoy for the transcription factors that are mandatory to trigger the transcription of the target gene. It has been suggested that the transcription factors bind to the decoys instead of the promoter of the faulty gene, which reduces the transcription of the target gene, and finally lowering of gene expression. Moreover, single-stranded DNA oligonucleotides have been used to direct a single base change within a mutant gene. The oligonucleotide is planned to the target gene with the exception of a central base, the target base, which serves as the template base for repair. This technique is called oligonucleotide-mediated gene repair or targeted gene repair.

10.7.6.6 Lipoplexes and polyplexes

To make DNA delivery most effective, DNA molecules must be protected from any structural and functional damage. In the beginning, anionic and neutral lipids are used to protect DNA from damage by construction of lipoplexes and, consequently, cationic lipids are first used to condense negatively charged DNA molecules so as to facilitate the encapsulation of DNA into liposomes. The use of cationic lipids significantly enhanced the stability of lipoplexes and also as a result of their charge, cationic liposomes network with the cell membrane. Furthermore, endocytosis is generally believed as the major route by which cells uptake lipoplexes. Endosomes are formed as the consequences of endocytosis. Nevertheless, if genes cannot be released into cytoplasm by breaking the membrane of endosome, they will be sent to lysosomes where all DNA will be broken before they attain their functions.

Even though cationic liposomes have been widely used as an alternative for delivery of gene, a dose-dependent toxicity of cationic lipids is also observed which could limit their therapeutic practices. It has been reported that the most common use of lipoplexes is its use in gene transfer into cancer cells, where the supplied genes are known to activate tumor suppressor genes in the cell and decrease the activity of oncogenes. Recently it has been shown that the use of lipoplexes in transfecting respiratory epithelial cells, can be used in the treatment of genetic respiratory diseases. In addition to lipoplexes, there are complexes that can also be used in gene transfection, such as polyplexes. Most polyplexes consist of cationic polymers and their production is regulated by ionic interactions. One of the major differences between the methods of action of polyplexes and lipoplexes is that polyplexes cannot release their DNA load into the cytoplasm of host cells.

10.7.6.7 Dendrimer

A dendrimer is a highly branched macromolecule which can be used in gene transfection as its having a spherical shape and it has been reported that it is possible to construct a cationic dendrimers such as, one with a positive surface charge. In a condition, genetic material such as DNA or RNA charge complementarity leads to a temporary association of the nucleic acid with the cationic dendrimer. Subsequently, the dendrimer–nucleic acid complex is then taken into the cell through the endocytosis process. In recent times, the best approach to transfect the cells are by using cationic lipids. It has been found that there are some limitations associated with competing reagents which include the absence of ability to transfect a number of cell types and the absence of robust active targeting capabilities, and also unsuitability with animal models. It has been reported that dendrimers offer robust covalent construction and extreme control over molecular structure, and together they have compelling advantages compared to existing approaches. Moreover, producing dendrimers has been a slow and expensive process consisting of numerous slow chemical reactions that have severely reduced their commercial development.

10.7.6.8 Hybrid methods

In view of having various shortcomings in gene transfer technologies, there have been efforts to make hybrid technology that combines two or more techniques together. It has been reported that virosomes are a hybrid that is developed by combining liposomes with an inactivated HIV or influenza virus. This hybrid method has shown to have more efficient gene transfer in respiratory epithelial cells than either by viral or by liposomal methods alone.

10.7.6.9 Challenges of nonviral-mediated gene therapy

Nonviral-mediated gene transfer was used in human gene therapy clinical trials that dealt with the treatment of inherited or acquired genetic disorders and cancer. Several preclinical (animal) studies are currently ongoing to employ nonviral vectors in genetic immunization programs for a variety of infectious diseases. The interest in nonviral-mediated gene transfer is motivated by two main reasons: (a) nonviral-based vectors do not derive from infectious agents and are minimally toxic; and (b) they can be easily produced in large quantities. However, the main drawbacks of nonviral-mediated gene transfer is related to the low transfection efficiency of target cells, especially *in vivo*, and to the transient nature of transgene expression. These drawbacks render nonviral-mediated gene transfer not particularly suitable for the treatment of pathological conditions that require long-term transgene expression, such as neurodegenerative disorders and inherited or acquired genetic diseases. On these grounds, the optimal application of nonviral-mediated gene transfer is in immunotherapy for cancer and infectious diseases, as a transient expression of the transgene might be sufficient to trigger effective and durable host immune responses.

10.8 Applications of gene therapy

It has been reported that the first approved gene therapy case took place in 1999, where gene therapy was performed on a four-year-old girl named Ashanti DeSilva as she was suffering from immune system deficiency. The gene therapy was conducted, though benefits were only temporary, but it created lots of interest among the scientific community around the world. A new gene therapy approach has been reported that can repair errors in mRNA derived from defective genes. This technique has the potential to treat blood disorders such as cystic fibrosis, thalassemia, and some cancers.

Furthermore, researchers are able to create tiny liposomes (25 nm) that can carry therapeutic DNA through pores in the nuclear membrane. In 1992, gene therapy trials were carried out using hematopoietic stem cells as vectors to deliver genes intended to correct hereditary diseases. Later on, this work was published indicating the first successful gene therapy treatment for adenosine deaminase (ADA) deficiency.

Gene therapy can also be used in the treatment of immune disease such as severe combined immune deficiency (SCID). The patients were treated with stem cells isolated from umbilical cord immediately after birth and the allele that codes for ADA was obtained and was inserted into a retrovirus. Later on retroviruses and stem cells were mixed, after which they entered and inserted the gene into the stem cell's chromosomes. Moreover, stem cells containing the ADA gene were injected into patients body through injections and ADA enzyme injections were also administered on a weekly basis. After 4 more years, treatment was given but that could not save the life of the patients and they died in 1999. The failure of the gene therapy experiment resulted in a significant setback in the research in the United States which has resulted in suspension by the US FDA of several clinical trials. In 2003, a research team successfully inserted genes into the brain using liposomes coated in a polymer called polyethyleneglycol. Furthermore, the transfer of genes into the brain is a noteworthy accomplishment because viral vectors are too big to get across the blood–brain barrier and this method has potential candidate for treating brain diseases including Parkinson's. Additionally, RNA interference (RNAi) or gene silencing technology may be used to treat Huntington's disease.

In addition to the above-mentioned techniques, researchers also successfully treated metastatic melanoma in two patients with genetically designed cells to specifically kill the cancer cells. Moreover, in an another research study, it has been shown that the gene can be delivered without being rejected by the body. So far, delivery of the normal gene has been difficult as the immune system recognizes the new gene as foreign and rejects the cells carrying it. To overcome such problems, researchers were able to uncover a network of genes regulated by molecules known as microRNAs that are known to selectively turn off the identity of their beneficial gene in cells of the immune system and prevent the gene from being found and destroyed. In order to prove this hypothesis, the researchers injected mice with the gene containing an immune-cell microRNA target sequence, and it was observed that the mice did not reject the gene.

In 2006, a new gene therapy trial has been tested with VRX496, a gene-based immunotherapy for the treatment of HIV. This new procedure used a lentiviral vector for delivery of an antisense gene against the HIV envelope. Moreover, in the phase I trial, five patients with chronic HIV infection were treated with a single intravenous infusion of autologous CD4 T cells, which are genetically modified with VRX496; this infusion was found safe and well tolerated. Moreover, all five patients were found stable and showed increased immune response to HIV antigens and other pathogens. This was the first clinical trial of a lentiviral vector administered in the USFDA-approved human clinical trials for any disease.

In 2007, researchers announced the world's first gene therapy trial for inherited retinal disease. The first operation was carried out on a 23-year-old man suffering from Leber's congenital amaurosis, which basically is an inherited blinding disease caused by mutations in the RPE 65 gene. The results were published and suggested that subretinal delivery of recombinant AAV carrying RPE65 gene, had positive results as a patient's vision has been improved with any apparent side effects. Later on in 2009, the researchers were able to give trichromatic vision to squirrel monkeys using gene therapy. In the same year researchers succeeded in halting a fatal brain disease which is known as adrenoleukodystrophy, by using a vector derived from HIV to deliver the gene for the missing enzyme.

10.9 Gene therapy clinical trials: The US scenario

10.9.1 Accomplished clinical trials

10.9.1.1 Gene therapy for ADA–SCID

This study involves investigating the safety and efficacy of different gene therapy techniques used for SCID caused by the deficiency of ADA enzyme. It has been reported that this is a severe condition that can be treated by HLA matched sibling donor bone marrow transplantation. The trial was initiated by enrolling patients in which HLA-identical sibling donors were not available and the patient showed evidence of enzyme replacement therapy failure. The primary aim of the trial was to assess the safety and efficacy of the procedure and to identify the relative role of peripheral blood lymphocytes and hematopoietic stem cells and progenitor cells in the long-term reconstitution of immune functions after retroviral vector-mediated ADA gene transfer.

10.9.1.2 Liver transplantation with ADV-TK gene therapy

The liver cancer disease with advanced hepatocellular carcinoma (HCC) can be treated with ADV-TK gene therapy highlight its potentiality as adjuvant treatment for HCC patients after liver transplant. It has been reported as an improved method outcome of liver transplant with the combined treatment of ADV-TK gene therapy in patients with intermediate or advanced HCC. The overall survival in the liver transplant with ADV-TK gene therapy group was found around 55% at 3 years. The patient with nonvascular invasion condition, treated with liver transplant plus ADV-TK therapy should 100% survival and recurrence-free survival than those with vascular invasion subgroup.

10.9.1.3 Gene therapy for chronic granulomatous diseases

To treat chronic granulomatous diseases (CGD), researchers have developed an *ex vivo* gene therapy method. As CGD is an inherited immune deficiency in which patients blood neutrophils and monocytes fail to produce superoxide and other antimicrobial oxidants, patients are prone to repeated life-threatening infections. Patients were given subcutaneous injections of the combination of flt3-ligand (flt3 L) along with CD34+ stem cells and the efficacy was tested by measuring NADPH oxidase-positive neutrophils.

10.9.1.4 Gene therapy for Alzheimer's disease: Clinical trial

Alzheimer's disease (AD) is caused due to abnormal accumulation of extracellular amyloid in the brain, the formation of intra-neuronal neurofibrillary tangles, synapse loss, and neuronal degeneration. In addition to drug therapy, researchers are also interested in finding out the cure for AD by using gene therapy. It has been reported that among the neuronal populations that degenerate in AD, loss of basal forebrain cholinergic neurons is particularly severe and loss of cholinergic neurons in AD is correlated with severity of dementia. The gene therapy is developed to prevent the cholinergic neurons from being destroyed due to Alzheimer's disease.

The trial was attempted to protect cholinergic neurons from degeneration, and to augment the function of remaining cholinergic neurons by directly uplifting choline acetyltransferase function of neurons. These two therapeutic interventions are being assessed by delivery of human NGF to the brain. Moreover, NGF has been shown to prevent both brain lesions, and age-related degeneration of basal forebrain cholinergic neurons. It has been shown that NGF infusions can reverse both lesions-induced memory loss and spontaneous, age-related memory loss in animal studies. It has been suggested that grafts of primary fibroblasts transduced to express human NGF have been shown to sustain NGF *in vivo* gene expression for at least 18 months in animal studies. Moreover, in primate, *ex vivo* NGF gene therapy has been demonstrated to sustain NGF protein production in the brain for at least 24 months.

10.9.1.5 Gene therapy in patients with severe angina pectoris

The aim of this study was to evaluate the mobilization of nonhematopoietic mesenchymal and hematopoietic stem cells from the bone marrow with granulocyte colony stimulating factor (G-CSF) treatment alone and in combination with vascular endothelial growth factor (VEGF) gene therapy in patients with severe chronic occlusive coronary artery disease. In recent clinical trials, VEGF delivered as plasmid DNA percutaneously by a catheter-based, intra-myocardial approach, have been demonstrated to be safe and are associated with a reduction in angina and an increase in exercise time or an improvement in regional wall motion in "no-option patients" with chronic myocardial ischemia. It has been demonstrated, that BM-derived stem cells mobilized by cytokines as G-CSF were capable of regenerating the myocardial tissue, leading to improve the survival and cardiac function after myocardial infarction. These data suggested that a combination therapy with exogenous administration of gene vascular growth factor combined with G-CSF mobilization of bone marrow stem cells might induce both angiogenesis and vasculogenesis in ischemic myocardium.

10.9.2 Terminated clinical trials

It has been found that during the process of clinical trials using gene therapy, if the expected results are not obtained the clinical trials were discontinued and terminated.

10.10 Ethical issues in gene therapy

There are ethical issues which are associated with gene therapy that we have discussed in a balanced way to put across both views received from pro-gene therapy and antigene therapy groups.

10.10.1 Ethical issue with gene therapy

With a view to maximize the success of gene therapy, National Health Institute (NIH), US has created Recombinant DNA Advisory Committee (RAC) to anticipate and address ethical concerns pertaining to gene therapy. The RAC was responsible for what some consider one of the most important milestones in the history of medicine namely, the endorsement of a human gene transfer study and human gene therapy protocols. It has been reported that currently gene therapy protocols involve only somatic (adult) cell gene therapy and somatic cell gene therapy denotes the insertion of new DNA into a particular tissue such as bone marrow of a sick individual. Moreover, the human reproductive system does not come under current gene therapy, so the new DNA material serves the individual only and is not transmitted to progeny. And debate is still going on about the use of viruses in the gene therapy, and how this gene therapy is effective in curing the genetic disorders. Extensive research is required to prove that gene therapy is safe and effective in patients.

10.11 Technical and regulatory issues with gene therapy

You might be surprised to know that the US Food and Drug Administration (FDA) has not yet approved any human gene therapy product for sale. It has been reported that current gene therapy is experimental and has not proven very successful in clinical trials. We have listed a few technical issues which need to be addressed before making gene therapy more acceptable for human treatments.

10.11.1 Short-lived nature of gene therapy

One of the major problems of the gene therapy is that clinically beneficial DNA introduced into target cells must remain functional and the cells containing the therapeutic DNA must be long-lived and stable gene. Another issue is that while integrating therapeutic DNA into the host genome and the rapidly dividing nature of many cells prevent gene therapy from achieving any long-term benefits, in that condition, patients will have to undergo multiple rounds of gene therapy that would not only be a painful process, but prove to be expensive.

10.11.2 Immune response

Anytime a foreign DNA is introduced into human tissues, the body's immune system is intended to attack the invader and this responsive immune system is known to reduce gene therapy effectiveness.

10.11.3 Problems with viral vectors

In gene therapy, genes are delivered through viral vectors and use of viral vectors may pose potential problems to the patient health, and may trigger immune and inflammatory responses. In addition, there is always the fear that the viral vector once inside the patient's body, may recover its ability to cause disease.

10.11.4 Multigene disorders

Most of the disorders such as high blood pressure, Alzheimer's disease, arthritis, heart disease, and diabetes are caused by the multiple gene dysfunction and it is very difficult to treat multigene or multifactorial disorders by using single gene therapy.

10.12 Summary

It has been suggested that each of us carries about half a dozen defective genes which can cause diseases and it has been reported that approximately 2800 specific conditions are known to be caused by genetic defects. Moreover, some single gene disorders are quite common, for example, cystic fibrosis is found in one out of every 2500 children born in Western countries. This disease which causes single gene defects accounts for about 5% of all admissions to children's hospitals. Over past few decades enormous efforts have been made to develop treatment for genetic disorders; however, not much success is achieved due to some technical or ethical issues. Nevertheless, genetic disorders can be treated by correcting the faulty genes, which is also called as gene therapy. It has been reported that gene therapy is a technique whereby the absent or faulty gene is replaced by a working gene, consequently that the body can make the correct enzyme or protein and consequently eliminate the root cause of the disease.

10.13 Scholar's achievements

Mendelian: Gregor Johann Mendel (1822–1884) was a German scientist who gained posthumous fame as the founder of the new science of genetics. Mendel demonstrated that the inheritance of certain traits in pea plants follows particular patterns, now referred to as the laws of Mendelian inheritance. The profound significance of Mendel's work was not recognized until the turn of the twentieth century, when the independent rediscovery of these laws initiated the modern science of genetics.

10.14 Knowledge builder

Monogenetic Inheritance: Monogenetic inheritance refers to the kind of inheritance whereby a trait is determined by the expression of a single gene or allele, not by several genes as in polygenic inheritance.

Huntington's Disease: Huntington's disease is a neurodegenerative genetic disorder that affects muscle coordination and leads to cognitive decline and psychiatric problems. It normally becomes conspicuous in mid-adult life. Huntington's disease is the most common genetic cause of abnormal involuntary writhing movements called chorea, which is why the disease used to be called Huntington's chorea.

Hemochromatosis: Hemochromatosis is an inherited disease in which too much iron builds up in your body and is one of the most common genetic diseases in the United States.

Marfan Syndrome: The Marfan syndrome is a genetic syndrome of the connective tissue in the body and people with Marfan syndrome tend to be unusually tall, with long limbs and long, thin fingers. The syndrome is inherited as a dominant trait, carried by the gene FBN1, which encodes the connective protein fibrillin-1. People have a pair of FBN1 genes. Because it is dominant, people who have inherited one affected FBN1 gene from either parent will have Marfan syndrome.

Down Syndrome: Down syndrome also known as trisomy 21, is a genetic disorder caused by the presence of all or part of a third copy of chromosome 21. Down syndrome is the most common chromosome abnormality in humans. It is typically associated with a delay in cognitive ability (mental retardation, or MR) and physical growth, and a particular set of facial characteristics.

Turner Syndrome: Turner syndrome also known as gonadal dysgenesis, 45 X, encompasses several conditions in human females, of which monosomy X (absence of an entire sex chromosome, the Barr body) is most common. It is a chromosomal abnormality in which all or part of one of the sex chromosomes is absent or has other abnormalities (unaffected humans have 46 chromosomes, of which two are sex chromosomes).

Klinefelter Syndrome: Klinefelter syndrome is 47, XXY or XXY syndrome, is a genetic disorder in which there is at least one extra X chromosome to a standard human male karyotype, for a total of 47 chromosomes rather than the 46 found in genetically normal humans.

Cri Du Chat Syndrome: Cri du chat syndrome, also known as chromosome 5p deletion syndrome, 5p minus syndrome, or Lejeune's syndrome, is a rare genetic disorder due to a missing part of chromosome 5. Its name is a French term (cat-cry or call of the cat) referring to the characteristic cat-like cry of affected children. The condition affects an estimated 1 in 50,000 live births, strikes all ethnicities, and is more common in females with a 4:3 ratio.

Duchenne Muscular Dystrophy: Duchenne muscular dystrophy (DMD) is a recessive X-linked form of muscular dystrophy, affecting around 1 in 3600 boys, which results in muscle degeneration and eventual death. The disorder is caused by a mutation in the dystrophin gene, the largest gene located on the human X chromosome, which codes for the protein dystrophin, an important structural component within muscle tissue that provides structural stability to the dystroglycan complex (DGC) of the cell membrane. While both sexes can carry the mutation, females rarely exhibit signs of the disease.

Reverse Transcriptase: Reverse transcriptase (RT) is an enzyme used to generate complementary DNA (cDNA) from an RNA template, a process termed reverse transcription. RT is needed for the replication of retroviruses (e.g., HIV), and RT inhibitors are widely used as antiretroviral drugs. RT activity is also associated with the replication of chromosome ends (telomerase) and some mobile genetic elements (retrotransposons).

Integrase Enzyme: Integrase is the enzyme that splices the viral DNA into a cellular chromosome.

Oncoviruses: Oncovirus is a virus that can cause cancer. This term originated from studies of acutely transforming retroviruses in the 1950–1960s, often called oncorna viruses to denote their RNA virus origin. It now refers to any virus with a DNA or RNA genome causing cancer and is synonymous with "tumor virus" or "cancer virus." The vast majority of human and animal viruses do not cause cancer, probably because of long-standing coevolution between the virus and its host.

Lentiviruses: Lentivirus is a genus of viruses of the Retroviridae family, characterized by a long incubation period. Lentiviruses can deliver a significant amount of viral RNA into the DNA of the host cell and have the unique ability among retroviruses of being able to infect nondividing cells, so they are one of the most efficient methods of a gene delivery vector. FIV, HIV, and SIV are all examples of lentiviruses.

Viral Protein: The viral proteins are basically a protein produced by a virus and these proteins are structural, forming the viral envelope and capsid. However, there are also viral nonstructural proteins and viral regulatory and accessory proteins.

Electron-Avalanche Transfection: A novel method for nonviral DNA transfer, called electron-avalanche transfection, was used that involved microsecond electric plasma-mediated discharges applied via microelectrode array. This transfection method, which produces synchronized pulses of mechanical stress and high electric field, was first applied to chorioallantoic membrane as a model system and then to rabbit RPE *in vivo.*

Cd4+ T: CD4+ T helper cells are white blood cells that are an essential part of the human immune system. They are often referred to as CD4 cells, T-helper cells, or T4 cells. They are called helper cells because one of their main roles is to send signals to other types of immune cells, including CD8 killer cells. CD4 cells send the signal and CD8 cells destroy and kill the infection or virus. If CD4 cells become depleted, for example, in untreated HIV infection, or following immune suppression prior to a transplant, the body is left vulnerable to a wide range of infections that it would otherwise have been able to fight.

Adv-Tk Gene Therapy: Adenovirus (Adv)-mediated herpes simplex virus thymidine kinase (adv/tk) gene therapy.

NADPH Oxidase: NADPH oxidase is an enzyme that catalyzes the production of superoxide from oxygen and NADPH. It is a complex enzyme consisting of two membrane-bound components and the three components in the cytosol, plus rac 1 or rac 2. The activation of the oxidase involves the phosphorylation of one of the cytosolic components.

Choline AcetylTransferase: Choline acetyltransferase is an enzyme that is synthesized within the body of a neuron. It is then transferred to the nerve terminal via axoplasmic flow. The role of choline acetyltransferase is to join acetyl-CoA to choline, resulting in the formation of the neurotransmitter acetylcholine.

NGF: Nerve growth factor (NGF) is a small secreted protein that is important for the growth, maintenance, and survival of certain target neurons.

Ischemic Myocardium: Myocardial ischemia is the pathological state underlying ischemic heart disease. It can lead to myocardial infarction (commonly known as heart attack) which in its acute form can lead to the death of the affected person. Myocardial ischemia is actually the restriction of blood supply thus causing lack of oxygen supply to the heart caused by rupture of an artery due to collection of fats and cholesterol on the walls of the artery.

Further reading

Abbott A. 1992. Gene therapy. Italians first to use stem cells. *Nature* 356 (6369): 465–199. doi:10.1038/356465a0. PMID 1560817. edit.

Baum C, Düllmann J, Li Z et al. 2003. Side effects of retroviral gene transfer into hematopoietic stem cells. *Blood* 101 (6): 2099–114. doi:10.1182/blood-2002-07-2314. PMID 12511419.

Brown BD, Venneri MA, Zingale A, Sergi SL, and Naldini L May 2006. Endogenous microRNA regulation suppresses transgene expression in hematopoietic lineages and enables stable gene transfer. *Nat Med* 12 (5): 585–91. doi:10.1038/nm1398. PMID 16633348.

Cavazzana-Calvo M, Thrasher A, and Mavilio F 2004. The future of gene therapy. *Nature* 427 (6977): 779–81. doi:10.1038/427779a. PMID 14985734.

Choi CQ 2006. The scientist: RNA can be hereditary molecule. The Scientist. http://www.the-scientist.com/?articles.view/articleNo/24011/title/RNA-can-be-heredity-molecule/. Retrieved 2006.

Cox BS 1965. [PSI], a cytoplasmic suppressor of super-suppression in yeast. *Heredity* 20 (4): 505–21. doi:10.1038/hdy.1965.65.

Durai S, Mani M, Kandavelou K, Wu J, Porteus MH, and Chandrasegaran S 2005. Zinc finger nucleases: Custom-designed molecular scissors for genome engineering of plant and mammalian cells. *Nucl Acids Res* 33 (18): 5978–90. doi:10.1093/nar/gki912. PMC 1270952. PMID 16251401. http://www.pubmedcentral.nih.gov/articlerender.fcgi?tool=pmcentrez&artid=1270952.

Friedman RC, Farh KK, Burge CB, and Bartel DP 2009. Most mammalian mRNAs are conserved targets of microRNAs. *Genome Res* 19 (1): 92–105. doi:10.1101/gr.082701.108. PMID 18955434.

Friedmann T and Roblin R 1972. Gene therapy for human genetic disease? *Science* 175 (25): 949. doi:10.1126/science.175.4025.949. PMID 5061866. edit.

Gaetano Romano 2007. Current development of nonviral-mediated gene transfer. *Drug News Perspect* 2007, 20 (4): 227.

Gardlík R, Pálffy R, Hodosy J, Lukács J, Turna J, and Celec P April 2005. Vectors and delivery systems in gene therapy. *Med Sci Monit* 11 (4): RA110–21. PMID 15795707. http://www.medscimonit.com/fulltxt.php?ICID=15907.

Gene therapy first for poor sight. BBC News. May 1, 2007. http://news.bbc.co.uk/1/hi/health/6609205.stm. Retrieved May 3, 2010.

Goll MG and Bestor TH 2005. Eukaryotic cytosine methyltransferases. *Annu Rev Biochem* 74:481–514. PMID 15952895.

Horn PA, Morris JC, Neff T, and Kiem HP 2004. Stem cell gene transfer efficacy and safety in large animal studies. *Mol Ther* 10 (3): 417–31. doi:10.1016/j.ymthe.2004.05.017. PMID 15336643.

Howden BP, Beaume M, Harrison PF et al. August 2013. Analysis of the small RNA transcriptional response in multidrug-resistant *Staphylococcus aureus* after antimicrobial exposure. *Antimicrob Agents Chemother* 57 (8): 3864–74. doi:10.1128/AAC.00263-13. PMC 3719707. PMID 23733475.

Kaiser J. 2009. Gene therapy halts brain disease in two boys—*ScienceNOW*. Sciencenow.sciencemag.org. http://sciencenow.sciencemag.org/cgi/content/full/2009/1105/1. Retrieved 2010-08-17.

Komáromy A, Alexander, J, Rowlan, J et al. 2010. Gene therapy rescues cone function in congenital achromatopsia. *Hum Mol Genet* 19 (13): 2581–93. doi:10.1093/hmg/ddq136. PMC 2883338.

PMID 20378608. http://www.pubmedcentral.nih.gov/articlerender.fcgi?tool=pmcentrez&artid=2883338. edit.

Lacroute F May 1971. Non-Mendelian mutation allowing ureidosuccinic acid uptake in yeast. *J Bacteriol* 106 (2): 519–22. PMC 285125. PMID 5573734.

Lee D and Shin C 2012. MicroRNA-target interactions: New insights from genome-wide approaches. *Ann N Y Acad Sci* 1271:118-28. doi: 10.1111/j.1749-6632.2012.06745.x. Review. PMID 23050.

Levine BL, Humeau LM, Boyer J et al. 2006. Gene transfer in humans using a conditionally replicating lentiviral vector. *Proc Natl Acad Sci USA* 103 (46): 17372–7. doi:10.1073/pnas.0608138103. PMC 1635018. PMID 17090675. http://www.pubmedcentral.nih.gov/articlerender.fcgi?tool=pmcentrez&artid=1635018.

Liebman SW and Sherman F. September 1979. Extrachromosomal psi+ determinant suppresses nonsense mutations in yeast. *J Bacteriol* 139 (3): 1068–71. PMC 218059. PMID 225301.

Lim LP, Lau NC, Garrett-Engele P, Grimson A, Schelter JM, Castle J, Bartel DP, Linsley PS, and Johnson JM 2005. Microarray analysis shows that some microRNAs downregulate large numbers of target mRNAs. *Nature* 433 (7027): 769–73. PMID 15685193.

Maguire AM, Simonelli F, Pierce EA et al. 2008. Safety and efficacy of gene transfer for Leber's congenital amaurosis. *N Engl J Med* 358 (21): 2240–8. doi:10.1056/NEJMoa0802315. PMC 2829748. PMID 18441370. http://content.nejm.org/cgi/content/full/NEJMoa0802315.

Mattick JS, Amaral PP, Dinger ME, Mercer TR, and Mehler MF 2009. RNA regulation of epigenetic processes. *BioEssays* 31 (1): 51–9. doi:10.1002/bies.080099. PMID 19154003.

Morgan RA, Dudley ME, Wunderlich JR et al. 2006. Cancer regression in patients after transfer of genetically engineered lymphocytes. *Science* 314 (5796): 126–9. doi:10.1126/science.1129003. PMC 2267026. PMID 16946036. http://www.pubmedcentral.nih.gov/articlerender.fcgi?tool=pmcentrez&artid=2267026.

Morris KL 2008. Epigenetic regulation of gene expression. *RNA and the Regulation of Gene Expression: A Hidden Layer of Complexity*. Norfolk, England: Caister Academic Press. ISBN 1-904455-25-5. [page needed].

Ott MG, Schmidt M, Schwarzwaelder K et al. 2006. Correction of X-linked chronic granulomatous disease by gene therapy, augmented by insertional activation of MDS1-EVI1, PRDM16 or SETBP1. *Nat Med* 12 (4): 401–9. doi:10.1038/nm1393. PMID 16582916.

Perez EE, Wang J, Miller JC et al. 2008. Establishment of HIV-1 resistance in CD4+ T cells by genome editing using zinc-finger nucleases. *Nat Biotechnol* 26 (7): 808–16. doi:10.1038/nbt1410. PMID 18587387.

Salmons B and Günzburg WH 1993. Targeting of retroviral vectors for gene therapy. *Hum Gene Ther* 4 (2): 129–41. doi:10.1089/hum.1993.4.2–129. PMID 8494923.

Shorter J and Lindquist S June 2005. Prions as adaptive conduits of memory and inheritance. *Nat Rev Genet* 6 (6): 435–50. doi:10.1038/nrg1616. PMID 15931169.

Subtle gene therapy tackles blood disorder—11 October 2002. *New Scientist*. http://www.newscientist.com/article/dn2915-subtle-gene-therapy-tackles-blood-disorder.html. Retrieved 2010-08-17.

Thrasher AJ, Gaspar HB, Baum C et al. 2006. Gene therapy: X-SCID transgene leukaemogenicity. *Nature* 443 (7109): E5–6; discussion E6–7. doi:10.1038/nature05219. PMID 16988659.

True HL and Lindquist SL. September 2000. A yeast prion provides a mechanism for genetic variation and phenotypic diversity. *Nature* 407 (6803): 477–83. doi:10.1038/35035005. PMID 11028992.

Urnov FD, Rebar EJ, Holmes MC, Zhang HS, and Gregory PD. 2010. Genome editing with engineered zinc finger nucleases. *Nat Rev Genet* 11 (9): 636–46. doi:10.1038/nrg2842. PMID 20717154.

Wang Z, Yao H, Lin S, Zhu X, Shen Z, Lu G, Poon WS, Xie D, Lin MC, and Kung HF. 2012. Transcriptional and epigenetic regulation of human microRNAs. *Cancer Lett* 331 (1): 1–10. doi: 10.1016/j.canlet.2012.12.006. PMID 3246373. http://www.mirbase.org/cgi-bin/browse.pl.

Woods NB, Bottero V, Schmidt M, von Kalle C, and Verma IM. 2006. Gene therapy: Therapeutic gene causing lymphoma. *Nature* 440 (7088): 1123. doi:10.1038/4401123a. PMID 16641981.

chapter eleven

Synthetic biology and nanomedicine

11.1 Introduction

Synthetic biology is a scientific discipline that combines knowledge of science with engineering tools in order to design and build novel biological tissues and systems. The application includes the design and construction of new biological parts of the human body, devices to be used in the human body, and systems required to perform human body function. Subsequently, synthetic biology has been known to produce diagnostic tools for various diseases such as HIV and hepatitis viruses. Furthermore, the term "synthetic biology" was first used on genetically engineered bacteria that were created by using recombinant DNA technology. Synthetic biology is used as a means to design human body parts using biomimetic chemistry, where organic molecules are used to generate artificial molecules that mimic natural molecules, such as enzymes. Recently, the engineering community is seeking to extract components of the biological systems to be reassembled in a way that can copycat the living body. Additionally, the biological information can be used to design products that can be used in various ways. For example, DNA which is basically located in the nucleus of a cell, consists of double-stranded antiparallel strands each having four various nucleotides assembled from bases, sugars, and phosphates. These combinations can be easily synthetically designed in the lab. In contrast, this is not true for a protein molecule, which is normally more complex and sometimes unpredictable.

11.2 Significance of synthetic biology

Recent advancements in recombinant DNA technology have revolutionized biological and medical science, including the synthetic biology field. These technologies refer to techniques by which DNA molecules that code for a protein of interest are synthesized using the blueprint of a known genetic sequence. Thereafter, by employing a variety of enzymatic techniques, these genetic sequences or genes are transferred into another organism and this bioengineered organism then uses its own genetic information together with the inserted gene to produce the protein of interest for human use. The whole concept of using genetic engineering is to enhance the production of biomolecules outside the human body (Figure 11.1).

The main reason synthetic biology came to an existence was the approval of human insulin, which was the first medicine made by using recombinant DNA technology; later came the development of the first recombinant vaccine. Researchers were also able to successfully synthesize the entire genome of *Mycoplasma mycoides* based on the known sequence of the microbe, and could replace the DNA from the bacterium *Mycoplasma capricolum* with this synthetic genome, and produce functional bacterial cells that are similar to natural *Mycoplasma mycoides.* There are various applications of synthetic biology that create new organisms for biofuel production, degrading biowastes, and enhancing the productivity of agriculture and food production.

Furthermore, over the past six decades, several crucial advances have been made that completely transformed the life science field, which include the discovery of the DNA

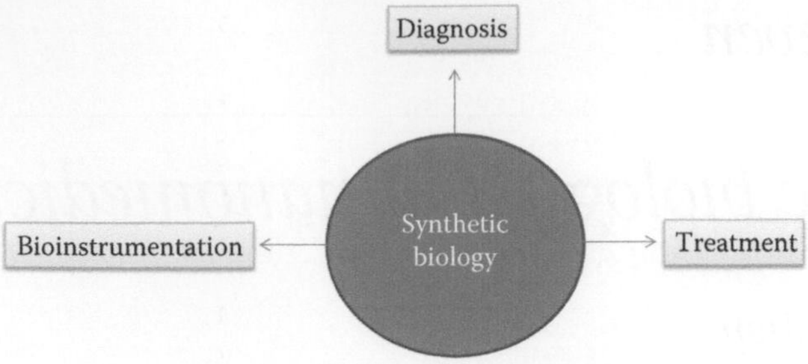

Figure 11.1 Significance of synthetic biology.

structure, decoding of the genetic information, the growth of recombinant DNA technology, and the decoding of the human genome. In addition, researchers have also made possible to design and construct human or animal body components by using biological information integrated with engineering field. The field of synthetic biology has also been revolutionized after creating synthetic DNA and the application of synthetic biology includes the creation of bioengineered microorganisms that can produce useful products such as pharmaceutical chemicals, to identify toxic chemicals, to break down pollutants and toxins, to repair defective genes, and to kill cancerous cells. Over a period of a few years, the synthetic biology field is considered an engineering discipline where human body parts or components are designed and manufactured (Figure 11.2).

Before 2004, the field of synthetic biology was only limited to laboratory levels. There was an international attempt to bring all synthetic biologists to one platform by conducting the first synthetic biology international conference conducted at the Massachusetts

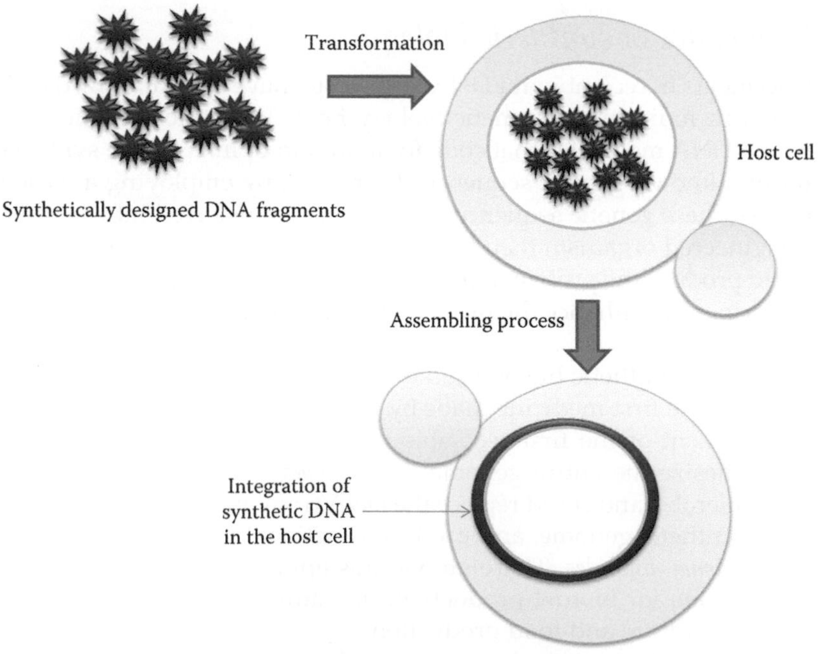

Figure 11.2 Applications of synthetic biology.

Institute of Technology (MIT), Cambridge, US. The whole purpose of organizing such an event is to bring together all researchers who are working to design and build biological parts, devices, and integrated biological systems that are useful for human benefits. This conference was a milestone in establishing synthetic biology as a separate and independent field of research as various universities started interdisciplinary research toward synthetic biology and teaching life sciences along with engineering subjects.

Moreover, there are many technologies that are related with synthetic biology which have existed for several years. For example, the application of metabolic engineering of bacteria used for natural product synthesis was first realized in 1970, and engineered bacterial plasmids for biotechnology were established in 1980. Moreover, the main difference between genetic engineering and synthetic biology is that though the former involves the transfer of individual genes from one organism to another, the latter comprises the assembly of distinctive microbial genomes from a set of standardized genetic parts and these components can be natural genes that are being applied for a new application. Furthermore, natural genes that are redesigned can proficiently work. In different parts of the world, it has been reported that the current research on synthetic biology is taking place mostly in the United States, Europe, Israel, and Japan. Additionally, there are also some leading U.S. companies (Amyris Biotechnologies of Emeryville, Codon Devices of Cambridge, Massachusetts, California, and Synthetic Genomics of Rockville, Maryland) which are involved in synthetically designed product development and manufacturing.

11.3 *Applications of synthetic biology*

There are various applications of synthetic biology that we briefly describe next.

11.3.1 *Genome design and construction*

One of the important applications of synthetic biology is to restructure the genomes of existing microbes to make them more effective to carry out new functions. In 2005, it was reported that researchers could simplify the genome of a bacteriophage called T-7 by separating overlapping genes and removal of nonessential DNA sequences to facilitate future modifications. Moreover, another group of researchers redesigned the bacterium *Mycoplasma genitalium*, which has the smallest known bacterial genome studied so far, and has all of the biochemical pathways needed to metabolize, grow, and reproduce. Furthermore, efforts have also been made to develop a synthetic version of the *Mycoplasma genitalium* genome that has the minimum number of genes required to support independent life. Moreover, the primary goal of this minimum genome project was to build a basic microbial platform to which new genes can be added, and also create synthetic organisms with known characteristics and functionality.

11.3.2 *Synthetic genome*

Synthetic genome basically refers to the set of technologies that makes it possible to construct any specified gene from short strands of synthetic DNA called oligonucleotides, which are normally produced chemically and have 50 and 100 base pairs in length. In August 2002, Eckard Wimmer, a virologist, announced that his research team had developed a live infectious *poliovirus* from customizing oligonucleotides viral genome. Similarly in 2003, researchers at the Center Institute developed a quick method for genome assembly by using synthetic oligonucleotides to construct a bacteriophage

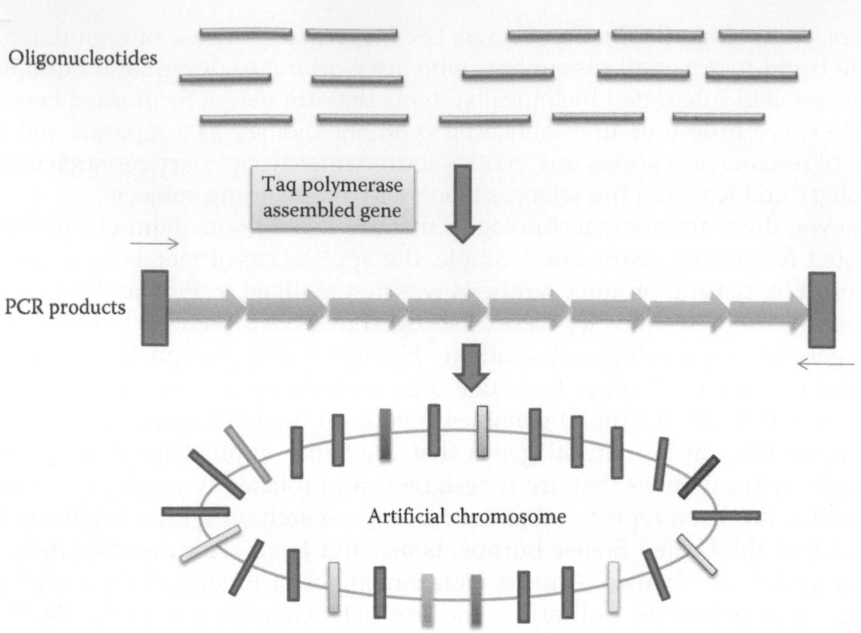

Figure 11.3 Development of artificial chromosome by synthetic biology tools.

called lambda X174 in 2 weeks' time. Additionally, in 2005, scientists at the US Centers for Disease Control and Prevention synthesized the Spanish *influenza virus*, which was responsible for the 1918 flu pandemic that killed 50–100 million people worldwide. Considering the various benefits of synthetic biology, it is also possible to reconstruct any existing virus for which the complete DNA sequence is known. The arrival of high-throughput DNA synthesis machines has sharply reduced the cost of DNA, and in 2000, it was shown that the price of customized oligonucleotides was as low as $1.00 per base pairs but in 2004, researchers from Harvard Medical School, USA invented a new multiplex DNA synthesis technique that finally reduced the cost of DNA synthesis to 20,000 base pairs for $1.00 (Figure 11.3).

11.3.3 Applied protein design

In addition to synthetically designed genes and DNA molecules, scientists are also working to make synthetic proteins. This idea was first proposed in 1980 by the Genex Corporation, which had suggested that synthetic proteins can be achieved by systematically altering the genes that code for certain proteins. After that, efforts have been made to develop protein-engineering technology to improve catalytic efficiency or to alter substrate specificity, or a protein that can tolerate high temperatures as well. It has been suggested that engineered enzymes are being utilized as laundry detergents and in various industrial applications. Researchers have also been working to design proteins that are present in the human body; these bioengineered proteins can be used to treat various diseases. Moreover, scientists have decoded the genetic code of an organism to specify unnatural amino acids, which can be replaced by natural proteins to change their strength as well as their catalytic and binding properties. This technique has made it possible to design protein-based drugs that can fight the rapid degradation of proteins in the body (Figure 11.4).

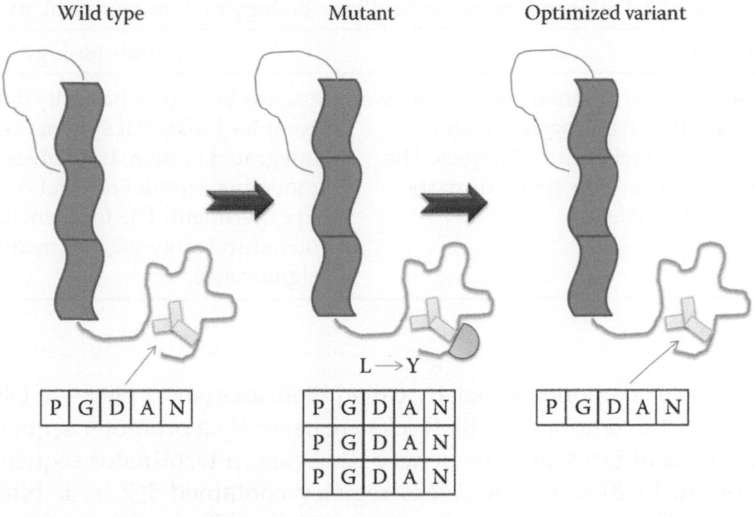

Figure 11.4 Computational protein design.

11.3.4 Natural product synthesis

Molecular cloning by using recombinant DNA technology has been used for making multiple copies of a single gene. These multiple copies of genes are later used for making specific types of protein. It has been observed that useful proteins such as human insulin can also be produced realistically by this technique. Presently, with the advent of synthetic biology, scientists can bioengineer microbes to perform complex multistep syntheses of natural products by assembling components of animal or plant genes that code for all the enzymes in a synthetic pathway. Furthermore, the method of using synthetic biology techniques to program yeast cells to manufacture the drug artemisinin, a natural product that is extremely effective in treating malaria. Currently, this compound can be extracted chemically from the sweet wormwood plant. The extraction of artemisinin is tough and costly, which causes a reduction in its availability and affordability in developing countries of the world. Interestingly, researchers have found a method to reduce the cost of the drug by using bioengineered metabolic pathway of yeast for the synthesis of precursor (artemisinic acid). The scientists have also assembled a group of several genes from sweet wormwood that code for the series of enzymes needed to make artemisinic acid, and inserted this cassette into yeast *Saccharomyces cerevisiae*. Later on, scientists analyzed the expression levels of each gene so that the entire multienzyme pathway can function competently. Once the engineered yeast cells have been coaxed into producing high yields of the artemisinin precursor, it becomes conceivable to manufacture this compound economically in large magnitudes by using fermentation technology. A similar approach can be to mass produce other drugs that are currently available in limited quantities from natural sources, such as the anticancer drugs and the anti-HIV compounds.

11.3.5 Creation of standardized biological parts and circuits

In addition to designing DNA and protein molecules, researchers have been working to create biological parts and circuit to simulate biological functions. For instance, researchers

Table 11.1 Difference between Synthetic Biology and Systems Biology

Synthetic biology	Systems biology
It has been shown that synthetic biology shows how to build artificial biological systems using engineering tools and techniques. The main interest is to develop synthetic parts using a biological system.	Systems biology is basically dealing with complex biological systems as an integrated system. It involves the use of modeling, simulation, and comparison to experiment. The focus inclines to be on natural systems with medical significance.

have made biological components that are called BioBricks (short pieces of DNA) that contain functional genetic components. BioBricks are basically a promoter sequence that initiate the transcription of DNA into messenger RNA, and a terminator sequence that stops RNA transcription. In 2006, the BioBricks registry contained 167 basic biological parts, including sensors, actuators, input and output devices, and regulatory elements. In addition to these parts, BioBricks registries contained 421 composite parts, and an additional 50 fragments were being created.

These synthetic product registries can be accessible through a public website that also invites interested researchers to use the existing knowledge and contribute to it. The main goal of such effort is to develop a methodology for the assembly of BioBricks into circuits with practical applications. Interestingly, these BioBricks have been gathered into a few simple genetic circuits and one such circuit condenses a film of bacteria that are highly sensitive to light, so that it can capture an image like a photographic negative. Furthermore, it is anticipated that the long-term goal of this kind of work is to convert bioengineered cells into tiny programmable chips or computers, so that it becomes possible to direct their operations by means of chemical signals or light. The difference between synthetic biology and systems biology is explained in Table 11.1.

11.4 Challenges in synthetic biology

In addition to the various useful applications of synthetic biology, there are technical problems associated with synthetic biology-based products. There are reports that suggest many synthetically designed biological parts have not been fully tested and characterized. Performances especially are not tested for long periods of time in order to know its longevity. In this direction, efforts have been made to optimize lactose production by using synthetic designed microbes, but show little success without much documentation. Moreover, it has been reported that about 1500 registry parts have been known to be in working condition, but there are 50 parts that fail while performing the activities. In order to improve the quality and performances of the synthetically designed products, the registry has been stepping up efforts to encouraging contributors to include documentation on part function and performances. The new project is proposed to reduce some of the variability in measurements from different laboratories and some researchers have found that it could eliminate half of the variations arising from experimental conditions and instruments. Measurements are tricky to standardize, however, in mammalian cells. For example, genes introduced into a cell integrate unpredictably into the cell's genome, and neighboring regions often affect expression. It has been suggested that this type of complexity is very difficult to capture by standardized characterization.

11.4.1 Unpredictable circuit

One of the major problems with synthetically designed parts is that these parts do not show any function when they are assembled together. Synthetic biologists are caught in a laborious process of testing as these synthetically designed bioparts are not predictable like other modern engineering products. Computer modeling could help reduce this guesswork. In 2009, Collins and his colleagues created several slightly different versions of two promoters; they used one version of each to create a genetic timer, a system that would cause cells to switch from expressing 1 gene to another gene after a certain interval time. Later on, they tested the timer, and fed the results back into a computer system and predicted how timers built from other versions would behave. Furthermore, by using such modeling techniques, researchers could improve computationally rather than test every version of a network. Nonetheless, designs cannot work perfectly all the time, but can be refined. This refining process is called directed evolution. It has been suggested that directed evolution is generally involved in mutating DNA sequences, screening their performance, selecting the best candidates, and repeating the process until the system is optimized.

11.4.2 Complexity of circuit

Other issues that are related to synthetically designed parts are their complexity and physical size, as during construction, the circuits get bigger and the process of constructing and testing them becomes more daunting. A system was developed, which uses about a dozen genes to produce a precursor of the antimalarial compound artemisinin in microbes. It has been estimated that it will roughly take 150 years of work to uncover genes involved in the pathway and to develop or refine parts to control their expression. It has been further stated that researchers had to test many part variations before they found a configuration that sufficiently increased the production of an enzyme needed to consume a toxic intermediate molecule. Additionally, another research group had created a system to combine genetic parts through automation as these parts have predefined flanking sequences, verbalized by a set of guidelines called the "BioBrick standard," and can be assembled by robots. Moreover, another research group had developed a system that caused engineered *Escherichia coli* cells, which are called assembler cells, and are being equipped with enzymes that can cut and stitch together DNA parts. Moreover, *E. coli* cells can be engineered to act as selective cells that can sort out the completed products from the surplus parts.

11.5 Health risk and ethical issues associated with synthetic biology

Synthetic biologists have accomplished a great deal of success in a short period of time, but major difficulties remain to be overcome before the actual applications of the technology can be realized. Interestingly, the behavior of bioengineered systems remains unpredictable and it has been suggested that genetic circuits can also tend to mutate quickly and become nonfunctional in time. It has been hypothesized that synthetic biology will not achieve its potential until investigators can accurately predict how a new genetic circuit will perform inside a living cell or living organism. Another issue that needs to be considered is that most of the bioengineered biological systems remain costly, unreliable, and unplanned because scientists do not understand the molecular processes of cells well enough to manipulate them reliably.

There are also risks involved in synthetic biology research, which need to be discussed because engineered microorganisms are self-replicating and they are associated with a different risk category than toxic chemicals or radioactive materials. Additionally, there are three main areas of risk in synthetic biology: first, synthetically designed microorganisms might escape from a research laboratory facility and cause environmental damage or threaten public life and population; second, synthetically designed microorganism developed for some applied purpose might cause destructive side effects after being intentionally released into the open environment; and third, fanatics and militants might exploit synthetic biology for hostile or hateful purposes.

11.5.1 *Risk of testing in the open environment*

One of the major applications of synthetic biology is the development of synthetic microorganisms to be used as biosensing, cleaning up soil contaminated with toxic chemicals. These synthetic microorganisms can also cause harmful effects on the natural flora and fauna. This problem is mainly associated with genetically modified organisms or crops, where it has been cautioned that extensive use of genetically modified organisms or crops may lead to health and environmental problems. Moreover, environmental safety agencies require a severe risk assessment before it can approve genetically modified organisms. Even though few genetically modified organisms have been synthesized for this purpose, including genetically modified strains of soil bacterium *Pseudomonas putida*. In that experiment, scientists used and monitored bioengineered bacteria, while they degraded a toxic chemical. Hypothetically, there could be three negative effects that are associated with synthetic biology products; first, synthetic microorganisms when released into the natural environment could interrupt local environment by means of competition or infection that, in the worst case, could lead to the extinction of one or more natural species or organism. The second negative effect would be once a synthetic organism has colonized in a locality, it might become widespread and thus impossible to eradicate. The third negative effect would be the synthetic organism might disrupt some aspect of the habitat into which it was presented first, upsetting the natural balance and caused the degradation or destruction of the local environment.

11.5.2 *Risk of deliberate misuse*

In 1972, the use and development of biological war weapons was banned by the Biological War Convention (BWC) held in the United States. In addition, the BWC modestly prohibits the synthesis of known or novel microorganisms for intimidating purposes. Additionally, if synthetic organisms are designed to produce chemical toxins, then the development and production of these poisons for weapons purposes can be prohibited as per the regulations of BWC. Nevertheless, one potential misuse of synthetic biology would be to recreate known pathogens such as the *Ebola virus* in the laboratory to cause an intimidating activity. Definitely, the viability of collecting an entire infectious viral genome from synthetic oligonucleotides has already been established for *poliovirus* and the Spanish *influenza virus*.

11.5.3 *Online selling of oligonucleotides*

With the rapid advancement of information technology tools, it becomes possible to buy genetically engineered molecules such as oligonucleotides and genes online. These oligonucleotide producers have emerged in several countries around the world and have started selling these oligonucleotides. A US-based company voluntarily uses special software to screen all oligonucleotide and gene orders for the presence of DNA sequences from select agents of harmful activities, and when such a sequence is detected, the request is denied. However, oligonucleotide suppliers are currently under no legal obligation to screen their orders, and because many clients value privacy, companies might put them in a difficulty in doing so. Furthermore, there are two possible solutions to this problem. First, the US Congress could pass a law requiring suppliers to check all oligonucleotide and gene orders for the presence of pathogenic DNA sequences. Otherwise, suppliers could agree among themselves to screen orders willingly.

11.6 Nanomedicine

Mankind is fighting against many complex illnesses such as cancer, multiple sclerosis, cardiovascular diseases, Alzheimer's and Parkinson's diseases, diabetes, as well as some inflammatory or infectious diseases such as HIV. It has been suggested that nanotechnology raises hopes and expectations for millions of patients that suffer from such diseases. For instance, it is estimated that clinicians will be able to terminate the very first cancer cells and thus stop the disease from growing using nanomaterials. Nanomedicine is a subfield of nanotechnology, which is regularly defined as the repair, construction, and control of human biological organs and systems. Basically, nanomedicine is the medical application of nanotechnology and over the last few years, the field of nanomedicine has created huge financial success; the sales of nanomedicine-based products reached a staggering $7 billion in 2004. In the United States, there are eight nanomedicine development centers that are staffed by multidisciplinary research teams established by the National Institutes of Health (NIH), including biologists, physicians, mathematicians, engineers, and computer scientists. Moreover, the initial phase of this program is directed toward gathering extensive information about the properties of nanoscale biomaterials. These biomaterials have the ability to be used in both diagnostic and therapeutic applications. It has been reported that there are over 100 nanotechnologies-based companies existing worldwide and the nanomedicine industry is expected to continue to rise in the coming years (Figure 11.5).

11.7 Nanomaterial

Nanomaterial is the material used to make or construct biomaterials with nanomorphological features and these biomaterials can be used for various applications. These nanomaterials are basically smaller than 1/10th of a micrometer in at least one dimension; however, this term is occasionally used for materials smaller than 1 μm.

11.7.1 Classification of nanomaterials

Based on physical and structural characteristics, nanomaterials are generally classified into two categories described below.

11.7.1.1 Fullerenes

Nanomaterials are a class of carbon molecule allotropes, which theoretically are graphene sheets rolled into tubes or spheres. These fullerenes comprise the carbon nanotubes or silicon nanotubes because of their mechanical strength and also because of their electrical properties. In research, it has been shown that fullerenes have the chemical and physical properties to become valuable materials to be used in the healthcare sector. Besides,

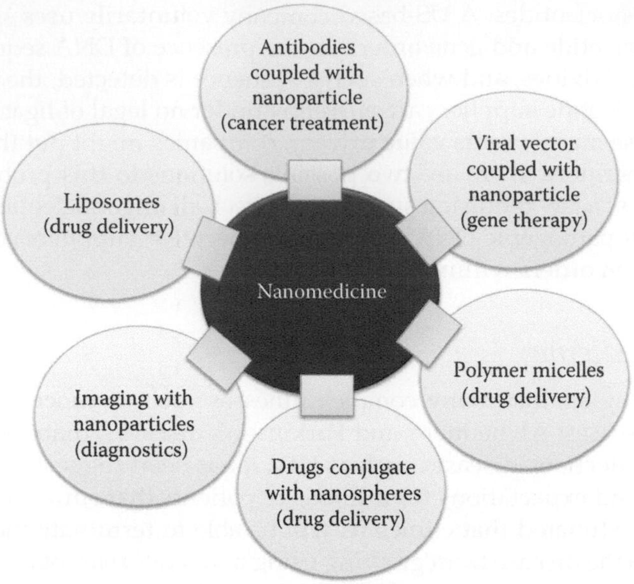

Figure 11.5 Applications of nanotechnology in medicine.

fullerenes can be used to bind specific antibiotics to bacteria (drug resistance) and even target certain types of cancer cells such as melanoma. New research finding suggests the use of fullerenes as light-activated antimicrobial agents.

11.7.1.2 Nanoparticles

Nanoparticles are generally made of metals, semiconductors, or oxides because of their mechanical, electrical, magnetic, optical, and chemical properties. It has been reported that nanoparticles can be used as quantum dots and as chemical catalysts to diagnose disease progression. Furthermore, these nanoparticles are of great scientific interest as they are effectively a bridge between bulk materials and atomic or molecular structures. Bulk material should have constant physical properties regardless of its size, but at the nanoscale, this is often not the case. Moreover, size-dependent properties are observed such as quantum confinement in semiconductor particles, surface plasmon resonance in some metal particles, and superparamagnetism in magnetic materials. Nanoparticles have unexpected visual properties because these materials are small enough to confine their electrons and produce quantum effects. For instance, gold nanoparticles appear deep red to black in the solution and they often have a very high surface-area-to-volume proportion of nanoparticles providing a tremendous driving force for diffusion, especially at elevated temperatures.

11.7.1.3 Solution–Gel

The solution–gel, also known as sol–gel, process is a wet-chemical technique widely used in the fields of materials science and ceramic engineering. Such methods are used primarily for the fabrication of materials starting from a chemical solution, which acts as the precursor for a combined network or gel of either distinct particles or network polymers. Typical precursors are metal alkoxides and metal chlorides, which undergo hydrolysis and polycondensation reactions to form either a network elastic solid or a colloidal suspension system composed of discrete (often amorphous) submicrometer particles dispersed to various degrees in a host fluid. The formation of a metal oxide involves connecting the metal centers with oxo (M–O–M) or hydroxo (M–OH–M) bridges, thereby generating metal-oxo or metal-hydroxo polymers in solution. The solution gel evolves toward the formation of a gel-like diphasic system containing both a liquid phase and a solid phase whose morphologies range from discrete particles to continuous polymer networks.

In the situation of the colloid, the volume fraction of particles can be low so that a significant amount of fluid may need to be removed initially from the gel-like properties to be recognized and this can be achieved in any number of ways. It has been recommended that the simplest method is to allow time for sedimentation to occur, and then decant the remaining liquid. Moreover, centrifugation can also be used to accelerate the process of phase separation. Furthermore, elimination of the remaining liquid phase requires a drying process, which is typically complemented by a significant amount of shrinkage and densification and the rate at which the solvent can be removed is eventually determined by the distribution of porosity in gel. Subsequently, a thermal treatment, or firing process, is often needed in order to make polycondensation and enhance mechanical properties and structural stability of the materials. One of the distinct advantages of using this methodology is that densification is often achieved at a much lower temperature. Furthermore, the sol–gel approach is an inexpensive and low-temperature technique that allows for the fine control of the product's chemical alignment and even small quantities of organic dyes and rare earth metals can be introduced in the solution and end up uniformly dispersed in the final product. These solutions gels can be used in ceramics processing and manufacturing as casting material, or in the process of producing thin films of metal oxides for various purposes. Moreover sol–gel-derived materials have diverse applications in optics, electronics, energy, space, biosensors, and separation technology.

11.8 Application of nanomaterials in medicine

11.8.1 Therapeutic delivery

Recent efforts have been made to improve drug bioavailability, and nanomaterials play an important role in it. The word "bioavailability" denotes the presence of drug molecules where they are needed in the body and perform normal body function. It has been reported that drug needs to be transported well in the body to easily reach the target site and there are times some drugs are not able to reach to target sites and get lost in the process. Furthermore, billions of dollars are wasted each year due to poor bioavailability of drug to target sites. Nanoparticles can also be used as contrastagents, to take ultrasound and magnetic resonance imaging (MRI) pictures. Additionally, polymer-based nanoparticles can be designed to improve the pharmacological and therapeutical properties of drugs. The strength of drug delivery systems is their ability to modify the pharmacokinetics and biodistribution of the drug. It has been suggested that nanoparticles have rare properties that can be used to increase drug delivery. These nanoparticles can be used to deliver complex drugs which cannot be easily transported inside cells especially inside the cell membranes and into the cell cytoplasm. Furthermore, drug delivery efficiency is important because many diseases depend upon processes within the cell and can only be obstructed by drugs that make their way into the cell. Another way to improve the drug action is by triggering response that happens when drugs placed in the body get activated only on encountering a particular signal; otherwise, they remain in an inactive state without losing its functionality. For example, a drug with poor solubility can be replaced by a drug delivery system where both hydrophilic and hydrophobic environments exist enhancing the drug solubility.

11.8.2 Biopharmaceutical drug delivery

Therapeutic proteins and peptides have great clinical application since they can be used for treating various diseases and disorders; these proteins and peptides are known as biopharmaceuticals. The function or action of these biopharmaceuticals can be enhanced by using nanomaterials such as nanoparticles and dendrimers. These nanoparticles and dendrimers are an emerging field, also called nanobiopharmaceutics, and these products are called nanobiopharmaceuticals.

11.8.2.1 Cancer

One of the best applications of nanoparticles is to precisely diagnose cancer diseases by using the small size of nanoparticles, which are known as quantum dots along with MRI. This combination of quantum dots and MRI usually produces an exceptional image of the tumor. It has been suggested that these nanoparticles are brighter than organic dyes and only need one light source for excitation and visualization, which also means that the use of quantum dots could produce a higher-contrast image at a lower cost when compared to organic dyes. Additionally, other nanomaterials with high surface area to volume ratio permits many functional groups to be attached to a nanoparticle, which can seek out and bind to certain tumor cells.

The small size of nanoparticles also allows them to accumulate at tumor sites. More recently, exciting research is starting to develop these imaging nanoparticles to diagnose and to treat cancer. It is thought that a promising new cancer treatment can one day replace existing radiation and chemotherapy. Furthermore, sensor test chips containing thousands of nanowires can detect proteins and other biomarkers left behind by cancer cells, and could permit the detection and diagnosis of cancer in the early stages from minute quantity of a patient's blood. Furthermore, the success of any therapy is primarily based on the way drugs are going to be delivered inside the human body and drug delivery is based upon three facts such as (i) efficient formulation of the drug molecules, (ii) successful delivery of said drugs to the targeted region of the body, and (iii) finally the successful release of that drug at the target site. The help of nanoparticles with 120 nm diameter nanoshells coated with gold, has been used to kill cancer tumors in animals (mice). Moreover, the nanoshells/capsule can be targeted to bind to cancerous cells by conjugating antibodies or peptides to the nanoshell surface. Furthermore, these nanoparticles can also be used to destroy cancer cells by irradiating the area of the tumor with infrared lasers.

Nanoparticles of cadmium selenide are also known as quantum dots. These quantum dots glow when exposed to ultraviolet light. When injected, they enter into cancer tumors and the physician can see the shining tumor and use it as a guide for more precise tumor elimination. In the case of photodynamic therapy, a nanoparticle is placed inside the body and is illuminated with light from the outside and the light gets absorbed by the particle. Furthermore, light can be used to produce high-energy oxygen particles, which will chemically react with cells and destroy most organic molecules that are next to them. It has been suggested that this therapy is appealing for many reasons as it does not have a toxic effect of reactive molecules throughout the body. Iit is directed where only the light is shown and the particles exist, and moreover, photodynamic therapy has the potential for a noninvasive procedure in dealing with tumors.

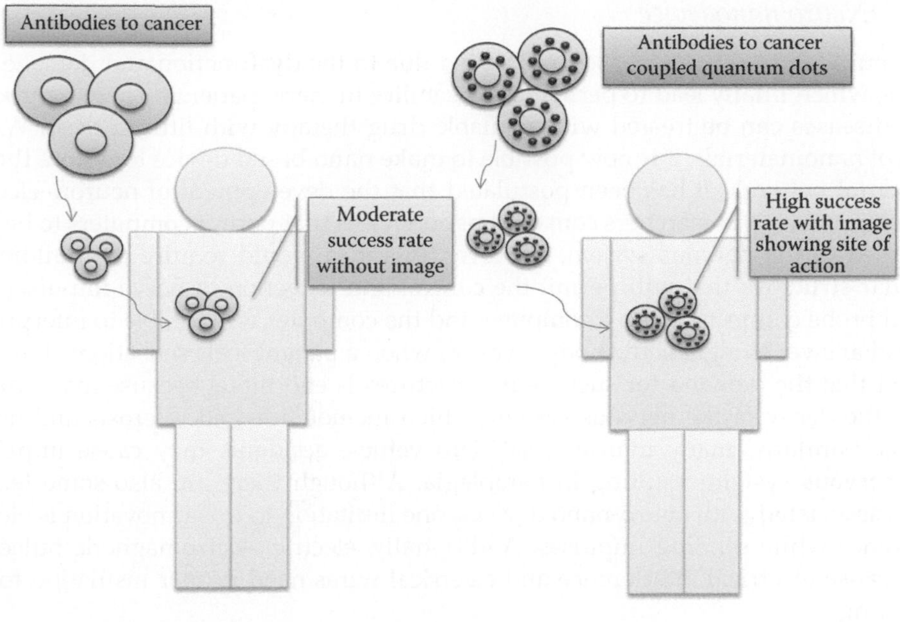

Figure 11.6 The application of quantum dots in medicine and how the use of quantum dots improves the diagnostics and treatment modalities in the patient.

11.8.2.2 Visualization

One of the major problems of current drug therapy is to visualize biomolecules in the body because it is difficult to track a small group of cells throughout the body, so researchers have been using different tracers to dye the cells. It has been suggested that these dyes require to be enhanced by light of a certain wavelength in order for them to brighten up. Whereas different color dyes absorb different frequencies of light, there was a need for light sources to be able to glow. This problem is solved by using nano-based tracking molecules known as quantum dots (Figure 11.6). These quantum dots can be anchored to proteins that penetrate cell membranes. These dots can be random in size and can be made of bioinert or biodegradable materials.

11.8.2.3 Nanoparticle targeting

It has been reported that nanoparticles can also be used for drug delivery, medical imaging, and as diagnostic sensors. One of the major issues with current drug therapy is to take the drug to the right site without losing functionality. This problem can be solved if we use the right drug delivery. However, the biodistribution of nanoparticles is mostly unknown due to the difficulty in targeting specific organs in the body. Present research in the excretory systems of mice shows the ability of gold amalgams to selectively target certain human body organs based on their size and charge. These gold composites are condensed by a dendrimer and assigned a specific charge and size. While positively charged gold nanoparticles were found to enter the kidneys, negatively charged gold nanoparticles remained in the liver and spleen. Furthermore, it has been suggested that the positive surface charge of the nanoparticle decreases the rate of release of nanoparticles in the liver, thus affecting the excretory pathway.

11.8.3 Neuro nanodevice

Many neurodegenerative diseases are caused due to the dysfunction and damage of the neurons, which finally lead to permanent disability in many patients. These neurodegenerative diseases can be treated with available drug therapy with little success. With the advent of nanomaterials, it is now possible to make nano-based device to restore the damaged neural network. It has been postulated that the development of neuron–electronic interfacing can help researchers construct nanodevices that permit computers to be joined and linked to the nervous system. However, this idea would require the building of a molecular structure that will permit the control and detection of nerve impulses by an external probe connected with a computer and the computer will be able to interpret, register, and answer to signals the body gives off when a patient feels sensations. It has been reported that the demand for such neurostructures is enormous because many diseases include the decay of the nervous system, which include amyloid sclerosis and multiple sclerosis. Similarly, many injuries related to vehicle accidents may cause impairment of the nervous system resulting in paraplegia. Although there are also some technical glitches associated with neuro-nano devices, one limitation to this innovation is electrical interference while sending impulses. Additionally, electric electromagnetic pulse fields can all cause electrical interference and electrical wires need proper insulation to avoid overheating.

11.8.4 Nanorobots

With the help of nanotechnology, it is becoming possible to make nanorobots, which can be introduced into the human body and repair or detect damages and infections. It has been suggested that a nanorobot with a size between 0.5 and 3.0 μm can be used in typical bloodborne medical treatment. It has been suggested that the carbon molecule could be the primary element that is used to build nanorobots. Also, owing to the intrinsic strength and characteristics of some forms of carbon, nanorobots can be fabricated in nanofactories specialized for this purpose. Therapeutic nanodevices would first be injected into a human body, and would then go travel to reach a specific organ or tissue mass for its action. The doctor/physician can monitor the progress of the nanodevice action and make sure that the nanodevices have reached the correct target site. The doctor/physician would also be able to scan a section of the body and actually see the nanodevices congregating neatly around their target so that he or she can be sure that the procedure was successful.

11.8.5 Nanocell repair

With the help of nanoparticles, it would be possible to repair an individual cell effectively. It has been reported that there is a great possibility to access the cells without killing them and it is possible to insert molecular machines inside the cell. Similarly, all specific biochemical interactions show that molecular systems can identify other molecules by touch, build, or rebuild every molecule in a cell. With the help of existing knowledge of cell function, it is possible to make a nanomachine to be able to guide and execute cell function. It has been suggested that the healthcare possibilities of these cell repair machines are impressive as these nanomachines can be able to accurately correct a single molecular disorder, which is caused due to DNA damage or enzyme deficiency.

11.8.6 Nanonephrology

Nanoparticles can also help in the diagnosis of renal diseases called nanonephrology. Nanonephrology is a branch of nanomedicine and nanotechnology that deals with the kidney. With the help of nanoparticles, it is possible to get nanoscale information on the cellular molecular mechanism involved in normal kidney processes and in pathological conditions. It has been suggested that by understanding the physical and biochemical characteristics of proteins and other macromolecules at the atomic level in various cells in the kidney, novel therapeutic methods can be designed to combat major renal diseases. Furthermore, the nanoscale artificial kidney is a goal that many physicians dream of making in the near future. Nanoscale engineering advances can permit programmable and controllable nanoscale robots to execute beneficial and reconstructive measures in the human kidney. Moreover, the ability to direct events in a skillful fashion at the cellular level has the potential of considerably improving the lives of patients with kidney diseases.

11.9 Safety issues associated with nanomaterials

Besides having so many useful benefits, there are safety issues related to nanomaterials that need to be addressed before making this technology public. It has been suggested that these nanomaterials might have possible adverse health and environmental impacts mostly due to the unknown physicochemical properties of materials at the nanoscale. Among all environmental, health, and safety issues, it has been reported that nanomaterials in particular cause the highest concern because of their potential of rapid uptake by the biological system in the living organisms. There is also concern due to their unidentified distribution pathways inside the body and potential interactions with various components of the biological system. Furthermore, nanoparticles are reported to be present in the air atmosphere, especially the area where the nanomaterials are being manufactured. It has been suggested that the production of nanomaterials requires high energy involving organic or inorganic chemicals and all these chemicals have the potential of producing ultrafine particles as one of the by-products, which can be inhaled by humans and as well as animals. These nanoparticles have unique physicochemical properties that are not found in the natural environment. Nanomaterials have a much higher reactivity, and because of their ultrasmall size, they can easily penetrate skin or cells, rapidly distribute into the human body, and even directly interact with organelles within cells. Furthermore, the surface area of a biological system can increase the chemical activities and, therefore, allow them to become efficient catalysts. These improved chemical and biological activities resulted in many engineered nanoparticles being considered for specific functions, including diagnostic or therapeutic medical uses that require the introduction of these nanometers inside the human body.

In addition to this, nanomaterials have devastating adverse health effects as the rapid uptake through the skin and epithelial cells could lead to severe health problems. For example, the use of carbon nanomaterials (fullerenes), which consist of repeating hexagonal and pentagonal rings of carbon atoms. However, recent studies found that buckyballs have considerable water solubility, and can cause lipid peroxidation in the fish brain after 48 h at a concentration of 500 parts per billion and this kind of oxidative stress is typically a first sign of biological damage. Moreover, a single-wall nanotube has been found to cause free radical formation and depletion of antioxidants in cells. Furthermore, metal impurity in the synthesis of nanotubes may also add to the toxicity. In addition, physical appearance of some nanotubes may cause pulmonary fibrosis and cancer. Additionally, quantum dots are made of a cadmium–selenium core with a zinc sulfide shell. All three metals are known to be toxic to different extents and the high surface area and rapid distribution of the ultrasmall particles are expected to further escalate the potential adverse health effects.

There are other nanoparticles that have already found their way into commercial products, such as titanium oxide for photochemical oxidation, self-cleaning paints, zinc oxide in cosmetics, iron particles for oxidation of contaminants in groundwater, copper oxide for antimicrobial activities, and iron oxide as a contrast agent for magnetic resonance imaging. Although most of these parent materials are not considered to be significantly toxic, the formation nanomaterials dusts may create unknown toxicity or environmental impacts. Moreover, it has been shown that the toxicity of nanosize titanium oxide can cause toxicity.

Another issue with regard to nanomaterials is the effect on individuals who are directly exposed to nanomaterials on a daily basis, such as researchers and manufacturing workers. It has been reported that the practice of occupational health may also face many challenges as for many conventional workplace contaminants; airborne route is considered the most crucial for worker protection. The shape and size of airborne nanoparticles and the conglomeration status are some of the main factors determining the hazard. Furthermore, nanoparticles in a liquid stage may serve as a carrier that facilitates skin penetration and can affect the overall hazard. In either the airborne or liquid phase, the nanomaterials have the potential to unfavorably influence the environment if they are not properly controlled during practice and disposed of afterwards.

11.9.1 Solutions for safety issues associated with nanomaterials

One of the major challenges in evaluating and treating hazards posed by nanoparticles is to find a suitable sampling and analytical method to evaluate the gravity of the impact. It is essential to consider the concentration of nanoparticles and surface area involved, instead of mass concentration, and moreover, the reliability of the detection technology is also one of the main concerns to be addressed. At least one passive sampling method coupled with a scanning electron microscope can be developed to assess and evaluate the gravity of toxicity. In addition, there are traditionally, high-efficiency particulate air (HEPA) filters used for removing airborne particulates to avoid air pollution, but for nanoparticles it has never been proved whether the HEPA filter can capture nanoscale particles. Recent research showed that HEPA filter is capable of removing more than 99.97% of particles down to the range of 2–4 nm.

11.10 Ethical issues related to nanomaterials

Besides environmental, health, and safety issues associated with nanomaterials, the threat of nanomachines will become real not only in war situations but also in case they were produced and used by miscreants in everyday life. As far as an ethical viewpoint, it is not desirable to create autonomous nanomachines as they could become not only out of human control but also cause damage to humanity and its environment. Another ethical issue that needs to be addressed before these nanomaterials are manufactured and sold at international markets is to create laws and regulations that govern the making of nanomaterials on a similar line with nuclear technology. The people who make and manufacture nanomaterials will also get exposed to nanoparticles and might also develop some health-related issues on a long-term basis; this also needs to be addressed before making these technologies available for mass production. Furthermore, the ethical limits of human body repair arise at the moment when such changes become a threat to human health and survival. More research is required to make this technology free from such manifestation.

11.11 Summary

The term "synthetic biology" defines research that combines biology with the principles of engineering to design and build standardized, interchangeable biological DNA building blocks. In synthetic biology, the DNA is artificially designed to create artificial biological systems of higher-order function. Nanomedicine is the application of nanoparticles in the medicine. Nanomedicine ranges from the medical applications of nanomaterials to nanoelectronic business, and even possible future applications of molecular nanotechnology. In this chapter, we discussed the significance of synthetic biology and nanomedicine and explained how these fields have revolutionized the modern treatment modalities in various ways.

11.12 Scholar's achievements

Eckard Wimmer: Eckard Wimmer (born 22 May, 1936) is a German American virologist, organic chemist, and distinguished professor of molecular genetics and microbiology at Stony Brook University. He is best known for his seminal work on the molecular biology of poliovirus and the first chemical synthesis of a viral genome capable of infection and subsequent production of live viruses.

Collins: James J. Collins (June 26, 1965) is an American bioengineer, professor of biomedical engineering at Boston University, and a Howard Hughes Medical Institute (HHMI) Investigator. He is one of the founders of the emerging field of synthetic biology, and a pioneering researcher in systems biology, having made fundamental discoveries regarding the actions of antibiotics and the emergence of antibiotic resistance.

11.13 Knowledge builder

Bioengineered organism: Bioengineered organisms are those organisms whose DNA has been manipulated to produce useful products, for example, genetically modified bacteria are used to produce the protein insulin to treat diabetes. Similar bacteria have been used to produce clotting factors to treat hemophilia, and human growth hormones to treat various forms of dwarfism transgenic fruit flies (*Drosophila melanogaster*) are used as genetic models to study the effects of genetic changes on development. Genetically modified plants tolerant to the herbicides glufosinate or glyphosate, and producing the Bt toxin, an insecticide, have dominated the agricultural seed market for corn and other crops. A tomato (called Flavr Savr) made by the Californian company Calgene is resistant to rot. Soybeans resistant to herbicides (trade name Roundup Ready) were developed by Monsanto. A sweet corn that produces its own insecticide (trade name Bt corn) from a gene extracted from the bacteria *Bacillus thuringiensis* and also golden rice, genetically modified to contain high amounts of vitamin A (beta-carotene), implanted with three new genes, two from daffodils and the third from a bacterium.

Mycoplasma mycoides: Mycoplasma mycoides is a bacterial species of the genus *Mycoplasma* in the class Mollicutes. This microorganism is a parasite that lives in ruminants (cattle and goats), causing lung disease.

Synthetic DNA: Artificial gene synthesis is a method in synthetic biology that is used to create artificial genes in the laboratory. Based on solid-phase DNA synthesis, it differs from molecular cloning and polymerase chain reaction (PCR) in that the user does not have to begin with preexisting DNA sequences. Therefore, it is possible to make a completely synthetic double-stranded DNA molecule with no apparent limits on either nucleotide sequence or size. The method has been used to generate functional bacterial chromosomes containing approximately 1 million base pairs.

Lambda X174: The phi X 174 bacteriophage was the first DNA-based genome to be sequenced. This work was completed by Fred Sanger and his team in 1977. In 1962, Walter Fiers and Robert Sinsheimer had already demonstrated the physical, covalently closed circularity of phi X 174 DNA. Nobel prize winner Arthur Kornberg used phi X 174 as a model to first prove that DNA synthesized in a test tube by purified enzymes could produce all the features of a natural virus, ushering in the age of synthetic biology in 2003, it was reported by Craig Venter's group that the genome of ΦX174 was the first to be completely assembled *in vitro* from synthesized oligonucleotides.

DNA synthesis machines: Artificial gene synthesis is a method in synthetic biology that is used to create artificial genes in the laboratory. Based on solid-phase DNA synthesis, it differs from molecular cloning and PCR in that the user does not have to begin with preexisting DNA sequences. Therefore, it is possible to make a completely synthetic double-stranded DNA molecule with no apparent limits on either nucleotide sequence or size. The method has been used to generate functional bacterial chromosomes containing approximately one million base pairs.

Protein-engineering technology: Protein engineering is the process of developing useful or valuable proteins. It is a young discipline, with much research taking place in the understanding of protein folding and recognition for protein design principles. There are two general strategies for protein engineering, "rational" protein design and directed evolution. These techniques are not mutually exclusive; researchers will often apply both. In the future, more detailed knowledge of protein structure and function, as well as advancements in high-throughput technology, may greatly expand the capabilities of protein engineering.

BioBricks: BioBrick standard biological parts are DNA sequences of defined structure and function; they share a common interface and are designed to be composed and incorporated into living cells such as *E. coli* to construct new biological systems. BioBrick parts represent an effort to introduce the engineering principles of abstraction and standardization into synthetic biology. The trademarked words BioBrick and BioBricks are correctly used as adjectives (not nouns) and refer to a specific brand of open-source genetic parts as defined via an open technical standards setting process that is led by the BioBricks Foundation. BioBrick parts were introduced by Tom Knight at MIT in 2003. Drew Endy, now at Stanford, and Christopher Voigt, at MIT, are also involved in the project in a big way. A registry of several thousand public domain BioBrick parts is maintained by Randy Rettberg team at http://partsregistry.org. The annual iGEM competition promotes the BioBrick parts concept by involving undergraduate and graduate students in the design of biological systems.

Biosensing: A biosensor is an analytical device, used for the detection of an analyte, that combines a biological component with a physicochemical detector and the process of such sensing is called biosensing. The sensitive biological element (e.g., tissue, microorganisms, organelles, cell receptors, enzymes, antibodies, and nucleic acids), a biologically derived material or biomimetic component that interacts (binds or recognizes) the analyst under study. The biologically sensitive elements can also be created by biological engineering.

Nanomaterials: Nanomaterials is a field that takes a materials science-based approach on nanotechnology. It studies materials with morphological features on the nanoscale, and especially those that have special properties stemming from their nanoscale dimensions. Nanoscale is usually defined as smaller than one-tenth of a micrometer in at least one dimension, though sometimes includes up to a micrometer.

Graphene: Graphene is an allotrope of carbon. In this material, carbon atoms are arranged in a regular hexagonal pattern. Graphene can be described as a one-atom-thick layer of the mineral graphite (many layers of graphene stacked together effectively form crystalline flake graphite). Among its other well-publicized superlative properties, it is very light, with a 1-m^2 sheet weighing only 0.77 mg.

Drug bioavailability: In pharmacology, bioavailability (BA) is a subcategory of absorption and is the fraction of an administered dose of unchanged drug that reaches the systemic circulation, one of the principal pharmacokinetic properties of drugs. By definition, when a medication is administered intravenously, its bioavailability is 100%. However, when a medication is administered via other routes, its BA generally decreases (due to incomplete absorption and first-pass metabolism) or may vary from patient to patient. BA is one of the essential tools in pharmacokinetics, as BA must be considered when calculating dosages for nonintravenous routes of administration.

High-efficiency particulate air: High-efficiency particulate air or HEPA is a type of air filter. Filters meeting the HEPA standard have many applications, including use in medical facilities, automobiles, aircraft, and homes.

Further reading

Allen TM and Cullis PR 2004. Drug delivery systems: Entering the mainstream. *Science* 303 (5665): 1818–1822. doi:10.1126/science.1095833. PMID 15031496.

Animal and Plant Health Inspection Service, U.S. Department of Agriculture, Questions and Answers on General Regulatory Policy under 7 CFR 340, http://www.aphis.usda.gov/brs/qagen.html (accessed April 10, 2006).

Benner SA and Sismour MA 2005. Synthetic biology. *Nat Rev Genet* 6 (7): 533–543.

Cavalcanti A, Shirinzadeh B, Freitas RA Jr, and Hogg T 2008. Nanorobot architecture for medical target identification. *Nanotechnology* 19 (1): 015103 (15pp). doi:10.1088/0957-4484/19/01/015103.

Couzin J 2002. Active poliovirus baked from scratch. *Science* 297 (5579): 174–175.

Editorial. 2006. Nanomedicine: A matter of rhetoric? *Nat Mater* 5 (4): 243. doi:10.1038/nmat1625. PMID 16582920.

Ferber D 2004. Microbes made to order. *Science* 303 (5655): 158–161.

Freitas RA Jr. 2005. What is nanomedicine? *Nanomedicine Nanotech Biol Med* 1 (1): 2–9.

Freitas RA Jr. and Ilkka H 2005. Current status of nanomedicine and medical nanorobotics. *J Comp Theor Nanosci* 2: 1–25. doi:10.1166/jctn.2005.001.

Glass JI, Assad-Garcia N et al. 2006. Essential genes of a minimal bacterium. *Proc Natl Acad Sci* 103 (2): 425–430.

Hamilton O, Clyde A, Hutchison, III et al. 2003. Generating a synthetic genome by whole genome assembly φX174 bacteriophage from synthetic oligonucleotides. *Proc Natl Acad Sci* 100 (26): 15440–15445.

Hasty J, McMillen D, and Collins JJ 2002. Engineered gene circuits. *Nature* 420 (6912): 224–230.

Katz R. and Raymond AZ (eds.) 2011. *Encyclopedia of Bioterrorism Defense,* 2nd Edition, Hoboken, NJ: John Wiley and Sons, Inc.

LaVan DA, McGuire T, and Langer R 2003. Small-scale systems for in vivo drug delivery. *Nat Biotechnol* 21 (10): 1184–1191. doi:10.1038/nbt876. PMID 14520404.

Levskaya A, Chevalier AA, Jeffrey J et al. 2005. Engineering *Escherichia coli* to see light. *Nature* 438 (7067): 441–442.

Loo C, Lin A, Hirsch L, Lee MH, Barton J, Halas N, West J, and Drezek R 2004. Nanoshell-enabled photonics-based imaging and therapy of cancer. *Technol Cancer Res Treat* 3 (1): 33–40. PMID 14750891.

Ro D-K, Paradise EM, Ouellet M, Fisher KJ, Karyn L et al. 2006. Production of the antimalarial drug precursor artemisinic acid in engineered yeast. *Nature* 440 (7086): 940–943.

Rod M 2008. Sizing up targets with nanoparticles. *Nature Nanotechnol* 3 (1): 12–13. doi:10.1038/nnano.2007.433. PMID 18654442.

Shuming N, Xing Y, Kim GJ, and Simmons JW 2007. Nanotechnology applications in cancer. *Annu Rev Biomed Eng* 9: 257. doi:10.1146/annurev.bioeng.9.060906.152025. PMID 17439359.

Synthetic Biology Research Community. 2004. Synthetic Biology 1.0: The First International Meeting on Synthetic Biology held at MIT, Cambridge, Massachusetts, on June 10–12, 2004, http://www.syntheticbiology.org/Synthetic_Biology_1.0.html (accessed January 21, 2006).

Tumpey TM, Basler CF, Aguilar PV, Zeng H et al. 2005. Characterization of the reconstructed 1918 Spanish influenza pandemic virus. *Science* 310 (5745): 77–80.

Ulmer KM 1983. Protein engineering. *Science* 219 (4585): 666–671.

United States Arms Control and Disarmament Agency. 1993. The Convention on the Prohibition of the Development, Production, Stockpiling and Use of Chemical Weapons and on Their Destruction (Washington, D.C.: U.S. Arms Control and Disarmament Agency). Treaty text available online: http://dosfan.lib.uic.edu/acda/treaties/cwctext.htm.

United States Arms Control and Disarmament Agency. 1996. The Convention on the Prohibition of the Development, Production and Stockpiling of Bacteriological (Biological) and Toxin Weapons and on Their Destruction, in Arms Control and Disarmament Agreements: Text and Histories of the Negotiations (Washington, D.C.: U.S. Arms Control and Disarmament Agency), pp. 98–104. Treaty text available online: http://dosfan.lib.uic.edu/acda/treaties/bwc1.htm.

Wagner V, Dullaart A, Bock AK, and Zweck A 2006. The emerging Nanomedicine landscape. *Nat Biotechnol* 24 (10): 1211–1217. doi:10.1038/nbt1006-1211. PMID 17033654.

Wang L, Brock A, Herberich B, and Schultz PG 2001. Expanding the genetic code of *Escherichia coli*. *Science* 292 (5516): 498–500.

Zheng G, Patolsky F, Cui Y, Wang WU, and Lieber CM 2005. Multiplexed electrical detection of cancer markers with nanowire sensor arrays. *Nat Biotechnol* 23 (10): 1294–1301. doi:10.1038/nbt1138. PMID 16170313.

chapter twelve

Pharmacogenomics and predictive medicine

12.1 Introduction

Most of the drugs we use today are primarily tested in a selected group of people, and not in all the people, because it is impossible to test drugs in each and every person. However, the drug regulators or controllers approve the drugs to be used by patients on the pretext that the intended drug will not cause any side effects in the large population of patients; however, it has been reported that some of the drugs could cause severe side effects. Moreover, it has been reported that more than two million fell seriously ill and over 100,000 deaths occurred due to adverse drug reactions (ADRs), making ADRs one of the leading causes of hospitalization and death in the United States alone. Currently, there is no simple way to determine whether people will respond well, badly, or not at all to a medication; therefore, pharmaceutical companies are limited to developing drugs based on random clinical trials. It has been found that the manner a person responds to a drug is a complex characteristic that is swayed by many different genes, and without knowing all of the genes involved in drug response, investigators have found it difficult to develop genetic tests that could predict a person's response to a particular drug. Additionally, once investigators discover small variations in the person's nucleotide content, genetic testing for predicting drug response is now conceivable.

12.2 Drug development

Before we learn about pharmacogenomics, let us briefly discuss a conventional drug development pathway to understand the various components of drug development.

12.2.1 Drug discovery

The use of pharmacogenomics in health care, especially in the drug discovery process, has been extensively anticipated, and one of the reasons why most of the pharmaceutical companies choose to work in the pharmacogenomics field is that it helps and expedites the process and development of new drug candidates. Before learning the significance of pharmacogenomics in the drug discovery pathway, it is important to know the normal drug discovery pathway and issues associated with it. Moreover, drug discovery is the process by which drugs are discovered and/or designed, and in the past, most drugs have been discovered either by identifying the active ingredient from traditional remedies (plants) or by an accidental discovery. Now, a new approach has been initiated to understand how disease and infection are controlled or regulated at the molecular and physiological levels. Furthermore, the process of drug discovery involves the identification of drug candidates, synthesis, characterization, screening, and assays for therapeutic efficacy. When a drug

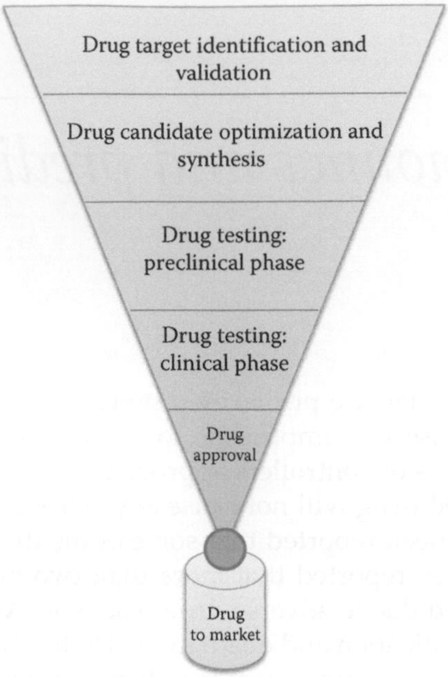

Figure 12.1 Drug development process.

compound has shown its value in these *in vitro* tests, it can be taken up for preclinical and clinical trials followed by industrial-level production (Figure 12.1).

12.2.1.1 Drug targets

The drug target is the naturally existing cellular or molecular structure located in the cells that are known to involve in the pathology of disease and these targets can be used by pharmaceutical companies to treat or cure the diseases. These targets are basically receptors that are located in the cell membrane. Moreover, there are two types of targets: one is new and the other is old (established target), and the distinction between a new and established target can be made by pharmaceutical companies engaged in the discovery and development of therapeutics. For example, established targets are those targets for which a good scientific understanding is available, supported by a concrete research publication track record. However, this does not imply that the mechanism of action of drugs that are thought to act through established targets is fully understood. But considering that established targets provide concrete proof of information, pharmaceutical companies would have to invest less money compared with new targets. The process of gathering such functional information from target sites is called target validation in the pharmaceutical industry. Additionally, established targets also include those targets that the pharmaceutical industry had been tested to check the effectiveness of drug molecules. In contrast to established targets, new targets are all those that are not tested and analyzed using any drug candidates. The new targets are those newly discovered proteins whose functions have now become clear due to scientific research. Furthermore, the majority of targets currently selected for drug discovery efforts are proteins that are G-protein-coupled receptors (GPCRs) and protein kinases. The process of drug discovery, including target discovery and validation of final product development, is illustrated in Figure 12.2.

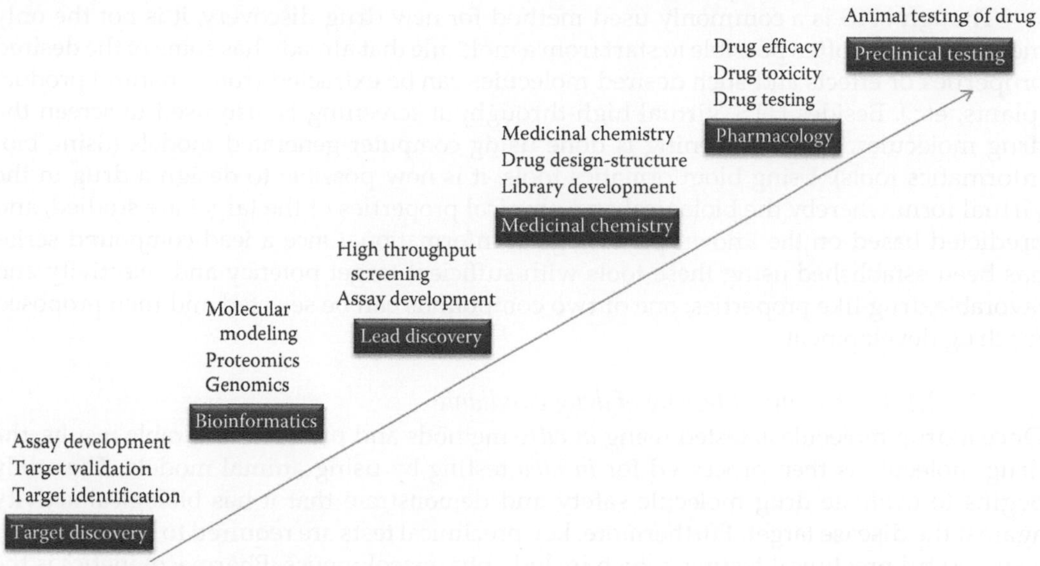

Figure 12.2 Pathway of drug discovery.

12.2.1.2 *Drug screening*

The process of finding a new drug using known targets is called drug screening. With the advent of technology, it is now possible to screen many drug molecules using high-throughput screening (HTS) method, where large libraries of drug compounds are tested for their ability to modify the target sites. For instance, if the target is novel GPCRs, drug compounds will be screened for their capacity to inhibit or stimulate that receptor; in case the target is a protein kinase, then the chemicals will be tested for their ability to inhibit that kinase. Another significant function of HTS is to show how selective the drug compounds are for the chosen target. It has been suggested that ideally a drug molecule should be highly specific in binding to target sites. Moreover, cross-screening is also important because sometimes drug molecules can also hit unrelated targets.

Furthermore, it is very unlikely that a perfect drug candidate can emerge from these screening methods. It has been observed that several drug compounds are found to have some degree of activity, and if these drug compounds share common chemical features, one or more pharmacophores (active drug chemical) can then be developed. During the screening process, the researchers can use also structure–activity relationships using bioinformatics tools to improve certain features of the lead compound. Interestingly, this process can require several screening runs, to obtain the molecule of interest, which can be later processed for *in vitro* and *in vivo* testing, respectively. Furthermore, it has been shown that the physical–chemical properties of a drug are checked by analyzing drug solubility, absorption, distribution, action, metabolism, and drug elimination parameters in both animals and humans. Drug permeability can be determined by PAMPA testing and Caco-2 testing, whereas PAMPA is attractive as an early screen due to the low intake of drug and lowest price compared to tests such as Caco-2. Furthermore, a range of parameters can be employed to assess the quality of a compound as proposed in the Lipinski's rule, which include calculation of drug lipophilicity, drug molecular weight, polar surface area, and measured properties, such as drug potency. Other parameters such as ligand efficiency and lipophilic efficiency can also be used to assess drug candidates.

Though HTS is a commonly used method for new drug discovery, it is not the only method and it is often possible to start from a molecule that already has some of the desired properties or effects and such desired molecules can be extracted from a natural product (plants, etc.). Besides HTS, virtual high-throughput screening is also used to screen the drug molecules, where screening is done using computer-generated models (using bioinformatics tools). Using bioinformatics tools, it is now possible to design a drug in the virtual form whereby the biological and physical properties of the target are studied, and predicted based on the known physiological information. Once a lead compound series has been established using these tools with sufficient target potency and selectivity and favorable drug-like properties, one or two compounds can be selected and then proposed for drug development.

12.2.1.3 Preclinical testing of drug candidate

Once a drug molecule is tested using *in vitro* methods and produces desirable results, the drug molecule is then processed for *in vivo* testing by using animal models. The study begins to evaluate drug molecule safety and demonstrate that it has biological activity against the disease target. Furthermore, key preclinical tests are required to be fulfilled for a successful preclinical testing, which include pharmacokinetics. Pharmacokinetics is the study of how drugs move through living organisms to safeguard that the intended drug candidate reaches its intended target and passes through the body properly. Additionally, researchers also conduct a number of other preclinical studies to establish the compound's purity, stability, and drug shelf life. Finally, the main objective of preclinical studies is to rigorously assess the safety profile of the drug candidate before human tests begin and this can take anywhere from 3 to 6 years. Moreover, some preclinical safety tests continue even after the start of human trials to determine if there are any long-term adverse effects.

12.2.1.4 Clinical testing of drug candidate

After the successful completion of the preclinical trial with the desirable results obtained, a drug candidate can be processed for human trails, which are also known as clinical trials (Figure 12.3). Before starting the clinical trials, the manufacturers need to obtain necessary approvals from the appropriate regulatory agency. Furthermore, in the United States, an Investigational New Drug (IND) application can be filed with the FDA before initiating human clinical trials. The main objective of an IND is to provide data (both *in vitro* and *in vivo*) to the FDA showing that a new drug candidate has satisfied both safety measures and effective measures. It has been suggested that the IND is not an application for marketing approval to launch a drug. The clinical trial starts with Phase 1 trials, which is the first trial in which a new drug candidate is tested in normal or healthy human subjects.

Phase 1 clinical trials are typically planned to evaluate the safety, acceptability, and pharmacokinetics of a drug candidate. Interestingly, Phase 1 clinical trials are generally conducted in a small group of healthy volunteers, though actual patients with disease may be used in certain conditions. In a distinctive Phase 1 study design, humans are administered a single dose of the new drug and the response is detected over a period of time. If the humans do not display or report any adverse side effects, then pharmacokinetics-based results are in line with expected safety values. In addition to this, the dose is also escalated until intolerable side effects appear and at this point, the drug is said to have reached the maximum tolerated dose. This testing of a single dose is known as a single-ascending dose study and after completing this study, multiple-ascending dose studies are conducted to better comprehend the pharmacokinetics and safety profile of multiple doses of the drug. In these studies, a group of humans receives multiple doses of the drug and

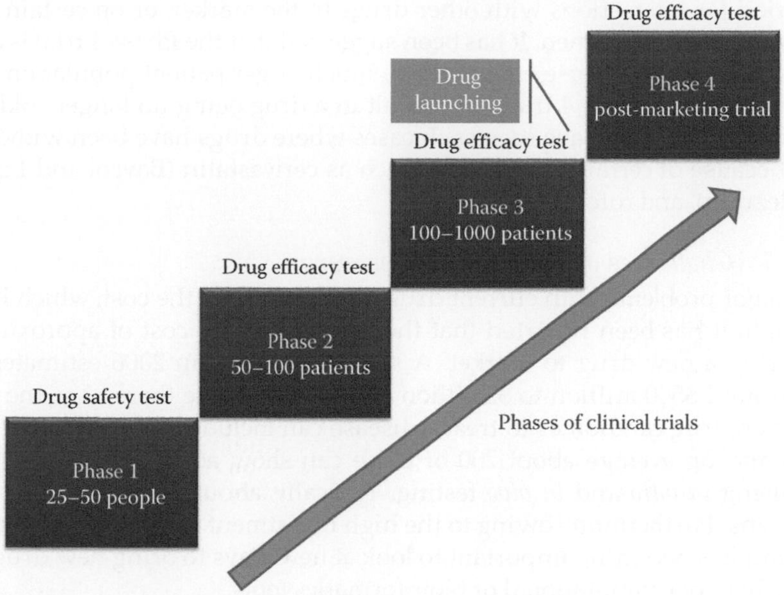

Figure 12.3 Different phases of clinical trials.

at various time intervals; blood samples and other fluids can be collected and analyzed to understand how the drug is processed within the body. The dose is subsequently escalated up to a predetermined level.

After the successful completion of Phase 1 trial, Phase 2 clinical trials are conducted to evaluate how well the drug works in patients with a particular disease. It has been reported that Phase 2 clinical trials include a larger group of patients and typically test different dose levels. Along with the effectiveness of the drug, the safety assessments are also continuing in the Phase 2 trial. Moreover, Phase 2 clinical trials are typically divided into Phase 2a and Phase 2b trials, whereas Phase 2a is specifically designed to assess dosage requirements, and Phase 2b is specifically designed to study the efficacy of the drug. Some trials combine both Phase 1 and Phase 2 together to obtain early results. Most Phase 2 trials are designed as randomized clinical trials, where few patients receive the drug and others receive a placebo tablet (containing no drug molecule).

The Phase 3 clinical trials are randomized and conducted in multicenters to finally assess how effective a drug is to treat a particular disease. It has been reported that Phase 3 clinical trials are the most expensive trials to design and run because of the huge number of patients studied and comparatively long duration, especially in therapies for chronic medical conditions and diseases. Moreover, certain Phase 3 trials are often called registrational trials, which can be submitted to support initial approval of the drug for marketing. Normally other Phase 3 clinical trials to be continued though the regulatory submission for marketing authorization are pending. During the Phase 3 trial, the patients continue to receive life-saving drugs until the new drug are marketed.

Once the drugs are successfully tested, the regulatory authority gives the permission to make the drugs in large quantity to be sold in the market. The Phase 4 trial is known as the Post-Marketing Surveillance Trial; also as pharmacovigilance. It has been reported that Phase 4 studies can be required by regulatory authorities or may be undertaken by the sponsoring company for competitive or other reasons; for example, the drug may not have been tried for interactions with other drugs in the market, or on certain population groups such as pregnant women. It has been suggested that the Phase 4 trial is designed to detect rare or long-term adverse effects over a much larger patient population. The harmful effects revealed by Phase 4 trials can result in a drug being no longer sold for certain uses and more recently we have seen such cases where drugs have been withdrawn from the market because of certain side effects. Such as cerivastatin (Baycol and Lipobay), troglitazone (Rezulin), and rofecoxib (Vioxx).

12.2.1.5 Challenges of current drug discovery

One of the major problems with current drug development is the cost, which is unexpectedly very high. It has been reported that there is an average cost of approximately $800 million to bring a new drug to market. A study published in 2006 estimates that costs vary from around $500 million to $2 billion depending on the therapy or the developing firm. Moreover, drug candidates to treat a disease can include more than 10,000 chemical compounds and on average about 200 of these can show adequate promise for further evaluation using *in vitro* and *in vivo* testing. Typically, about 10 of these can qualify for tests on humans. Furthermore, owing to the high investment cost, the drug becomes more expensive, and it is becoming important to look at new ways to bring new drug molecules and with the help of computational or bioinformatics tools.

Infectious diseases are now the world's biggest killers of children and young adults. They account for more than 13 million deaths a year and one out of two deaths in developing countries as reported by the WHO. Furthermore, most deaths from infectious diseases occur in developing countries and the main cause for this has been attributed to the unavailability of efficient drugs and if at all available, they are very expensive and poor people cannot afford to buy them. Henceforth, the development of cheap and efficient drugs for a disease is one of the major difficulties faced by mankind. The solution to this problem could be from balanced drug design using bioinformatics tools and over few years, for the focus of the pharmaceutical industry to shift from the trial-and-error method of drug discovery to a rational and structure-based drug design (Figure 12.4).

With the advent of information technology, it becomes easy for the drug designers to design the drug virtually with more economical ways and the whole idea of drugs is based on the structure of molecules. These structural-based drug designs are used for the prediction of drug identification and elimination of candidate molecules that are unlikely to survive the later stages of discovery and development. The drug candidates could be predicted by genetic algorithm and neural network-based methods. Furthermore, researchers have been working on constructing effective algorithms and improved energy functions to predict protein structures and interaction of small molecules. The use of bioinformatics tools can also reduce the number of trials in the screening of drug compounds and in identifying prospective drug targets for a particular disease using high-power computing information. Profound applications of bioinformatics in genome sequence have led to a new area in pharmacology, called pharmacogenomics, which is the study of the genetic basis for the differences between individuals in response to drugs and this difference is mainly due to single nucleotide polymorphisms (SNPs). These SNPs can be used to check the drug response and recently enormous efforts have been made to map human SNPs by major pharmaceutical companies in which IBM is also a member. It has been suggested that in the future, drug design is going to rely on the variation in SNPs and in fact SNPs with combinatorial chemistry option can speed up the process of drug discovery and can also end up in identifying a new set of target proteins. Furthermore, by considering all these mentioned factors that have involved in developing effective drugs, there has been a

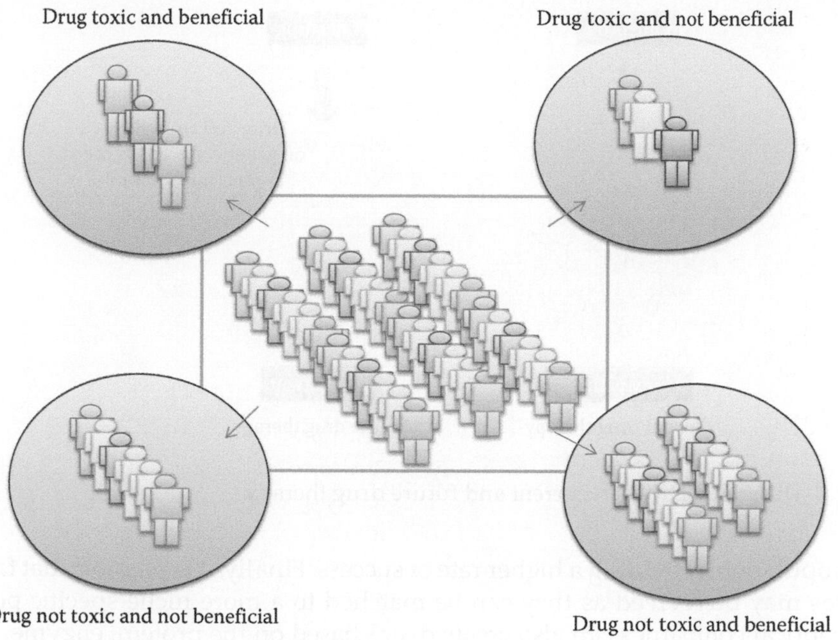

Figure 12.4 Issues related to current drug therapy.

strong urge to start the Human Proteomics Initiative. This initiative aims at identifying the functions and polymorphism of all the proteins coded in the human genome and predicts their structure, and cracks the structure of these proteins if conceivable, so that these could be used as potential targets for developing new drugs. Moreover, rapid advances in the field of information technology have revolutionized drug discovery pathways and there are several databases available to help and expedite the drug discovery.

12.3 Pharmacogenomics and drug discovery process

Pharmacogenomics plays an important role throughout the development of biotherapeutics, from target identification through clinic trials, followed by patient care. In addition to speeding up drug discovery, it can aid in increasing the therapeutic efficacy while decreasing the risks of toxicity. Moreover, pharmaceutical companies can now use pharmacogenomics to identify new drug targets and to create drugs based on the proteins, enzymes, and RNA molecules associated with specific genes and diseases. Subsequently, it has been studied that drug efficacy is influenced by genetic variation; drug discovery now includes pharmacogenomics screens to identify common genetic polymorphisms as part of the drug development process and this provides pharmaceutical companies with the potential to develop therapeutics that target populations that have specific genetic history (Figure 12.5).

As the development of a potential drug moves into the clinical trial stages, earlier work from preclinical stages can be used to help identify trial participants. Simple molecular diagnostic genotyping assays have been used to qualify participants for trials. The cost and risk of clinical trials can be reduced by only selecting the participants with genotypes that are likely to respond positively to the drug. The process of obtaining regulatory approval should also be simplified as tailored drugs are targeted toward a specific

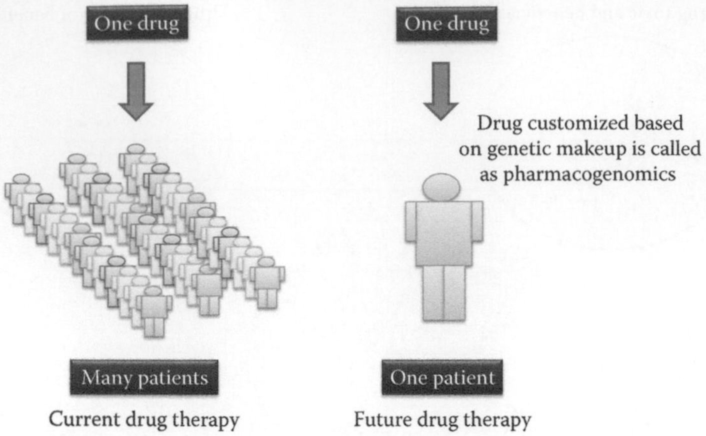

Figure 12.5 Difference between current and future drug therapy.

genetic population, providing a higher rate of success. Finally, it is possible that failed drug candidates may be revived as they can be matched to a more niche-specific population. Pharmaceutical companies can also create drugs based on the protein, enzyme, and RNA molecules, which are linked with genes and diseases, and this will allow the companies to produce a therapy more targeted to specific diseases. Furthermore, this accuracy of drug target not only maximizes therapeutic effects but also decreases damage to nearby healthy cells. Pharmaceutical companies are now able to discover probable therapies more easily using genome targets. Finally, the cost and risk involved in clinical trials will be condensed by targeting only those persons capable of responding to a drug.

12.3.1 *Better and safer drugs*

With the help of pharmacogenomics, it would be possible for the doctors to be able to examine a patient's genetic profile and recommend the best available drug therapy from the commencement of the treatment. Pharmacogenomics can also speed up recovery time and minimize the chances of adverse reactions. It has been reported that pharmacogenomics can potentially reduce the estimated many thousand deaths and couple of millions of hospitalizations that occur each year in the United States as the result of adverse drug responses.

12.3.2 *Determining accurate drug dosages*

Current methods of drug dosages that are based on the weight and age of the patient will be replaced in future with dosages based on a person's genetic profile and the time it takes to metabolize it. The patient-specific drug therapy can also maximize the therapy's value and decrease the occurrence of overdose.

12.3.3 *Advanced screening for diseases*

Interestingly, knowing a person's genetic code will allow a person to make adequate lifestyle changes at an early age so as to avoid or lessen the severity of genetic disorders. Similarly, advance knowledge of a particular genetic disease will allow careful monitoring, and treatments can be introduced at the most appropriate stage to avoid further complications.

12.3.4 Improved vaccines development

Vaccines made of genetic material, either from DNA or RNA promise all the benefits of existing vaccines without all the risks. The vaccines activate the immune system, but will be unable to cause infections. They are inexpensive, stable, easy to store, and capable of being engineered to carry several strains of a pathogen at once.

12.3.5 Decrease in the overall cost of health care

It has been suggested that the use of pharmacogenomics decreases the number of ADRs, the number of failed drug trials, and the time it takes to get a drug approved. The use of pharmacogenomics also reduces the length of time patients are on medication, and possibly detects the disease early and accurately.

12.4 Current application of pharmacogenomics

The cytochrome P450 (CYP) is an enzyme present in the liver, which is responsible for metabolizing more than 30 different classes of drugs. DNA variations in genes that code for these enzymes can affect their capability to metabolize certain drugs. It has been reported that inactive forms of CYP enzymes are unable to break down the drugs and also efficiently eliminate drugs from the body can cause drug overdose in patients (Figure 12.6). Today, clinical trial researchers use genetic tests for identifying variations in cytochrome

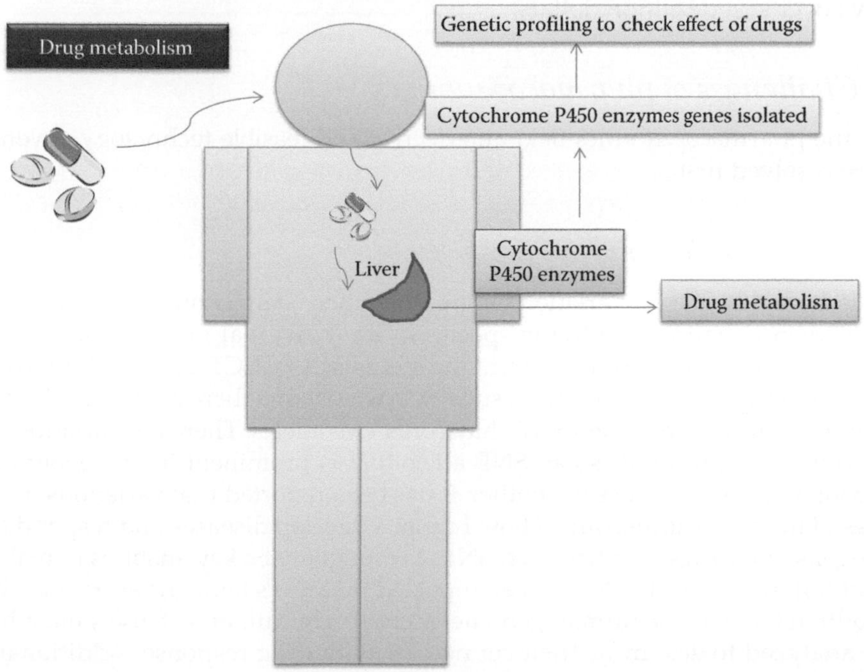

Figure 12.6 Drug metabolism with the help of CYP450 enzymes.

P450 genes to screen and monitor patients. In addition, many pharmaceutical companies screen their chemical compounds to see how well they are metabolized by variant forms of CYP enzymes.

There is another enzyme called TPMT (thiopurine methyl-transferase) that plays a vital role in the treatment of common childhood leukemia by metabolizing a class of therapeutic compounds called thiopurines. Furthermore, a small fraction of the Caucasian population have genetic variants that prevent them from producing an active form of this protein As a consequence, thiopurines rise to toxic levels in the patient because the inactive form of TMPT is unable to break down the drug. Today, physicians can use a genetic test to screen patients for this deficiency, and the TMPT action is checked to determine appropriate thiopurine dosage levels.

The biotechnology company Pharmigene, a leader in advancing tailored medicine through genetic-based diagnostic solutions, had announced a new milestone in the practice of pharmacogenomics and personalized medicine by partnering with over 50 hospitals across Taiwan. It has been reported that health care centers in Taiwan are now using Pharmigene's genetic test used to detect the presence of a key human leukocyte antigen, in individual patients being considered for treatment with the anticancer drug carbamazepine. Furthermore, patients who have the allele and are clinically treated with drug carbamazepine have been linked to a higher risk of developing Stevens Johnson syndrome. In order to prevent exposing these particular patients to the risks of these diseases, Pharmigene has developed a genetic test kit that physicians can use to find which patients have a significantly higher risk of developing this syndrome after taking carbamazepine. With the help of this genetic test, physicians have several choices of prescription drugs to treat these symptoms; nevertheless, carbamazepine has the best efficacy and is the least expensive. Moreover, the use of the companion diagnostics model, combining the use of genetic test kits plus carbamazepine for the treatment of several thousand new patients, could save over several billion dollars.

12.5 Challenges of pharmacogenomics

To make the pharmacogenomics field an effective and feasible technology, several issues need to be resolved first.

12.5.1 Gene variations and drug response

An SNP is a DNA sequence variation happening when a single nucleotide in the genome differs between members of a living species in an individual person. For instance, two sequenced DNA fragments from different individuals [AAGCCTA to AAGCTTA] contain a difference in a single nucleotide and in such case we say that there are two *alleles* [C and T]. Furthermore, almost all common SNPs have only two alleles. There are variations of allele between human populations, so an SNP allele that is prominent in one geographical or ethnic group may be much less in another. It has been reported that variations in the DNA sequences of humans can also affect how humans develop diseases and respond to different pathogens and drugs. Furthermore, SNPs is thought to be key enablers in realizing the concept of tailored medicine. It has been reported that SNPs happens every 100–300 bases along 3 billion bases in the human genome; accordingly, millions of SNPs must be identified and analyzed to determine their connection with drug response. Additionally, there is also no clarity of the precise role of each gene in the disease development.

12.5.2 *Limited drug options*

Only one or two approved drugs are currently available for the treatment of a particular disease condition. Moreover, if patients have genetic variations that prevent them using these drugs, they may be left without any treatment.

12.5.3 *Disincentives for drug companies*

Most pharmaceutical companies have been successful with their one-size-fits-all approach to drug development. Subsequently, it costs hundreds of millions of dollars to bring a drug to market, and now the question is, will these pharmaceutical or drug companies be willing to develop customized drugs that serve only a small portion of the population?

12.5.4 *Educating health care providers*

Another issue with regard to patient-tailored drug is that the company needs to introduce multiple pharmacogenomics products to treat the same condition for different population subsets and that would certainly complicate the process of prescribing and dispensing drugs in the clinics and hospitals. Additionally, doctors or physicians will have to take an extra diagnostic step to determine which drug is best appropriate for each patient. Furthermore, to interpret the diagnostic data accurately, each patient will need a better understanding of genetics.

12.6 *Predictive medicine*

Over the past few years, predictive medicine has been the most rapidly emerging field of health science, which involves predicting disease to either prevent the disease altogether or significantly decrease its impact upon patient mortality. Although different diagnostic methods exist, which are based on genomics and proteomics techniques, the most important way to predict future disease is based on the genetics. Moreover, proteomics-based techniques can allow for an early detection of disease, and most of the time those detect biological markers that happen because a disease process has already started. Inclusive genetic testing by using DNA arrays or genome sequencing allows the estimation of disease risk several years before any disease even happens. Furthermore, persons who are more vulnerable to disease in the future can be advised to alter his/her lifestyle with an aim to prevent the predicted illness. Interestingly, modern genetic testing techniques supported by the physicians discourage predictive genetic testing of minors and infant until they reach adult age to understand the significance of genetic screening. Genetic screening of newborns or children in the field of predictive medicine is thought appropriate if there is a convincing clinical intention to do so, such as the availability of prevention or treatment as a child that would prevent future disease.

12.6.1 *Benefits of predictive medicine*

There are several benefits of predictive medicine, for example, with the help of predictive medicine, it is possible for physicians to be proactive in introducing lifestyle modifications to minimize the risk of developing some diseases. Moreover, predictive medicine is envisioned not for patients but more so for healthy persons, its purpose being to decide whether susceptibility to a particular disease is increased or not in a healthy person. More recently, an incredible number of research studies have been published in scientific literature that shows associations between specific genetic variants in a person's genetic code and a specific disease. These studies have found that a female individual with a mutation in the "BRCA1" gene has a 65% higher risk of developing breast cancer. Genetic diagnostic testing is already generating income for BRCA1 and BRCA2 gene examination.

Unlike many preventive interventions, prophetic medicine is conducted on an individualized basis. For instance, glaucoma is a monogenetic disease whose early detection can allow preventing permanent loss of vision. Predictive medicine is expected to be most effective when applied to polygeneric multifactorial disease such as diabetes mellitus, hypertension, and myocardial infarction. Furthermore, predictive diagnostics such as genetic screens can help to diagnose inherited genetic disease caused by problems with a single gene such as cystic fibrosis. It can help in early treatment and some types of cancer and heart disease that can be inherited as single gene diseases. Some people in these high-risk families may also benefit from access to genetic tests. In the future, as more and more genes related to increased vulnerability to certain diseases are reported, predictive medicine can become more useful and successful. It has been reported that direct-to-consumer genetic testing allows a consumer to screen his or her own genes without the need to go through a physician. Various other benefits associated with predictive medicine are described in brief.

12.6.1.1 *Newborn screening*

Newborn screening is done just after birth to identify any genetic disorders or defects that can be treated early in life. This newborn screening for certain genetic disorders is one of the most widespread uses of genetic screening for phenylketonuria and congenital hypothyroidism conditions. Furthermore, in the United States and other countries, it becomes mandatory to collect a blood from a newborn baby to perform genetic screening.

12.6.1.2 *Diagnostic testing*

The use of predictive approach improves the specificity of diagnosis or detection of a disease. Moreover, it is frequently used to confirm a particular diagnosis when some condition is based on the patient's genetic mutations and physical symptoms.

12.6.1.3 *Medical bioinformatics*

Medical bioinformatics involves determining individual cell and molecular parameters by using cytomics and single-cell-based microarrays. This information can be used by a bioinformatician to analyze the genetic data using computer-assisted identification and characterization of a particular populations or gene clusters of interest.

12.6.1.4 *Prenatal testing*

Many governmental agencies are now recommending mandatory prenatal tests for all pregnant mothers and the information gained from this test can be used to identify genetic diseases in a fetus before it is born. Furthermore, this prenatal testing is offered for couples who have an increased risk of having a baby with genetic or chromosomal abnormalities. One of the technical issues about screening method that has raised concern is to also identify the sex of the fetus before its born and that sex determination before birth is considered to be unlawful in many countries, because a lot of female infanticides is reported in many countries around the world after obtaining the information of sex determination. Furthermore, prenatal testing can aid a couple to decide whether to abort the pregnancy or not. Corresponding to diagnostic testing, prenatal testing can be noninvasive. This noninvasive technique includes examinations of the mother's womb through ultrasonography or maternal serum screens. Furthermore, these noninvasive techniques can evaluate the risk of a condition, but cannot determine with surety if the fetus has some problems, so that it has been recommended to go for invasive prenatal methods that are somewhat more dangerous for the fetus and involve needles being introduced into the placenta for sampling purposes.

12.6.1.5 Genetic disease carrier testing

To find out whether some genetic-disease-prone individuals can develop the disease in the later part of their life; the carrier testing can be done to identify people who carry one copy of a gene of mutation that, when present in two copies, causes a genetic disorder. Moreover, this type of testing is offered to individuals who have a genetic disorder in their family history with greater possibility of certain genetic diseases. Henceforth, both parents can be tested to find out about a couple having a risk of having a child with a genetic disorder.

12.6.2 Limitations of predictive medicine

Interestingly, having the faulty gene still does not necessarily mean someone will contract the disease. The diseases can happen not only due to genetic difficulties but due to external causes such as lifestyle and environment so therefore, genes are not perfect interpreters of the future health of an individual and it has been reported that individuals with both high-risk form of the gene and those without, are all candidates to get the disease in different stages of life. There are multiple environmental factors such as diet, exercise, infection, and pollution that can lead to the development of genetic disease. Additionally, the potential incorrect positives or incorrect negatives that may arise from a predictive genetic screen can cause substantial redundant strain on the individual patients. In addition, there is another potential downfall of commercially available genetic testing which can cause psychological and emotional reactions. One of the key parts of genetic treatment is to deliver counseling to all patients; however, adequate individual counseling cannot be possible for a large proportion of the population having a high risk of common complex diseases. Furthermore, some patients are susceptible to adverse psychological reactions to genetic predictions of fears such as cancer or mental illness.

12.6.3 Ethical issues associated with predictive medicine

Like other medical treatment, the predictive medicines do have some legal and ethical issues. There are several organizations that believe that information pertaining to predictive genetic tests can be used to decide who gets an insurance or a job. Moreover, the consequences for patients with respect to health insurance and employment are also of the utmost importance, which may result into stigma and discrimination in the workplace. Furthermore, in the future, there is the possibility that it may be mandatory for persons to reveal his/her genetic information about his/her health to their employers or health insurance companies. It has been cautioned that the unattractive prospect of discrimination based on a person's genetic makeup can lead to a genetic outcry, which does not receive equal opportunity for insurance and employment. Presently, in the United States, health insurance companies do not require applicants (patients) for coverage to undergo genetic testing as the genetic information of an individual is under the same protection of confidentiality as other medical health care sectors. Interestingly, Genetic Information Non-Discrimination Act, signed in 2008, which in fact prohibits health insurance companies from rejecting coverage or charging differentials in premiums, and bars employers from making job placement or hiring decisions based on the person's genetic profile.

12.7 Summary

Confrontational or ADRs are one of the most serious problems of current drug therapy and it has been reported that ADRs cause serious illness in millions of patients across the world and 100,000 patients lost their lives because of ADRs in the United States alone. At present, there is no method to determine whether people will respond well, badly, or not at all to a drug treatment, so therefore, pharmaceutical companies have been developing drugs by using a one-size-fit for all patients. Moreover, the current drug therapy allows the development of drugs that only an average patient can respond; nonetheless, the statistics suggests that one size does not fit all, and infrequently gives devastating results and side effects. Henceforth, it is important to have a system where the drug can be properly checked and verified based on individual requirement and needs, the study of the drug response on an individual's genetic makeup is called pharmacogenomics. It has been suggested that pharmacogenomics is a branch of medical science that examines the inherited variations in genes that command drug response and explores the ways these variations can be used to predict whether an individual will have a good response to a drug, a bad response to a drug, or no response at all. In this chapter, we discussed the significance of pharmacogenomics, explained the difference between pharmacogenetics and pharmacogenomics, and described how this emerging field can really help pharmaceutical companies to make effective and safe drugs.

12.8 Knowledge builder

Pharmacogenomics: Pharmacogenomics is the technology that analyzes how the genetic makeup affects an individual's response to drugs. It deals with the influence of genetic variation on drug response in patients by correlating gene expression or SNPs with a drug's efficacy or toxicity. By doing so, pharmacogenomics aims to develop a rational means to optimize drug therapy, with respect to the patients' genotype, to ensure maximum efficacy with minimal adverse effects.

Drug screening: The method by which a drug candidate is tested on the animals or cells or tissue to check their effectiveness or any toxicological effect is called drug screening.

G-protein-coupled receptors: GPCRs, also known as seven-transmembrane domain receptors, 7TM receptors, heptahelical receptors, serpentine receptor, and G protein-linked receptors, constitute a large protein family of receptors that senses molecules outside the cell and activates inside signal transduction pathways and, ultimately, cellular responses. They are called transmembrane receptors because they pass through the cell membrane, and they are called seven-transmembrane receptors because they pass through the cell membrane seven times.

Bioinformatics: Bioinformatics is an interdisciplinary field that develops and improves the methods for storing, retrieving, organizing, and analyzing biological data. A major activity in bioinformatics is to develop software tools to generate useful biological knowledge. Bioinformatics has become an important part of many areas of biology. In experimental molecular biology, bioinformatics techniques such as image and signal processing allow extraction of useful results from large amounts of raw data. In the field of genetics and genomics, bioinformatics uses many areas of computer science, mathematics, and engineering to process biological data. Complex machines are used to read biological data at a much faster rate than before. Databases and information systems are used to store and organize biological data.

PAMPA testing: PAMPA (parallel artificial membrane permeability assay) is a method that determines the permeability of substances from a donor compartment, through a lipid-infused artificial membrane into an acceptor compartment. A multiwell microtiter plate is used for the donor and a membrane/acceptor compartment is placed on top; the whole assembly is commonly referred to as a "sandwich." At the beginning of the test, the drug is added to the donor compartment, and the acceptor compartment is drug-free.

Caco-2 testing: Caco-2 permeability assay uses an established method for predicting the *in vivo* absorption of drugs across the gut wall by measuring the rate of transport of a compound across the Caco-2 cell line. The Caco-2 cell line is derived from a human colon carcinoma. The cells have characteristics that resemble intestinal epithelial cells such as the formation of a polarized monolayer, well-defined brush border on the apical surface, and intracellular junctions.

Pharmacokinetics: Pharmacokinetics, sometimes abbreviated as PK, is a branch of pharmacology dedicated to the determination of the fate of substances administered externally to a living organism. The substances of interest include pharmaceutical agents, hormones, nutrients, and toxins. Pharmacokinetics describes how the body affects a specific drug after administration through the mechanisms of absorption and distribution, as well as the chemical changes of the substance in the body.

Safety profile of the drug: The process by which a drug candidate is tested to study its effects on the body tissues, function, and physiology is called the safety profile of the drug and clinical trial Phase 1 is the time when the drug safety profile is checked and evaluated.

Pharmacovigilance: Pharmacovigilance (abbreviated PV or PhV), also known as drug safety, is the pharmacological science relating to the collection, detection, assessment, monitoring, and prevention of adverse effects with pharmaceutical products.

BRCA1: BRCA1 is a human caretaker gene that produces a protein called breast cancer type 1 susceptibility protein, responsible for repairing DNA. BRCA1 is expressed in the cells of breast and other tissues, where it helps repair damaged DNA, or destroy cells if the DNA cannot be repaired. If BRCA1 is damaged, the damaged DNA is not repaired properly and this increases the risk for cancers.

BRCA2: BRCA2 (breast cancer type 2 susceptibility protein) is a protein found inside cells. In humans, it is encoded by the gene BRCA2. BRCA2 belongs to the tumor suppressor gene family, and orthologs have been identified in most mammals for which complete genome data are available. The protein encoded by this gene is involved in the repair of chromosomal damage with an important role in the error-free repair of DNA double strand breaks.

Cytomics: Cytomics is the study of cell systems (cytomes) at a single cell level. It combines all the bioinformatic knowledge to attempt to understand the molecular architecture and functionality of the cell system (cytome). Much of this is achieved by using molecular and microscopic techniques that allow the various components of a cell to be visualized as they interact *in vivo*.

Microarray: A microarray is a multiplex lab-on-a-chip. It is a 2D array on a solid substrate (usually a glass slide or silicon thin-film cell) that assays large amounts of biological material using HTS methods. The concept and methodology of microarrays was first introduced and illustrated in antibody microarrays (also referred to as antibody matrix) in 1983 in a scientific publication and a series of patents. As the "gene chip" industry started to grow in the 1990s, with the establishment of companies, such as Affymetrix, Illumina, and others, the technology of DNA microarrays has become more sophisticated and the most widely used.

Prenatal test: Prenatal diagnosis or prenatal screening is testing for diseases or conditions in a fetus or embryo before it is born. The aim is to detect birth defects such as neural tube defects, Down syndrome, chromosome abnormalities, genetic diseases, and other conditions, such as spina bifida, cleft palate, Tay Sachs disease, sickle cell anemia, thalassemia, cystic fibrosis, muscular dystrophy, and fragile X syndrome. Screening can also be used for prenatal sex discernment. Common testing procedures include amniocentesis, ultrasonography, including nuchal translucency ultrasound, serum marker testing, or genetic screening.

Predictive genetic test: Predictive testing is a form of genetic testing. It is also known as presymptomatic testing. These types of tests are used to detect gene mutations associated with disorders that appear after birth, often later in life. These tests can be helpful to people who have a family member with a genetic disorder, but who have no features of the disorder themselves at the time of testing. Predictive testing can identify mutations that increase a person's risk of developing disorders with a genetic basis, such as certain types of cancer. For example, an individual with a mutation in BRCA1 has a 65% cumulative risk of breast cancer. Presymptomatic testing can determine whether a person will develop a genetic disorder, such as hemochromatosis (an iron overload disorder), before any signs or symptoms appear. The results of predictive and presymptomatic testing can provide the information about a person's risk of developing a specific disorder and help with making decisions about medical care.

Adverse drug reaction: An ADR is an expression that describes harm associated with the use of medications at a normal dosage during normal use. ADRs may occur following a single dose or prolonged administration of a drug or result from the combination of two or more drugs. The meaning of this expression differs from the meaning of side effect, as this last expression might also imply that the effects can be beneficial.

Further reading

Adams C and Brantner V 2006. Estimating the cost of new drug development: Is it really 802 million dollars? *Health Aff (Millwood)* 25(2): 420–428. doi:10.1377/hlthaff.25.2.420. PMID 16522582.

Antoniou A, Pharoah PD, Narod S et al. 2003. Average risks of breast and ovarian cancer associated with BRCA1 or BRCA2 mutations detected in case series unselected for family history: A combined analysis of 22 studies. *Am J Hum Genet* 72(5): 1117–1130. doi:10.1086/375033. PMC 1180265. PMID 12677558. http://linkinghub.elsevier.com/retrieve/pii/S0002-9297(07)60640-5.

Baird P 2001. The Human Genome Project, genetics and health. *Commun Genet* 4(2): 77–80. doi:10.1159/000051161. PMID 12751482. http://content.karger.com/produktedb/produkte.asp?DOI=CMG2001004002077&typ=pdf.

Borry P, Evers-Kiebooms G, Cornel MC, Clarke A, and Dierickx K 2009. Genetic testing in asymptomatic minors: Background considerations towards ESHG Recommendations. *Eur J Hum Genet* 17(6): 711–719. doi:10.1038/ejhg.2009.25. PMC 2947094. PMID 19277061. http://www.pubmedcentral.nih.gov/articlerender.fcgi?tool=pmcentrez&artid=2947094.

Cheraskin E, Ringsdorf WM, Setyaadmadja AT, and Barrett RA 1967. Biochemical profile in predictive medicine. *Biomed Sci Instrum* 3: 3–15. PMID 5582616.

Dausset J 1997. Predictive medicine and its ethics (in French). *Pathol Biol* 45(3): 199–204. PMID 9296063.

DiMasi J 2002. The value of improving the productivity of the drug development process: Faster times and better decisions. *Pharmacoeconomics* 20 (Suppl 3): 1–10. PMID 12457421.

DiMasi J, Hansen R, and Grabowski H 2003. The price of innovation: New estimates of drug development costs. *J Health Econ* 22(2): 151–185. doi: 10.1016/S0167-6296 (02)00126-1. PMID 12606142.

GeneWatch UK 2001. Genetic Testing in Insurance and Employment: A New Form of Discrimination. Briefing 15, June 2001.
Hodgson J and Marshall A 1998. Pharmacogenomics: Will the regulators approve? *Nat Biotechnol* 16: 243–246.
Lazarou J, Pomeranz BH, and Corey PN 1998. Incidence of adverse drug reactions in hospitalized patients: A meta-analysis of prospective studies. *JAMA* 279(15): 1200–1205.
Marteau TM and Lerman C 2001. Genetic risk and behavioural change. *BMJ* 322(7293): 1056–1059. doi:10.1136/bmj.322.7293.1056. PMC 1120191. PMID 11325776. http://bmj.com/cgi/pmidlookup?view=long&pmid=11325776.
Redei GP 2003. *Encyclopedia Dictionary of Genetics, Genomics, and Proteomics* (2nd Edition). 1024 pp., UK: Wiley-Liss.
Schulte PA, Lomax GP, Ward EM, and Colligan MJ 1999. Ethical issues in the use of genetic markers in occupational epidemiologic research. *J Occup Environ Med* 41(8): 639–646. doi:10.1097/00043764-199908000-00005. PMID 10457506. http://meta.wkhealth.com/pt/pt-core/template-journal/lwwgateway/media/landingpage.htm?issn=1076-2752&volume=41&issue=8&spage=639.
Valet GK and Tarnok A 2003. Cytomics in predictive medicine. *Cytometry B Clin Cytom* 53(1): 1–3. doi:10.1002/cyto.b.10035. PMID 12717684.
Vineis P, Schulte P, and McMichael AJ 2001. Misconceptions about the use of genetic tests in populations. *Lancet* 357(9257): 709–712. doi:10.1016/S0140-6736(00)04136-2. PMID 11247571. http://linkinghub.elsevier.com/retrieve/pii/S0140-6736(00)04136-2.
Weber TB 1967. Instrumentation and prospects for predictive medicine. *Biomed Sci Instrum* 3: 55–61. PMID 5582617.

chapter thirteen

Bioethics

13.1 Introduction

Bioethical issues have been debated since ancient times, and public attention has always been present for the use of human in any kind of medical research. It all started with regulatory agencies that have asked the drug manufacturing companies to test the drug first in both animals and humans before marketing the drugs. The use of humans in clinical trials has been the main criteria to obtain approval from US FDA. Ethical people are concerned about the extensive use of humans in such biomedical research and drug trials, which may cause some physical, mental, emotional, and genetic disabilities related to the drug tested upon them.

13.2 Bioethics in historical perspective

The field of bioethics has addressed a broad band of human investigation, extending from debates over the boundaries of life such as abortion or euthanasia. Moreover, bioethicists often disagree among themselves over the accuracy limits of their discipline, debating whether the field should concern itself with the ethical evaluation of all questions involving biology and medicine. Interestingly, some bioethicists are considering only the morality of medical treatments or technological innovations, and the timing of medical treatment of humans rather than other aspects. It all started with the formation of a code of ethics written by the physician Thomas Percival in the eighteenth century. It provided a foundation for the first code of ethics, established in 1846 by the American Medical Association, and the Nuremberg Code for research ethics on human subjects, which was established during the war crime trials at the close of World War II. Later on, the advent of new medical technologies further complicated the moral and societal issues related to biomedical research and medical practice. The efforts are being made to better evaluate biomedical research ethics. One system developed in the late 1970s by Tom Beauchamp and James Childress is known as principlism, or the four principles approach. This system works by considering the importance of four separate elements: (1) respecting individuals' autonomy and their right to their own decisions and beliefs; (2) the principle of beneficence, with helping people as the primary goal; (3) the related principle of nonmaleficence, or refraining from harming people; and (4) justice, or distributing burdens and benefits fairly (Figure 13.1).

The roots of bioethics is associated with the field of philosophy, but today's bioethics requires collaboration among many additional areas of study, which include pharmaceuticals, law, medicine, stem cell research, biotechnology, politics, sociology, genetics, environmental toxicology, and public health. Interestingly, bioethical quandaries, once occasional, now are commonplace, in part because new medical technologies have overtaken our ability to understand their repercussions. Conventionally, bioethicists are known to deal with difficult medical decisions, but their role has stretched with the explosion of knowledge in the fields of genetics and biotechnology. Ethical decisions are required for issues as diverse as human cloning, the use of human embryonic stem cells, and the genetic-engineered crops. Recent growth in the fields of biomedical, bioengineering, and biotechnology

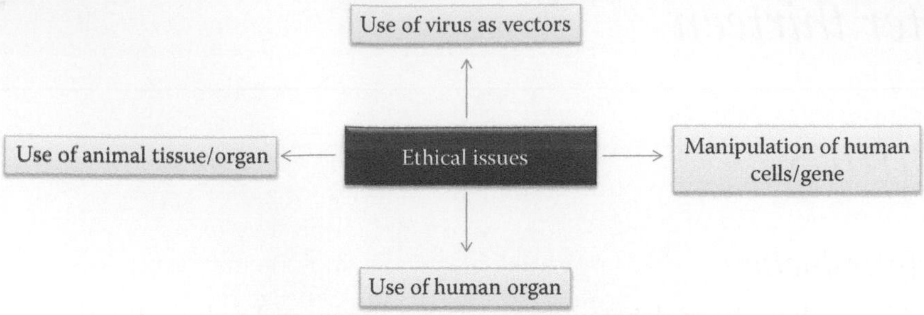

Figure 13.1 Implications of ethical issues on medical health care.

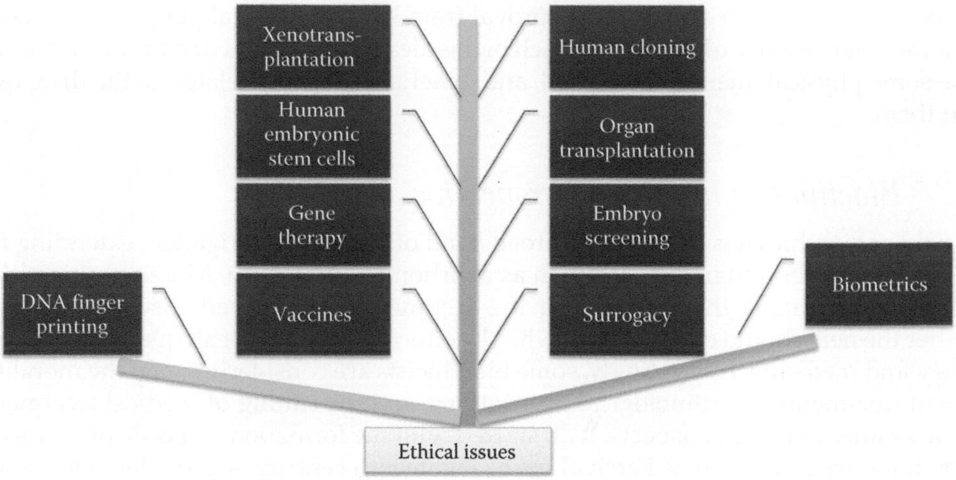

Figure 13.2 Major ethical issues of modern times.

research has created an unparalleled need for our society to oppose the new and challenging ethical implications that arise. Moreover, it has been suggested that bioethics consists of identifying emerging moral issues related to human health and biological systems and analyzing them according to the principles determined by the value system of the community. The ethical issues kept haunting the health care and biotechnology industries over the last few decades, which resulted in the involvement of both private and government sectors and is debated in both public and congressional levels. Some of the major issues as shown in Figure 13.2 are considered major bioethical concerns affecting the diagnostics and treatment developments.

13.3 Human cloning

Human cloning is the creation of a genetically identical copy of a human by using genetic tools and it does not follow the natural process of fertilization and birth. The ethics of cloning is an extremely controversial issue in the present scenario (the term "cloning" is generally used to refer to artificial human cloning). There are two types of human cloning: therapeutic cloning and reproductive cloning. Therapeutic cloning involves cloning cells from an adult for use in medicine and is an active area of research, whereas reproductive cloning is involved in making cloned humans. Interestingly, such reproductive cloning has not been performed or attempted so far and is illegal in many countries around the world. A third type of cloning, which is called as replacement cloning, is a theoretical possibility, though not much research has been conducted in this field, and can be a combination of therapeutic and reproductive cloning. Furthermore, replacement cloning would involve the replacement of comprehensively damaged, dysfunctional body parts through transplantation.

Those who profess human therapeutic cloning believe that genetically identical cells could be used to treat various diseases and conditions. It is expected that such bioengineered cells, tissues, and organs will neither trigger an immune response nor require the use of immunosuppressive drugs. In contrast to this, it has been argued that children cloned for therapeutic purposes such as to donate bone marrow to a sibling with leukemia might someday be viewed as heroes. It has also been suggested that human cloning might prevent the human aging process. Furthermore, human cloning also raises implications of a social-ethical nature, particularly concerning the role of that cloning might play in changing the shape of the family structure by complicating the kinship relationships. For instance, a female DNA donor would be the clone's genetic donor, rather than the mother, complicating the genetic and social relationships between mother and child as well as the relationships between other family members and the clone. Therefore, various laws have been crafted to deal with bioethical considerations.

13.3.1 Government response

13.3.1.1 United Nations

The United Nations General Assembly has elaborated an international convention against the reproductive cloning of humans. Moreover, a broad coalition of countries including Italy, Philippines, Spain, the United States, and Costa Rica wanted to extend the debate to ban all forms of human cloning. Furthermore, Costa Rica proposed the adoption of an international convention to ban all forms of human cloning. Finally, after having an extensive debate and discussion, nonbinding countries of the United Nations Declaration on human cloning called for the ban on all forms of human cloning.

13.3.1.2 Australia

In recent years, Australia had also prohibited the development of human cloning, but had brought a bill that legalized therapeutic cloning, creation of human embryos for stem cell research made its way through the House of Representatives and within certain regulatory restrictions, therapeutic cloning is now legal in some parts of Australia.

13.3.1.3 European Union

It has been reported that the European Convention on Human Rights and Biomedicine prohibits human cloning in one of its additional protocols, but this protocol has been sanctioned only by Spain, Greece, and Spain. Furthermore, the charter is legally binding for the institutions of the European Union under the Treaty of Lisbon.

13.3.1.4 United States of America

In the United States, a bill [HR 4808, 2010] was introduced by a section banning federal funding for human cloning and such law shall not prevent research work that is going on in private institutions such as universities that have both private and federal funding. There are currently no federal laws in the United States that ban cloning completely.

Furthermore, about 13 American states have already banned reproductive cloning and three states prohibits the use of public funds for such research.

13.3.1.5 *United Kingdom*

The British government also passed "The Human Fertilization and Embryology Regulations" in 2001 to alter the "Human Fertilization and Embryology Act" of 1990 by extending permissible reasons for embryo research and to permit research around stem cells and cell nuclear replacement, which allow therapeutic cloning. However, in the same year 2001, a pro-life group won a legal battle, which struck down the regulation and effectively left all forms of cloning to be unregulated. The first license was granted in 2004 to researchers of the University of Newcastle, which allowed them to examine treatments for Parkinson's disease, diabetes, and Alzheimer's disease.

13.3.2 *Religious views*

In addition to legal issues, there are religious issues that are haunting the biomedical research and biomedical product development. For example, the Roman Catholic Church, under the papacy of Benedict (XVI) has condemned the practice of human cloning, stating that it signifies a serious misconduct to the dignity of that person as well as to the fundamental equality of all people. Similarly, Islam has also forbidden human cloning and the Islamic Fiqh Academy, in its 10th Conference chronicles, which was convened in Saudi Arabia in the year 1997, had issued a Fatwa (a religious decree) stating that human cloning is prohibited.

13.4 *Organ transplantation*

Over the last few decades, there has been a tremendous demand of human organs worldwide to save the lives of millions of patients. Organ donation is basically the donation of biological tissue from a living or deceased person to a living recipient. The organs that need to be transplanted can be removed in a surgical procedure following a determination, based on the donor's medical and social history, which are suitable for transplantation. The transplantation of organs from one human to another human is called allotransplantation, whereas the transplantation of organs from animal to human is called xenotransplantation. Over the past couple of decades, organ donation has become an important bioethical issue from a social perspective as well. Though most developed countries have a legal system for organ transplantation, the fact remains that the demand far exceeds the supply and the human organ issues are considered to be highly controversial by many ethical experts. Furthermore, organ transplantation will exploit those humans who are in desperate need for money and they will sell their organs for monetary gains. On the other hand, some believe that human organ transplantation is morally preferable to death; one can save the life of a fellow citizen by donating the organs.

Surveys conducted among living donors who had donated their organs have shown extreme guilt in a majority of the donors; additionally, many study participants reported that their economic condition has worsened ever since they donated the organs. In most of the country, the transplantation of kidneys is permissible as per the law, which has really caused the creation of the black market for organs. Bioethical experts cautioned that such kind of market to sell human organs for the sake of monetary gains would encourage offenders by making it easier for them to claim that their stolen organs were legal.

On the other hand, it has been recommended that legalization of the international organ trade could lead to increased supply, lowering prices so that persons outside the developed countries could also afford such organs as well. There could be serious exploitation of donors as the donor would agree to donate the organs without undergoing physical examination by the trained doctors. There is also the possibility that the donors are not paid enough for the organ. It has been reported that the city of Chennai, India, has one of the largest black markets for organ sale with organ selling price starts with little over $1000.

13.4.1 Sociopolitical reasons

A healthy and normal human has two kidneys. It has been reported that humans can survive with only one kidney and the one kidney can be donated to someone who needs it. A kidney can be transplanted to close relatives, but other people can also benefit. The lowest type of donation is the direction donation whereby a donor gives a kidney to a stranger. In recent times, searching for donors using the Internet has also become a way to find lifesaving organs. But Internet advertising for organs is a highly controversial practice, as some scholars consider it undercuts the traditional list-based allocation system. Moreover, the Spanish transplant system is one of the most successful in the world, but it still cannot meet the demand, as 10% of those needing a transplant die while still on the transplant list. As per Spanish law, every cadaver can provide organs unless the dead person particularly rejected it, because family members still can prohibit the donation. Moreover, in the majority of cases, organ donation is not possible for reasons of recipient safety, HLA match failures, or clinically the organ condition is not good.

13.4.2 Religious understanding

All major religions of the world including Christianity and Islam accept organ donation and among Christians, the Roman Catholic Church also supports organ donation on the basis that it constitutes an act of charity and provides a means of saving a life. Some religions impose certain restrictions on the types of organs that may be donated and/or on the means by which organs may be harvested and/or transplanted. For example, Jehovah's Witnesses require that organs be drained of any blood due to their interpretation of the Hebrew Bible or Christian Old Testament as prohibiting blood transfusion, and Muslims require that the donor have provided written consent in advance. Moreover, few groups dislike organ transplantation or donation; in particular the Shinto and those who follow the customs of the Gypsies, whereas Orthodox Judaism considers organ donation obligatory if it will save a life and the donor is considered dead as defined by Jewish law. Furthermore, in both Orthodox Judaism and non-Orthodox Judaism religion, the mainstream view holds that organ donation is allowable in the case of permanent cardiac rhythm cessation.

13.5 Embryo screening

Another field that gets lots of attention is the embryo screening to know more about the genetic makeup of the fetus. In medicine field, preimplantation genetic diagnosis (PIGD), also known as embryo screening, denotes procedures that are performed on embryos prior to implantation, occasionally even on sites prior to fertilization. It has been reported that PIGD is considered another way to prenatal diagnosis; its main advantage is that it avoids selective pregnancy termination. Furthermore, PIGD is basically an assistant to reproductive technology and requires *in vitro* fertilization to obtain oocytes or embryos for evaluation. Moreover, the word preimplantation genetic screening is used to signify procedures that do not look for a specific disease, but use PIGD techniques to identify embryos at threat. PIGD is always misunderstood with the diagnosis, because in medication to diagnose means to identify an illness or determine its cause. Moreover, as an oocyte or early-stage embryo has no symptoms of disease, PIGD cannot be considered a diagnostic tool.

In spite of having various attributes, PIGD has raised ethical issues as this technique can be used to determine the gender of the embryo, and thus can be used to differentiate male and female fetuses. Though PIGD is a controversial procedure, this approach is less destructive than fetal deselection during pregnancy. Furthermore, PIGD has the prospective to screen for genetic issues unrelated to medical requirements and there is also the possibility of a designer baby by using the PIGD technique. Religious organizations have already disapproved this procedure.

13.6 Xenotransplantation

The transplantation of living cells, tissues, or organs from one species to another, such as from pigs to humans is called xenotransplantation. Moreover, such kinds of cells, tissues, or organs are called xenografts or xenotransplants. Recent advances in the field have brought science to a stage where it is sensible to consider that organs from other species (sheep or goat) may soon be engineered to minimize the risk of rejection and used as an alternative to human tissues, possibly ending organ scarcities in the near future. The cells derived from other species like animals could be used to treat life-threatening and devastating illnesses such as diabetes, liver failure, cancer, and Parkinson's disease. The xenotransplants could save the life of thousands of patients who are awaiting organ donation worldwide.

Moreover, the organs from a pig or baboon could be genetically altered with human genes to pretend a patient's immune system into accepting it as a part of its own body. Similarly, xenotransplantation of ovarian tissue into immunodeficient nude mice is already used in research to study the development of ovarian follicles. It has been reported that mature follicles can be developed, and both host and graft vessels can contribute to the revascularization of xenografted human ovarian tissue in mice. Besides having so many beneficial applications of xenotransplantation, this procedure is also considered a controversial procedure because religious groups considered transplanting animal organ inside human body might create unwarranted social implications.

13.7 Human embryonic stem cells

The human embryonic stem cells are the most talked about, discussed, and debated topic both in published forums and in the government. As the name suggests, human embryonic stem cells are a novel type of cells that can be derived from embryos and most embryonic stem cells are derived from embryos donated by patients for research purposes with informed consent of the donors. There are many applications of human embryonic stem cells as studies of human embryonic stem cells can yield information about the complex events that occur during human development. The human embryonic stem cells are basically pluripotent stem cells, which means these cells can be differentiated into all types of body cells and organs. With the help of *in vitro* cell culture, it is now possible to grow human embryonic stem cell in the laboratory and these stem cells can be stored for a long period of time. These embryonic stem cells can be used to treat various diseases. In addition, some of the most serious medical conditions, such as cancer and natal deficiencies, are due to abnormal cell division and differentiation, they can also be diagnosed by studying the stem cells. Conceivably, the most important potential application of human stem cells is the derivation of cells and tissues that could be used for cell-based therapies.

Donated organs and tissues are frequently used to replace ailing or damaged tissue. These stem cells can be differentiated into specific cell types and offer the possibility of a renewable source of replacement cells and tissues to treat diseases, including spinal cord injury, stroke, burns, heart disease, Alzheimer's diseases, diabetes, osteoarthritis, and rheumatoid arthritis. Besides having so many applications, human embryonic stem cell raises some ethical issues and the fundamental proclamation of those who oppose embryonic stem cell research is the belief that human life is sacred. Combined with the fact that human life begins when a sperm cell fertilizes an egg cell to form a single cell, yet an embryo is only human once it has developed cells that perform human functions. The ethical experts believe the generation of human embryonic stem cells would escalate the killing of human embryos for monetary reasons and will have serious implications on the social structure and human dignity.

13.8 Gene therapy

Human genes are located on chromosomes and these genes carry specific sequences of bases that encode instructions on how to make proteins so that the body functions properly. Although genes get a lot of attention, it is the proteins that execute most body functions and even make up the majority of cellular structures. Once genes are altered so that the encoded proteins are unable to carry out their normal functions, genetic disorders can result. Furthermore, genetic alteration can be corrected by gene therapy, which is basically the insertion, alteration, or removal of genes within an individual's cells and biological tissues to treat disease. It is a technique for correcting defective genes that are responsible for disease development. In general form, the gene therapy involves the insertion of functional genes into an unspecified genomic location to substitute or an altered gene, but other forms of gene therapy involve direct correction of the mutation that enables a viral infection.

Since gene therapy involves making changes to the body's set of basic instructions, it raises many unique ethical concerns. Interestingly, public debate over the ethics of using gene technology to treat human beings fumed when recombinant DNA research began in the 1960s. The viewpoint of altering human gene what many noticed as the blueprint of human life raised questions about tampering with God's creation. Whereas some had hopes of eliminating virtually all disease, others saw the specter of eugenics and catastrophic unintended consequences. Furthermore, there was something unique, something ground breaking about this new science and technology. Progressively, the debate moved from general philosophical and theological echo to attempt to develop a practical review process for research protocols. Many felt that somatic (adult) cell gene therapy is purely an extension of conventional therapies, posing few if any new ethical problems. Another more serious issue that has been raised is the use of the virus as a vector to transport the genetic materials, which is still considered to be an unsafe and unethical way to treat patients. Bioethical experts also cautioned that the viral vectors may also trigger viral-mediated diseases in humans.

13.9 Vaccines

Vaccines are considered to be some of the most powerful health care tools of this century as they are known to improve body immunity against a variety of diseases. In a general sense, a vaccine typically contains an agent that resembles a disease-causing microorganism in the body, and is often made from weakened or killed forms of the microbe or its toxins. Furthermore, this agent stimulates the body's immune system to recognize the agent as foreign, destroy it, and recall it, so that the immune system can more easily recognize and destroy any of these microbes that later come across. In spite of high use of vaccines, there are technical and ethical issues associated with the concept of vaccines and their benefits. For example, more and more vaccines are coming on the market; the opposition to vaccines has also increased. Bioethical experts claim that vaccines do not work, that they are or may be dangerous, that individuals should trust on individual hygiene instead, and also suggested that mandatory vaccinations violate individual rights or religious principles. However, these arguments have succeeded in reducing vaccination rates in a few communities, leading to increased eruptions of preventable, and sometimes fatal, childhood illnesses.

Furthermore, vaccines can cause side effects, and the success of immunization programs are based on public self-confidence. Vaccination has been opposed on religious grounds ever since it was introduced. Moreover, some vaccines are derived from tissues taken from therapeutic abortions performed in the 1960s, leading to moral questions. Furthermore, the American Chiropractic Association and the International Chiropractic Association support individual exemptions to compulsory vaccination laws, and in a survey conducted in the US, chiropractors found that there was no scientific proof that immunization prevents disease. Moreover, critics have indicted the vaccine industry of distorting the safety and efficiency of vaccines, covering up and suppressing information, and influencing health policy decisions for financial gain.

13.10 DNA fingerprinting

The chemical structure of everyone's DNA is the same and the only difference between people is the order of the basepairs. It has been reported that there are millions of base pairs in each person's DNA that every person has a different sequence. By using these sequences, every person could be identified solely by the sequence of their base pairs. Still, here are so many millions of base pairs; the task would be very daunting. DNA fingerprinting is one of the best ways to solve questions of human identity. It has been reported that everyone has a particular DNA structure, which is as distinctive as an actual fingerprint and can have amazing accuracy. Nevertheless, issues concerning the pros and cons of DNA fingerprinting have been argued about for some time. Moreover, DNA fingerprinting is also known as genetic fingerprinting and can pinpoint a person's unique DNA structure. DNA genetic fingerprinting is an identifying method popularly used in forensics, medicine, and paternity testing.

There are many ethical issues associated with DNA fingerprinting. It has been argued that DNA is a blueprint of the makeup of one's body, and it is not correct to keep such sensitive material on file as discrimination could occur in many forms. Moreover, people can be rejected from certain health care if his DNA reveals something about him. Another issue is it's an individual's choice to undergo genetic fingerprinting. For example, if a child has his DNA fingerprinted during his youth, he may not want such information on file once he is an adult. DNA fingerprinting is not necessary in the cognizance of many who think basic fingerprinting works with great accuracy.

13.11 Biometrics

Biometrics are automated methods of recognizing a person based on an anatomical or structural characteristic, which include face, fingerprints, hand geometry, handwriting, iris, retinal, vein, voice, and so on. Over the last few years, biometric technologies are becoming the foundation of a widespread array of highly secure identification and personal verification solutions. Moreover, biometric-based solutions are able to provide confidential financial transactions and personal data privacy within seconds. Nowadays, you may find biometrics machines in all offices of federal, state, and local governments to control attendance. A variety of ethical concerns with biometric identification methods has been registered by users such as (i) some biometric identification methods are relatively invasive (like retina scans); (ii) the gathering of biometric information like fingerprints is associated with criminal behavior in the minds of many people; (iii) traditionally, detailed biometric information has been gathered by large institutions, like the military or police; people may feel a loss of privacy or personal dignity; (iv) people feel embarrassed when rejected by a public sensor; and (v) automated face recognition in public places could be used to track everyone's movements without their knowledge or consent. There are also many questions about how these data are stored and used and various issues associated with biometrics that need to be resolved ethically as well as technically.

13.12 Nanomedicine

There are various benefits of nanoparticles and nanomaterials especially in water purification systems, energy systems, physical enhancement, nanomedicine, better food production and nutrition, and large-scale infrastructure auto-fabrication. In spite of all these benefits, there are several issues that are associated with nanomaterials and their products that need to be resolved. It has been suggested the use of nanomaterials may cause health problems in humans, as the dust of nanomaterials can enter the human body through the skin and respiratory tract, which can cause irritation, inflammation, and severe health problems.

13.13 Summary

Bioethics, in general form, is a science to ensure that any type of technology or treatment does not cause any harm to any form of life, especially to animals and humans. This field is multidisciplinary that extends far beyond the scopes of health care and medical ethics. It includes a wide range of ethical problems associated with life sciences, which include cloning and genetics, theories of human development, and behavioral psychology. It has been reported that the rapid developments in the field of biomedical technology and biomedical research have caused the ethical to be more proactive as they fear too much technological manipulation may affect the human body and its environment. The field of bioethics has addressed a broad spectrum of human inquiry, ranging from human cloning, embryonic stem cell research, gene therapy, nanomedicine, xenotransplantation, and organ donation.

13.14 Scholar's achievement

Tom L. Beauchamp: Tom L. Beauchamp is an American philosopher specializing in moral philosophy, bioethics, and animal ethics. He is a professor of philosophy at Georgetown University, and a senior research scholar at the university's Kennedy Institute of Ethics.

Beauchamp is the author or coauthor of several books on ethics, and on the philosophy of David Hume, including *Hume and the Problem of Causation* (1981, with Alexander Rosenberg), *Principles of Biomedical Ethics* (1985, with James F. Childress), and *The Human Use of Animals* (1998, with F. Barbara Orlans et al.). He is the coeditor with R.G. Frey of *The Oxford Handbook of Animal Ethics* (2011). He is also the coeditor of the complete works of Hume, *The Critical Edition of the Works of David Hume* (1999), published by Oxford University Press.

James Franklin Childress: James Franklin Childress (born October 4, 1940) is a philosopher and theologian mainly concerned with ethics, particularly biomedical ethics. Currently, he is the John Allen Hollingsworth Professor of Ethics in the Department of Religious Studies at the University of Virginia. He is also a professor of medical education at this university and directs its Institute for Practical Ethics. He has obtained a BA from Guilford College, a BD from Yale Divinity School, and an MA and a PhD from Yale University. He was vice chair of the National Task Force on Organ Transplantation, and has also served on the board of directors of the United Network for Organ Sharing (UNOS), the UNOS Ethics Committee, the Recombinant DNA Advisory Committee, the Human Gene Therapy Subcommittee, the Biomedical Ethics Advisory Committee, and several Data and Safety Monitoring Boards for NIH clinical trials. From 1996 to 2001, he served on the presidentially appointed National Bioethics Advisory Commission. He is a fellow of the Hastings Center, an independent bioethics research institution.

13.15 Knowledge builder

USFDA: The Food and Drug Administration (FDA or USFDA) is an agency of the United States Department of Health and Human Services, one of the U.S. federal executive departments. The FDA is responsible for protecting and promoting public health through the regulation and supervision of food safety, tobacco products, dietary supplements, prescription and over-the-counter pharmaceutical drugs (medications), vaccines, biopharmaceuticals, blood transfusions, medical devices, electromagnetic radiation emitting devices (ERED), and veterinary products.

Euthanasia: Euthanasia refers to the practice of intentionally ending a life to relieve pain and suffering. Euthanasia is categorized in different ways, which include voluntary, nonvoluntary, or involuntary. Voluntary euthanasia is legal in some countries and the United States. Nonvoluntary euthanasia is illegal in all countries. Involuntary euthanasia is usually considered murder.

Therapeutic cloning: In genetics and developmental biology, somatic-cell nuclear transfer is a laboratory technique for creating a clone embryo with a donor nucleus (see the process below). It can be used in embryonic stem cell research, or, potentially, in regenerative medicine, where it is sometimes referred to as "therapeutic cloning." It can also be used as the first step in the process of reproductive cloning.

Reproductive cloning: Reproductive cloning is the production of a genetic duplicate of an existing organism. A human clone would be a genetic copy of an existing person. Somatic-cell nuclear transfer (SCNT) is the most common cloning technique. SCNT involves putting the nucleus of a body cell into an egg from which the nucleus has been removed. This produces a clonal embryo, which is triggered to begin developing with chemicals or electricity. Placing this cloned embryo into the uterus of a female animal and bringing it to term creates a clone, with genes identical to those of the animal from which the original body cell was taken.

Allotransplantation: Allotransplantation is the transplantation of cells, tissues, or organs, to a recipient from a genetically nonidentical donor of the same species. The transplant is called an allograft, allogeneic transplant, or homograft. Most human tissues and organ transplants are allografts.

Xenotransplantation: Xenotransplantation is the transplantation of living cells, tissues, or organs from one species to another. Such cells, tissues, or organs are called xenografts or xenotransplants. In contrast, the term "allotransplantation" refers to a same-species transplant. Human xenotransplantation offers a potential treatment for end-stage organ failure, a significant health problem in parts of the industrialized world. It also raises many novel medical, legal, and ethical issues. A continuing concern is that many animals, such as pigs, have shorter lifespan than humans, meaning that their tissues age at a quicker rate.

Further reading

Allen A 2007. Epilogue: Our best shots. *Vaccine: The Controversial Story of Medicine's Greatest Lifesafer.* New York: W. W. Norton & Company, Inc. pp. 421–42. ISBN 0-393-05911-1.

Allhoff F and Lin P 2008. *Nanotechnology & Society: Current and Emerging Ethical Issues.* Dordrecht: Springer.

Allhoff F, Lin P, Moor J, and Weckert J 2007. *Nanoethics: The Ethical and Societal Implications of Nanotechnology.* Hoboken: John Wiley & Sons.

Baylor N, Egan W, and Richman P 2002. Aluminum salts in vaccines. US perspective. *Vaccine* 20: S18–x20. doi:10.1016/S0264-410X(02)00166-4. PMID 12184360.

Bowman D and Fitzharris, M 2007. Too small for concern? Public health and nanotechnology. *Aust NZ J Public Health* 31(4): 382–384. doi:10.1111/j.1753-6405.2007.00092.x. PMID 17725022.

Bowman D and Hodge G 2006. Nanotechnology: Mapping the wild regulatory frontier. *Futures* 38(9): 1060–1073. doi:10.1016/j.futures.2006.02.017.

Bowman D and Hodge G 2007. A small matter of regulation: An international review of nanotechnology regulation. *Colum Sci Technol Law Rev* 8: 1–32.

Brain Death and Transplantation: The Japanese. *Medscape*. 2000-04-25. http://www.medscape.com/viewarticle/408769. Retrieved 2010-02-17.

Brown AS 2006. Prenatal infection as a risk factor for schizophrenia. *Schizophr Bull* 32(2): 200–202. doi:10.1093/schbul/sbj052. PMC 2632220. PMID 16469941. http://schizophreniabulletin.oxfordjournals.org/cgi/content/full/32/2/200.

Busse JW, Morgan L, and Campbell JB 2005. Chiropractic antivaccination arguments. *J Manipulative Physiol Ther* 28(5): 367–373. doi:10.1016/j.jmpt.2005.04.011. PMID 15965414. http://jmptonline.org/article/S0161-4754(05)00111-9/fulltext.

Busse JW, Wilson K, and Campbell JB 2008. Attitudes towards vaccination among chiropractic and naturopathic students. *Vaccine* 26(49): 6237–6242. doi:10.1016/j.vaccine.2008.07.020. PMID 18674581.

Campbell JB, Busse JW, and Injeyan HS 2000. Chiropractors and vaccination: A historical perspective. *Pediatrics* 105(4): e43. doi:10.1542/peds.105.4.e43. PMID 10742364. http://pediatrics.aappublications.org/cgi/content/full/105/4/e43.

Carson SA, Gentry WL, Smith AL, and Buster JE 1993. Trophectoderm microbiopsy in murine blastocysts: Comparison of four methods. *J Assist Reprod Genet* 10(6): 427–433. doi:10.1007/BF01228093. PMID 8019091.

Colgrove J and Bayer R 2005. Manifold restraints: Liberty, public health, and the legacy of Jacobson v Massachusetts. *Am J Public Health* 95(4): 571–576. doi:10.2105/AJPH.2004.055145. PMC 1449222. PMID 15798111. http://ajph.aphapublications.org/cgi/content/full/95/4/571.

Coutelle C, Williams C, Handyside A, Hardy K, Winston R, and Williamson R 1989. Genetic analysis of DNA from single human oocytes: A model for preimplantation diagnosis of cystic fibrosis. *BMJ* 299(6690): 22–24. doi:10.1136/bmj.299.6690.22. PMC 1837017. PMID 2503195. http://www.pubmedcentral.nih.gov/articlerender.fcgi?tool=pmcentrez&artid=1837017.

Deer B 2011. How the case against the MMR vaccine was fixed. *BMJ* 342: c5347. doi:10.1136/bmj.c5347. PMID 21209059. http://www.bmj.com/content/342/bmj.c5347.full.

Demko Z, Rabinowitz M, and Johnson D 2010. Current methods for preimplantation genetic diagnosis. *J Clin Embryol* 13(1): 6–12. http://www.genesecurity.net/wp-content/uploads/2010/04/Current-Methods-for-Preimplantation-Genetic-Diagnosis.pdf.

Edwards RG and Gardner RL 1967. Sexing of live rabbit blastocysts. *Nature* 214(5088): 576–577. doi:10.1038/214576a0. PMID 6036172.

Ernst E 2001. Rise in popularity of complementary and alternative medicine: Reasons and consequences for vaccination. *Vaccine* 20 (Suppl 1): S89–S93. doi:10.1016/S0264-410X(01)00290-0. PMID 11587822.

Fine PE and Clarkson JA 1986. Individual versus public priorities in the determination of optimal vaccination policies. *Am J Epidemiol* 124(6): 1012–1020. PMID 3096132.

Fiore AE, Shay DK, Haber P et al. 2007. Prevention and control of influenza: Recommendations of the Advisory Committee on Immunization Practices (ACIP), 2007. *MMWR Recomm Rep* 56(RR–6): 1–54. PMID 17625497. http://www.cdc.gov/mmwr/preview/mmwrhtml/rr5606a1.htm.

Freitas RA Jr. 2005. What is nanomedicine? *Nanomed: Nanotech Biol Med* 1(1): 2–9. doi:10.1016/j.nano.2004.11.003. PMID 17292052.

Gardner RL and Edwards RG 1968. Control of the sex ratio at full term in the rabbit by transferring sexed blastocysts. *Nature* 218(5139): 346–349. doi:10.1038/218346a0. PMID 5649672.

Gianaroli L, Magli MC, Ferraretti AP, and Munné S 1999. Preimplantation diagnosis for aneuploidies in patients undergoing *in vitro* fertilization with a poor prognosis: Identification of the categories for which it should be proposed. *Fertil Steril* 72(5): 837–844. doi:10.1016/S0015-0282(99)00377-5. PMID 10560987. http://linkinghub.elsevier.com/retrieve/pii/S0015-0282 (99)00377-5.

Godlee F, Smith J, and Marcovitch H 2011. Wakefield's article linking MMR vaccine and autism was fraudulent. *BMJ* 342: c7452: c7452. doi:10.1136/bmj.c7452. http://www.bmj.com/content/342/bmj.c7452.full.

Goyal M, Mehta RL, Schneiderman LJ, and Sehgal AR 2002. Economic and health consequences of selling a kidney in India. *JAMA* 288(13): 1589–1593. doi:10.1001/jama.288.13.1589. PMID 12350189. http://jama.ama-assn.org/cgi/pmidlookup?view=long&pmid=12350189.

Grabenstein JD 1999. Moral considerations with certain viral vaccines (PDF). *Christ Pharm* 2(2): 3–6. ISSN 1094-9534. http://www.immunizationinfo.org/files/nnii/files/Moral_Considerations_With_Certain_Viral_Vaccines.pdf. Retrieved 2009-05-11.

Handyside AH, Lesko JG, Tarín JJ, Winston RM, and Hughes MR 1992. Birth of a normal girl after *in vitro* fertilization and preimplantation diagnostic testing for cystic fibrosis. *N Engl J Med* 327(13): 905–909. doi:10.1056/NEJM199209243271301. PMID 1381054.

Holding C and Monk M 1989. Diagnosis of beta-thalassaemia by DNA amplification in single blastomeres from mouse preimplantation embryos. *Lancet* 2(8662): 532–535. doi:10.1016/S0140-6736(89)90655-7. PMID 2570237. http://linkinghub.elsevier.com/retrieve/pii/S0140-6736(89) 90655-7.

Honey K 2008. Attention focuses on autism. *J Clin Invest* 118(5): 1586–1587. doi:10.1172/JCI35821. PMC 2336894. PMID 18451989. http://jci.org/articles/view/35821.

Kahraman S, Bahçe M, Samli H et al. 2000. Healthy births and ongoing pregnancies obtained by preimplantation genetic diagnosis in patients with advanced maternal age and recurrent implantation failure. *Hum Reprod* 15(9): 2003–2007. doi:10.1093/humrep/15.9.2003. PMID 10967004. http://humrep.oxfordjournals.org/cgi/pmidlookup?view=long&pmid= 10967004.

Kearnes M, Grove-White R, Macnaghten P, Wilsdon J, and Wynne B 2006. From bio to nano: Learning lessons from the UK agricultural biotechnology controversy. *Sci Culture (Routledge)* 15(4): 291–307. December 2006. doi:10.1080/09505430601022619. http://www.informaworld.com/smpp/content?content=10.1080/09505430601022619. Retrieved 2007-10-19.

Kelly A 2009. Child sacrifice and ritual murder rise as famine looms. *The Guardian*. http://www.guardian.co.uk/world/2009/sep/06/uganda-child-sacrifice-ritual-murder (retrieved 2011-03-31).

Kerr MA 2009. Movement impact (PDF). The Autism Spectrum Disorders/vaccine link debate: A health social movement (PhD thesis). University of Pittsburgh. pp. 194–203. http://etd.library.pitt.edu/ETD/available/etd-04302009-115908/unrestricted/Kerr_FINAL.pdf. Retrieved 2010-02-25.

Lewis CM, Pinêl T, Whittaker JC, and Handyside AH 2001. Controlling misdiagnosis errors in preimplantation genetic diagnosis: A comprehensive model encompassing extrinsic and intrinsic sources of error. *Hum Reprod* 16(1): 43–50. doi:10.1093/humrep/16.1.43. PMID 11139534. http://humrep.oxfordjournals.org/cgi/pmidlookup?view=long&pmid=11139534.

Li M, DeUgarte CM, Surrey M, Danzer H, DeCherney A, and Hill DL 2005. Fluorescence in situ hybridization reanalysis of day-6 human blastocysts diagnosed with aneuploidy on day 3. *Fertil Steril* 84(5): 1395–1400. doi:10.1016/j.fertnstert.2005.04.068. PMID 16275234.

May T and Silverman RD 2005. Free-riding, fairness and the rights of minority groups in exemption from mandatory childhood vaccination (PDF). *Hum Vaccin* 1(1): 12–15. PMID 17038833. http://landesbioscience.com/journals/vaccines/article/mayHV1-1.pdf.

McArthur SJ, Leigh D, Marshall JT, de Boer KA, and Jansen RP 2005. Pregnancies and live births after trophectoderm biopsy and preimplantation genetic testing of human blastocysts. *Fertil Steril* 84(6): 1628–1636. doi:10.1016/j.fertnstert.2005.05.063. PMID 16359956.

Montag M, van der Ven K, Dorn C, and van der Ven H 2004. Outcome of laser-assisted polar body biopsy and aneuploidy testing. *Reprod Biomed* Online 9(4): 425–429. doi:10.1016/S1472-6483(10)61278-3. PMID 15511343. http://openurl.ingenta.com/content/nlm?genre=article&issn= 1472-6483&volume=9&issue=4&spage=425&aulast=Montag.

More countries hope to copy Spain's organ-donation success 2011. Canadian Medical Association. 29 September 2003. http://www.cmaj.ca/news/29_09_03.shtml (retrieved 2011-03-31).

Munné S, Chen S, Fischer J et al. 2005. Preimplantation genetic diagnosis reduces pregnancy loss in women aged 35 years and older with a history of recurrent miscarriages. *Fertil Steril* 84(2): 331–335. doi:10.1016/j.fertnstert.2005.02.027. PMID 16084873.

Munné S, Cohen J, and Sable D 2002. Preimplantation genetic diagnosis for advanced maternal age and other indications. *Fertil Steril* 78(2): 234–236. doi:10.1016/S0015-0282(02)03239-9. PMID 12137856. http://linkinghub.elsevier.com/retrieve/pii/S0015028202032399.

Munné S, Dailey T, Sultan KM, Grifo J, and Cohen J 1995. The use of first polar bodies for preimplantation diagnosis of aneuploidy. *Hum Reprod* 10(4): 1014–1020. PMID 7650111. http://humrep.oxfordjournals.org/cgi/pmidlookup?view=long&pmid=7650111.

Munné S, Magli C, Cohen J et al. 1999. Positive outcome after preimplantation diagnosis of aneuploidy in human embryos. *Hum Reprod* 14(9): 2191–2199. doi:10.1093/humrep/14.9.2191. PMID 10469680. http://humrep.oxfordjournals.org/cgi/pmidlookup?view=long&pmid=10469680.

Navidi W and Arnheim N 1991. Using PCR in preimplantation genetic disease diagnosis. *Hum Reprod* 6(6): 836–849. PMID 1757524. http://humrep.oxfordjournals.org/cgi/pmidlookup?view=long&pmid=1757524.

Offit P and Moser C 2009. The problem with Dr Bob's alternative vaccine schedule. *Pediatrics* 123(1): e164–e169. doi:10.1542/peds.2008-2189. PMID 19117838. Edit lay summary.

Platteau P, Staessen C, Michiels A, Van Steirteghem A, Liebaers I, and Devroey P 2005. Preimplantation genetic diagnosis for aneuploidy screening in women older than 37 years. *Fertil Steril* 84(2): 319–324. doi:10.1016/j.fertnstert.2005.02.019. PMID 16084871.

Russell ML, Injeyan HS, Verhoef MJ, and Eliasziw M 2004. Beliefs and behaviours: Understanding chiropractors and immunization. *Vaccine* 23(3): 372–379. doi:10.1016/j.vaccine.2004.05.027. PMID 15530683.

Sandalinas M, Sadowy S, Alikani M, Calderon G, Cohen J, and Munné S 2001. Developmental ability of chromosomally abnormal human embryos to develop to the blastocyst stage. *Hum Reprod* 16(9): 1954–1958. doi:10.1093/humrep/16.9.1954. PMID 11527904. http://humrep.oxfordjournals.org/cgi/pmidlookup?view=long&pmid=11527904.

Schmidt K and Ernst E 2003. MMR vaccination advice over the Internet. *Vaccine* 21(11–12): 1044–1047. doi:10.1016/S0264-410X(02)00628-X. PMID 12559777.

Sheridan C 2009. Vaccine market boosters. *Nat Biotechnol* 27(6): 499–501. doi:10.1038/nbt0609-499. PMID 19513043.

Shkumatov A, Kuznyetsov V, Cieslak J, Ilkevitch Y, and Verlinsky Y 2007. Obtaining metaphase spreads from single blastomeres for PGD of chromosomal rearrangements. *Reprod Biomed* Online 14(4): 498–503. doi:10.1016/S1472-6483(10)60899-1. PMID 17425834. http://openurl.

ingenta.com/content/nlm?genre=article&issn=1472-6483&volume=14&issue=4&spage=498&aulast=Shkumatov.

Skowronski DM and De Serres G 2009. Is routine influenza immunization warranted in early pregnancy? *Vaccine* 27(35): 4754–4770. doi:10.1016/j.vaccine.2009.03.079. PMID 19515466.

Staessen C, Platteau P, Van Assche E et al. 2004. Comparison of blastocyst transfer with or without preimplantation genetic diagnosis for aneuploidy screening in couples with advanced maternal age: A prospective randomized controlled trial. *Hum Reprod* 19(12): 2849–2858. doi:10.1093/humrep/deh536. PMID 15471934.

Verlinsky Y, Ginsberg N, Lifchez A, Valle J, Moise J, and Strom CM 1990. Analysis of the first polar body: preconception genetic diagnosis. *Hum Reprod* 5(7): 826–829. PMID 2266156. http://humrep.oxfordjournals.org/cgi/pmidlookup?view=long&pmid=2266156.

Verlinsky Y, Rechitsky S, Schoolcraft W, Strom C, and Kuliev A 2001. Preimplantation diagnosis for Fanconi anemia combined with HLA matching. *JAMA* 285(24): 3130–3133. doi:10.1001/jama.285.24.3130. PMID 11427142. http://jama.ama-assn.org/cgi/pmidlookup?view=long&pmid=11427142.

Wagner V, Dullaart A, Bock AK, and Zweck A 2006. The emerging nanomedicine landscape. *Nat Biotechnol* 24(10): 1211–1217. doi:10.1038/nbt1006-1211. PMID 17033654.

Wolfe R and Sharp L 2002. Anti-vaccinationists past and present. *BMJ* 325(7361): 430–432. doi:10.1136/bmj.325.7361.430. PMC 1123944. PMID 12193361. http://www.pubmedcentral.nih.gov/articlerender.fcgi?tool=pmcentrez&artid=1123944.

Zargooshi J 2001. Quality of life of Iranian kidney "donors." *J Urol* 166(5): 1790–1799. doi:10.1016/S0022-5347(05)65677-7. PMID 11586226. http://linkinghub.elsevier.com/retrieve/pii/S0022-5347(05)65677-7.

chapter fourteen

Biobusiness and intellectual property rights

14.1 Introduction

It has been anticipated that the market for biotechnology-based drugs will change significantly by the year 2015, when many patent protections will expire on a number of biotechnology drugs. Biotechnology-based drugs are a class of drugs that is created through biological rather than chemical processes and they represent an annual market of $60 billion approximately. The end of these patents represents a huge opportunity for biotechnology companies able to produce generic biotechnology drugs. Over two decades, the field of biotechnology has been growing very rapidly and its development has benefited almost every part of human life. The importance and significance of biotechnology products can be understood by the fact that their benefits have been widely observed in various fields, which include agriculture, environment, and animal welfare. The important role of biotechnology is to find out the best conceivable technological measure that does not disturb nature's biodiversity considerably and at the same time proves to be constructive for mankind. It has been suggested that there are various kinds of microorganisms that are beneficial to mankind in various ways; for example, they can help to make drugs by recombinant DNA technology or to make desirable vaccines. Before discussing the biobusiness pathway, let us first try to understand how business in general is done.

14.2 What is business?

A business can be defined as an organization that provides goods and services to others in exchange for financial compensation. There are various components of businesses, which have been described below.

14.2.1 Business plan

One of the first steps taken by any biotechnology company is to make a feasible and viable business plan. A business plan is basically a formal statement of business goals, the reasons why they are thought realizable, and the plan for making those goals succeed. The business plan also contains background information about the organization or business experts who make an attempt to reach those goals. The outcome of the business plans mainly helps biotechnology companies to make a conscious decision to start or not to start new product development. Though there is no permanent content for a business plan, the content and format of the business plan are generally determined by the goals and product demands. In brief, a business plan mainly consists of the vision and strategy of the company about marketing, finance, operations, human resources, as well as a legal plan. A business plan also helps the organization to rethink about various strategies based on past mistakes and past marketing flaws. In case the company wants to get a financal loan from banks, one of the major criteria for banks to give the loan is to know about the business plan; the better the business plan, the greater the chances of getting the loan sanctioned. In the same way, venture investment agencies would also know the business plan before investing in the company. In addition, preparing a business plan also creates knowledge for many different business disciplines such as finance, human resource, intellectual property rights, marketing, and operations issues. Business plans include an executive report, business description, business environment analysis, industry background, competitor background analysis, market research analysis, marketing plan, operations plan, and financial plan. We have briefly described the various components of business plans in this section.

14.2.2 Executive report

It is a term used in business as a small document that reviews a longer report, proposal, or group of related reports in such a way that business executives can quickly become conversant with a large body of material without having to read it all. It usually contains a brief account of the proposal enclosed in the major document. The report is intended to help the business managers take a quick decision.

14.2.3 Competitor analysis

This is very important to any industry player and helps the company to know the strengths and weaknesses of current and impending competitors. This kind of competitive analysis provides both aggressive and self-protective strategies for the company to deal with its competitors. It has been observed that the competitor analysis report is an essential component of corporate strategy around the world.

14.2.4 Market analysis

This is another documented report that is prepared to enlist all the issues related to biotechnology product marketing planning, lab inventory, purchase, human resource hiring, facility expansion, and many other aspects of a company. The main goal of a market analysis is to determine the potentials of a market, both locally and globally. It has been found that some organizations evaluate the future potentials of a market examining its own strengths and weaknesses. The marketing report also helps the organizations to guide the investment decisions they make to advance their success in the market. The findings of a market analysis are known to motivate an organization to change various aspects of its investment strategy. One of the first things any company does is to make the marketing plan to know the market demand of the product and its value. In most organizations, especially biotechnology and pharmaceutical companies, strategic planning is an annual process to ensure that the company is moving toward the right direction as far as marketing demand is concerned. Sometimes, some organizations also look into the marketing plan, which is extended from 3 to 5 years. Perhaps the most important factor in successful marketing biotechnology or health care product is the corporate image and its brand image. If the organization in general has a strong vision, then there is a better chance that the organization can achieve a strong market position. The list of "P" that is important for a successful business is shown in Table 14.1.

Table 14.1 List of "P" That Are Important for a Successful Business

1.	Price—The amount of money needed to buy products
2.	Product—The actual product
3.	Promotion (advertising)—Getting the product known
4.	Placement—Where the product is located
5.	People—Represent the business
6.	Physical environment—The ambiance, mood, or tone of the environment
7.	Process—How do people obtain your product
8.	Packaging—How the product will be protected

14.2.5 *Financial plan*

The most important aspect of any business is finance and it is true for biotechnology or health care-related sectors as well. In a broad sense, a financial plan can be an annual budget for future revenue and profits and this plan allocates future income to various types of heads such as rent or utilities, and also reserves some income for short-term and long-term savings. Moreover, a financial plan can also be an investment plan, which allocates savings to various projects expected to produce future income, such as a new product line and shares from existing business. Additionally, in business, a financial plan can denote the three primary financial statements, which are balance sheet, income statement, and cash flow statement. Financial forecasts or financial plans can also refer to an annual projection of income and expenses for a company.

14.3 *Business of biotechnology*

Like other product development such as mobiles, iPhone, or iPad, and health care products, biotechnology products are based on the investment and profit concepts. The investors fund the research projects, which eventually lead to the development of new or novel products, and marketing such novel products brings revenue and profits to the investors. The whole process of the development of a biotechnology product requires team efforts from investors, scientists, engineers, and financial, marketing, and legal experts. Such product development processes are known as biobusiness (Figure 14.1), which means the business of making by-products that include medicine, diagnostic machines, diagnostic kits, and reagents. The process of biotechnology product development has been illustrated in Figure 14.2.

14.4 *Benefits of biotechnology*

It has been suggested that business in biotechnology is primarily to use living organism (microorganism) processes to develop technologies and products that help improve human life and the environment. In biotechnology business, the biological processes have been used to develop bioproducts such as bread, cheese, and dairy products. In the modern era of biotechnology, the main focus is on products and technologies such as health care products to combat devastating and rare diseases, products related to reducing environmental footprint, improving crop quantity and yield, and biofuel. It has been estimated that currently there are more than 255 biotechnology health care products and vaccines available to patients, many for previously untreatable diseases and conditions. Furthermore, it has been

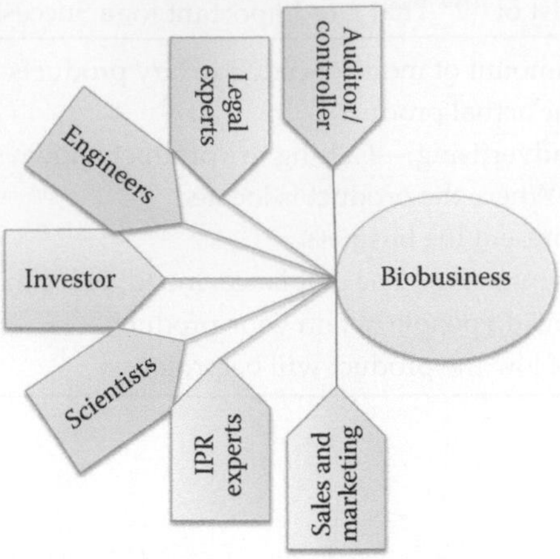

Figure 14.1 Components of biobusiness.

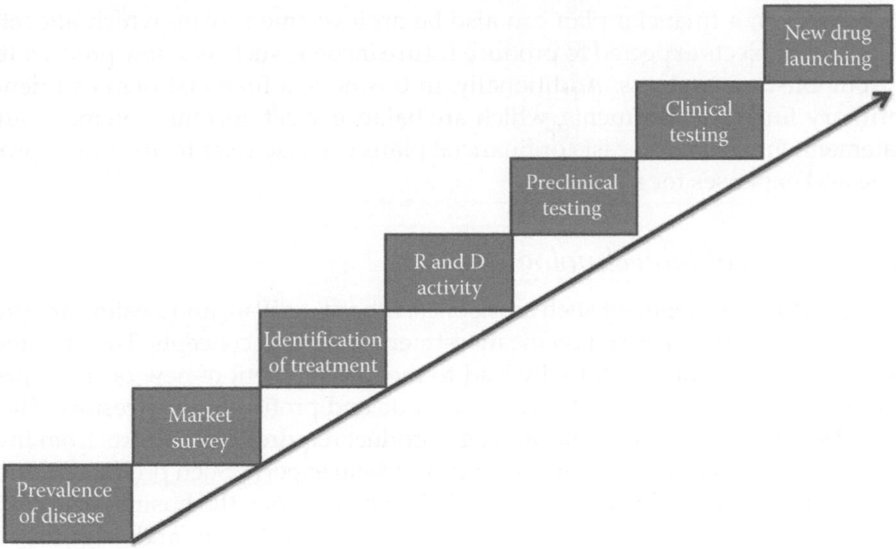

Figure 14.2 Pathway of biobusiness.

reported that more than 13 million farmers around the world use agricultural biotechnology to increase crop yields and prevent crops from being damaged by insects and pests. Owing to depleting natural oil reservoirs, efforts have been made to find an alternative energy source, and it has been reported that there are more than 50 biorefineries being built across North America to test and refine technologies and to produce biofuels and chemicals from biomass, which can help reduce greenhouse gas emissions and chemical pollutions.

14.4.1 *Heal the world*

The field of biotechnology is helping to heal the world by harnessing nature's own toolbox and using our own genetic makeup by: (i) reducing rates of infectious disease; (ii) saving millions of children's lives; (iii) changing the odds of serious, life-threatening conditions affecting millions around the world; (iv) tailoring treatments to individuals to minimize health risks and side effects; (v) creating more precise tools for disease detection; and (vi) combating serious illnesses and everyday threats confronting the developing world.

14.4.2 Fuel the world

The use of biological processes such as fermentation and the use of biocatalysts such as enzymes, yeast, and other microbes to make biological active molecules, are basically biotechnology product developments. It has been suggested that biotechnology is helping the world by (i) streamlining the steps in chemical manufacturing processes by 80% or more; (ii) lowering the temperature for cleaning clothes and potentially saving $4.1 billion annually; (iii) improving manufacturing process efficiency to save 50% or more on operating costs; (iv) reducing use of and reliance on petrochemicals; (v) using biofuels to cut greenhouse gas emissions by 52% or more; (vi) decreasing water usage and waste generation; and (vi) tapping into the full potential of traditional biomass waste products.

14.4.3 Feed the world

The field of biotechnology improves insect resistance of crops, enhances herbicide tolerance of crops, and facilitates the use of more environmentally sustainable farming practices. It has been reported that the products of biotechnology are helping the world by (i) generating higher crop yields with fewer inputs; (ii) lowering volumes of agricultural chemicals required by crops—limiting the run-off of these products into the environment; (iii) using biotech crops that need fewer applications of pesticides and that allow farmers to reduce tilling farmland; (iv) developing crops with enhanced nutrition profiles that solve vitamin and nutrient deficiencies; (v) producing foods free of allergens and toxins such as mycotoxin; and (vi) improving food and crop oil content to help improve cardiovascular health.

14.5 Investment in biotechnology business?

The enormous financial benefits of biotechnology products such as vaccines or antibiotics have attracted a lot of investors in the development of new therapy and treatment. The global life sciences or biotechnology industry is one of the largest sources of innovation available today. It has been reported that life science-related research has resulted in scores of therapies and new methods for the early detection of disease. It has been reported that life science research has also improved agricultural yields to meet increasing demands for food worldwide, reduced pesticide use in farming, and introduced new methods of environmental cleaning by bioremediation. It has been estimated there would be a worldwide increase in the population of humans over the age of 60, which will also increase the demand for the health care products and food supply. It has been suggested that the healthcare markets today represent a unique opportunity to invest in companies at varying stages of development.

14.5.1 Benefits of investing in biotechnology business

Those who are seriously considering making investments in biotechnology business or product development need to consider the five critical points before making any investment.

14.5.1.1 *Job satisfaction*

Biotechnology jobs in the United States pay double the national median salary, suggesting a demand for educated, ambitious employees who seeks a challenging career in the field of biotechnology. In *Fortune* magazine's survey of the 100 Best Companies to Work for the year 2006, where two-thirds of the scoring weight was based on employee evaluation, Genentech was listed the No. 1 company in the United States.

14.5.1.2 *Fastest-growing job sector*

With today's aging population, the life sciences or health care industry is expected to continue to be one of the fastest-growing job sectors in future as there is continued demand for the medicine and diagnostics tools in the coming years.

14.5.1.3 *Available funding*

In order to find cures for many diseases such as Parkinson's, cancer, and diabetes, enormous research is going on in both public universities and private biotechnology companies, which has attracted lots of finance from different sectors. The National Health Institute of the United States has allocated more than 26.5 billion dollars in 2013 on research and development projects. Research in the field of biotechnology is also happening in other parts of the world, and especially countries like India, China, Italy, and Israel are among those countries showing the most growth in this sector.

14.6 *Financial stocks and biotechnology business*

It has been reported that the biotechnology industry is one of the most unstable sectors in the stock market, with stocks rising and falling by large margins. It is largely due to the success and failures of clinical trials, and companies that are investing in this sector generally prepare for such situations. However, experienced traders or investors who specialize in this sector are substantially rewarded at the end of the day. For example, in less than 2 months in 2009, shares of cancer researcher "Dendreon" exploded from less than $3 per share to nearly $20.

14.7 *Regulatory and compliance issues in biobusiness*

The regulation of therapeutic goods such as drugs and therapeutic devices varies by jurisdiction. In some countries, such as the United States, they are regulated at the national level by a single agency like the USFDA, therapeutic goods in Australia are regulated by the Therapeutic Goods Administration (TGA), and therapeutic goods in Brazil are regulated by the Brazilian Health Ministry, through its Sanitary Surveillance Agency. In Canada, regulation of therapeutic goods is governed by the Food and Drug Act and associated regulations. Moreover, the regulation of drugs in China is governed by the State Food and Drug Administration, whereas in the United Kingdom, they are regulated by the Medicines and Healthcare Products Regulatory Agency (MHRA). Furthermore, MHRA also approves marketing authorization of the medicine. Whereas in Switzerland, medicines are regulated by SwissMedic Company. This country is not part of the European Union and is regarded by many as one of the stress-free places to conduct clinical trials of new drug compounds. Additionally, the development of new medicines in India is regulated by the Central Drugs Standard Control Organization (CDSCO), which is basically a federal government agency that works under the Ministry of Health and Family Welfare. This organization is headed by a Directorate General of Health Services, and it

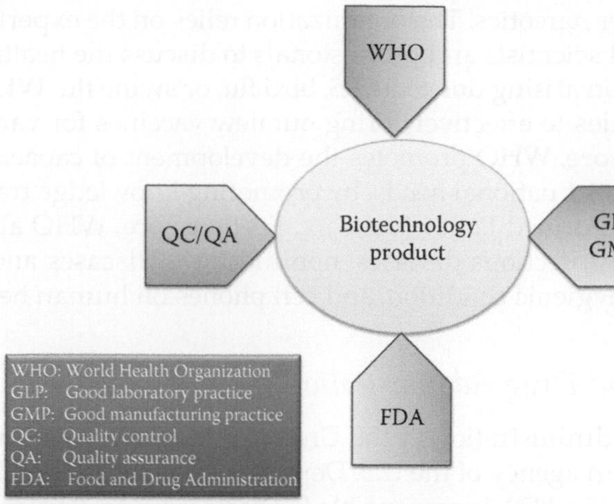

Figure 14.3 Role of regulators in biotechnology product development.

has been reported that CDSCO regulates the medicinal products through the Controller General of India. The role of therapeutic products regulation is designed mainly to protect the health and safety of the population and these regulations are aimed at ensuring the safety, quality, and efficacy of the therapeutic products. In most jurisdictions, it has been recommended that these therapeutic products must be registered before they are allowed to be manufactured and marketed. In the next section, we discuss some of the well-known regulating agencies in order to understand their roles in health care products, including biotechnology products (Figure 14.3).

14.7.1 World Health Organization

As you are aware the World Health Organization (WHO) is a specialized agency of the United Nations (UN) that acts as a coordinating authority to look after international public health and safety, and disease prevention issues? WHO was established on April 7, 1948, with headquarters in Geneva, Switzerland, and the agency got the mandate and resources of its antecedent, the Health Organization, which was an agency of the League of Nations before the formation of WHO. Besides being involved in various health-related issues internationally, WHO also coordinates international efforts to control outbreaks of infectious disease, such as malaria, tuberculosis, SARS, influenza, HIV, and AIDS. Moreover, the WHO sponsors programs to prevent and treat such diseases especially in developing countries. Furthermore, the WHO also supports the development and distribution of safe and effective vaccines, diagnostic help, and drugs to patients in various parts of the world. Interestingly, in 1980, the WHO declared that chicken pox was the first disease that had been eradicated completely and efforts are going on to eradicate polio within the next few years. The organization also develops and promotes the use of well-tested and well-validated health care products and policies to support all UN member countries to improve public condition across the globe. WHO also regularly publishes a World Health Report to describe the condition or prevalence of various diseases. Furthermore, the organization has published tools for monitoring the ability of national health systems and health workforces to meet population health needs. The WHO also carries out various health awareness campaigns to enhance the intake of fruits and vegetables worldwide and to discourage the use of tobacco and other narcotics. The organization relies on the expertise and experience of many world-reputed scientists and professionals to discuss the health issues, especially to deal with the situation arising due to SARS, bird flu, or swine flu. WHO also encourages biotechnology companies to effectively bring out new vaccines for various diseases such as swine flu. Furthermore, WHO promotes the development of capacities in countries to do research that addresses national needs, by promoting knowledge translation platforms such as the Evidence Informed Policy Network. Furthermore, WHO also conducts health research in the field of infectious diseases, noninfectious diseases and to determine the effects of drugs, poor hygienic condition, and cell phones on human health.

14.7.2 U.S. Food and Drug Administration

The Food and Drug Administration of the United States, which is commonly known as the FDA or USFDA, is an agency of the U.S. Department of Health and Human Services. It has been reported that the FDA is responsible for protecting and promoting public health through the regulation and supervision of food safety, vaccines, biopharmaceuticals, blood transfusions, medical devices, electromagnetic radiation-emitting devices, tobacco products, dietary supplements, pharmaceutical drugs, veterinary products, and cosmetic products. Moreover, the FDA also imposes other laws such as section (361) of the "Public Health Service Act" and related regulations, many of which are not directly related to food or drug products. The FDA is led by the commissioner of Food and Drugs. It has been reported that the FDA regulates more than $1 trillion worth of consumer goods related to health care, food, and cosmetics; this includes $466 billion in food sales, $275 billion in drugs, $60 billion in cosmetics, and $18 billion in vitamin supplements.

14.7.2.1 Drug regulations

The Center for Drug Evaluation and Research has different requirements for the three types of drug products, which include new drugs (under patent), generic drugs (do not come under patent), and over-the-counter (OTC) drugs. Moreover, a drug is considered new if it is made by a different manufacturer by using different ingredients, and for a different purpose. Additionally, new drug molecules undergo the most rigorous testing phase and new drug molecules receive wide-ranging inspection before FDA approval in a process called New Drug Application (NDA) and moreover, new drugs are available only by prescription. A change to OTC status is a separate process, and the drug must be approved through an NDA first. Moreover, a drug that is approved is believed to be safe and effective when used as directed by the manufacturer.

The FDA also reviews and regulates prescription drug advertisements and promotions; the drug advertising regulations contain two key requirements and under most conditions, a company can only advertise a drug for the specific indication for which it was approved by the FDA. An advertisement needs to contain a fair balance between the benefits and risks of a drug. After getting an approval of an NDA, the sponsor must review and report to the FDA every patient's adverse drug experience which it encounters, and moreover, unexpected serious and fatal adverse drug events must be reported within 15 days of the clinical trials. The FDA can also receive adverse drug reports directly through its MedWatch program and the reports filed by consumers and health professionals on a voluntary basis. This kind of reporting is called postmarked safety surveillance. In a few cases, the FDA requires risk management plans for some drugs to check drug safety and effective profiles.

Generic drugs are those drugs that do not come under the patent law, where patent effectiveness has expired and in a general sense these generic drugs are less expensive and are manufactured and marketed by other companies. In the 1990s, about one-third of all prescriptions written in the United States were generic in nature. In order to get an approval of a generic drug, the USFDA requires scientific evidence that the generic drug is therapeutically equivalent to the originally approved drug; this type of application is called an "abbreviated new drug application."

14.7.2.2 Biotechnology product regulations

The Center for Biologics Evaluation and Research is the branch of the FDA that is responsible for ensuring the safety and efficacy of biological therapeutic agents; these include vaccines, cell, blood and blood products, tissue-based products, and gene therapy products. Furthermore, new biologics are required to undergo a premarket approval process similar to that for drugs. The original authority for government regulation of biological products was established by the 1902 Biologics Control Act, with additional regulations established in the 1944 Public Health Service Act. Initially, the unit responsible for the regulation of biological products exists under the National Institutes of Health (NIH) of the United States.

14.7.3 International Conference on Harmonization

Besides having WHO and FDA as the drug regulators, we have another regulatory body called the International Conference on Harmonization (ICH), which is the regulatory authorities of Japan, Europe, and the United States. The experts from these three regions discuss scientific and technical aspects of pharmaceutical product registration. Henceforth, the purpose of ICH is to reduce the need to duplicate the testing carried out in different parts of the world to avoid further delay in releasing drugs into the market. Moreover, the process of harmonization can lead to a more economical use of human, animal, and material resources, the elimination of unnecessary deferment in the worldwide development, and availability of new medicines while at the same time maintaining safeguards on safety, quality, and efficacy. Interestingly, ICH guidelines have been adopted as law in several countries; however, they are only used as guidance for the USFDA.

14.8 Intellectual property rights in health care business

Intellectual property (IP) is a term referring to a number of distinct types of creations or discoveries made by humans, which brings a set of exclusive rights. Moreover, under intellectual property law, owners (inventors) are granted certain exclusive rights to a variety of medical treatments, therapies, and diagnostic tests or machines. Though many of the legal principles governing intellectual property rights have evolved over centuries, it was not until the nineteenth century that the term intellectual property began to be used, and not until the late twentieth century that it became commonplace in the United States. The British Statute of Anne-1710 and the Statute of Monopolies-1623 are now understood as the origins of copyright and patent law, respectively. Moreover, common types of intellectual property include patents and trademarks.

14.8.1 Patents

A patent is basically a legal document that allows an inventor to exclude others to work, sell, and manufacture the same for at least 17–20 years. The patent application can be filed in the respective country as well as another country based on the scope of benefits. Furthermore, a patent application can include one or more claims defining the invention, which must be a novelty, utility, and commercial application. It has been reported that the exclusive right granted to an inventor in most countries is the right to prevent others from making, using, selling, or marketing the patented invention without permission and, in brief, patent is nothing but the legal right to prevent others to use it. Furthermore, under the World Trade Organization's (WTO) Agreement on Trade Related Aspects of Intellectual Property Rights, patents should be available to all WTO member states for any inventions and the maximum term of protection available should be 20 years.

With regard to patenting the biotechnology products, though human beings have been using and making biotechnology products for ages, there was no system of patenting a discovery related to biotechnology before the nineteenth century. With the advent of patent rights, scientists started using the rights, to patent the biotechnology-related discovery and invention. Intellectual property protection for biotechnology products is currently in a state of change as the field of biotechnology keeps evolving with time; there is also an enormous increase in a number of new techniques and new ways of making biotechnology products being observed, which has affected patenting the biotechnology rights. Genetically modified crops/organism, cloning, and stem cell therapy are among the most widely patented areas of biotechnology. These changes have been largely seen in the United States and other industrialized countries, but as other countries wish to compete in the new market associated with biotechnology products, they are likely to change their national laws in order to protect and encourage investment in biotechnology. Moreover, at the moment no clear international agreement on how biotechnology products should be treated. Bodies such as the World Intellectual Property Organization (WIPO), which is basically the United Nations permanent body primarily responsible for international cooperation in intellectual property, and the Organization for Economic Cooperation and Development have conducted separate studies and produced various reports about biotechnology.

14.8.1.1 Intellectual property protection in biotechnology

The products of biotechnology can be patented like other products and patent rights can be obtained based on the type of products such as plant-based patents and healthcare-based patents. Both systems provide exclusive, time-limited rights of exploitation. Keeping biotechnology "secret" can also be a valuable form of protection. Previously, various laws were formed to protect the rights of patent holders, but all attempts to harmonize trade secret laws in Europe were not very successful. It has been observed that most jurisdictions do provide some form of safeguard against those who steal or use others trade secrets unethically. Nevertheless, the problem with this form of protection is that it becomes public once the biotechnology product is used commercially and thus the protection is lost.

Additionally, patents provide a wide range of legal rights, including the right to possess, use, transfer by sale or gift, and to exclude others from similar rights and duration can be for around 20 years whereas in the case of the United States its only 17 years. Moreover, these rights are generally restricted to the territorial jurisdiction of the country granting the patent and in case an inventor who wishes to protect inventions in different countries need to apply separately in each of those countries. There are countries that have special laws to protect biotechnology patent rights, which include Czechoslovakia, Hungary, Romania, Japan, Australia, Bulgaria, and Canada. Furthermore, it has been reported that in all the National Patent Offices where patents are granted for biotechnology products, there is a considerable accumulation of pending applications to be processed.

14.8.1.2 Rights in plant varieties

During the mid-1960s, only a handful of countries such as Germany and the United States gave any intellectual property protection to plant varieties and this happened because of pressure from their plant breeding industries as 10 western European countries entered into a diplomatic process in 1960. This eventually led to the formation of the International Union for the Protection of New Varieties of Plants (UPOV) and the signing of a convention started; after that, a number of other countries have become parties to the UPOV Convention. Additionally, a few amendments were made to the UPOV Convention in 1978, principally to facilitate the entry of the United States. It has been reported that the UPOV Convention basically requires that a country that has signed the convention must adopt national legislation to give at least 24 plant species within 8 years of signing. Moreover, a plant variety is protectable under the UPOV system if it is different, uniform, and stable, and satisfies a novelty requirement.

It has been reported that the duration of patent protection depends on national legislation and on the plant species to which the variety belongs, but it is generally for 20 years and the patent is generally granted the exclusive right to sell the reproductive material such as seed, cuttings, and whole plants of the protected variety. Nevertheless, these rights do not extend to vegetables such as fruit, and wheat seed grown for milling flour, and more importantly the exclusive rights outline what others (farmers) may or may not do in relation to the protected varieties. It has been observed that plant breeders of different countries were dissatisfied with the protection provided by the UPOV system and this ultimately resulted in a major diplomatic conference in 1991 in which the UPOV regulations were substantially revised. Interestingly, the revised UPOV systems provide far superior protection system and most notably by requiring that all member countries can apply the convention to all types and species by extending the exclusive rights to include harvested material such as fruit and wheat grown for milling into flour.

14.8.1.3 International treaties

There are three different international intellectual property treaties that have been signed relating to the protection of the biotechnology field. One treaty is the Paris Convention for the Protection of Industrial Property, also known as the Paris Convention; the second one is the Budapest Treaty on the International Recognition of the Deposit of Microorganisms for the Purposes of Patent Procedure; and the third one is the Patent Cooperation Treaty also known as the PCT. It has been reported that the Paris Convention was originally signed in 1883 by just 11 countries, but now almost all countries that have some form of intellectual property law are affiliated to it. The biotechnology patent applications often face considerable difficulties in describing the nature of the invention adequately, whereas the Deposit Treaty is a means of solving these problems, primarily through the formation of a series of International Depository Authorities (IDA) and through the recognition by all member countries. Moreover, the PCT simplifies the process of filing patent applications simultaneously in a number of countries. Under the PCT, a single application can be filed in one of the official offices, designating any number of PCT member countries, which can finally result in a national patent being granted in each of the designated countries. The application is generally granted based on the novelty and usefulness in different countries.

14.9 Patenting and partnership in biotechnology industries

The success of a biotechnology company also depends on its patent portfolio and licensing revenue. The patents on biological inventions were not allowed before 1980, and became necessary only with the advent of biotechnology. Subsequently, patents are now allowed for biological inventions involving microorganisms, vectors, DNA/RNA, proteins, monoclonal antibodies and hybridoma, isolated antigens, vaccine compositions, and transgenic animals and plants. Patents have also been allowed for methods involving (i) isolation or purification of biological material, (ii) gene cloning and production of proteins, (iii) diagnosis, (iv) treatment and use of a product, and (v) screening methods. These patent issues in biotechnology have been discussed in some detail. The development of biotechnology industry partly depends on its licensing revenue, which stems from a good patent portfolio.

Similarly, the success of a pharmaceutical company partly depends upon its revenue that is generated from the marketing of compounds that are licensed by a biotechnology company. The revenue generated by pharmaceutical companies from licensing compounds is estimated to have increased from 24% in 1992 to 35% in 2002 and is expected to grow in coming years. Similarly, the licensing revenue in the biotechnology industry has increased from $5.7 billion in 1998 to more than $6.4 billion in 2000, which is expected to rise in coming years. Biogen, for example, made about $600 million from its licensing activity during 1991–1995, which was a prerequisite for licensing its first product Avonex in 1996. For example, in 2000, licensing revenue of Biogen was about 18% of its total revenue. This example suggests that the biotechnology industry depends heavily on a long-term deal with their pharmaceutical partners, which not only determines the total revenue but also the company's share price in the stock market. For instance, the very news that Curagen, US, had entered into a deal for drug development alliance with Bayer, Germany sent Curagen's share price up 35% to around $36. This illustrates that the survival of biotechnology companies sometimes depends on successful deals with pharmaceutical and other companies.

Success depends on the deals with pharmaceutical and other companies. Successful deals depend on finding the right partner and the postdeal governance. The selection of the right partner in the biotechnology industry involves three steps: (i) designing of search criteria, which should include scientific data; (ii) large and diverse database about biotechnology companies, which meet the search criteria and therefore could be prospective partners; and (iii) screening process, which involves the negotiation of the terms of the deal. Once a deal has materialized following the above three steps, it is necessary to nurture and improve the relationship between partners, since there are examples of bad relationships affecting businesses adversely and also those of good relationships boosting the business. For instance, Johnson and Johnson and Amgen entered into a deal for marketing erythropoietin (EPO) for anemia and had serious problems affecting business. In controls, the productive relationship between Pfizer and Neurogen, which involved licensing the drug for the treatment of Alzheimer's disease, led to further fruitful collaboration, since both partners invested heavily in building trust in the partnership.

14.10 Biotechnology capital market in the United States

The first biotechnology company in the United States to make an initial public offering (IPO) in the capital market was Genentech (San Francisco, USA), which made an offer of $35 million at the rate of $35 per share. This share soared to $88 within the first 20 min and closed at the end of the day at $56 per share, thus giving the company a valuation of $400 million. Similarly, in March 1981, Cetus's gross IPO was $120 million giving a valuation of approximately $500 million to this company. However, this trend in the United States did not continue later in the 1980s and 1990s. The average IPO raised by an individual company during 1980–2000 did not exceed $20–30 million per year, although the total capital raised due to the biotechnology business improved significantly due to an increase in the number of biotechnology companies. In 1986 (the best year for the biotechnology business in the 1980s), the U.S. biotechnology industry raised $900 million, which steadily improved over the years, reaching a level of several billion dollars per year during the 1990s. However, in general, the biotechnology industry did not attract investors very much during the 1990s, except toward the end of the twentieth century. For instance, in 1999, the share price of Tularik (a biotechnology company) improved from $11 to $13 per share in October 1999 to $90 in February, 2000, and the company's valuation improved from $500 million to $4 billion during the same period. Other companies, impressed by the performance of Tularik, suddenly began filing for IPOs, so that 2000 was a record year for biotechnology financing, with 63 IPOs completed and $5.4 billion (with an average IPO proceeds of an individual company rising from $30 million to $85 million) raised for the biotechnology industry. As many as 37 new biotechnology companies were floated in the area of genomics research alone, although most of them may not be able to sustain and therefore may merge with or be acquired by other successful companies. The revival of the biotechnology industry was also witnessed in Europe, as suggested by several European biotechnological companies such as Neurotech, Transgene, NicOx, and Cytomix, which raised a total of $194 million in the month of May in 2001 alone.

14.11 Mergers and acquisitions of biotechnology companies

Another feature witnessed in the biotechnology industry around the globe during 1990–2000 was the merger and or acquisition of biotechnology companies. In most cases, this was due to the inability of several companies to retain their independent existence. For instance, Celera Genomics announced the acquisition of Axys Pharmaceuticals, and Lexicon Genetics announced the purchase of Coelacanth. Many more mergers, acquisitions, and collaborations took place in the first decade of the twenty-first century. One of the noteworthy examples of mergers is the merger of Sequinom and Gemini Genomics, both specializing in information mining in the Human Genome Project. While Sequenom has mass spectrometry-based genetic analysis system, Gemini Genomics specialized in clinical population genomics. The purpose of the merger was to combine the human genetic resources with the rapid analytical system to generate a more powerful data generating machine. This merger is seen as a synergistic effort, where two youthful and vigorous companies, which raised $250 million in IPO, decided to merge, not due to poverty, but due to well thought-out strategy.

During the span of 10 years ending in 2009, there was a total of 11,100 mergers and acquisitions of biotechnology companies worldwide, with revealed prices totaling more than $300 billion. Furthermore, each of the 25 largest biotechnology mergers and acquisitions was valued at $1.5 billion and leading scorers for that decade include AstraZeneca, GlaxoSmithKline, Roche, Amgen, Eli Lilly Company, and Genzyme. Interestingly, the largest deal by far among biotechnology mergers and acquisitions declared was acquired by Roche at the price of $46.8 billion and the next largest among biotechnology mergers and acquisitions announced was AstraZeneca's $15 billion acquisition of mid-Immune, which was announced in 2007.

All of the top 25 biotechnology mergers and acquisitions announced within 10 years ending in 2009 involved a publicly traded entity as the seller and also as the buyer. In more

Table 14.2 List of Mergers and Acquisitions during 2000–2009

Year	Amount	Number of mergers
2009	$47,523,349,040	193
2008	$93,879,257,347	148
2007	$42,105,127,700	145
2006	$36,407,170,500	115
2005	$23,196,902,050	113
2004	$6,764,873,000	96
2003	$16,681,231,200	168
2002	$3,274,727,708	96
2001	$20,150,840,000	85
2000	$5,076,797,094	52
Total	$295,060,275,639	1171

than 76% of the 25 largest biotechnology mergers and acquisitions announced, the target was a revenue-producing biotechnology company. However, among all 1171 biotechnology mergers and acquisitions announced from 2000 to 2009, only about 18% of the companies targeted were producing any disclosed revenue at the time of acquisition. Moreover, among the top 25 largest biotechnology mergers and acquisitions announced from 2000 through 2009, four companies announced multiple acquisitions: GlaxoSmithKline (four acquisitions), Amgen, Inc. (two acquisitions), Eli Lilly & Co. (two acquisitions), and Genzyme Corporation (two acquisitions). Furthermore, GlaxoSmithKline has announced its $3 billion acquisition of the license for Almorexant (a sleeping pill) in 2008, and also paid over $2 billion to acquire the rights of HuMax-CD20 (a leukemia drug) in 2006. Additionally, in 2007, GlaxoSmithKline also forged a $2.0 billion alliance with Galapagos NV to develop anti-infective drugs. The list of company mergers and acquisitions during the period between 2000 and 2009 is listed in Table 14.2.

In 2009, the highest number of company acquisitions happened with various states of the United States, which included Maryland, Pennsylvania, North Carolina, California, New York, Massachusetts, New Jersey, Washington, and Texas. The greatest numbers of biotechnology mergers and acquisitions happened in England, the Netherlands, Japan, Canada, Switzerland, Germany, France, Australia, England, and Denmark. As far as the product selling trends are concerned, the maximum numbers of biotechnology mergers and acquisitions that happened in the United States included Maryland, New York, New Jersey, Washington, California, Massachusetts, Pennsylvania, North Carolina, and Texas, whereas in other countries, the greatest numbers of biotechnology mergers and acquisitions happened in Canada, England, Switzerland, Germany, and France.

14.11.1 Merger trends in India

The Indian pharmaceutical sector is currently the largest among the developing nations. Looking at its current momentum of growth, the Indian pharmaceutical (generic drug development) market is expected to expand with great volume and number. The key factors that drive the Indian pharmaceutical sectors are trained and skilled human resources and easy investment opportunities. Additionally, profit margins of Indian pharmaceutical companies are on the rise and the recent trend of mergers and acquisitions by Indian pharmaceuticals with multinational companies are likely to provide an upside to the growing numbers. The total Indian pharmaceutical market is valued at $1.0 billion with a growth rate of 8.5%. As indicated, the market is predominantly a branded generic market with more than 20,000 domestic manufacturers of pharmaceuticals, whereas in the organized sector of the Indian pharmaceutical industry, there are about 300 companies dealing with pharmaceutical products.

With regard to biotechnology research and product development in India, it is interesting to know that most of the pharmaceutical companies that only deal with synthetic drug development have now opened a biotechnology research and production wing in their companies. The prominent Indian biotechnology companies are working with vaccines and biotherapeutics or therapeutic proteins such as insulin and growth hormones. This sector has evolved continuously, giving tremendous business opportunities for the investors. Some of the major players that have recently focused on biotechnology product development are Reliance Life Sciences, Dr. Reddy's Laboratories, Ranbaxy Laboratories Limited, Wockhardt, Cadila Pharmaceuticals, and Shantabiotech. In addition, there are also acquisitions and mergers happening with mainly European and U.S.-based companies, such as the acquisitions of RPG Aventis (acquired by Ranbaxy) and Alpharma (acquired by Cadila) in France. These are clear samples of acquisitions. Furthermore, in several other cases, acquisitions by Indian generic companies are small and have been primarily to expand the geographical reach while at the same time, shifting production from the acquired units to their cost-effective Indian plants such as Wockhardt's acquiring of CP Pharma and Esparma.

14.12 Summary

Like other product development sectors, which include electronics and automobiles, biotechnology products do have the same ingredients, which include investment, loss and profit, and compliance components. In fact, biotechnology product development is one of the most expensive, lengthy, and highly regulated process of all product development. Biotechnology companies that make vaccines, drugs, and monoclonal antibodies primarily work on the profit and loss basics called biobusiness. The main components of biobusiness are novel ideas, finance, investment, research and development, manufacturing and product development, animal and human trials, regulation and compliance, patents and intellectual property right, sales, and marketing. In addition to these topics, in this chapter, we have discussed the issues related to biotechnology company mergers, acquisitions, patent disputes, financial stocks, and pipeline products.

14.13 Knowledge builder

Biorefineries: A biorefinery is a facility that integrates biomass conversion processes and equipment to produce fuels, power, heat, and value-added chemicals from biomass. The biorefinery concept is analogous to today's petroleum refinery, which produces multiple fuels and products from petroleum. The International Energy Agency Bioenergy Task 42 on Biorefineries has defined bargaining as the sustainable processing of biomass into a spectrum of bio-based products (food, feed, chemicals, materials) and bioenergy (biofuels, power, and/or heat).

Biofuels: A biofuel is a fuel that uses energy from a carbon fixation. These fuels are produced from living organisms. Examples of this carbon fixation are plants and microalgae. These fuels are made from biomass conversion. Biomass refers to recently living organisms, most often referring to plants or plant-derived materials. This biomass can be converted to energy in three different ways: thermal conversion, chemical conversion, and biochemical conversion. This biomass conversion can be in solid, liquid, or gas form. This new biomass can be used for biofuels. The popularity of biofuels has increased because of rising oil prices and the need for energy security. However, according to the European Environment Agency, biofuels address global warming concerns only in specific cases.

Biomass: Biomass is the biological material derived from living or recently living organisms. It most often refers to plants or plant-derived materials, which are specifically called lignocellulosic biomass. As a renewable energy source, biomass can either be used directly via combustion to produce heat, or indirectly after converting it to various forms of biofuel. The conversion of biomass to biofuel can be achieved by different methods, which are broadly classified into thermal, chemical, and biochemical methods.

Greenhouse Gas Emissions: A greenhouse gas (sometimes abbreviated GHG) is a gas in an atmosphere that absorbs and emits radiation within the thermal infrared range. This process is the fundamental cause of the greenhouse effect. The primary greenhouse gases in the earth's atmosphere are water vapor, carbon dioxide, methane, nitrous oxide, and ozone. Annual per capita emissions in the industrialized countries is typically as much as 10 times the average in developing countries. Since the beginning of the industrial revolution, the burning of fossil fuels has contributed to a 40% increase in the concentration of carbon dioxide in the atmosphere from 280 to 400 ppm.

Biocatalysts: Biocatalysis is the use of natural catalysts, such as protein enzymes, to perform chemical transformations on organic compounds. Both enzymes that have been more or less isolated and enzymes still residing inside living cells are employed for this task.

SARS: Severe acute respiratory syndrome (SARS) is a viral respiratory disease in humans that is caused by the SARS coronavirus (SARS-CoV). It is not clear how a virus came to be named after a syndrome but the term was rapidly taken up by the media. Between November 2002 and July 2003, an outbreak of SARS in South China and then Hong Kong nearly became a pandemic, with 8273 cases and 775 deaths worldwide (9.6% fatality) according to the WHO.

Biologic: A medicinal preparation created by a biological process.

Company Mergers: Mergers and acquisitions (abbreviated M&A) are an aspect of corporate strategy, corporate finance, and management dealing with the buying, selling, dividing, and combining of different companies and similar entities that can help an enterprise grow rapidly in its sector or location of origin, or a new field or new location, without creating a subsidiary or another child entity, or using a joint venture.

Patent Disputes: Patent infringement or dispute is the commission of a prohibited act with respect to a patented invention without permission from the patent holder. Permission may typically be granted in the form of a license. The definition of patent infringement may vary by jurisdiction, but it typically includes using or selling the patented invention.

Pipeline Products: A product pipeline is a series of products developed and sold by a company, ideally in different stages of their life cycle. The goal is having at any point in a company's life, some products in the growth and mature stage of the life cycle.

Further reading

Chronicle of the World Health Organization 1947. http://whqlibdoc.who.int/hist/chronicles/chronicle_1947.pdf. Retrieved July 18, 2007.

Constitution of the World Health Organization 2007. World Health Organization. http://whqlibdoc.who.int/hist/official_records/constitution.pdf. Retrieved July 18, 2007. For an easier-to-read

version, see Constitution of the World Health Organization (English only version). World Health Organization. http://www.who.int/entity/governance/eb/who_constitution_en.pdf. Retrieved February 11, 2008.
FDA Centennial 1906–2006. US FDA. http://www.fda.gov/centennial/. Retrieved September 13, 2008.
FDA Commissioner. US FDA. http://www.fda.gov/oc/commissioners/hamburg.html. Retrieved May 27, 2009.
FDA's International Posts: Improving the Safety of Imported Food and Medical Products. USFDA. http://test.fda.gov/ForConsumers/ConsumerUpdates/ucm185769.htm. Retrieved April 10, 2010.
FDA Website: Expanded Access and Expedited Approval of New Therapies Related to HIV/AIDS.
Frum D 2000. *How We Got Here: The '70s*. New York: Basic Books. p. 180. ISBN 0465041957.
Handbook on Monitoring and Evaluation of Human Resources for Health 2009. Geneva: World Health Organization.
Harris G 2008. The safety gap. *New York Times Magazine*. http://www.nytimes.com/2008/11/02/magazine/02fda-t.html.
Health Canada: Drugs and Health Products. Ottawa, Ontario: Health Canada. 2000. ISBN 0-662-29208-1. http://www.hc-sc.gc.ca/dhp-mps/index-eng.php. Retrieved July 2, 2010.
Iriye A 2002. *Global Community: The Role of International Organizations in the Making of the Contemporary World*. Berkeley: University of California Press. ISBN 052023179.
Karki L 2005. Review of FDA law related to pharmaceuticals: The Hatch–Waxman Act, regulatory amendments and implications for drug patent enforcement. *J Patent Trademark Office Soc* 87: 602–620.
League of Nations: Health Organization. http://whqlibdoc.who.int/hist/chronicles/health_org_1931.pdf
MedWatch 2007. The FDA Safety Information and Adverse Event Reporting Program. Accessed October 9, 2007.
Members of the World Health Organization 2009. Appendix 1, World Health Organization. http://apps.who.int/gb/bd/PDF/bd47/EN/members-en.pdf. Retrieved November 18, 2010.
Orlando V 1999. The FDA's accelerated approval process: Does the pharmaceutical industry have adequate incentives for self-regulation? *Am J Law Med* 25(4): 543–568. PMID 10629734.
Ross G 2006. A perspective on the safety of cosmetic products: A position paper of the American Council on Science and Health. *Int J Toxicol* 25(4): 269–277. doi:10.1080/10915810600746049. PMID 16815815.
Temple R 2002. Policy developments in regulatory approval. *Statistics Med* 21 (19): 2939–2948. doi:10.1002/sim.1298. PMID 12325110.
Therapeutic Equivalence of Generic Drugs 2007. U.S. Food and Drug Administration. 1998. Archived from the original on September 9, 2007. http://web.archive.org/web/20070909162853/http://www.fda.gov/cder/news/nightgenlett.htm. Retrieved October 10, 2007.
United Nations General Assembly Resolution 61 Session 1 Establishment of the World Health Organization on 14 December 1946.

chapter fifteen

Career opportunities

15.1 Introduction

As we have seen in the previous chapters about the various applications of biotechnology and considering its enormous impact on human life, this field is considered to be one of the most rapidly developed and promising health science fields. To a great extent, the biotechnology field is mainly known for the manipulation of genetic materials to make products for healthcare, diagnostics, agriculture, and environment. Biotechnology offers outstanding prospects and opportunities, primarily in the domains of medicine, environmental, biopharmaceutical, biofuel, agriculture, and related fields. As you have learnt in the previous chapters, biotechnology is a highly diverse field of applied science where different disciplines such as genetics, molecular biology, biochemistry, microbiology, pathology, immunology, virology, chemistry, bioinformatics, agriculture and animal science, ecology, cell biology, soil science and soil conservation, biostatistics, and plant physiology integrate and provide a range of applications. Among all applications, the field of biotechnology has been extensively used in developing healthcare products such as antibiotics, vaccines, and therapeutic proteins, monoclonal antibodies and also in the areas of transgenic plants, animals, genetically modified crops, and biofuels. In addition to this, biotechnology is also useful in animal husbandry and animal breeding, the improvement of quality seeds, insecticides, and fertilizers, in controlling pollution, and in wastewater management. In fact, biotechnology-based products are in all aspects of human life (Figure 15.1).

15.2 Research and development jobs

Biotechnology is a research-oriented or research-intensive field that provides ample opportunities for those candidates who want to shape their careers in drug discovery. The people who work hard to help make technology successful are researchers or scientists. Tthese researchers or scientists work in the respective labs located in the universities or companies bringing interesting and challenging discoveries. There is a great scope for individuals who hold a PhD degree in life or health science and are keen to pursue a career in research and development. The company generally looks for trained doctoral candidates who have experience in biotechnology-related laboratory techniques such as molecular and genetic techniques with a proven research track record of publication. Doctoral candidates with postdoctoral experience in cell tissue culture, recombinant DNA technology, or therapeutic proteins, and bioengineering fields hold a better chance of getting jobs in the biotechnology industry. There are various levels of jobs available in the research and development segment of any biotechnology industry, which is broadly classified into basic research laboratories, formulation research laboratories, preclinical testing laboratories, clinical testing, and bioassay laboratories.

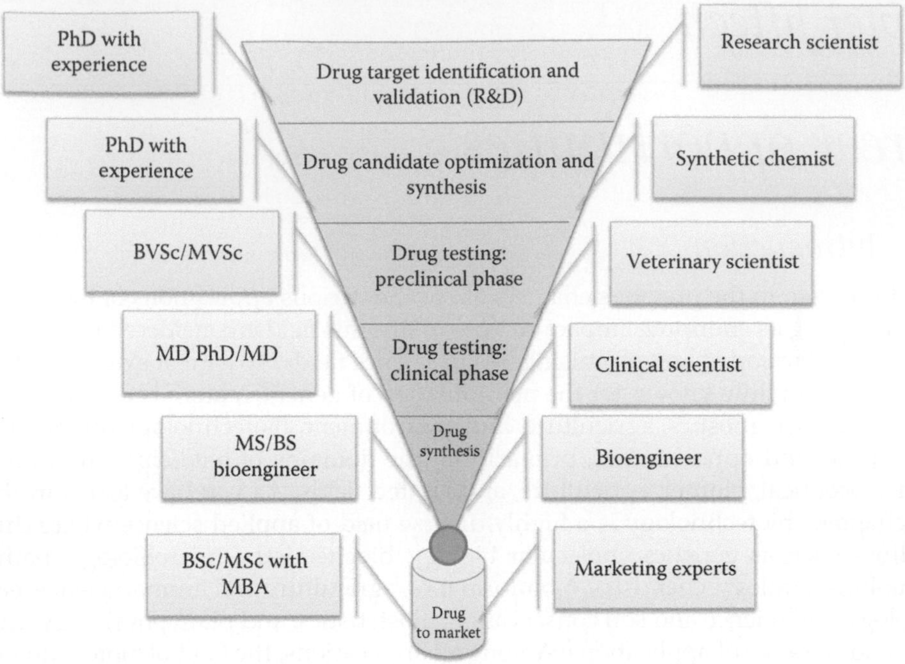

Figure 15.1 Careers in biotechnology.

15.2.1 *Basic research labs*

In any field, basic research is very segmented to bring out new ideas, new technology, and new products. In biotechnology companies, basic research labs are called drug discovery labs whereas in universities, they are usually called basic or fundamental research labs. The main objective of any biotechnology company is to bring out novel and effective products. To achieve this they need a team of researchers and scientists who are not only theoretical experts of the field but also possess laboratory skills to bring out new discoveries. Doctorates in the fields of microbiology, biotechnology, immunology, molecular biology, pharmacology, and human genetics are widely accepted in most of the biotechnology-based universities or companies.

15.2.2 *Preclinical labs*

This is the most important phase that any drug or biomolecule producing or manufacturing company needs to undergo for checking the toxic effects of the drugs before moving to human trials. After completing the initial phase of research and development, biotechnology products such as drugs or hormones are being tested for their efficacy and toxicity using *in vitro* and *in vivo* models, which basically allows the biotechnology company to short list the drug or hormones they want to use for further testing. One of the interesting aspects of any drug testing is to test the drug candidate in animals and such studies conducted in animals are called preclinical studies. In general, preclinical is a stage of research that begins before testing in humans that is also known as clinical testing. During animal testing, scientists or researchers generally collected data based on efficacy and toxicity results. The main objectives of preclinical studies are to determine a biotechnology product's safety profile and as per the drug regulators all class of biotechnology products must undergo different types of preclinical testing phase. During preclinical testing, drugs are tested in animals to check the effect of the drugs on body (pharmacodynamics) and also the effect of body on the drugs (pharmacokinetics). The data collected from animal testing allow researchers to carefully estimate a safe dose of the drug for clinical trials in humans. In contrast, medical devices that are being only used for diagnostics purposes that do not have a drug attached would not undergo these additional tests and may go directly to good laboratory practices (GLP) testing for the safety of the device and its components. Some diagnostic devices may also undergo biocompatibility testing, which helps to show whether a component of the device is viable in a living system such as the human body.

Typically, in preclinical testing, there are two different kinds of tests that can be performed, known as *in vitro* and *in vivo* tests. In *in vitro* testing, the drug is tested outside a living organism, such as kidney cells or pancreatic cells, whereas in *in vivo* testing, the drug is tested inside a living organism (animals) through injection. The information collected from these animal studies is vital so that safe human testing can begin. Normally, in drug development, animal testing involves mainly rodent species, which include rats, mouse, guinea pigs, and so on. The initial stage of any animal trial is generally to study the efficacy and toxicity of the drug molecules. The most commonly used models are rodents, although primate and pigs are also used. Also, there is a need to consider the differences between animals and human with regard to enzyme activity and the circulatory system. In addition, other considerations make certain models more suitable based on the dosage form and site of activity. For instance, dogs will not be good models for solid oral dosage forms because the characteristic dog intestine is underdeveloped compared to the omnivores. Also, rodents cannot be good models for antibiotic drugs because of the differences in the intestinal flora, which may result in adverse effects. There are reports that suggest animal testing in the pharmaceutical and biotechnology industry has been reduced for ethical and cost reasons. Nevertheless, most research still involves animal testing for efficacy and toxicity. In order to do all those things that have been described above, organizations are required to employ individuals with a qualification of a bachelor's or master's degree in veterinary science or animal studies. Senior positions individuals should have a doctorate degree in veterinary science or animal studies plus 10–15 years of experience in laboratory animal handling and knowledge of GLP guidelines.

15.2.3 Formulation labs

Once a drug is tested in animals for its efficacy and toxicity, the next step is to test it in humans. But before testing it in humans, it is very important to know how this drug can be given to patients and in what form. Formulation scientists design to find out through which route (oral, intravenous, intra muscular, etc.) a medicine can be delivered to patients and in what compositions (tablet, injection, or syrups). It is imperative to know what variety of other substances the drug contains apart from the drug itself, and studies have to be carried out to ensure that the drug is compatible with other substances. It has been suggested that the first step in the formulation of a drug is to fully characterize the drug's physical, chemical, and mechanical properties in order to select what other constituents can be used in the preparation. While making protein-based drug formulation, the formulation scientist also investigates the effect of stress conditions such as freeze and thaw, and temperature on drug formulation, and also studies particle size, polymorphism, pH, solubility, and bioavailability a drug. The formulation scientist ensures that the drug be combined with inactive additives by a method that ensures the quantity of drug present is consistent in each dosage. In addition, the formulation scientist also ensures that the dosage should have a uniform appearance with a satisfactory taste. Companies look for candidates who have either a master's degree in medicinal chemistry and pharmacology, or a doctorate degree in medicinal chemistry and pharmacology.

15.2.4 Clinical research

Clinical research is a branch of medical science that determines the efficacy and safety of drug molecules that are intended to be used in humans. There are four phases of testing drugs, namely, phase I, phase II, phase III, and phase IV. Ample job opportunities are available in the clinical research domain, and these jobs are available to those individuals who have obtained specialized training on human subjects besides having a basic degree in medical science such as an MBBS, MD, or a doctorate in clinical pharmacology. Candidates who do not have a medical or doctorate degree wishing to pursue their career in clinical research need to do a postgraduate certificate course in clinical research from a reputed organization offered in many countries. Trials are generally conducted in a designated medical hospital or centers approved by the drug regulators of each country.

15.2.5 Production and manufacturing

Once the drugs or therapeutic molecules are successfully synthesized or tested at both preclinical and clinical levels, the next step would be to synthesize the molecules at a large scale. To produce a large volume or quantity of therapeutic molecules, specialized equipment is required such as bioreactors and other equipment and accessories. The operation of the whole process of biotechnology products such as therapeutic proteins, vaccines, and antibiotics requires individuals with special qualifications and experiences. These individuals should have a bachelor's or master's degree in the field of microbial biotechnology or industrial biotechnology, and for a senior position, the candidate should preferably have a doctorate degree in microbial or industrial biotechnology. Most of the biotechnology manufacturers normally have product development specialists, a production manager, a plant supervisor, production workers, raw materials manager, a store man, formulation and packaging supervisor, and so on. The candidates may join the manufacturing plant based on his/her qualification and expertise. If someone would like to pursue a career in the production division, then the candidate must have both theoretical and practical knowledge of biotechnology product development and bioreactor design and function, plus possess engineering degrees in industrial biotechnology.

15.2.6 Quality assurance

Quality assurance (QA) is the methodology that guarantees a manufactured product such as a drug or medicine, consistently meet the mandatory quality standards. The QA team usually aims to ensure that the intended drug fulfills all the quality requirements suggested by drug controllers and regulators; for example, in the United States, the Food and Drug Administration (FDA) regulates drug development. Pharmaceutical and biotechnology companies must have a separate department of QA to assure the quality of their products. The company needs to have individuals who can work for the QA. These individuals should be trained and scientists and technologists should know the FDA guidelines about the quality of products. Individuals with a doctorate degree in life sciences, a proven track record of quality of publications, and experience in a QA lab are desirable. There are several activities described briefly, which are associated with QA.

15.2.6.1 Improve quality

QA professionals are involved in all critical activities of organizations such as design, manufacturing, material procurement, packaging, and logistics. When all the processes are being tracked and monitored properly, there are fewer chances of non-FDA compliance of products with respect to the requirements.

15.2.6.2 Low cost

QA not only ensures the quality of drugs but also reduces the overall costs of product development. If the product is developed in a right and proper way from the beginning, there will be less chance of failure and there will be no wastage of materials with no financial loss in the production process. Finally, QA reduces the operating costs of the organizations and, hence, results in increased operating profits for any pharmaceutical and biotechnology company.

15.2.6.3 Reputation

Biotechnology or pharmaceutical companies that are able to manufacture good-quality products according to the requirements of the customers as well as per the standards of the USFDA, grow by reputation. This helps the organization to maintain existing customers and get more business from them, and at the same time, also helps in attracting new customers. Finally, this will in turn increase the revenue and profit of the organization.

15.2.6.4 Reduce execution time

The QA team also helps the biotechnology and pharmaceutical company to reduce the time taken for the execution of the orders. For instance, if the quality of a drug is not up to the standard of the customer, there will be more grievances and that would result in huge financial and time losses. Therefore, if the QA guidelines are implemented appropriately in the organization, the order execution time automatically gets reduced.

15.2.6.5 Compliance to standards

The QA system also ensures that the organization meets all the standard requirements for different quality management systems present in different parts of the world. For example, to meet customer requirements efficiently and constantly, it is vital for biotechnology or pharmaceutical companies to have a QA department. The QA team will ensure that cautions and measures are adhered to, enabling the company to make the product as per customers' expectations.

15.2.6.6 Difference between quality control and quality assurance

It has been suggested that many people, including some quality professionals, do not know what quality control is or what QA is, and many times both these terms are used interchangeably. Nevertheless, both terms are different in meaning as well as purpose and function. It has been suggested that quality guarantee or assurance is based on the process and approach to make a product, whereas quality monitoring and its assurance ensure that the processes and systems are developed and adhered to in such a way that the intended products are of good quality. Moreover, the process is meant to produce defect-free goods or services, which means being right the first time with no rework. It has been suggested that quality control is a product-based approach to check whether the planned product satisfies the quality requirements as well as the specifications of the customers or not. Based on the reports, suitable corrective action is taken by quality control personnel. Another major difference between quality control and QA is that the confirmation of quality is done before starting a project whereas the quality control initiates once the product has been manufactured. It has been suggested that during quality process assurance, the requirements of the customers are defined, and based on those requirements, the processes and systems are established and documented. It has been reported that after manufacturing the product, the quality control process begins. Customer requirements and standards are developed during the quality making process; the quality control personnel check whether the manufactured product meets all those requirements or not. Accordingly, QA starts a preventive process to avoid defects, whereas quality control is a remedial process to identify the defects in order to correct them during manufacturing.

It has been suggested that most activities falling under the purview of QA are performed by managers, customers, and third-party companies or auditors, and these activities include process documentation, creating standards, conducting internal audits, conducting external audits, and developing checklists, whereas engineers, inspectors, and supervisors can perform quality control activities. Their job activities include performing and receiving inspection reports, and final inspection report. Both quality control and assurance of quality individuals are largely interdependent and the QA department depends on the feedback provided by the quality control department. For instance, if there are frequent problems with the quality of the product, then the quality control department provides feedback to the QA personnel that there is an issue in the process that is affecting product quality. Later on, the assurance staff of the quality department determines the source of the problem and brings changes to the process to ensure that there are no quality problems in future. Correspondingly, the quality control department follows the guidelines and standards established by assurance of the quality department to check whether the developed products meet the quality requirements or not. Therefore, both these departments are essential to maintain good quality of the products.

15.2.6.7 Jobs opportunities

Abundant job opportunities are available in the biotechnology and pharmaceutical industry for QA experts. For example, a QA manager is the main position involved in a QA team. This QA individual in pharmaceutical and biotechnology companies is responsible for developing and implementing quality management procedures and systems, which means that this person in charge of quality monitoring and assurance has to ensure that all products manufactured or marketed by a company are free from any defects and meet the highest quality as per international standards.

It has been seen that the role of a quality manager in a company is determined by the type of industry. Nevertheless, the QA job description in many industries may feature certain similarities. The main responsibility of a QA manager is to ensure the even progress of manufacturing and marketing products. The QA manager should appreciate the processes in the company and then establish a relationship with the line man to get the inside knowledge of the various processes involved, such as how they work and what could possibly go wrong at different steps. This information would help the QA manager to gain an insight of the maximum amount of work to be done in minimum time.

Besides these, the QA team is also involved in designing and defining quality policies, which in fact ensures that the existing standards of production are satisfactory and follow safety regulations. A quality manager generally verifies the past records of production to assess if the existing standards can enhance customer numbers. The basic responsibilities handled by QA managers involves reviewing business statistics of product development, to determine and document any areas that may need improvement, sampling the entire manufacturing process, reviewing the current policies in order to to improve the existing quality standards, to ensure that all procedures within the company follow health and safety regulations, and to educate the sales and marketing departments regarding the specific requirements of clients.

QA managers unquestionably play a key role in the success of a company. The interested candidate for a QA position should have experience in testing and examining the products. A QA manager is quite a responsible position, as this is the point where the QA manager could stop a product or service that is not up to the required standard. It has been suggested that the reputation or the popularity of the product is totally dependent on its quality. QA managers are involved in several functionalities, which include gathering sample data from the production site and also test or examine the quality of product. QA managers also monitor the production unit to maintain the standard of production and QA managers also find out methods of product improvement. The QA managers are totally responsible for promoting perfection throughout the organization. To apply for these QA jobs in pharmaceutical or biotechnology industries, the candidate should have a bachelor's in biotechnology or pharmaceutical sciences and a postgraduate certificate course on quality control will be an added qualification for these jobs. In addition to these, the candidate should have excellent analytical skills and power to motivate other people.

15.2.7 *Patent and intellectual property rights*

Any pharmaceutical or biotechnology company needs to have an excellent patent and intellectual property rights team to maintain their unique market position. The intellectual property (IP) laws include patent, copyright, trademark, and trade secret laws, which typically protect the IP rights of an assigned company. Patents, copyrights, and trademarks are basically law, where the government/federal authorities recognize an original idea in the form of a patent for a limited period of time. Likewise, trade secrets, recognized by federal law, can protect IP rights. In the United States, IP laws exist at both the state and federal levels and these laws vary from state to state. The federal government is authorized under the constitution to deal with patents and copyrights, and partially with trademarks. IP law is extremely complex, and by its very nature, constantly evolving. Tremendous job opportunities are available for those who have a basic degree in science and a law degree along with a postgraduate diploma in intellectual property rights (IPR).

15.2.7.1 *Job opportunities in IP law*

The increasing numbers of biotechnology products in daily life and the escalating numbers of biotechnology companies around the world have caused a high demand for patent attorney or lawyers with scientific backgrounds to fill patents and to fight IP infringement cases. Biotechnology and pharmaceutical companies really want to have a competent team of IP attorneys to safeguard the company's position in the market against their competitors. The candidate should have a bachelor's degree in science and a degree in law or a basic degree in law and a postgraduate degree in IPR. These candidates can work as a technical specialist or associate, patent attorney, or legal advisor. The patent attorney will find out about the product and its copyright violations and who has infringed the rights and make a legal case against such companies. In the same fashion, the competitors against which the legal case was filed can also defend his case by appointing a patent attorney. A combined science and law degree provides an essential platform to launch you for lucrative jobs in biotechnology and pharmaceutical companies. Though it is not all glamor and courtroom sessions, the majority of the routine work involves attending client meetings, reading research literature, writing letters, and reviewing contracts and other documents. While preparing the patent application, the patent attorney must ensure that an invention that has been previously described in the literature (publications, patent offices), or something that has been on the market for years, cannot be patented, and the company needs to hire a patent attorney to examine the facts, decipher the legal position, establish precedence, and defend their case in court.

It has been found that sometimes biotechnology and pharmaceutical companies have a hard time finding experts with sound knowledge and understanding of biotechnology and legal laws. Owing to the enormous commercialization of biotechnology products, many companies are hiring legal experts to safeguard their market positions. The candidates seeking a position as a life science specialist should have a BS in science or any life science and excellent communication and writing skills. Qualified candidates should have strong technical skills and preferably a doctorate degree in life science or biotechnology. Upon getting a job, successful candidates can work with more senior members of the organization on a variety of IP matters, including patent application writing, patent application filing, patent prosecution, and general IP counseling.

15.2.8 Financial management

Biotechnology companies have grown quickly over the past two decades, and there is a great demand for individuals who have degrees in finance or economics with a sound knowledge of the biotechnology industry and product development. Companies utilize the experience of business management to facilitate an efficient biotechnology product development.

15.2.8.1 Biotechnology management course of study

Biotechnology companies require skilled individuals to handle financial and business-related issues efficiently on a regular basis. The candidate with a bachelor's degree in science or biotechnology and with a postgraduate degree in business administration, finance, operation, and marketing would help them secure jobs in biotechnology industries. Candidates pursuing an MBA degree find it hard to distinguish biotechnology-related specialized management with the usual business administration programs. Based on the demand of biotechnology companies, biotechnology-related management could be divided into equally important specialized areas such as marketing management of biopharmaceuticals or biotechnology, human resource management in biotechnology companies, financing and venture capital funding management, and IPR management in biotechnology.

It has been found that the biotechnology industry needs qualified professionals at both the technical and administrative levels. The most promising segments of the biotechnology industry that need financial or business executives are molecular biology, recombinant DNA technology, agricultural biotechnology, industrial biotechnology, marine biotechnology, food biotechnology, medical biotechnology, nanobiotechnology, biotechnology intellectual property (IPR issues), and regulatory affairs. It has been found that those who are trained in the biotechnology industry as financial and marketing experts are known to create commercial success.

15.2.8.2 Biotechnology management career opportunities

It has been reported that the manager of a biotechnology startup company faces the challenge of creating a strong scientific team that can bring intended products on time, and the key role of financial management in a biotechnology company is a demand for individuals with proven financial qualification and expertise. Also, the potential for knowledge of biotechnology-related finance, marketing, and competitors are an added advantage. Financial managers will also play a key role attracting venture capitalists, and investment bankers for the benefits of biotechnology.

15.2.8.3 Postgraduate diploma and postgraduate courses

After completing a bachelor's degree, the candidate can also do a postgraduate diploma in various financial and marketing sections such as management information systems, logistics and supply chain management, decision science, sales and distribution, business and financial management, business communication, managerial economics, fundamentals of marketing, research methodology, principles of management, marketing management, strategic management, product and brand management, project management, taxation, quantitative models in marketing, human resource management, financial and cost accounting, intellectual property rights, rural marketing, international business, marketing strategy, integrated marketing communications, consumer, and industrial.

Additionally, a course in biotech management is generally available at the postgraduate level and preference is given to students who have completed their bachelor's in biotechnology, biology, biochemistry, botany, chemistry, microbiology, physics, zoology, agriculture, biomedical sciences, and pharmacy. It has been reported that the biotech management course not only provide students with a broad-based introduction to biotechnology companies but also introduces the theories and practices of management and managerial skills. Subsequently, over the years, this field has emerged as an attractive career option for opportunities at the management level in biotechnology and pharmaceutical industries. It has been shown that candidates with graduate or equivalent postgraduate degrees in management can become part of the biotechnology management team. Furthermore, candidates with work experience in the biotechnology industry and a degree in relevant study disciplines like life science can also join the biotechnology industry as a management manager in the field of finance, economics, human resources, strategy, and other disciplines. Moreover, biotechnology management professionals or managers can find work opportunities in biotechnology, biochemical, pharmaceutical, clinical research, hospital, environment, and academic centers.

15.2.8.4 Biotechnology management career prospects

As the field of biotechnology is still expanding, there will be tremendous demand for management trainees or managers in the biotechnology industry, and having an MBA degree in biotechnology will be on high demand to manage core industrial issues, technical and nontechnical and human resources. Global economies have generated vast opportunities for the world biotechnology industry through joint ventures, mergers, and acquisitions. Recently, the biotechnology industry introduced several hundred products to the market, which caused a severe demand for financial, marketing, and sales experts, as marketing and sales experts are needed to study and develop markets and eventually enable the delivery of products to the consumers.

15.2.8.5 *Biotechnology management program*

The management program in biotechnology (MBA in biotechnology or postgraduate diploma in biobusiness) is aimed at equipping students to turn into management-savvy professionals for the services of the biotechnology industry. Moreover, it also deals with managerial and entrepreneurial aspects in biotechnology, chemical, pharmaceutical, and allied industries. Additionally, the qualities of biotechnology management professionals include effective and optimum utilization of revenue, resource, and space, and biotechnology managers generally focus on socioeconomic and ethical issues, so that the technology is applied for the universal betterment of mankind.

15.2.8.6 *Self-employment biotechnology*

Biotechnology business can also be initiated on your own provided you have the funds and required qualification and experience of biotechnology product development. One who has a master's degree in biotechnology management can now gain access to the industry's specific companies, top jobs, as well as network and become a leader in this exciting sector. After getting a basic degree in biotechnology, individuals can also start their own company in various fields such as food and agriculture by employing biotechnology tools. In recent times, biotechnology is seen as a new hope for knowledge development because of several discoveries made in this field.

15.3 *Top biotechnology companies: Global scenario*

We have listed the world's top biotechnology companies and their financial status in Table 15.1, which are revised up to 2006, as an example to show the financial investment information made by each and every company, along with the number of employees working in biotechnology companies.

15.4 *Emerging technologies of biotechnology*

We have listed in Table 15.2 some of the emerging technologies related to biotechnology fields and these emerging technologies are those technical innovations that represent progressive developments.

15.5 *Online biotechnology career information*

We have listed below some of the biotechnology-related career opportunities in and around the world; these web-based sites are very informative in providing job descriptions and future openings, and information on how to become a member of scientific societies related to the biotechnology field.

- Access Excellence (http://www.accessexcellence.org)
- ActionBioScience.org (www.aibs.org)
- Adsumo: A Life Sciences Career Website (www.adsumo.com)
- America's Job Bank (www.ajb.com)
- America's Recruiting, Inc. (www.amrecruit.com)
- American Society for Microbiology (www.asm.org)
- American Society of Plant Biologists (www.aspb.org)
- Bio.Com (http://www.bio.com)

Table 15.1 List of the World's Top Biotechnology Companies

Rank 2006	Company	Country	Revenue in 2006 (USD millions)	R&D in 2006 (USD millions)	Net income/ (loss) in 2006 (USD millions)	Employees in 2006
1	Amgen	USA	14,268.0	3366.0	2950.0	20,100
2	Genentech	USA	11,724.0	2995.0	2740.0	10,001+
3	Genzyme	USA	3187.0	650.0	(16.8)	9000+
4	UCB	Belgium	3169.6	772.6	461.1	8477
5	Gilead Sciences	USA	3026.1	383.9	(1190.0)	7575
6	Serono	Switzerland	2804.9	560.5	735.4	4775
7	Biogen Idec	USA	2683.0	718.4	217.5	3750
8	CSL	Australia	2148.3	119.1	86.8	2895
9	Cephalon	USA	1764.1	403.4	144.8	2515
10	MedImmune	USA	1276.8	448.9	48.7	2359
11	Celgene	USA	898.9	258.6	69.0	1864
12	Abraxis BioScience	USA	765.5	96.9	(46.9)	1734
13	Actelion	Switzerland	754.6	169.0	192.4	1550
14	ImClone Systems	USA	677.8	112.1	370.7	1287
15	Amylin Pharmaceuticals	USA	510.9	222.1	(218.9)	1100
16	Millennium Pharmaceuticals	USA	486.8	318.2	(44.0)	1073
17	PDL BioPharma	USA	414.8	260.7	(130.0)	993
18	OSI Pharmaceuticals	USA	375.7	176.7	(582.2)	962
19	MGI Pharma	USA	342.8	100.1	(40.2)	947
20	Pharmion	USA	238.6	70.1	(91.0)	793
21	Nektar Therapeutics	USA	217.7	149.4	(154.8)	770
22	Vertex Pharmaceuticals	USA	216.4	371.7	(206.9)	760
23	Biocon	India	200.3	30.5	43.5	1838
24	Cubist Pharmaceuticals	USA	194.7	57.4	(0.4)	746
25	Enzon Pharmaceuticals	USA	185.7	43.5	21.3	722
26	QLT	Canada	175.1	56.4	(101.6)	653
27	ViroPharma	USA	167.2	19.2	66.7	651
28	Alkermes	USA	166.6	89.1	3.8	617
29	Crucell	Netherlands	165.3	84.9	(110.0)	611
30	United Therapeutics	USA	159.6	57.6	74.0	585
31	LifeCell	USA	141.7	16.5	20.5	573
32	Ligand Pharmaceuticals	USA	141.0	41.9	(31.7)	540
33	Myriad Genetics	USA	114.3	83.8	(38.2)	511
34	Exelixis	USA	98.7	185.5	(101.5)	500
35	Cangene	Canada	96.8	22.1	11.6	498
36	InterMune	USA	90.8	103.8	(107.2)	492
37	Nabi Biopharmaceuticals	USA	89.9	37.6	(58.7)	487
38	BioMarin Pharmaceutical	USA	84.2	66.7	(28.5)	417

continued

Table 15.1 (continued) List of the World's Top Biotechnology Companies

Rank 2006	Company	Country	Revenue in 2006 (USD millions)	R&D in 2006 (USD millions)	Net income/ (loss) in 2006 (USD millions)	Employees in 2006
39	Lexicon Pharmaceuticals	USA	72.8	106.7	(54.3)	410
40	Progenics Pharmaceuticals	USA	69.9	61.7	(21.6)	410
41	Innogenetics	Belgium	67.5	32.1	(31.5)	371
42	Idenix Pharmaceuticals	USA	67.4	96.1	(75.1)	359
43	MorphoSys	Germany	66.6	21.9	7.6	336
44	Omrix Biopharmaceuticals	USA	63.8	3.4	23.1	335
45	Regeneron Pharmaceuticals	USA	63.4	137.1	(102.3)	323
46	Acambis	UK	57.0	68.2	(30.4)	285
47	Tanox	USA	56.1	53.4	(2.6)	285
48	ViaCell	USA	54.4	14.0	(21.0)	282
49	Indevus Pharmaceuticals	USA	50.5	43.2	–50.6	279
50	Medarex	USA	48.6	194.5	(181.7)	277
51	NPS Pharmaceuticals	USA	48.5	68.4	(112.7)	276
52	Monogram Biosciences	USA	48.0	19.0	(38.7)	274
53	Oscient Pharmaceuticals	USA	46.2	12.4	(78.5)	267
54	Array BioPharma	USA	45.0	33.4	(39.6)	263
55	AEterna Zentaris	Canada	41.4	28.7	33.4	260
56	IsoTis	Switzerland	40.7	7.7	(18.5)	255
57	Enzo Biochem	USA	39.8	7.9	(15.7)	255
58	CuraGen	USA	39.6	58.5	(59.8)	254
59	Neurocrine Biosciences	USA	39.2	97.7	(107.2)	254
60	MediGene	Germany	38.4	26.7	(8.7)	248
61	Life Therapeutics	Australia	37.6	0.1	(31.2)	245
62	Inspire Pharmaceuticals	USA	37.1	42.5	(42.1)	238
63	CV Therapeutics	USA	36.8	135.3	(274.3)	233
64	Cerus	USA	35.6	29.5	(4.8)	208
65	SciClone Pharmaceuticals	USA	32.7	14.1	0.7	197
66	ImmunoGen	USA	32.1	40.9	(17.8)	197
67	Protherics	UK	30.9	11.8	(16.5)	196
68	Arena Pharmaceuticals	USA	30.6	103.4	(88.3)	195
69	Vernalis	UK	30.1	71.7	(78.2)	192
70	Bavarian Nordic	Denmark	29.5	19.9	(27.1)	191
71	Xoma	USA	29.5	52.1	(51.8)	189
72	GPC Biotech	Germany	28.5	81.3	(80.4)	180

Table 15.1 (continued) List of the World's Top Biotechnology Companies

Rank 2006	Company	Country	Revenue in 2006 (USD millions)	R&D in 2006 (USD millions)	Net income/ (loss) in 2006 (USD millions)	Employees in 2006
73	Micromet	USA	27.6	28.3	0.0	171
74	Targacept	USA	27.5	21.8	(1.2)	170
75	Carrington Laboratories	USA	27.4	5.8	(7.6)	166
76	Acorda Therapeutics	USA	27.4	12.1	(60.0)	158
77	Anika Therapeutics	USA	26.8	3.6	4.6	156
78	Human Genome Sciences	USA	25.8	209.2	(251.2)	151
79	Dusa Pharmaceuticals	USA	25.6	6.2	(31.3)	150
80	ZymoGenetics	USA	25.4	128.5	(130.0)	150
81	Maxygen	USA	25.0	49.1	(16.5)	147
82	Isis Pharmaceuticals	USA	24.5	80.6	(45.9)	133
83	Genmab	Denmark	23.9	90.6	(77.4)	128
84	BioSciMed	USA	23.9	11.6	(1.0)	126
85	Bioniche Life Sciences	Canada	24.1	11.9	(1.0)	127
86	Vitrolife	Sweden	23.2	3.3	2.1	124
87	Coley Pharmaceutical Group	USA	20.2	40.9	(29.4)	122
88	Palatin Technologies	USA	19.7	41.0	(29.0)	116
89	Encysive Pharmaceuticals	USA	19.0	64.4	(109.3)	109
90	GenVec	USA	18.9	29.6	(19.3)	95
91	Medivir Group	Sweden	18.8	39.7	(29.7)	88
92	Peptech	Australia	18.7	4.6	3.8	85
93	Ambrilia Biopharma	Canada	17.4	8.3	(2.1)	85
94	Cytogen	USA	17.3	7.3	(15.1)	85
95	Replidyne	USA	16.0	38.3	(34.6)	79
96	Sinovac Biotech	China	15.4	0.3	(0.7)	67
97	Trimeris	USA	15.2	18.3	7.4	64
98	Avanir Pharmaceuticals	USA	15.2	29.2	(62.6)	64
99	Adolor	USA	15.1	56.7	(69.7)	51

- BioCareer Center (http://www.bio-career.com/)
- BioChem Net (http://biochemhub.com/biochem/jobs.cfm)
- Biocom (www.biocom.org)
- Biocom Workforce (www.biocomworkforce.com)
- BioHealthRx (www.biohealthrx.com)
- BioJobNet (www.biojobnet.com
- Biojobnetwork (www.biojobnetwork.net)
- Bio-Link (www.biolink.com)
- BioSpace (www.biospace.com)
- BioTactics (http://www.biotactics.com)

Table 15.2 List of Emerging Technologies in Biotechnology

Emerging technology	Status	Main industries	Applications
Genetic engineering	Trials are done successfully	Animal husbandry, plant breeding	Creating and modifying species, biomachines, and eliminating genetic disorders
Synthetic biology, synthetic genomics	Research, development, first synthetic bacteria created in May 2010	Chemical industry, petroleum industry, process manufacturing	Creating infinitely scalable production processes based on programmable species of bacteria and other life forms
Artificial photosynthesis	Research, experiments are performed		Replicate the natural process of photosynthesis, converting sunlight, water, carbon dioxide into carbohydrates and oxygen
Antiaging drugs (e.g., resveratrol)	Animal testing are performed	Existing treatments for age-related diseases	Life extension
Vitrification or cryoprotectant	Theory, some experiments are performed	Ischemic damages	Organ transplantation
Hibernation	Research, development, animal trials are performed	Surgical anesthesia	Organ transplantation, space travel, prolonged surgery, emergency care
Stem cell therapy	Research, experiments, phase I human trial spinal cord injury treatment, cultured cornea transplants	Other therapies	Treatment for a wide range of diseases and injuries
Personalized medicine	Research is going on	Orphan drugs	Cancer management and preventive treatment; genetic disorders
Body implants, prosthesis	Clinical trials are successfully conducted	Various fields of medicine	Brain implant, retinal implant
In vitro meat	Research is conducted	Animal husbandry, livestock, poultry, and fishing	Cruelty free and inexpensive meat to consume
Regenerative medicine	Some laboratory trials are performed		Life extension

- Biotech Jobs (http://www.medzilla.com/biotech-jobs/)
- Biotechfind (http://www.biotechfind.com)
- Biotechnology Industry Organization (http://www.bio.org/)
- Biotechnology Jobs, Seattle, WA (www.seattlebiotechjobs.com)
- Hire Health (www.hirehealth.com)
- Massachusetts Biotechnology Council (http://www.massbio.org)
- Medzilla (www.medzilla.com)
- Nature Jobs (www.nature.com)
- NIH Careers (www.jobs.nih.gov)
- Pharmaopportunities Biotech Jobs (www.pharmaopprtunities.com)
- ScienceJobs (www.sciencejobs.com)
- TinyTechJobs (www.tinytechjobs.com)
- Vault (www.vault.com)
- WetFeet (www.wtefeet.com)

15.6 *Professional associations for networking*

- American Association of Clinical Chemists (http://www.aacc.org)
- American Chemical Society (http://www.acs.org)
- American Society of Clinical Pathologists (www.ascp.org)
- American Society of Microbiology (http://www.asm.org)
- Biotechnology Industry Organization (http://www.bio.org)
- Clinical Ligand Assay Society (http://www.clas.org)
- Massachusetts Biotechnology Council (http://www.massbio.org)
- Medical Device Associations (www.biotechmedia.com/Associations-MedDevice_Instr.html)

15.7 *Summary*

The revolution in the biotechnology field has generated tremendous job opportunities in various parts of the world, especially in developed countries. The application of biotechnology can be found in healthcare, environmental, and agricultural sectors. The science of biotechnology is also used to alter the genetic information in both animals and plants to improve them in a way that benefits mankind. It has been advocated that biotechnology is one of the most important applied sciences of the twenty-first century. On the one hand biotechnology provides an excellent platform to discover new treatment methods for various diseases and on other hand gives immense job opportunities in various fields not limited to research and development, formulation, animal testing and clinical trials, manufacturing and production of biotherapeutics, regulatory affairs, and sales and marketing segments of biotechnology products. In this chapter, we discussed various career opportunities available in the biotechnology field, more specifically in the medical or healthcare science field.

Further reading

Biotech100 Stock Index Class A. http://www.biotech100.com/index_stocks/index_classA.htm

DePalma A 2005. Twenty-five years of biotech trends. *Genetic Engineering News (Mary Ann Liebert)* 25(14): 1, 14–23, ISSN 1935-472X, http://www.genengnews.com/articles/chitem.aspx?aid=1005&chid=0, retrieved 2008-08-17

Genetic test could be used to 'personalize' drugs, say scientists 2011. *The Independent*. March 1, 2010. http://www.independent.co.uk/news/science/genetic-test-could-be-used-to-personalise-drugs-say-scientists-1913662.html. Retrieved April 16, 2011.

International Congress Innovation and Technology XXI: Strategies and Policies towards the XXI Century, & Soares, O. D. D. 1997. *Innovation and Technology: Strategies and Policies*. Dordrecht: Kluwer Academic.

Top 100 biotechnology companies, *MedAdNews*, June 2007.

Glossary

Abiotic stress: Abiotic stress is defined as the negative impact of nonliving factors on the living organisms in a specific environment.

Acclimatization: Acclimatization or acclimation is the process of an individual organism adjusting to a gradual change in its environment (such as a change in temperature, humidity, photoperiod, or pH) allowing it to maintain performance across a range of environmental conditions.

Acellular: Containing no cells; not made of cells.

Acentric chromosome: An acentric fragment is a segment of a chromosome that lacks a centromere.

Acetyl coenzyme A; acetyl CoA: Acetyl coenzyme A or acetyl-CoA is an important molecule in metabolism, used in many biochemical reactions. Its main function is to convey the carbon atoms within the acetyl group to the citric acid cycle to be oxidized for energy production.

Acrocentric: A chromosome (one of the microscopically visible carriers of the genetic material DNA) with its centromere (the "waist" of the chromosome) located quite near one end of the chromosome.

Acrylamide gels: A polyacrylamide gel is a separation matrix used in electrophoresis of biomolecules, such as proteins or DNA fragments. Traditional DNA sequencing techniques such as Maxam–Gilbert or Sanger methods used polyacrylamide gels to separate DNA fragments differing by a single base pair in length so that the sequence could be read. Most modern DNA separation methods now use agarose gels, except for particularly small DNA fragments.

Actin: Actin is a globular, roughly 42-kDa moonlighting protein found in all eukaryotic cells (the only known exception being nematode sperm) where it may be present at concentrations of over 100 µM. It is also one of the most highly conserved proteins, differing by no more than 20% in species as diverse as algae and humans.

Activated charcoal: Activated carbon, also called activated charcoal or activated coal, is a form of carbon that has been processed to make it extremely porous and thus to have a very large surface area available for adsorption or chemical reactions.

Activated macrophage: Macrophages are components of the monocyte–macrophage system. Macrophages are usually immobile but become actively mobile when stimulated by inflammation, immune cytokines, and microbial products. They are an important class of antigen-presenting cells (APCs).

Activated sludge system: Activated sludge is a process for treating sewage and industrial wastewaters using air and a biological floc composed of bacteria and protozoans.

Activator: A DNA-binding protein that regulates one or more genes by increasing the rate of transcription.

Active site: In molecular biology the active site is part of an enzyme where substrates bind and undergo a chemical reaction. The majority of enzymes are proteins but RNA enzymes called ribozymes also exist. The active site of an enzyme is usually found in a cleft or pocket that is lined by amino acid residues (or nucleotides in ribozymes) that participates in recognition of the substrate. Residues that directly participate in the catalytic reaction mechanism are called active site residues.

Adaptation: Adaptation is the evolutionary process whereby a population becomes better suited to its habitat. This process takes place over many generations, and is one of the basic phenomenon in biology.

Adaptor: An adaptor in genetic engineering is a short, chemically synthesized, double-stranded DNA molecule which is used to link the ends of two other DNA molecules. It may be used to add sticky ends to cDNA allowing it to be ligated into the plasmid much more efficiently.

Additive gene effects: When the combined effects of alleles at different loci are equal to the sum of their individual effects. In this type of inheritance, there is no sharp distinction between genotypes, but there are many gradations between the two extremes. An example of how additive genes express themselves may be illustrated by imagining a large glass cylinder of clear water on a desk top. The water would represent genes on the chromosomes that are neutral (have no expression). If a red pill is added to the water it begins to turn pink. If another pill is added it turns light red, add another pill and it turns red. The point is as the neutral genes on the chromosomes are replaced with genes that have additive expression and the phenotype of the individual changes. Thus, each pill added changes the water color in a linear manner. The same would be true when replacing neutral alleles on the chromosomes with additive alleles.

Adenine: Adenine (A, Ade) is a nucleobase (a purine derivative) with a variety of roles in biochemistry including cellular respiration, in the form of both the energy-rich adenosine triphosphate (ATP) and the cofactors nicotinamide adenine dinucleotide (NAD) and flavin adenine dinucleotide (FAD), and protein synthesis, as a chemical component of DNA and RNA. The shape of adenine is complementary to either thymine in DNA or uracil in RNA.

Adenosine diphosphate: Adenosine diphosphate, abbreviated ADP, is a nucleotide. It is an ester of pyrophosphoric acid with the nucleoside adenosine. ADP consists of the pyrophosphate group, the pentose sugar ribose, and the nucleobase adenine.

Adenosine triphosphate: A nucleotide of fundamental importance as a carrier of chemical energy in all living organisms. It consists of adenosine with three phosphate groups, linked together linearly. ATP is regenerated by rephosphorylation of AMP and ADP, using chemical energy derived from the oxidation of food.

Adenovirus: Adenoviruses are medium-sized (90–100 nm), nonenveloped (without an outer lipid bilayer) icosahedral viruses composed of a nucleocapsid and a double-stranded linear DNA genome. There are 55 described serotypes in humans, which are responsible for 5–10% of upper respiratory infections in children, and several infections in adults as well.

Adenylate cyclase: Adenylate cyclase is a lyase enzyme. It is a part of the cAMP-dependent pathway.

Adhesion: Adhesion is any attraction process between dissimilar molecular species that can potentially bring them in "direct contact." By contrast, cohesion takes place between similar molecules.

A-DNA: A-DNA is one of the many possible double helical structures of DNA. A-DNA is thought to be one of three biologically active double helical structures along with B- and Z-DNA. It is a right-handed double helix fairly similar to the more common and well-known B-DNA form, but with a shorter more compact helical structure.

Adsorption: Adsorption is the adhesion of atoms, ions, biomolecules or molecules of gas, liquid, or dissolved solids to a surface. This process creates a film of the adsorbate (the molecules or atoms being accumulated) on the surface of the adsorbent. It differs from absorption, in which a fluid permeates or is dissolved by a liquid or solid.

Aerobic: Aerobic is an adjective that means "requiring air," where "air" usually means oxygen.

Aerobic bacteria: Bacteria which require oxygen in order to grow and survive.

Aerobic respiration: Respiration is a process which releases energy inside each of the body's cells.

Affinity chromatography: A method of separating biochemical mixtures and based on a highly specific biological interaction such as that between antigen and antibody, enzyme and substrate, or receptor and ligand. Affinity chromatography combines the size fractionation capability of gel permeation chromatography with the ability to design a chromatography that reversibly binds to a known subset of molecules. The method was discovered and developed by Pedro Cuatrecasas and Meir Wilchek for which the Wolf Prize in Medicine was awarded in 1987.

Aflatoxin: Aflatoxins are naturally occurring mycotoxins that are produced by many species of *Aspergillus*, a fungus, most notably *Aspergillus flavus* and *Aspergillus parasiticus*. Aflatoxins are toxic and among the most carcinogenic substances known.

Agar: Agar or agar-agar is a gelatinous substance derived from a polysaccharide that accumulates in the cell walls of agarophyte red algae.

Agarose: Agarose is a polysaccharide obtained from agar that is used for a variety of life science applications especially in gel electrophoresis. Agarose forms an inert matrix utilized in separation techniques.

Agrobacterium: *Agrobacterium* is a genus of Gram-negative bacteria established by H. J. Conn that uses horizontal gene transfer to cause tumors in plants. *Agrobacterium tumefaciens* is the most commonly studied species in this genus. *Agrobacterium* is well known for its ability to transfer DNA between itself and plants, and for this reason it has become an important tool for genetic engineering.

Agrobacterium tumefaciens: *Agrobacterium tumefaciens* (updated scientific name: *Rhizobium radiobacter*) is the causal agent of crown gall disease (the formation of tumors) in over 140 species of dicots. It is a rod-shaped Gram-negative soil bacterium (Smith et al., 1907). Symptoms are caused by the insertion of a small segment of DNA (known as the T-DNA, for "transfer DNA") into the plant cell, which is incorporated at a semi-random location into the plant genome.

Albinism: Albinism is a congenital disorder characterized by the complete or partial absence of pigment in the skin, hair and eyes due to absence or defect of an enzyme involved in the production of melanin.

Allele: An allele is one of two or more forms of a gene. Sometimes, different alleles can result in different traits, such as color. Other times, different alleles will have the same result in the expression of a gene.

Allele frequency: Allele frequency is the proportion of all copies of a gene that is made up of a particular gene variant (allele). In other words, it is the number of copies of a particular allele divided by the number of copies of all alleles at the genetic place (locus) in a population. It can be expressed for example as a percentage.

Allergen: An allergen is any substance that can cause an allergy. Technically, an allergen is a nonparasitic antigen capable of stimulating a type-I hypersensitivity reaction in atopic individuals.

Allogamy: Allogamy (cross-fertilization) is a term used in the field of biological reproduction describing the fertilization of an ovum from one individual with the spermatozoa of another. By contrast, autogamy is the term used for self-fertilization. In humans, the fertilization event is an instance of allogamy.

Allopolyploid: Allopolyploids are hybrids that have a chromosome number double than their parents. Some of these are created via selective breeding to produce new varieties of plants from previously sterile species.

Allosteric control: Allosteric control, in enzymology, inhibition or activation of an enzyme by a small regulatory molecule that interacts at a site (allosteric site) other than the active site (at which catalytic activity occurs). The interaction changes the shape of the enzyme so as to affect the formation at the active site of the usual complex between the enzyme and its substrate (the compound upon which it acts to form a product).

Allosteric enzyme: Allosteric enzymes are enzymes that change their conformation upon binding of an effector. An allosteric enzyme is an oligomer whose biological activity is affected by altering the conformation(s) of its quaternary structure. Allosteric enzymes tend to have several subunits. These subunits are referred to as protomers.

Allosteric regulation: In biochemistry, allosteric regulation is the regulation of an enzyme or other protein by binding an effector molecule at the protein's allosteric site (i.e., a site other than the protein's active site). Effectors that enhance the protein's activity are referred to as allosteric activators, whereas those that decrease the protein's activity are called allosteric inhibitors.

Alternative mRNA splicing: Alternative splicing (or differential splicing) is a process by which the exons of the RNA produced by transcription of a gene (a primary gene transcript or pre-mRNA) are reconnected in multiple ways during RNA splicing. The resulting different mRNAs may be translated into different protein isoforms; thus, a single gene may code for multiple proteins.

Ambient temperature: Ambient temperature simply means "the temperature of the surroundings" and will be the same as room temperature indoors.

Aminoacyl site: A nucleotide sequence near the 5′ terminus of mRNA required for binding of mRNA to the small ribosomal subunit.

Aminoacyl tRNA synthetase: An aminoacyl tRNA synthetase (aaRS) is an enzyme that catalyzes the esterification of a specific amino acid or its precursor to one of all its compatible cognate tRNAs to form an aminoacyl-tRNA. This is sometimes called "charging" the tRNA with the amino acid. Once the tRNA is charged, a ribosome can transfer the amino acid from the tRNA onto a growing peptide, according to the genetic code.

Amitosis: Direct division of the nucleus and cell, without the complicated changes in the nucleus that occur during the ordinary process of cell reproduction.

Amniocentesis: Amniocentesis (also referred to as amniotic fluid test or AFT), is a medical procedure used in prenatal diagnosis of chromosomal abnormalities and fetal infections, in which a small amount of amniotic fluid, which contains fetal tissues, is extracted from the amnion or amniotic sac surrounding a developing fetus, and the fetal DNA is examined for genetic abnormalities. A procedure for obtaining amniotic fluid from a pregnant mammal for the diagnosis of some diseases in the unborn fetus.

Amnion: The amnion is a membrane building the amniotic sac that surrounds and protects an embryo. It is developed in reptiles, birds, and mammals, which are hence called "Amniota"; but not in amphibians and fish which are consequently termed "Anamniota."

Amniotic fluid: Amniotic fluid is the nourishing and protecting liquid contained by the amniotic sac of a pregnant woman.

Amorph: A mutant gene that produces no detectable phenotypic effect.

Amphidiploid: An organism or individual having a diploid set of chromosomes derived from each parent.

Amphimixis: The union of the sperm and egg in sexual reproduction.

Ampicillin: Ampicillin is a beta-lactam antibiotic that has been used extensively to treat bacterial infections since 1961. Until the introduction of ampicillin by the British company Beecham, penicillin therapies had only been effective against Gram-positive organisms such as staphylococci and streptococci.

Amplification: A mechanism leading to multiple copies of a chromosomal region within a chromosome arm. The DNA amplification technique of the polymerase chain reaction (PCR) in molecular biology is a laboratory method for creating multiple copies of small segments of DNA.

Amplified fragment-length polymorphism (AFLP): Amplified fragment-length polymorphism PCR (or AFLP-PCR or just AFLP) is a PCR-based tool used in genetics research, DNA fingerprinting, and in the practice of genetic engineering. AFLP uses restriction enzymes to digest genomic DNA, followed by ligation of adaptors to the sticky ends of the restriction fragments. A subset of the restriction fragments is then selected to be amplified.

Amylase: Amylase is an enzyme that catalyzes the breakdown of starch into sugars. Amylase is present in human saliva, where it begins the chemical process of digestion.

Amylopectin: Amylopectin is a soluble polysaccharide and highly branched polymer of glucose found in plants. It is one of the two components of starch, the other being amylose.

Amylose: Amylose is a linear polymer made up of D-glucose units. This polysaccharide is one of the two components of starch, making up approximately 20–30% of the structure. The other component is amylopectin, which makes up 70–80% of the structure.

Anabolic pathway: The series of chemical reactions that constructs or synthesizes molecules from smaller units, usually requiring input of energy (ATP) in the process.

Anaerobic: Anaerobic is a technical word which literally means without oxygen, as opposed to aerobic. In wastewater treatment the absence of oxygen is indicated as anoxic; and anaerobic is used to indicate the absence of a common electron acceptor such as nitrate, sulfate, or oxygen. An anaerobic adhesive is a bonding agent that does not cure in the presence of air.

Anaerobic digestion: Anaerobic digestion is a series of processes in which microorganisms break down biodegradable material in the absence of oxygen, used for industrial or domestic purposes to manage waste and/or to release energy.

Anaerobic respiration: Anaerobic respiration is a form of respiration using electron acceptors other than oxygen. Although oxygen is not used as the final electron acceptor, the process still uses a respiratory electron transport chain; it is respiration without oxygen. In order for the electron transport chain to function, an exogenous final electron acceptor must be present to allow electrons to pass through the system.

Anaphase: Anaphase is the stage of mitosis or meiosis when chromosomes separate in an eukaryotic cell. Each chromatid moves to opposite poles of the cell, the opposite ends of the mitotic spindle, near the microtubule organizing centers. During this stage, anaphase lag could happen.

Anchor gene: A gene that has been positioned on both the physical map and the linkage map of a chromosome, and thereby allows their mutual alignment.

Aneuploidy: Aneuploidy is an abnormal number of chromosomes, and is a type of chromosome abnormality. An extra or missing chromosome is a common cause of genetic disorders (birth defects). Some cancer cells also have abnormal numbers of chromosomes. Aneuploidy occurs during cell division when the chromosomes do not separate properly between the two cells.

Animal cloning: Animal cloning is the process by which an entire organism is reproduced from a single cell taken from the parent organism and in a genetically identical manner. This means the cloned animal is an exact duplicate in every way of its parent; it has the exact DNA.

Annealing temperature: The reaction temperature is lowered to 50–65°C for 20–40 s allowing annealing of the primers to the single-stranded DNA template. Typically the annealing temperature is about 3–5°C below the T_m of the primers used. Stable DNA–DNA hydrogen bonds are only formed when the primer sequence very closely matches the template sequence. The polymerase binds to the primer–template hybrid and begins DNA synthesis.

Antagonism: When a substance binds to the same site an agonist would bind to without causing activation of the receptor.

Antagonist: A chemical compound which reversed the effects of agonist is called as antagonist.

Anthocyanins: Anthocyanins are water-soluble vacuolar pigments that may appear red, purple, or blue according to pH. They belong to a parent class of molecules called flavonoids synthesized via the phenylpropanoid pathway; they are odorless and nearly flavorless, contributing to taste as a moderately astringent sensation. Anthocyanins occur in all tissues of higher plants, including leaves, stems, roots, flowers, and fruits.

Antiauxin: A substance that inhibits the growth-regulating function of an auxin.

Antibiotic: The term "antibiotic" was coined by Selman Waksman in 1942 to describe any substance produced by a microorganism that is antagonistic to the growth of other microorganisms in high dilution.

Antibiotic resistance: Antibiotic resistance is a type of drug resistance where a microorganism is able to survive exposure to an antibiotic. Genes can be transferred between bacteria in a horizontal fashion by conjugation, transduction, or transformation. Thus, a gene for antibiotic resistance which had evolved via natural selection may be shared. Evolutionary stress such as exposure to antibiotics then selects for the antibiotic-resistant trait.

Antibody: An antibody, also known as an immunoglobulin, is a large Y-shaped protein used by the immune system to identify and neutralize foreign objects such as bacteria and viruses.

Anticoding strand: The DNA strand that forms the template for both the transcribed mRNA and the coding DNA strand.

Anticodon: A sequence of three adjacent nucleotides located on one end of the transfer RNA. It binds to the complementary coding triplet of nucleotides in the messenger RNA during the translation phase of protein synthesis.

Antigen: An antigen is a substance/molecule that, when introduced into the body triggers the production of an antibody by the immune system, which will then kill or neutralize the antigen that is recognized as a foreign and potentially harmful invader.

Anti-idiotype vaccines: Anti-idiotypic vaccines comprise antibodies that have three-dimensional immunogenic regions, designated idiotopes that consist of protein sequences that bind to cell receptors. Idiotopes are aggregated into idiotypes specific of their target antigen.

Antimicrobial agent: An antimicrobial is a substance that kills or inhibits the growth of microorganisms such as bacteria, fungi, or protozoans. Antimicrobial drugs either kill microbes (microbiocidal) or prevent the growth of microbes (microbiostatic). Disinfectants are antimicrobial substances used on nonliving objects or outside the body.

Antioxidant: An antioxidant is a molecule capable of inhibiting the oxidation of other molecules. Oxidation is a chemical reaction that transfers electrons from a substance to an oxidizing agent.

Antiparallel orientation: Two strands of DNA arranged in opposite directions.

Antisense DNA: Antisense DNA: DNA normally has two strands, that is, the sense strand and the antisense strand. In double-stranded DNA, only one strand codes for the RNA that is translated into protein. This DNA strand is referred to as the antisense strand. The strand that does not code for RNA is called the sense strand.

Antisense gene: A gene that produces an mRNA complementary to the transcript of a normal gene (usually constructed by inverting the coding region relative to the promoter).

Antisense RNA: Antisense RNA is a single-stranded RNA that is complementary to a messenger RNA (mRNA) strand transcribed within a cell. Antisense RNA may be introduced into a cell to inhibit translation of a complementary mRNA by base pairing to it and physically obstructing the translation machinery.

Antisense therapy: Antisense therapy is a form of treatment for genetic disorders or infections. When the genetic sequence of a particular gene is known to be causative of a particular disease, it is possible to synthesize a strand of nucleic acid (DNA, RNA, or a chemical analogue) that will bind to the messenger RNA (mRNA) produced by that gene and inactivate it, effectively turning that gene "off." This is because mRNA has to be single stranded for it to be translated. Alternatively, the strand might be targeted to bind a splicing site on pre-mRNA and modify the exon content of an mRNA.

Antiseptic: Antiseptics are antimicrobial substances that are applied to living tissue/skin to reduce the possibility of infection, sepsis, or putrefaction. Antiseptics are generally distinguished from antibiotics by the latter's ability to be transported through the lymphatic system to destroy bacteria within the body, and from disinfectants, which destroy microorganisms found on nonliving objects.

Apoenzyme: The protein component of an enzyme, to which the coenzyme attaches to form an active enzyme.

Apomixis: Reproduction without meiosis or formation of gametes.

Apoptosis: The process of cell death by disintegration of cells into membrane-bound particles that are then eliminated by phagocytosis or by shedding.

Arabidopsis: Genus of the mustard family having white or yellow or purplish flowers; closely related to genus *Arabis*.

Artificial insemination: Introduction of animal semen into the uterus without sexual contact.

Artificial selection: Artificial selection (or selective breeding) describes intentional breeding for certain traits, or combination of traits. The term was used by Charles Darwin in contrast to natural selection, in which the differential reproduction of organisms with certain traits is attributed to improved survival or reproductive ability ("Darwinian fitness"). As opposed to artificial selection, in which humans favor specific traits, in natural selection the environment acts as a sieve through which only certain variations can pass.

Aseptic: Free from the living germs of disease, fermentation, or putrefaction.

Asexual reproduction: Asexual reproduction is a mode of reproduction by which offspring arise from a single parent, and inherit the genes of that parent only; it is reproduction which does not involve meiosis, ploidy reduction, or fertilization.

Attenuated vaccine: An attenuated vaccine is a vaccine created by reducing the virulence of a pathogen, but still keeping it viable (or "live"). Attenuation takes an infectious agent and alters it so that it becomes harmless or less virulent.

Autoclave: An autoclave is an instrument used to sterilize equipment and supplies by subjecting them to high-pressure saturated steam at 121°C for around 15–20 min depending on the size of the load and the contents. It was invented by Charles Chamberland in 1879.

Autoimmune disease: Autoimmune diseases arise from an overactive immune response of the body against substances and tissues normally present in the body. In other words, the body actually attacks its own cells. The immune system mistakes some part of the body as a pathogen and attacks it.

Autologous cells: Cells taken from an individual, cultured (or stored), and, possibly, genetically manipulated before being transferred back into the original donor.

Autonomous Replicating Sequence: An autonomously replicating sequence (ARS) contains the origin of replication in the yeast genome. It contains four regions (A, B1, B2, and B3), named in order of their effect on plasmid stability; when these regions are mutated, replication does not initiate.

Autopolyploid: An individual or strain whose chromosome complement consists of more than two complete copies of the genome of a single ancestral species.

Autoradiography: An autoradiograph is an image on an x-ray film or nuclear emulsion produced by the pattern of decay emissions (e.g., beta particles or gamma rays) from a distribution of a radioactive substance.

Autosome: An autosome is a chromosome that is not a sex chromosome, or allosome; that is to say, there are an equal number of copies of the chromosome in males and females. For example, in humans, there are 22 pairs of autosomes. In addition to autosomes, there are sex chromosomes, to be specific: X and Y. So, humans have 23 pairs of chromosomes.

Autotrophic: An autotroph[α], or producer, is an organism that produces complex organic compounds (such as carbohydrates, fats, and proteins) from simple inorganic molecules using energy from light (by photosynthesis) or inorganic chemical reactions (chemosynthesis).

Auxotrophy: Auxotrophy is the inability of an organism to synthesize a particular organic compound required for its growth (as defined by IUPAC). An auxotroph is an organism that displays this characteristic; auxotrophic is the corresponding adjective. Auxotrophy is the opposite of prototrophy, which is characterized by the ability to synthesize all the compounds that the parent organism could.

Bacillus thuringiensis: *Bacillus thuringiensis* (or Bt) is a Gram-positive, soil-dwelling bacterium, commonly used as a biological alternative to a pesticide; alternatively, the Cry toxin may be extracted and used as a pesticide. *B. thuringiensis* also occurs naturally in the gut of caterpillars of various types of moths and butterflies, as well as on the dark surface of plants.

Back mutation: The process that causes reversion of mutation.

Bacterial artificial chromosome: Bacterial artificial chromosome (BAC) is a DNA construct, based on a functional fertility plasmid (or F-plasmid), used for transforming and cloning in bacteria, usually *E. coli*. F-plasmids play a crucial role because they contain partition genes that promote the even distribution of plasmids after bacterial cell division. The BACs usual insert size is 150–350 kbp, but can be greater than 700 kbp.

Bacterial toxin: Bacterial toxin is a type of toxin that is generated by bacteria.

Bactericide: A bactericide or bacteriocide is a substance that kills bacteria and, ideally, nothing else. Bactericides are disinfectants, antiseptics, or antibiotics.

Bacteriocin: Bacteriocins are proteinaceous toxins produced by bacteria to inhibit the growth of similar or closely related bacterial strain(s). They are typically considered to be narrow-spectrum antibiotics, though this has been debated. They are phenomenologically analogous to yeast and paramecium killing factors, and are structurally, functionally, and ecologically diverse.

Bacteriophage: A bacteriophage is any one of a number of viruses that infect bacteria. Bacteriophages are among the most common biological entities on Earth. The term is commonly used in its shortened form, phage.

Bacteriostat: Bacteriostat is a biological or chemical agent that causes bacteriostasis. It stops bacteria from reproducing, while not necessarily harming them otherwise. Upon removal of the bacteriostat, the bacteria usually start to grow again. Bacteriostats are often used in plastics to prevent growth of bacteria on the plastic surface. This is in contrast to bacteriocides, which kill bacteria.

Balanced lethal system: An arrangement of alleles of two recessive lethal genes in repulsion phase that maintains a heterozygous chromosome combination whereas homozygotes for any lethal-bearing chromosome will be lethal.

Balanced polymorphism: Balanced polymorphism is an equilibrium mixture of homozygotes and heterozygotes maintained by natural selection against both homozygotes.

Barr body: Barr body (named after the discoverer Murray Barr) is the inactive X chromosome in a female somatic cell, rendered inactive in a process called lyonization, in those species (including humans) in which sex is determined by the presence of the Y or W chromosome rather than the diploidy of the X or Z.

Basal body: A basal body (also called a basal granule or kinetosome) is an organelle formed from a centriole, and a short cylindrical array of microtubules. It is found at the base of a eukaryotic undulipodium (cilium or flagellum) and serves as a nucleation site for the growth of the axoneme microtubules.

Base pair: In molecular biology and genetics, two nucleotides on opposite complementary DNA or RNA strands that are connected via hydrogen bonds are called a base pair (often abbreviated bp). In the canonical Watson–Crick DNA base pairing, adenine (A) forms a base pair with thymine (T) and guanine (G) forms a base pair with cytosine (C).

Basophil: Basophils are part of your immune system that normally protects your body from infection, but can also be partly responsible for your asthma symptoms. Basophils are a type of white blood cell that is involved in inflammatory reactions in your body, especially those related to allergies and asthma.

Batch culture: A large-scale closed system culture in which cells are grown in a fixed volume of nutrient culture medium under specific environmental conditions (e.g., nutrient type, temperature, pressure, aeration, etc.) up to a certain density in a tank or airlift fermenter, harvested and processed as a batch, especially before all nutrients are used up.

Batch fermentation: Fermentation the anaerobic enzymatic conversion of organic compounds, especially carbohydrates, to simpler compounds, especially to ethyl alcohol, producing energy in the form of ATP.

B cells: B cells are lymphocytes that play a large role in the humoral immune response (as opposed to the cell-mediated immune response, which is governed by T cells).

βeta-galactosidase: β-galactosidase, also called beta-gal or β-gal, is a hydrolase enzyme that catalyzes the hydrolysis of β-galactosides into monosaccharides. Substrates of different β-galactosidases include ganglioside GM1, lactosylceramides, lactose, and various glycoproteins. Lactase is often confused as an alternative name for β-galactosidase, but it is actually simply a sub-class of β-galactosidase.

βeta-lactamase: Beta-lactamases are enzymes (EC 3.5.2.6) produced by some bacteria and are responsible for their resistance to beta-lactam antibiotics such as penicillins, cephamycins, and carbapenems (ertapenem). (Cephalosporins are relatively resistant to beta-lactamase.)

Binary vector system: Binary vector systems include the most commonly used vectors devised for Agrobacterium gene transfer to plants. In these systems, the T-DNA region containing a gene of interest is contained in one vector and the vir region is located in a separate disarmed (without tumor-genes) Ti plasmid. The plasmids co-reside in *Agrobacterium* and remain independent.

Bioassay: Bioassay (commonly used shorthand for biological assay), or biological standardization is a type of scientific experiment. Bioassays are typically conducted to measure the effects of a substance on a living organism and are essential in the development of new drugs and in monitoring environmental pollutants. Both are procedures by which the potency or the nature of a substance is estimated by studying its effects on living matter.

Bio-augmentation: Bio-augmentation is the introduction of a group of natural microbial strains or a genetically engineered variant to treat contaminated soil or water. Usually the steps involve studying the indigenous varieties present in the location to determine if bio-stimulation is possible. If the indigenous variety do not have the metabolic capability to perform the remediation process, exogenous varieties with such sophisticated pathways are introduced.

Bioconversion: The term bioconversion, also known as biotransformation refers to the use of live organisms often microorganisms to carry out a chemical reaction that is more costly or not feasible nonbiologically. These organisms convert a substance to a chemically modified form. An example is the industrial production of cortisone. One step is the bioconversion of progesterone to 11-alpha-hydroxyprogesterone by *Rhizopus nigricans.*

Biodegradation: Biodegradation or biotic degradation or biotic decomposition is the chemical dissolution of materials by bacteria or other biological means. The term is often used in relation to ecology, waste management, biomedicine, and the natural environment (bioremediation) and is now commonly associated with environmentally friendly products that are capable of decomposing back into natural elements.

Biodiversity: Biodiversity is the degree of variation of life forms within a given ecosystem, biome, or an entire planet. Biodiversity is a measure of the health of ecosystems. Greater biodiversity implies greater health. Biodiversity is in part a function of climate. In terrestrial habitats, tropical regions are typically rich whereas Polar Regions support fewer species.

Bioenrichment: Adding nutrients or oxygen to increase microbial breakdown of pollutants.

Bioethics: Bioethics is the study of controversial ethics brought about by advances in biology and medicine. Bioethicists are concerned with the ethical questions that arise in the relationships among life sciences, biotechnology, medicine, politics, law, and philosophy.

Biofuel: Biofuel is a type of fuel which is in some way derived from biomass. The term covers solid biomass, liquid fuels, and various biogases. Biofuels are gaining increased public and scientific attention, driven by factors such as oil price spikes, the need for increased energy security, concern over greenhouse gas emissions from fossil fuels, and government subsidies.

Biogas: Biogas typically refers to a gas produced by the biological breakdown of organic matter in the absence of oxygen. Biogas originates from biogenic material and is a type of biofuel.

Bioinformatics: Bioinformatics is the application of statistics and computer science to the field of molecular biology. The primary goal of bioinformatics is to increase the understanding of biological processes.

Biolistics: Gene gun or a biolistic particle delivery system, originally designed for plant transformation, is a device for injecting cells with genetic information. The payload is an elemental particle of a heavy metal coated with plasmid DNA. This technique is often simply referred to as bioballistics or biolistics.

Biological containment: Biological containment (or biocontainment) describes measures aimed at preventing genetically modified organisms (GMOs) and their transgenes from spreading into the environment.

Biometric: Biometrics consists of methods for uniquely recognizing humans based upon one or more intrinsic physical or behavioral traits. In computer science, in particular, biometrics is used as a form of identity access management and access control. It is also used to identify individuals in groups that are under surveillance.

Biopesticide: Biopesticides are biochemical pesticides that are naturally occurring substances that control pests by nontoxic mechanisms.

Biopolymer: Biopolymers are polymers produced by living organisms. Since they are polymers, biopolymers contain monomeric units that are covalently bonded to form larger structures.

Bioprocess: A bioprocess is any process that uses complete living cells or their components (e.g., bacteria, enzymes, chloroplasts) to obtain desired products.

Bioreactor: A bioreactor may refer to any manufactured or engineered device or system that supports a biologically active environment. In one case, a bioreactor is a vessel in which a chemical process is carried out which involves organisms or biochemically active substances derived from such organisms. This process can either be aerobic or anaerobic. These bioreactors are commonly cylindrical, ranging in size from liters to cubic meters, and are often made of stainless steel.

Bioremediation: Bioremediation is the use of microorganism metabolism to remove pollutants. Technologies can be generally classified as in situ or ex situ. In situ bioremediation involves treating the contaminated material at the site, while ex situ involves the removal of the contaminated material to be treated elsewhere.

Biosensor: A biosensor is an analytical device for the detection of a chemical compound that combines a biological component with a physicochemical detector component.

Biosphere: Our biosphere is the global sum of all ecosystems. It can also be called the zone of life on Earth, a closed (apart from solar and cosmic radiation) and self-regulating system.

Biosynthesis: Biosynthesis (also called biogenesis) is an enzyme-catalyzed process in cells of living organisms by which substrates are converted into more complex products. The biosynthesis process often consists of several enzymatic steps in which the product of one step is used as substrate in the following step. Examples for such multi-step biosynthetic pathways are those for the production of amino acids, fatty acids, and natural products. Biosynthesis plays a major role in all cells, and many dedicated metabolic routes combined constitute general metabolism.

Biotic factor: A factor created by a living thing or any living component within an environment in which the action of the organism affects the life of another organism, for example, a predator consuming its prey.

Biotic stress: Biotic stress is stress that occurs as a result of damage done to plants by other living organisms, such as bacteria, viruses, fungi, parasites, beneficial and harmful insects, weeds, and cultivated or native plants.

Biotin: Biotin is a water-soluble B-complex vitamin (vitamin B7). It was discovered by Bateman in 1916. It is composed of a ureido (tetrahydroimidizalone) ring fused with a tetrahydrothiophene ring. A valeric acid substituent is attached to one of the carbon atoms of the tetrahydrothiophene ring. Biotin is a coenzyme in the metabolism of fatty acids and leucine, and it plays a role in gluconeogenesis.

Biotoxin: A toxic substance produced by a living organism.

Biotransformation: Biotransformation is the chemical modification (or modifications) made by an organism on a chemical compound. If this modification ends in mineral compounds like CO_2, NH_4+, or H_2O, the biotransformation is called mineralization.

Bivalent: A molecule formed from two or more atoms bound together as a single unit molecule.

β-Lactamase: β-lactamases are enzymes produced by some bacteria and are responsible for their resistance to beta-lactam antibiotics such as penicillins, cephamycins, and carbapenems.

Blastocyst: The blastocyst is a structure formed in the early embryogenesis of mammals, after the formation of the morula. It is a specifically mammalian example of a blastula.

Blastomere: A blastomere is a type of cell produced by division of the egg after fertilization.

Blastula: The blastula is a solid sphere of cells formed during an early stage of embryonic development in animals. The blastula is created when the zygote undergoes the cell division process known as cleavage.

Blot: Blot (biology), method of transferring proteins, DNA, RNA or a protein onto a carrier.

Blunt end: The end of a DNA fragment resulting from the breaking of DNA molecule in which there are no unpaired bases, hence, both strands are of the same length.

Blunt-end cut: To cut a double-stranded DNA with a restriction endonuclease which generates blunt ends.

B lymphocyte: B cells are lymphocytes that play a large role in the humoral immune response (as opposed to the cell-mediated immune response, which is governed by T cells).

Breed: A breed is a group of domestic animals or plants with a homogeneous appearance, behavior, and other characteristics that distinguish it from other animals of the same species.

Breeding: Breeding is the reproduction that is, producing of offspring, usually animals or plants.

Brewing: Brewing is the production of beer through steeping a starch source (commonly cereal grains) in water and then fermenting with yeast. Brewing has taken place since around the 6th millennium BC, and archeological evidence suggests that this technique was used in ancient Egypt.

Bovine spongiform encephalopathy: Bovine spongiform encephalopathy (BSE), commonly known as mad-cow disease is a fatal neurodegenerative disease in cattle that causes a spongy degeneration in the brain and spinal cord. BSE has a long incubation period, about 30 months to 8 years, usually affecting adult cattle at a peak age onset of four to five years, all breeds being equally susceptible.

Bubble column fermenter: A bioreactor in which the cells or microorganisms are kept suspended in a tall cylinder by rising air, which is introduced at the base of the vessel.

Buffer: Solution which reduces the change of pH upon addition of small amounts of acid or base, or upon dilution.

Buoyant density: A measure of the tendency of a substance to float in some other substance; large molecules are distinguished by their differing buoyant densities in some standard fluid.

CAAT box: In molecular biology, a CCAAT box (also sometimes abbreviated a CAAT box or CAT box) is a distinct pattern of nucleotides with GGCCAATCT consensus sequence that occur upstream by 75–80 bases to the initial transcription site. The CAAT box signals the binding site for the RNA transcription factor, and is typically accompanied by a conserved consensus sequence.

Callus culture: The callus culture is a technique of tissue culture; it is usually carried out on solidified gel medium in the presence of growth regulators and initiated by inoculation of small explants or sections from established organ or other cultures.

Calorie: The calorie is a pre-SI metric unit of energy. It was first defined by Nicolas Clément in 1824 as a unit of heat, entering French and English dictionaries between 1841 and 1867. In most fields its use is archaic, having been replaced by the SI unit of energy, the joule. However, in many countries it remains in common use as a unit of food energy.

Cancer: Cancer is the uncontrolled growth of abnormal cells in the body. Cancerous cells are also called malignant cells.

Candidate gene: A candidate gene is a gene, located in a chromosome region suspected of being involved in the expression of a trait such as a disease, whose protein product suggests that it could be the gene in question. A candidate gene can also be identified by association with the phenotype and by linkage analysis to a region of the genome.

Cap: The structure found on the 5′-end of eukaryotic mRNA, and consisting of an inverted, methylated guanosine residue is called as Cap.

Capsid: The protein coat of a virus.

Cap site: Gene translation initiation site.

Carcinogen: A carcinogen is any substance, radionuclide, or radiation that is an agent directly involved in causing cancer. This may be due to the ability to damage the genome or to the disruption of cellular metabolic processes.

Carcinoma: Carcinoma is the medical term for the most common type of cancer occurring in humans.

Carotene: The term carotene is used for several related hydrocarbon substances having the formula C40Hx, which are synthesized by plants but cannot be made by animals.

Carotenoids: Carotenoids are tetraterpenoid organic pigments that are naturally occurring in the chloroplasts and chromoplasts of plants and some other photosynthetic organisms such as algae, some types of fungus some bacteria and at least one species of aphid. Carotenoids are generally not manufactured by species in the animal kingdom, although one species of aphid is known to have acquired the genes for synthesis of the carotenoid torulene from fungi, by the known phenomenon of horizontal gene transfer.

Carrier DNA: DNA of undefined sequence which is added to the transforming (plasmid) DNA used in physical DNA-transfer procedures. This additional DNA increases the efficiency of transformation in electroporation and chemically mediated DNA delivery systems.

Carrier molecule: A molecule that plays a role in transporting electrons through the electron transport chain. Carrier molecules are usually proteins bound to a non-protein group; they can undergo oxidation and reduction relatively easily, thus allowing electrons to flow through the system.

Casein: Casein is the name for a family of related phosphor–protein proteins. These proteins are commonly found in mammalian milk, making up 80% of the proteins in cow milk and between 60% and 65% of the proteins in human milk.

Catabolic pathway: A sequence of degradative chemical reactions that break down complex molecules into smaller units, usually releasing energy in the process.

Catabolism: Catabolism is the set of pathways that break down molecules into smaller units and release energy. In catabolism, large molecules such as polysaccharides, lipids, nucleic acids, and proteins are broken down into smaller units such as monosaccharides, fatty acids, nucleotides, and amino acids, respectively.

Catabolite repression: Carbon catabolite repression, or simply catabolite repression, is an important part of global control system of various bacteria and other microorganisms. Catabolite repression allows bacteria to adapt quickly to a preferred (rapidly metabolizable) carbon and energy source first.

Catalysis: Catalysis is the change in rate of a chemical reaction due to the participation of a substance called a catalyst. Unlike other reagents that participate in the chemical reaction, a catalyst is not consumed by the reaction itself. A catalyst may participate in multiple chemical transformations. Catalysts that enhance the speed of the reaction are called positive catalysts.

Catalytic RNA: A ribozyme is an RNA molecule with a well-defined tertiary structure that enables it to catalyze a chemical reaction. Ribozyme means ribonucleic acid enzyme. It may also be called an RNA enzyme or catalytic RNA.

Cation: A positively charged ion.

cDNA library: A cDNA library is a combination of cloned cDNA (complementary DNA) fragments inserted into a collection of host cells, which together constitute some portion of the transcriptome of the organism. cDNA is produced from fully transcribed mRNA found in the nucleus and therefore contains only the expressed genes of an organism.

Cell culture: Cell culture is the complex process by which cells are grown under controlled conditions. In practice, the term "cell culture" has come to refer to the culturing of cells derived from multicellular eukaryotes, especially animal cells.

Cell cycle: The cell cycle, or cell-division cycle, is the series of events that takes place in a cell leading to its division and duplication (replication). In cells without a nucleus (prokaryotic), the cell cycle occurs via a process termed binary fission.

Cell fusion: Cell fusion is an important cellular process that occurs during differentiation of muscle, bone, and trophoblast cells, during embryogenesis, and during morphogenesis. Cell fusion is a necessary event in the maturation of cells so that they maintain their specific functions throughout growth.

Cell generation time: The doubling time is the period of time required for a quantity to double in size or value. It is applied to population growth, inflation, and resource extraction, consumption of goods, compound interest, the volume of malignant tumors, and many other things that tend to grow over time. When the relative growth rate (not the absolute growth rate) is constant, the quantity undergoes exponential growth and has a constant doubling time or period which can be calculated directly from the growth rate.

Cell hybridization: Fusion of two or more dissimilar cells, leading to formation of a synkaryon.

Cell line: A cell line is a product of immortal cells that are used for biological research. Cells used for cell lines are immortal, that happens if a cell is cancerous. The cells can perpetuate division indefinitely which is unlike regular cells which can only divide approximately 50 times. These cells are "useful" for experimentation in labs as they are always available to researchers as a product and do not require what is known as "harvesting" (the acquiring of tissue from a host) every time cells are needed in the lab.

Cell membrane: The cell membrane is a biological membrane that separates the interior of all cells from the outside environment. The cell membrane is selectively permeable to ions and organic molecules and controls the movement of substances in and out of cells.

Cell sap: The liquid inside the large central vacuole of a plant cell that serves as storage of materials and provides mechanical support, especially in nonwoody plants. It has also a vital role in plant cell osmosis.

Cell strain: A cell strain is derived either from a primary culture or a cell line by the selection or cloning of cells having specific properties or markers. In describing a cell strain, its specific features must be defined. The terms finite or continuous are to be used as prefixes if the status of the culture is known. If not, the term strain will suffice. In any published description of a cell strain, one must make every attempt to publish the characterization or history of the strain. If such has already been published, a reference to the original publication must be made. In obtaining a culture from another laboratory, the proper designation of the culture, as originally named and described, must be maintained and any deviations in cultivation from the original must be reported in any publication.

Cellular immune response: Cell-mediated immunity is an immune response that does not involve antibodies or complement but rather involves the activation of macrophages, natural killer cells (NK), antigen-specific cytotoxic T-lymphocytes, and the release of various cytokines in response to an antigen.

Cellulose: Cellulose is an organic compound with the formula (C6H10O5)n, a polysaccharide consisting of a linear chain of several hundred to over 10,000 $\beta(1 \rightarrow 4)$ linked D-glucose units.

Cellulose nitrate: Nitrocellulose (also: cellulose nitrate, flash paper) is a highly flammable compound formed by nitrating cellulose through exposure to nitric acid or another powerful nitrating agent.

Cellulosomes: Cellulosomes are complexes of cellulolytic enzymes created by bacteria such as *Clostridium* and *Bacteroides*. They consist of catalytic subunits such as glycoside hydrolases, polysaccharide lyases, and carboxyl esterases bound together by scaffoldins consisting of cohesins connected to other functional units such as the enzymes and carbohydrate binding modules via dockerins. They assist in digestion or degradation of plant cell wall materials, most notably cellulose.

Central dogma: The central dogma of molecular biology deals with the detailed residue-by-residue transfer of sequential information. It states that information cannot be transferred back from protein to either protein or nucleic acid.

Centrifugation: Centrifugation is a process that involves the use of the centrifugal force for the separation of mixtures with a centrifuge, used in industry and in laboratory settings. More-dense components of the mixture migrate away from the axis of the centrifuge, while less-dense components of the mixture migrate toward the axis.

Centromere: A centromere is a region of DNA typically found near the middle of a chromosome where two identical sister chromatids come closest in contact. It is involved in cell division as the point of mitotic spindle attachment. The sister chromatids are attached all along their length, but they are closest at the centromere.

Centrosome: In cell biology, the centrosome is an organelle that serves as the main microtubule organizing center (MTOC) of the animal cell as well as a regulator of cell-cycle progression.

Chain termination: Chain termination is any chemical reaction that ceases the formation of reactive intermediates in a chain propagation step in the course of a polymerization, effectively bringing it to a halt.

Charcoal: Charcoal is the dark-gray residue consisting of impure carbon obtained by removing water and other volatile constituents from animal and vegetation substances. Charcoal is usually produced by slow pyrolysis, the heating of wood or other substances in the absence of oxygen.

Chelate: A chemical compound in the form of a heterocyclic ring, containing a metal ion attached by coordinate bonds to at least two nonmetal ions.

Chemically defined medium: A chemically defined medium is a growth medium suitable for the *in vitro* cell culture of human or animal cells in which all of the chemical components are known.

Chemical mutagens: Chemical mutagens are defined as those compounds that increase the frequency of some types of mutations. They vary in their potency since this term reflects their ability to enter the cell, their reactivity with DNA, their general toxicity, and the likelihood that the type of chemical change they introduce into the DNA will be corrected by a repair system. Most of the following mutagens are used *in vivo* treatments, but some of them can also be used *in vitro*.

Chemiluminescence: Chemiluminescence (sometimes "chemoluminescence") is the emission of light with limited emission of heat (luminescence), as a result of a chemical reaction.

Chemostat: A chemostat (from chemical environment is static) is a bioreactor to which fresh medium is continuously added, while culture liquid is continuously removed to keep the culture volume constant. By changing the rate with which the medium is added to the bioreactor the growth rate of the microorganism can be easily controlled.

Chemotaxis: Chemotaxis is the phenomenon in which somatic cells, bacteria, and other single-cell or multicellular organisms direct their movements according to certain chemicals in their environment. This is important for bacteria to find food (e.g., glucose) by swimming toward the highest concentration of food molecules, or to flee from poisons (e.g., phenol).

Chemotherapy: Chemotherapy (sometimes cancer chemotherapy) is the treatment of cancer with an antineoplastic drug or with a combination of such drugs into a standardized treatment regimen.

Chimeric DNA: A molecule of DNA that has resulted from recombination, or has resulted from DNA from two sources being spliced together.

Chimeric gene: Chimeric genes form through the combination of portions of one or more coding sequences to produce new genes. These mutations are distinct from fusion genes which merge whole gene sequences into a single reading frame and often retain their original functions.

Chimeric protein: A hybrid protein encoded by a nucleotide sequence spliced together from 2+ complete or partial genes produced by recombinant DNA technology.

Chimeric selectable marker gene: A gene that is constructed from parts of two or more different genes and allows the host cell to survive under conditions where it would otherwise die.

Chi-squared: A chi-square test (also chi-squared test or χ^2 test) is any statistical hypothesis test in which the sampling distribution of the test statistic is a chi-square distribution when the null hypothesis is true, or any in which this is asymptotically true, meaning that the sampling distribution (if the null hypothesis is true) can be made to approximate a chi-square distribution as closely as desired by making the sample size large enough.

Chitin: Chitin is a long-chain polymer of *N*-acetylglucosamine, a derivative of glucose, and is found in many places throughout the natural world.

Chitinase: Chitinases are digestive enzymes that break down glycosidic bonds in chitin. Because chitin is a component of the cell walls of fungi and exoskeletal elements of some animals (including worms and arthropods), chitinases are generally found in organisms that either need to reshape their own chitin or to dissolve and digest the chitin of fungi or animals.

Chloramphenicol: Chloramphenicol (INN) is a bacteriostatic antimicrobial. It is considered a prototypical broad-spectrum antibiotic, alongside the tetracyclines.

Chlorenchyma: Plant tissue consisting of parenchyma cells that contain chloroplasts.

Chlorophyll: Chlorophyll is a green pigment found in almost all plants, algae, and cyanobacteria. Chlorophyll is an extremely important biomolecule, critical in photosynthesis, which allows plants to obtain energy from light.

Chloroplasts: Chloroplasts are organelles found in plant cells and other eukaryotic organisms that conduct photosynthesis. Chloroplasts capture light energy to conserve free energy in the form of ATP and reduce NADP to NADPH through a complex set of processes called photosynthesis.

Chromatid: A chromatid is one of the two identical copies of DNA making up a duplicated chromosome, which are joined at their centromeres, for the process of cell division (mitosis or meiosis). They are called sister chromatids as long as they are joined by the centromeres. When they separate (during anaphase of mitosis and anaphase 2 of meiosis), the strands are called daughter chromosomes.

Chromatin: Chromatin is the combination of DNA and other proteins that make up the contents of the nucleus. The primary functions of chromatin are; to package DNA into a smaller volume to fit in the cell, to strengthen the DNA to allow mitosis and meiosis and prevent DNA damage, and to control gene expression and DNA replication.

Chromatography: Chromatography is the collective term for a set of laboratory techniques for the separation of mixtures. It involves passing a mixture dissolved in a "mobile phase" through a stationary phase, which separates the analyte to be measured from other molecules in the mixture based on differential partitioning between the mobile and stationary phases. Subtle differences in a compound's partition coefficient result in differential retention on the stationary phase and thus changing the separation.

Chromosomal aberration: A chromosome anomaly, abnormality or aberration reflects an atypical number of chromosomes or a structural abnormality in one or more chromosomes. A karyotype refers to a full set of chromosomes from an individual which can be compared to a "normal" karyotype for the species via genetic testing. A chromosome anomaly may be detected or confirmed in this manner. Chromosome anomalies usually occur when there is an error in cell division following meiosis or mitosis. There are many types of chromosome anomalies. They can be organized into two basic groups, numerical and structural anomalies.

Chromosomal polymorphism: In genetics, chromosomal polymorphism is a condition where one species contains members with varying chromosome counts or shapes. Polymorphism is a general concept in biology where more than one version of a trait is present in a population. In some cases of differing counts, the difference in chromosome counts is the result of a single chromosome is undergoing fission, where it splits into two smaller chromosomes, or two undergoing fusion, where two chromosomes join to form one.

Chromosome banding: The banding patterns lend each chromosome a distinctive appearance so the 22 pairs of human nonsex chromosomes and the X and Y chromosomes can be identified and distinguished without ambiguity. Banding also permits the recognition of chromosome deletions (lost segments), chromosome duplications (surplus segments) and other types of structural rearrangements of chromosomes.

Chromosome jumping: Chromosome jumping is a tool of molecular biology that is used in the physical mapping of genomes. It is related to several other tools used for the same purpose, including chromosome walking.

Chromosome mutations: Chromosomal mutations take place when the number of chromosomes changes or when structural changes occur in the chromosomes. This process occurs generally during the formation of a zygote where changes in the number of chromosomes may result in fission (two into one or one into two) or fusion (two into one).

Chromosome theory of inheritance: The theory that chromosomes are linear sequences of genes and genes are located in specific sites on chromosomes.

Chromosome walking: Chromosome walking is a technique to clone a gene (e.g., a disease gene) from its known closest markers. The closest linked marker (e.g., EST or a known gene) to the gene is used to probe a genomic library. A restriction fragment isolated from the end of the positive clones is used to reprobe the genomic library for overlapping clones. This process is repeated several times to walk across the chromosome and reach the gene of interest.

Chymosin: Chymosin or rennin is an enzyme found in rennet. It is produced by cows in the lining of the abomasum (the fourth and final, chamber of the stomach). Chymosin is produced by gastric chief cells in infants to curdle the milk they ingest, allowing a longer residence in the bowels and better absorption.

Cistron: A cistron is a term used to describe the locus responsible for generating a protein. It can also be defined as the segment of DNA that contains all the information for production of single polypeptide.

Clonal propagation: Asexual propagation of many new plants (ramets) from an individual (ortet); all have the same genotype.

Clonal selection: The clonal selection hypothesis has become a widely accepted model for how the immune system responds to infection and how certain types of B and T lymphocytes are selected for destruction of specific antigens invading the body.

Cloning: Cloning in biology is the process of producing similar populations of genetically identical individuals that occurs in nature when organisms such as bacteria, insects, or plants reproduce asexually. Cloning in biotechnology refers to processes used to create copies of DNA fragments (molecular cloning), cells (cell cloning), or organisms. The term also refers to the production of multiple copies of a product such as digital media or software.

Cloning vector: A cloning vector is a small piece of DNA into which a foreign DNA fragment can be inserted. The insertion of the fragment into the cloning vector is carried out by treating the vehicle and the foreign DNA with a restriction enzyme that creates the same overhang, then ligating the fragments together. There are many types of cloning vectors. Genetically engineered plasmids and bacteriophages (such as phage λ) are perhaps most commonly used for this purpose. Other types of cloning vectors include bacterial artificial chromosomes (BACs) and yeast artificial chromosomes (YACs).

Co-culture: In the study of cell interaction co-culture is obviously necessary. In some cases actual contact with cells grown in a mixture is desired while in others the mutual effect of cell types on one another is of interest while the cells themselves are kept apart. In the former case the usual cell culture plastics are ideal while in the latter the use of cell culture inserts may allow control of both of the physical contact and also of the duration of that contact.

Coding sequence: The coding region of a gene is that portion of a gene's DNA or RNA, composed of exons, that codes for protein. The region is bounded nearer the 5′ end by a start codon and nearer the 3′ end with a stop codon. The coding region in mRNA is bounded by the five prime untranslated regions and the three prime untranslated regions, which are also parts of the exons.

Coding strand: When referring to DNA transcription, the coding strand is the DNA strand which has the same base sequence as the RNA transcript produced (although with thymine replaced by uracil). It is this strand which contains codons, while the non-coding strand contains anticodons.

Codon: A series of three adjacent bases in one polynucleotide chain of a DNA or RNA molecule, which codes for a specific amino acid.

Coenzyme: Coenzyme A (CoA, CoASH, or HSCoA) is a coenzyme, notable for its role in the synthesis and oxidation of fatty acids, and the oxidation of pyruvate in the citric acid cycle. All sequenced genomes encode enzymes that use coenzyme A as a substrate, and around 4% of cellular enzymes use it (or a thioester, such as acetyl-CoA) as a substrate. It is adapted from cysteamine, pantothenate, and adenosine triphosphate.

Cofactor: A cofactor is a nonprotein chemical compound that is bound to a protein and is required for the protein's biological activity. These proteins are commonly enzymes, and cofactors can be considered "helper molecules" that assist in biochemical transformations.

Cohesive ends: DNA end or sticky end refers to the properties of the end of a molecule of DNA or a recombinant DNA molecule. The concept is important in molecular biology, especially in cloning or when subcloning inserts DNA into vector DNA. All the terms can also be used in reference to RNA. The sticky ends or cohesive ends form base pairs. Any two complementary cohesive ends can anneal, even those from two different organisms. This bondage is temporary however, and DNA ligase will eventually form a covalent bond between the sugar–phosphate residues of adjacent nucleotides to join the two molecules together.

Cointegrate vector: Called cointegrated vectors or hybrid Ti plasmids, these vectors were among the first types of modified and engineered Ti plasmids devised for *Agrobacterium*-mediated transformation, but are not widely used today. These vectors are constructed by homologous recombination of a bacterial plasmid with the T-DNA region of an endogenous Ti plasmid in *Agrobacterium*. Integration of the two plasmids requires a region of homology present in both.

Colchicine: Colchicine is a medication used for gout. It is a toxic natural product and secondary metabolite, originally extracted from plants of the genus *Colchicum* (autumn crocus, *Colchicum autumnale*, also known as "meadow saffron").

Complementary DNA: In genetics, complementary DNA (cDNA) is DNA synthesized from a mature mRNA template in a reaction catalyzed by the enzyme reverse transcriptase and the enzyme DNA polymerase, cDNA is often used to clone eukaryotic genes in prokaryotes.

Dalton: Dalton (symbol: Da) is a unit that is used for indicating mass on an atomic or molecular scale. It is defined as one-twelfth of the rest mass of an unbound atom of carbon-12 in its nuclear and electronic ground state, and has a value of 1.660538291(73) × 10 – 27 kg. One Dalton is approximately equal to the mass of one proton or one neutron. The CIPM have categorized it as a "non-SI unit whose values in SI units must be obtained experimentally."

ddNTP: Dideoxy nucleoside triphosphates (ddNTPs).

Death phase: The final growth phase, during which nutrients have been depleted and cell number decreases.

Dedifferentiation: Regression of a specialized cell or tissue to a simpler, more embryonic, unspecialized form. Dedifferentiation may occur before the regeneration of appendages in plants and certain animals and in the development of some cancers.

Degeneration: Deterioration of a tissue or an organ in which its function is diminished or its structure is impaired.

Dehydrogenase: A dehydrogenase (also called DHO in the literature) is an enzyme that oxidizes a substrate by transferring one or more hydrides (H–) to an acceptor, usually NAD+/NADP+ or a flavin coenzyme such as FAD or FMN.

Deionized: Purified water is water from any source that is physically processed to remove impurities. Distilled water and deionized (DI) water have been the most common forms of purified water, but water can also be purified by other processes including reverse osmosis, carbon filtration, microfiltration, ultrafiltration, ultraviolet oxidation, or electrodialysis.

Denaturated DNA: The denaturation of nucleic acids such as DNA due to high temperatures is the separation of a double strand into two single strands, which occurs when the hydrogen bonds between the strands are broken. This may occur during polymerase chain reaction. Nucleic acid strands realign when "normal" conditions are restored during annealing. If the conditions are restored too quickly, the nucleic acid strands may realign imperfectly.

Denitrification: Denitrification is a microbially facilitated process of nitrate reduction that may ultimately produce molecular nitrogen (N2) through a series of intermediate gaseous nitrogen oxide products.

***De novo* synthesis:** *De novo* synthesis refers to the synthesis of complex molecules from simple molecules such as sugars or amino acids, as opposed to their being recycled after partial degradation. For example, nucleotides are not needed in the diet as they can be constructed from small precursor molecules such as formate and aspartate. Methionine, on the other hand, is needed in the diet because while it can be degraded to and then regenerated from homocysteine, it cannot be synthesized *de novo*.

Deoxyribonuclease: A deoxyribonuclease (DNase) is any enzyme that catalyzes the hydrolytic cleavage of phosphodiester linkages in the DNA backbone. Thus, deoxyribonucleases are one type of nuclease. A wide variety of deoxyribonucleases are known, which differ in their substrate specificities, chemical mechanisms, and biological functions.

Deoxyribonucleic acid: Deoxyribonucleic acid or DNA, is a nucleic acid that contains the genetic instructions used in the development and functioning of all known living organisms (with the exception of RNA viruses).

Derepression: In genetics and biochemistry, a repressor gene inhibits the activity of an operator gene. By inactivating the repressor, the operator gene becomes active again. This effect is called derepression.

Dessicator: Desiccators are sealable enclosures containing desiccants used for preserving moisture-sensitive items. A common use for desiccators is to protect chemicals which are hygroscopic or which react with water from humidity.

Desoxyribonucleic acid: DNA.

Detergent: A detergent is a surfactant or a mixture of surfactants having "cleaning properties in dilute solutions." Commonly, "detergent" refers to alkylbenzenesulfonates, a family of compounds that are similar to soap but are less affected by hard water. In most household contexts, the term detergent by itself refers specifically to laundry detergent or dish detergent, as opposed to hand soap or other types of cleaning agents. Detergents are commonly available as powders or concentrated solutions.

Determinate growth: In biology determinate growth means not continuing to grow indefinitely. Determinate growth describe a more or less rapid growth to a mature conclusive size, with no growth thereafter like in the animals and leaves that stop growing at the reaching of the adult final condition.

Deviation: The difference between the value of an observation and the mean of the population in mathematics and statistics.

Dextrins: Dextrins are a group of low-molecular-weight carbohydrates produced by the hydrolysis of starch or glycogen. Dextrins are mixtures of polymers of D-glucose units linked by α-(1 $\rightarrow$ 4) or α-(1 $\rightarrow$ 6) glycosidic bonds.

Diabetes: Diabetes is a chronic (lifelong) disease marked by high levels of sugar in the blood.

Diakinesis: The final stage of the prophase in meiosis, characterized by shortening and thickening of the paired chromosomes, formation of the spindle fibers, disappearance of the nucleolus, and degeneration of the nuclear membrane.

Dicentric chromosome: Dicentric chromosome is an aberrant chromosome having two centromeres. Dicentric chromosomes form when two chromosome segments (from different chromosomes or from the two chromatids of a single one), each with a centromere, fuse end to end, with loss of their acentric fragments.

Dichogamy: The maturing of pistils and stamens at different times, preventing self-pollination.

Di-deoxynucleotide: Dideoxynucleotides, or ddNTPs, are nucleotides lacking a 3′-hydroxyl (-OH) group on their deoxyribose sugar. Since deoxyribose already lacks a 2′-OH, dideoxyribose lacks hydroxyl groups at both its 2′ and 3′ carbons. The lack of this hydroxyl group means that, after being added by a DNA polymerase to a growing nucleotide chain, no further nucleotides can be added as no phosphodiester bond can be created based on the fact that deoxyribonucleoside triphosphates (which are the building blocks of DNA) allow DNA chain synthesis to occur through a condensation reaction between the 5′ phosphate (following the cleavage of pyrophosphate) of the current nucleotide with the 3′ hydroxyl group of the previous nucleotide.

Differential centrifugation: Differential centrifugation is a common procedure in microbiology and cytology used to separate certain organelles from whole cells for further analysis of specific parts of cells. In the process, a tissue sample is first homogenized to break the cell membranes and mix up the cell contents.

Differentiation: In developmental biology, cellular differentiation is the process by which a less specialized cell becomes a more specialized cell type. Differentiation occurs numerous times during the development of a multicellular organism as the organism changes from a simple zygote to a complex system of tissues and cell types. Differentiation is a common process in adults as well: adult stem cells divide and create fully differentiated daughter cells during tissue repair and during normal cell turnover.

Diffusion: Diffusion describes the spread of particles through random motion from regions of higher concentration to regions of lower concentration.

Digest: A restriction digest is a procedure used in molecular biology to prepare DNA for analysis or other processing. It is sometimes termed DNA fragmentation (this term is used for other procedures as well).

Dimer: A dimer is a chemical entity consisting of two structurally similar subunits called monomers joined by bonds that can be either strong or weak.

Dimethyl sulfoxide: Dimethyl sulfoxide (DMSO) is an organo-sulfur compound with the formula $(CH_3)_2SO$. This colorless liquid is an important polar aprotic solvent that dissolves both polar and nonpolar compounds and is miscible in a wide range of organic solvents as well as water.

Dimorphism: The existence of a part (as leaves of a plant) in two different forms.

Direct embryogenesis: The formation in culture, on the surface of zygotic or somatic embryos or on explant tissues (leaf section, root tip, etc.), of embryoids without an intervening callus phase.

Direct repeat: Direct repeats are nucleotide sequences present in multiple copies in the genome. There are several types of repeated sequences. Interspersed (or dispersed) DNA repeats (interspersed repetitive sequences) are copies of transposable elements interspersed throughout the genome. Flanking (or terminal) repeats (terminal repeat sequences) are sequences that are repeated on both ends of a sequence, for example, the long terminal repeats (LTRs) on retroviruses.

Directed mutagenesis: Site-directed mutagenesis, also called site-specific mutagenesis or oligonucleotide-directed mutagenesis, is a molecular biology technique in which a mutation is created at a defined site in a DNA molecule. In general, this form of mutagenesis requires that the wild-type gene sequence be known.

Directional cloning: DNA inserts and vector molecules are digested with two different restriction enzymes to create noncomplementary sticky ends at either end of each restriction fragment. This allows the insert to be ligated to the vector in a specific orientation and prevent the vector from self-ligation.

Disaccharide: A disaccharide or biose is the carbohydrate formed when two monosaccharides undergo a condensation reaction which involves the elimination of a small molecule, such as water, from the functional groups only. Like monosaccharides, disaccharides also dissolve in water, taste sweet and are called sugars.

Discontinuous variation: Discontinuous variation is a variation within a population of a characteristic that falls into two or more discrete classes. Classic examples include such things as eye color in animals and the tall and short pea phenotypes used by Austrian botanist Gregor Johann Mendel. Characteristics that display discontinuous variation are present in one state or another; there is no blending or merging of the different forms possible. Unlike continuous variation, discontinuous variation is displayed by characteristics that are usually controlled by only one or two genes and that have little or no environmental component in their expression.

Dissecting microscope: The stereo or dissecting microscope is an optical microscope variant designed for low magnification observation or a sample using incident light illumination rather than trans-illumination. It uses two separate optical paths with two objectives and two eyepieces to provide slightly different viewing angles to the left and right eyes. In this way it produces a three-dimensional visualization of the sample being examined.

Distillation: Distillation is a method of separating mixtures based on differences in their boiling points. Distillation is a unit operation, or a physical separation process, and not a chemical reaction.

Disulfide bond: In chemistry, a disulfide bond is a covalent bond, usually derived by the coupling of two thiol groups. The linkage is also called an SS bond or disulfide bridge.

Diurnal: Occurring or active during the daytime rather than at night.

DNA amplification: The polymerase chain reaction (PCR) is a scientific technique in molecular biology to amplify a single or a few copies of a piece of DNA across several orders of magnitude, generating thousands to millions of copies of a particular DNA sequence.

DNAase: Deoxyribonuclease I (DNase I) is a single, glycosylated polypeptide that degrades unwanted single- and double-stranded DNA. The enzyme works by cleaving DNA into 5′ phosphodinucleotide and small oligonucleotide fragments. DNase I is commonly added to cell lysis reagents to remove the viscosity caused by the DNA content in bacterial cell lysates or to remove the DNA templates from RNAs produced by *in vitro* transcription.

DNA chip: DNA microarray (also commonly known as gene chip, DNA chip, or biochip) is a collection of microscopic DNA spots attached to a solid surface. Scientists use DNA microarrays to measure the expression levels of large numbers of genes simultaneously or to genotype multiple regions of a genome. Each DNA spot contains picomoles (10–12 moles) of a specific DNA sequence, known as probes (or reporters). These can be a short section of a gene or other DNA element that are used to hybridize a cDNA or cRNA sample (called target) under high-stringency conditions.

DNA cloning: DNA cloning is a technique to reproduce DNA fragments. It can be achieved by two different approaches: (1) cell based, and (2) using polymerase chain reaction (PCR). In the cell-based approach, a vector is required to carry the DNA fragment of interest into the host cell.

DNA construct: A DNA construct (stress on first syllable) is an artificially constructed segment of nucleic acid that is going to be "transplanted" into a target tissue or cell. It often contains a DNA insert, which contains the gene sequence encoding a protein of interest that has been subcloned into a vector, which contains bacterial resistance genes for growth in bacteria, and promoters for expression in the organism.

DNA delivery system: Gene (DNA) delivery is the process of introducing foreign DNA into host cells. Gene delivery is, for example, one of the steps necessary for gene therapy and the genetic modification of crops. There are many different methods of gene delivery developed for various types of cells and tissues, from bacterial to mammalian. Generally, the methods can be divided into two categories, viral and nonviral.

DNA fingerprint: DNA profiling (also called DNA testing, DNA typing, or genetic fingerprinting) is a technique employed by forensic scientists to assist in the identification of individuals by their respective DNA profiles. DNA profiles are encrypted sets of numbers that reflect a person's DNA makeup, which can also be used as the person's identifier. DNA profiling should not be confused with full genome sequencing. It is used in, for example, parental testing and criminal investigation.

DNA helicase: The role of helicases is to unwind the duplex DNA in order to provide a single-stranded DNA for replication, transcription, and recombination for instance.

DNA hybridization: DNA–DNA hybridization generally refers to a molecular biology technique that measures the degree of genetic similarity between pools of DNA sequences. It is normally used to determine the genetic distance between two species. When several species are compared that way, the similarity values allow the species to be arranged in a phylogenetic tree; it is therefore one possible approach to carrying out molecular systematics.

DNA ligase: In molecular biology, DNA ligase is a specific type of enzyme, a ligase that repairs single-stranded discontinuities in double-stranded DNA molecules, in simple words strands that have double-strand break (a break in both complementary strands of DNA).

DNA marker: A genetic marker is a gene or DNA sequence with a known location on a chromosome that can be used to identify cells, individuals, or species. It can be described as a variation (which may arise due to mutation or alteration in the genomic loci) that can be observed. A genetic marker may be a short DNA sequence, such as a sequence surrounding a single base-pair change (single-nucleotide polymorphism, SNP), or a long one, like minisatellites.

DNA microarray: DNA microarray (also commonly known as gene chip, DNA chip, or biochip) is a collection of microscopic DNA spots attached to a solid surface. Scientists use DNA microarrays to measure the expression levels of large numbers of genes simultaneously or to genotype multiple regions of a genome. Each DNA spot contains picomoles (10–12 moles) of a specific DNA sequence, known as probes (or reporters). These can be a short section of a gene or other DNA element that are used to hybridize a cDNA or cRNA sample (called target) under high-stringency conditions. Probe–target hybridization is usually detected and quantified by detection of fluorophore-, silver-, or chemiluminescence-labeled targets to determine relative abundance of nucleic acid sequences in the target.

DNA polymerase: DNA polymerase is an enzyme that helps catalyze in the polymerization of deoxyribonucleotides into a DNA strand. DNA polymerases are best known for their feedback role in DNA replication, in which the polymerase "reads" an intact DNA strand as a template and uses it to synthesize the new strand. This process copies a piece of DNA.

DNA polymorphism: One of two or more alternate forms (alleles) of a chromosomal locus that differ in nucleotide sequence or have variable numbers of repeated nucleotide units.

DNA primase: DNA primases are enzymes whose continual activity is required at the DNA replication fork. They catalyze the synthesis of short RNA molecules used as primers for DNA polymerases.

DNA probe: A labeled segment of DNA used to find a specific sequence of nucleotides in a DNA molecule. Probes may be synthesized in the laboratory, with a sequence complementary to the target DNA sequence.

DNA repair: DNA repair refers to a collection of processes by which a cell identifies and corrects damage to the DNA molecules that encode its genome. In human cells, both normal metabolic activities and environmental factors such as UV light and radiation can cause DNA damage, resulting in as many as 1 million individual molecular lesions per cell per day.

DNA replication: DNA replication is a biological process that occurs in all living organisms and copies their DNA; it is the basis for biological inheritance. The process starts with one double-stranded DNA molecule and produces two identical copies of the molecule. Each strand of the original double-stranded DNA molecule serves as template for the production of the complementary strand.

DNA sequencing: DNA sequencing includes several methods and technologies that are used for determining the order of the nucleotide bases adenine, guanine, cytosine, and thymine in a molecule of DNA.

DNA transformation : In molecular biology transformation is the genetic alteration of a cell resulting from the direct uptake, incorporation and expression of exogenous genetic material (exogenous DNA) from its surrounding and taken up through the cell membrane(s). Transformation occurs most commonly in bacteria and in some species occurs naturally.

Dolly: Dolly was a female domestic sheep, and the first mammal to be cloned from an adult somatic cell, using the process of nuclear transfer. She was cloned by Ian Wilmut, Keith Campbell, and colleagues at the Roslin Institute near Edinburgh in Scotland. She was born on July 5, 1996 and she lived until the age of six.

Dominant gene: Gene that produces the same phenotype in the organism whether or not its allele is identical; "the dominant gene for brown eyes."

Dominant marker selection: Selection of cells via a gene encoding a product that enables only the cells that carry the gene to grow under particular conditions. For example, plant and animal cells that express the introduced neo gene are resistant to neomycin and analogous antibiotics, while cells that do not carry neo are killed.

Dominant selectable marker gene: Selectable marker is a gene introduced into a cell, especially a bacterium or to cells in culture that confers a trait suitable for artificial selection. They are a type of reporter gene used in laboratory microbiology, molecular biology, and genetic engineering to indicate the success of a transfection or other procedure meant to introduce foreign DNA into a cell. Selectable markers are often antibiotic-resistance genes; bacteria that have been subjected to a procedure to introduce foreign DNA are grown on a medium containing an antibiotic, and those bacterial colonies that can grow have successfully taken up and expressed the introduced genetic material.

Dormancy: Dormancy is a period in an organism's life cycle when growth, development, and (in animals) physical activity are temporarily stopped. This minimizes metabolic activity and therefore helps an organism to conserve energy. Dormancy tends to be closely associated with environmental conditions.

Double crossing-over: Chromosomal crossover (or crossing over) is an exchange of genetic material between homologous chromosomes. It is one of the final phases of genetic recombination, which occurs during prophase I of meiosis (pachytene) in a process called synapsis. Synapsis begins before the synaptonemal complex develops, and is not completed until near the end of prophase I. Crossover usually occurs when matching regions on matching chromosomes break and then reconnect to the other chromosome.

Double helix: The term double helix refers to the structure formed by double-stranded molecules of nucleic acids such as DNA and RNA. The double helical structure of a nucleic acid complex arises as a consequence of its secondary structure, and is a fundamental component in determining its tertiary structure.

Double recessive: A diploid individual homozygous for (containing two copies of) the same recessive allele of a gene, as indicated by the expression of the recessive allele in the phenotype.

Doubling time: The doubling time is the period of time required for a quantity to double in size or value. It is applied to population growth, inflation, and resource extraction, consumption of goods, compound interest, the volume of malignant tumors, and many other things which tend to grow over time. When the relative growth rate (not the absolute growth rate) is constant, the quantity undergoes exponential growth and has a constant doubling time or period which can be calculated directly from the growth rate.

Downstream processing: Downstream processing refers to the recovery and purification of biosynthetic products, particularly pharmaceuticals, from natural sources such as animal or plant tissue or fermentation broth, including the recycling of salvageable components and the proper treatment and disposal of waste. It is an essential step in the manufacture of pharmaceuticals such as antibiotics, hormones (e.g., insulin and human growth hormone), antibodies (e.g., infliximab and abciximab) and vaccines; antibodies and enzymes used in diagnostics; industrial enzymes; and natural fragrance and flavor compounds. Downstream processing is usually considered a specialized field in biochemical engineering, itself a specialization within chemical engineering, though many of the key technologies were developed by chemists and biologists for laboratory-scale separation of biological products.

Drug delivery: Drug delivery is the method or process of administering a pharmaceutical compound to achieve a therapeutic effect in humans or animals. Drug delivery technologies are patent-protected formulation technologies that modify drug release profile, absorption, distribution, and elimination for the benefit of improving product efficacy and safety, as well as patient convenience and compliance.

Most common routes of administration include the preferred noninvasive peroral (through the mouth), topical (skin), transmucosal (nasal, buccal/sublingual, vaginal, ocular, and rectal), and inhalation routes.

dscDNA: Double-stranded complementary DNA.

dsDNA: Double-stranded DNA.

***E. coli*:** *Escherichia coli.*

Ecology: Ecology is the scientific study of the relations that living organisms have with respect to each other and their natural environment. Variables of interest to ecologists include the composition, distribution, amount (biomass), number, and changing states of organisms within and among ecosystems.

Ecosystem: An ecosystem is a biological environment consisting of all the organisms living in a particular area, as well as all the nonliving, physical components of the environment with which the organisms interact, such as air, soil, water, and sunlight. It is all the organisms in a given area, along with the nonliving (abiotic) factors with which they interact; a biological community and its physical environment.

EDTA: Ethylene-diamine tetra-acetic acid.

Effector cells: The muscle, gland, or organ cell capable of responding to a stimulus at the terminal end of an efferent neuron or motor neuron.

Effector molecule: An effector is a molecule (originally referring to small molecules but now encompassing any regulatory molecule, including proteins) that binds to a protein and thereby alters the activity of that protein. A modulator molecule binds to a regulatory site during allosteric modulation and allosterically modulates the shape of the protein. An effector can also be a protein that is secreted from a pathogen, which alters the host organism to enable infection, for example, by suppressing the host's immune system capabilities.

Electroblotting: Electroblotting is a method in molecular biology to transfer proteins or nucleic acids onto a membrane by using PVDF or nitrocellulose, after gel electrophoresis. The protein or nucleic acid can then be further analyzed using probes such as specific antibodies, ligands like lectins, or stains. This method can be used with all polyacrylamide and agarose gels. An alternative technique for transferring proteins from a gel is capillary blotting.

Electron microscope: An electron microscope is a type of microscope that uses a particle beam of electrons to illuminate the specimen and produce a magnified image. Electron microscopes (EM) have a greater resolving power than a light-powered optical microscope, because electrons have wavelengths about 100,000 times shorter than visible light (photons), and can achieve better than 50 pm resolution and magnifications of up to about 10,000,000×, whereas ordinary, nonconfocal light microscopes are limited by diffraction to about 200 nm resolution and useful magnifications below 2000×.

Electrophoresis: Electrophoresis is the motion of dispersed particles relative to a fluid under the influence of a spatially uniform electric field. This electrokinetic phenomenon was observed for the first time in 1807 by Reuss (Moscow State University), who noticed that the application of a constant electric field caused clay particles dispersed in water to migrate. It is ultimately caused by the presence of a charged interface between the particle surface and the surrounding fluid.

Electroporation: Electroporation, or electro-permeabilization, is a significant increase in the electrical conductivity and permeability of the cell plasma membrane caused by an externally applied electrical field. It is normally used in molecular biology as a way of introducing some substance into a cell, such as loading it with a molecular probe, a drug that can change the cell's function, or a piece of coding DNA.

ELISA: Enzyme-linked immunosorbent assay (ELISA), also known as an enzyme immunoassay (EIA), is a biochemical technique used mainly in immunology to detect the presence of an antibody or an antigen in a sample. The ELISA technique has been used as a diagnostic tool in medicine and plant pathology, as well as a quality-control check in various industries. In simple terms, in ELISA, an unknown amount of antigen is affixed to a surface, and then a specific antibody is applied over the surface so that it can bind to the antigen. This antibody is linked to an enzyme, and in the final step a substance is added that the enzyme can convert into some detectable signal, most commonly a color change in a chemical substrate.

Elongation factors: Elongation factors are a set of proteins that facilitate the events of translational elongation, the steps in protein synthesis from the formation of the first peptide bond to the formation of the last one.

Embryo cloning: Artificial embryo splitting or embryo twinning may also be used as a method of cloning, where an embryo is split in the maturation before embryo transfer.

Embryo culture: Embryo culture has been used to produce plants from embryos that would not normally develop within the fruit. This occurs in early-ripening peaches and in some hybridization between species. Embryo culture can also be used to circumvent seed dormancy.

Embryogenesis: Embryogenesis is the process by which the embryo is formed and develops, until it develops into a fetus. Embryogenesis starts with the fertilization of the ovum (or egg) by sperm. The fertilized ovum is referred to as a zygote. The zygote undergoes rapid mitotic divisions with no significant growth (a process known as cleavage) and cellular differentiation, leading to development of an embryo.

Embryoid bodies: Embryoid bodies are aggregates of cells derived from embryonic stem cells, and have been studied for years with mouse embryonic stem cells. Cell aggregation is imposed by hanging drop, plating upon nontissue culture-treated plates or spinner flasks; either method prevents cells from adhering to a surface to form the typical colony growth. Upon aggregation, differentiation is initiated and the cells begin to a limited extent to recapitulate embryonic development.

Embryonic stem cells: Embryonic stem cells (ES cells) are pluripotent stem cells derived from the inner cell mass of the blastocyst, an early-stage embryo. Human embryos reach the blastocyst stage 4–5 days post fertilization, at which time they consist of 50–150 cells. Isolating the embryoblast or inner cell mass (ICM) results in destruction of the fertilized human embryo, which raises ethical issues?

Encapsidation: Process by which a virus' nucleic acid is enclosed in a capsid.

Encapsulation: Molecular encapsulation in supramolecular chemistry is the confinement of a guest molecule inside the cavity of a supramolecular host molecule (molecular capsule, molecular container, or cage compounds). Examples of supramolecular host molecule include carcerands and endohedral fullerenes.

Encode: ENCODE (the ENCyclopedia Of DNA Elements) is a public research consortium launched by the US National Human Genome Research Institute (NHGRI) in September 2003. The goal is to find all functional elements in the human genome, one of the most critical projects by NHGRI after it completed the successful Human Genome Project. All data generated in the course of the project will be released rapidly into public databases.

5′ end: The 5′ cap is a specially altered nucleotide on the 5′ end of precursor messenger RNA and some other primary RNA transcripts as found in eukaryotes. The process of 5′ capping is vital to creating mature messenger RNA, which is then able to undergo translation. Capping ensures the messenger RNA's stability while it undergoes translation in the process of protein synthesis, and is a highly regulated process that occurs in the cell nucleus.

Endangered species: An endangered species is a population of organisms which is at risk of becoming extinct because it is either few in numbers, or threatened by changing environmental or predation parameters. The International Union for Conservation of Nature (IUCN) has calculated the percentage of endangered species as 40% of all organisms based on the sample of species that have been evaluated through 2006.

End labeling: There are two ways to label a DNA molecule; by the ends or all along the molecule. End labeling can be performed at the 3′- or 5′ end. Labeling at the 3′ end is performed by filling 3′-end recessed ends with a mixture or labeled and unlabeled dNTPs using Klenow or T4 DNA polymerases.

Endocrine gland: Endocrine glands are glands of the endocrine system that secrete their products, hormones, directly into the blood rather than through a duct. The main endocrine glands include the pituitary gland, pancreas, ovaries, testes, thyroid gland, and adrenal glands. The hypothalamus is a neuroendocrine organ. Other organs which are not so well known for their endocrine activity include the stomach, which produces such hormones as ghrelin.

Endocytosis: Endocytosis is the process by which cells absorb molecules (such as proteins) by engulfing them. It is used by all cells of the body because most substances important to them are large polar molecules that cannot pass through the hydrophobic plasma or cell membrane. The process opposite to endocytosis is exocytosis.

Endoderm: Endoderm is one of the germ layers formed during animal embryogenesis. Cells migrating inward along the archenteron form the inner layer of the gastrula, which develops into the endoderm. The endoderm consists at first of flattened cells, which subsequently become columnar. It forms the epithelial lining of multiple systems.

Endodermis: The innermost layer of the cortex that forms a sheath around the vascular tissue of roots and some stems. In the roots the endodermis helps regulate the intake of water and minerals into the vascular tissues from the cortex.

Endogenous: Growing or developing from within; originating within the body or cell.

Endomitosis: Endomitosis is reproduction of nuclear elements not followed by chromosome movements and cytoplasmic division.

Endonuclease: Endonucleases are enzymes that cleave the phosphodiester bond within a polynucleotide chain, in contrast to exonucleases, which cleave phosphodiester bonds at the end of a polynucleotide chain. Typically, a restriction site will be a palindromic sequence four to six nucleotides long. Most restriction endonucleases cleave the DNA strand unevenly, leaving complementary single-stranded ends. These ends can reconnect through hybridization and are termed "sticky ends." Once paired, the phosphodiester bonds of the fragments can be joined by DNA ligase.

Endoplasmic reticulum: The endoplasmic reticulum (ER) is a eukaryotic organelle that forms an interconnected network of tubules, vesicles, and cisternae within cells. Rough endoplasmic reticula synthesize proteins, while smooth endoplasmic reticula synthesize lipids and steroids, metabolize carbohydrates and steroids (but not lipids), and regulate calcium concentration, drug metabolism, and attachment of receptors on cell membrane proteins. Sarcoplasmic reticula solely regulate calcium levels.

Endopolyploidy: An increase in the number of chromosome sets caused by replication without cell division.

Endosperm: Endosperm is the tissue produced inside the seeds of most flowering plants around the time of fertilization. It surrounds the embryo and provides nutrition in the form of starch, though it can also contain oils and protein. This makes endosperm an important source of nutrition in human diet. For example, wheat endosperm is ground into flour for bread (the rest of the grain is included as well in whole wheat flour), while barley endosperm is the main source for beer production. Other examples of endosperm that forms the bulk of the edible portion are coconut "meat" and coconut "water," and corn, including popcorn. Some plants, like the orchid, lack endosperm in their seeds.

Endotoxin: Endotoxins are toxins associated with certain Gram-negative bacteria. An "endotoxin" is a toxin that is a structural molecule of bacteria that is recognized by the immune system.

End-product inhibition: End-product inhibition is a negative feedback used to regulate the production of a given molecule.

Enhancer: In genetics, an enhancer is a short region of DNA that can be bound with proteins (namely, the *trans*-acting factors, much like a set of transcription factors) to enhance transcription levels of genes (hence the name) in a gene cluster. While enhancers are usually *cis*-acting, an enhancer does not need to be particularly close to the genes it acts on, and sometimes need not be located on the same chromosome.

Enterotoxin: An enterotoxin is a protein toxin released by a microorganism in the intestine. Enterotoxins are chromosomally encoded exotoxins that are produced and secreted from several bacterial organisms.

Enucleated ovum: Egg cell without nucleus.

Enzyme: Enzymes are proteins that catalyze (i.e., increase the rates of) chemical reactions. In enzymatic reactions, the molecules at the beginning of the process are called substrates, and they are converted into different molecules, called the products.

Enzyme Commission Number: The Enzyme Commission number (EC number) is a numerical classification scheme for enzymes, based on the chemical reactions they catalyze. As a system of enzyme nomenclature, every EC number is associated with a recommended name for the respective enzyme.

Epicotyl: In plant physiology, the epicotyl is the embryonic shoot above the cotyledons. In most plants, the epicotyl will eventually develop into the leaves of the plant. In dicots, the hypocotyl is what appears to be the base stem under the spent withered cotyledons, and the shoot just above that is the epicotyl. In monocot plants, the first shoot that emerges from the ground or from the seed is the epicotyl, from which the first shoots and leaves emerge.

Epidermis: The epidermis is the outer layer of the skin, which together with the dermis forms the cutis. The epidermis is a stratified squamous epithelium, composed of proliferating basal and differentiated suprabasal keratinocytes. The epidermis acts as the body's major barrier against an inhospitable environment.

Epigenesis: The unfolding development in an organism and in particular the development of a plant or animal from an egg or spore through a sequence of steps in which cells differentiate and organs form.

Epigenetic variation: In biology, and specifically genetics, epigenetics is the study of changes produced in gene expression caused by mechanisms other than changes in the underlying DNA sequence—hence the name epigenetics. Examples of such changes might be DNA methylation or histone deacetylation, both of which serve to suppress gene expression without altering the sequence of the silenced genes.

Epinasty: A downward bending of leaves or other plant parts, resulting from excessive growth of the upper side.

Epiphyte: An epiphyte (or air plants) is a plant that grows upon another plant (such as a tree) nonparasitically or sometimes upon some other object (such as a building or a telegraph wire), derives its moisture and nutrients from the air and rain and sometimes from debris accumulating around it, and is found in the temperate zone (as many mosses, liverworts, lichens, and algae) and in the tropics (as many ferns, cacti, orchids, and bromeliads).

Episome: A genetic element in bacteria that can replicate free in the cytoplasm (has a different number of copies) or can be inserted into the main bacterial chromosome and replicate with the chromosome. Plasmids are an example.

Epistasis: In genetics, epistasis is the phenomenon where the effects of one gene are modified by one or several other genes, which are sometimes called modifier genes. The gene whose phenotype is expressed is called epistatic, while the phenotype altered or suppressed is called hypostatic. Epistasis can be contrasted with dominance, which is an interaction between alleles at the same gene locus. Epistasis is often studied in relation to quantitative trait loci (QTL) and polygenic inheritance.

Epitope: An epitope, also known as antigenic determinant, is the part of an antigen that is recognized by the immune system, specifically by antibodies, B cells, or T cells. The part of an antibody that recognizes the epitope is called a paratope. Although epitopes are usually thought to be derived from nonself-proteins, sequences derived from the host that can be recognized are also classified as epitopes.

Epizootic: In epizoology, an epizootic is a disease that appears as new cases in a given animal population, during a given period, at a rate that substantially exceeds what is "expected" based on recent experience (i.e., a sharp elevation in the incidence rate).

Equational division: The second meiotic division is an equational division because it does not reduce chromosome numbers. A nuclear division that maintains the same ploidy level of the cell.

Equatorial plate: The plane located midway between the poles of a dividing cell during the metaphase stage of mitosis or meiosis. It is formed from the migration of the chromosomes to the center of the spindle.

Equilibrium: The state in which the concentrations of the reactants and products have no net change over time.

Equimolar: Having an equal number of moles.

Erlenmeyer flask: An Erlenmeyer, also known as a conical flask, is a widely used type of laboratory flask which features a flat bottom, a conical body, and a cylindrical neck. It is named after the German chemist Emil Erlenmeyer, who created it in 1861.

Essential amino acid: An essential amino acid or indispensable amino acid is an amino acid that cannot be synthesized de novo by the organism (usually referring to humans), and therefore must be supplied in the diet.

Established culture: Established cultures are those cultures which have been completely characterized and tested.

Estimated breeding value: An "estimated breeding value" (EBV) is a statistical numerical prediction of the relative genetic value of a particular dog (male or female) available for breeding. EBVs are used to rank breeding stock for selection, based upon the genetic risk of each dog with regard to one or more specified traits.

Estrogens: Estrogens are a group of compounds named for their importance in the estrous cycle of humans and other animals. They are the primary female sex hormones. Natural estrogens are steroid hormones, while some synthetic ones are nonsteroidal.

Ethanol: Ethanol, also called ethyl alcohol, pure alcohol, grain alcohol, or drinking alcohol, is a volatile, flammable, colorless liquid. It is a psychoactive drug and one of the oldest recreational drugs. Best known as the type of alcohol found in alcoholic beverages, it is also used in thermometers, as a solvent, and as a fuel. In common usage, it is often referred to simply as alcohol or spirits.

Ethidium bromide: Ethidium bromide is an intercalating agent commonly used as a fluorescent tag (nucleic acid stain) in molecular biology laboratories for techniques such as agarose gel electrophoresis. It is commonly abbreviated as "EtBr," which is also an abbreviation for bromoethane. When exposed to ultraviolet light, it will fluoresce with an orange color, intensifying almost 20-fold after binding to DNA.

Ethylenediamine tetraacetic acid: Ethylenediamine tetraacetic acid (EDTA) is a polyamino carboxylic acid and a colorless, water-soluble solid. It is widely used to dissolve limescale. Its usefulness arises because of its role as a hexadentate ligand and chelating agent, that is, its ability to "sequester" metal ions such as Ca^{2+} and Fe^{3+}. After being bound by EDTA, metal ions remain in solution, but exhibit diminished reactivity. EDTA is produced as several salts, notably disodium EDTA and calcium disodium EDTA.

Euchromatin: Euchromatin is a lightly packed form of chromatin (DNA, RNA, and protein) that is rich in gene concentration, and is often (but not always) under active transcription. Unlike heterochromatin, it is found in both cells, with nuclei (eukaryotes) and cells without nuclei (prokaryotes).

Eugenics: Eugenics is the "applied science or the bio-social movement which advocates the use of practices aimed at improving the genetic composition of a population," usually referring to human populations.

Eukaryote: A eukaryote is an organism whose cells contain complex structures enclosed within membranes. Eukaryotes may more formally be referred to as the taxon Eukarya or Eukaryota.

Euploid: The normal number of chromosomes for a species. In humans, the euploid number of chromosomes is 46 with the notable exception of the unfertilized egg and sperm in which it is 23.

Evolution: Evolution (also known as biological or organic evolution) is the change over time in one or more inherited traits found in populations of organisms. Inherited traits are particular distinguishing characteristics, including anatomical, biochemical, or behavioral characteristics that are passed on from one generation to the next. Evolution may occur when there is variation of inherited traits within a population.

Excinuclease: Excision endonuclease also known as "excinuclease" is a nuclease (enzyme) which excises a fragment of nucleotides during DNA repair. The excinuclease cuts out a fragment by hydrolyzing two phosphodiester bonds, one on either side of the lesion in the DNA. This process is part of "nucleotide excision repair," a mechanism that can fix specific damages to the DNA in the G1 phase of the eukaryotic cell cycle. Such damages can include the thymine dimers created by UV rays.

Excision: In surgery, the complete removal of an organ, tissue, or tumor from a body.

Excision repair: Excision repair mechanisms that remove the damaged nucleotide replacing it with an undamaged nucleotide complementary to the nucleotide in the undamaged DNA strand.

***Ex novo*:** From the beginning.

Exo III: Exonuclease III (ExoIII) is an enzyme that belongs to the exonuclease family. ExoIII catalyzes the stepwise removal of mononucleotides from 3′-hydroxyl termini of duplex DNA. A limited number of nucleotides are removed during each binding event, resulting in coordinated progressive deletions within the population of DNA molecules.

Exocrine gland: Exocrine glands are glands that secrete their products (including hormones and other chemical messengers) into ducts (duct glands) which lead directly into the external environment. They are the counterparts to endocrine glands, which secrete their products (hormones) directly into the bloodstream (ductless glands) or release hormones (paracrines) that affect only target cells nearby the release site.

Exogenous: Produced by growth from superficial tissue.

Exon: An exon is a nucleic acid sequence that is represented in the mature form of an RNA molecule either after portions of a precursor RNA (introns) has been removed by *cis*-splicing or when two or more precursor RNA molecules have been ligated by *trans*-splicing. The mature RNA molecule can be a messenger RNA or a functional form of a noncoding RNA such as rRNA or tRNA. Depending on the context, the exon can refer to the sequence in the DNA or its RNA transcript.

Exonuclease: Exonucleases are enzymes that work by cleaving nucleotides one at a time from the end (exo) of a polynucleotide chain. A hydrolyzing reaction that breaks phosphodiester bonds at either the 3′ or the 5′ end occurs. Its close relative is the endonuclease, which cleaves phosphodiester bonds in the middle (endo) of a polynucleotide chain.

Exonuclease III: Exonuclease III (ExoIII) is an enzyme that belongs to the exonuclease family. ExoIII catalyzes the stepwise removal of mononucleotides from 3′-hydroxyl termini of duplex DNA. A limited number of nucleotides are removed during each binding event, resulting in coordinated progressive deletions within the population of DNA molecules.

Exotoxin: An exotoxin is a toxin excreted by a microorganism, including bacteria, fungi, algae, and protozoa. An exotoxin can cause damage to the host by destroying cells or disrupting normal cellular metabolism. They are highly potent and can cause major damage to the host. Exotoxins may be secreted, or, similar to endotoxins, may be released during lysis of the cell.

Expected progeny difference: Expected progeny differences (EPDs) provide estimates of the genetic value of an animal as a parent. Specifically, differences in EPDs between two individuals of the same breed predict differences in performance between their future offspring when each is mated to animals of the same average genetic merit. EPDs are calculated for birth, growth, maternal, and carcass traits and are reported in the same units of measurement as the trait (normally pounds).

Explant: In biology, explant culture is a technique used for the isolation of cells from a piece or pieces of tissue. Tissue harvested in this manner is called an explant. It can be a portion of the shoot, leaves, or some cells from a plant, or can be any part of the tissue from an animal.

Exponential phase: A growth phase. In the exponential (log) phase, cells divide as fast as possible according to the growth medium, the microorganism itself, and environmental conditions. This phase has a limited duration.

Expressed sequence tag: An expressed sequence tag or EST is a short sub-sequence of a cDNA sequence. They may be used to identify gene transcripts, and are instrumental in gene discovery and gene sequence determination. The identification of ESTs has proceeded rapidly, with approximately 65.9 million ESTs now available in public databases (e.g., GenBank June 18, 2010, all species).

Expression library: Expression cloning is a technique in DNA cloning that uses expression vectors to generate a library of clones, with each clone expressing one protein. This expression library is then screened for the property of interest and clones of interest recovered for further analysis. An example would be using an expression library to isolate genes that could confer antibiotic resistance.

Expression system: Gene expression is the process by which information from a gene is used in the synthesis of a functional gene product. These products are often proteins, but in nonprotein coding genes such as ribosomal RNA (rRNA), transfer RNA (tRNA), or small nuclear RNA (snRNA) genes, the product is a functional RNA.

Expression vector: An expression vector, otherwise known as an expression construct, is generally a plasmid that is used to introduce a specific gene into a target cell. Once the expression vector is inside the cell, the protein that is encoded by the gene is produced by the cellular-transcription and translation machinery ribosomal complexes. The plasmid is frequently engineered to contain regulatory sequences that act as enhancer and promoter regions and lead to efficient transcription of the gene carried on the expression vector.

Extrachromosomal: Extrachromosomal DNA (sometimes called extranuclear DNA or nonchromosomal DNA) is DNA located or maintained in a cell apart from the chromosomes.

Extrachromosomal inheritance: Inheritance of traits through DNA that is not connected with the chromosomes but rather to DNA from organelles in the cell and it is also called cytoplasmic inheritance.

***Ex vitro*:** Grown in the natural condition, for example, *ex vitro* plant means field-grown plants.

***Ex vivo* gene therapy:** *Ex vivo* means that which take place outside an organism. In science, *ex vivo* refers to experimentation or measurements done in or on tissue in an artificial environment outside the organism with the minimum alteration of natural conditions. *Ex vivo* conditions allow experimentation under more controlled conditions than possible in *in vivo* experiments (in the intact organism), at the expense of altering the "natural" environment.

F factor: A sequence of bacterial DNA

F_1: The first filial generation.

F_2: The second filial generation.

FACS: Fluorescence-activated cell sorting (FACS) is a specialized type of flow cytometry. It provides a method for sorting a heterogeneous mixture of biological cells into two or more containers, one cell at a time, based upon the specific light scattering and fluorescent characteristics of each cell. It is a useful scientific instrument, as it provides fast, objective, and quantitative recording of fluorescent signals from individual cells as well as physical separation of cells of particular interest. The acronym FACS is trademarked and owned by Becton, Dickinson and Company.

Factorial mating: A mating scheme in which each male parent is mated with each female parent. It is made possible in animals by means of *in vitro* embryo production. Such a mating scheme substantially reduces the rate of inbreeding in a selection program.

False fruit: A fruit, as the apple, strawberry, or pineapple, that contains, in addition to a mature ovary and seeds, a significant amount of other tissue.

False negative: A result that appears negative but fails to reveal a situation. An example of a false negative: a particular test designed to detect cancer of the toenail is negative but the person has toenail cancer.

False positive: A result that is erroneously positive when a situation is normal. An example of a false positive: a particular test designed to detect cancer of the toenail is positive but the person does not have toenail cancer.

Fed-batch fermentation: A fed batch is a biotechnological batch process which is based on feeding of a growth limiting nutrient substrate to a culture. The fed-batch strategy is typically used in bio-industrial processes to reach a high cell density in the bioreactor. Mostly, the feed solution is highly concentrated to avoid dilution of the bioreactor. The controlled addition of the nutrient directly affects the growth rate of the culture and allows to avoid overflow metabolism (formation of side metabolites, such as acetate for *Escherichia coli*, lactic acid in cell cultures, ethanol in *Saccharomyces cerevisiae*), oxygen limitation (anaerobiosis).

Feedback inhibition: A cellular control mechanism in which an enzyme that catalyzes the production of a particular substance in the cell is inhibited when that substance has accumulated to a certain level, thereby balancing the amount provided with the amount needed.

Fermentation: In a general sense, fermentation is the conversion of a carbohydrate such as sugar into an acid or an alcohol. More specifically, fermentation can refer to the use of yeast to convert sugar into alcohol or the use of bacteria to create lactic acid in certain foods. Fermentation occurs naturally in many different foods given the right conditions, and humans have intentionally made use of it for many thousands of years.

Fermentation substrates: Substrate for fermentation is usually glucose. But depending on the yeast type it can be fructose or other monosaccharides too.

Fermenter: An apparatus for carrying out fermentation.

Fertilization: Fertilization (also known as conception, fecundation, and syngamy) is the fusion of gametes to produce a new organism. In animals, the process involves the fusion of an ovum with a sperm, which eventually leads to the development of an embryo. Depending on the animal species, the process can occur within the body of the female in internal fertilization, or outside (external fertilization). The entire process of development of new individuals is called reproduction.

Fertilizer: Fertilizer is any organic or inorganic material of natural or synthetic origin (other than liming materials) that is added to a soil to supply one or more plant nutrients essential to the growth of plants. A recent assessment found that about 40–60% of crop yields are attributable to commercial fertilizer use.

Feulgen's test: A test used to detect DNA in nuclei, especially during cell division. A section of tissue is first placed in dilute hydrochloric acid for 10 min at 60°C to hydrolyze DNA, removing the purine bases, and exposing the aldehyde groups of deoxyribose. When the tissue is soaked in Schiff's reagent the location of the DNA is shown by the development of a magenta color.

Filter bioreactor: A cell culture system, in which cells are grown on a fine mesh of an inert material, which allows the culture medium to flow past it but retains the cells. This is similar in idea to membrane and hollow fiber reactors, but can be much easier to set up, being similar to conventional tower bioreactors, but with the mesh replacing the central reactor space.

Filtration: Filtration is commonly the mechanical or physical operation which is used for the separation of solids from fluids (liquids or gases) by interposing a medium through which only the fluid can pass. Oversize solids in the fluid are retained, but the separation is not complete; solids will be contaminated with some fluid and the filtrate will contain fine particles (depending on the pore size and filter thickness).

Fission: In biology, fission is the carp of a body, population, or species into parts and the regeneration of those parts into separate individuals. Binary fission, or prokaryotic fission, is a form of asexual reproduction and cell division used by all prokaryotes, some protozoa, and some organelles within eukaryotic organisms.

Flagellum: flagellum is a tail-like projection that protrudes from the cell body of certain prokaryotic and eukaryotic cells, and functions in locomotion. There are some notable differences between prokaryotic and eukaryotic flagella, such as protein composition, structure, and mechanism of propulsion.

Flanking region: A region of DNA that is adjacent to the 5′ end of the gene. The 5′ flanking region contains the promoter, and may contain enhancers or other protein binding sites. It is the region of DNA that is not transcribed into RNA.

Flavin adenine dinucleotide: In biochemistry, flavin adenine dinucleotide (FAD) is a redox cofactor involved in several important reactions in metabolism. FAD can exist in two different redox states, which it converts between by accepting or donating electrons. The molecule consists of a riboflavin moiety (vitamin B2) bound to the phosphate group of an ADP molecule.

Floccule: A small, loosely held mass or aggregate of fine particles, resembling a tuft of wool and suspended in or precipitated from a solution.

Flow cytometry: Flow cytometry (abbreviated: FCM) is a technique for counting and examining microscopic particles, such as cells and chromosomes, by suspending them in a stream of fluid and passing them by an electronic detection apparatus. It allows simultaneous multi-parametric analysis of the physical and/or chemical characteristics of up to thousands of particles per second. Flow cytometry is routinely used in the diagnosis of health disorders, especially blood cancers, but has many other applications in both research and clinical practice.

Folded genome: The condensed state of the chromosomal DNA of a bacterium. The DNA is segregated into domains, and each domain is independently negatively supercoiled.

Follicle: A follicle is a small spherical or vase-like group of cells containing a cavity in which some other structure grows. Follicles are best known as the sockets from which hairs grow in humans and other mammals, but the bristles of annelid worms also grow from such sockets.

Follicle-stimulating hormone: Follicle-stimulating hormone (FSH) is a hormone found in humans and other animals. It is synthesized and secreted by gonadotrophs of the anterior pituitary gland. FSH regulates the development, growth, pubertal maturation, and reproductive processes of the body. FSH and luteinizing hormone (LH) act synergistically in reproduction.

Forced cloning: The insertion of foreign DNA into a cloning vector in a predetermined orientation.

Functional gene cloning: Gene therapy involves supplying a functional gene to cells lacking that function, with the aim of correcting a genetic disorder or acquired disease. Gene therapy can be broadly divided into two categories. The first is alteration of germ cells, that is, sperm or eggs, which results in a permanent genetic change for the whole organism and subsequent generations. This "germ line gene therapy" is considered by many to be unethical in human beings.

Fungicide: Fungicides are chemical compounds or biological organisms used to kill or inhibit fungi or fungal spores. Fungi can cause serious damage in agriculture, resulting in critical losses of yield, quality, and profit. Fungicides are used both in agriculture and to fight fungal infections in animals. Chemicals used to control oomycetes, which are not fungi, are also referred to as fungicides as oomycetes use the same mechanisms as fungi to infect plants.

Fusion gene: A fusion gene is a hybrid gene formed from two previously separate genes. It can occur as a result of a translocation, interstitial deletion, or chromosomal inversion. Often, fusion genes are oncogenes. Most fusion genes are found from hematological cancers, sarcomas, and prostate cancer.

Fusion protein: Fusion proteins or chimeric proteins are proteins created through the joining of two or more genes which originally coded for separate proteins. Translation of this fusion gene results in a single polypeptide with functional properties derived from each of the original proteins. Recombinant fusion proteins are created artificially by recombinant DNA technology for use in biological research or therapeutics.

Gamete: Gamete is a cell that fuses with another cell during fertilization (conception) in organisms that reproduce sexually.

Gastrula: An early metazoan embryo in which the ectoderm, mesoderm, and endoderm are established either by invagination of the blastula (as in fish and amphibians) to form a multilayered cellular cup with a blastopore opening into the archenteron or by differentiation of the blastodisc (as in reptiles, birds, and mammals) and inward cellular migration.

Gel electrophoresis: Gel electrophoresis refers to using a gel as an anticonvective medium and or sieving medium during electrophoresis. Gel electrophoresis is most commonly used for separation of biological macromolecules such as deoxyribonucleic acid (DNA), ribonucleic acid (RNA), or protein; however, gel electrophoresis can be used for separation of nanoparticles.

Gelatin: Gelatin is a translucent, colorless, brittle (when dry), tasteless solid substance, derived from the collagen inside animals' skin and bones. It is commonly used as a gelling agent in food, pharmaceuticals, photography, and cosmetic manufacturing.

Gene addition: Gene addition inserts a functioning copy of a misfunctioning or nonfunctional native gene. Viral-based gene addition involves the "domestication" of viral genomes as vectors.

Gene amplification: A cellular process characterized by the production of multiple copies of a particular gene or genes to amplify the phenotype that the gene confers on the cell. Drug resistance in cancer cells is linked to amplification of the gene that prevents absorption of the chemotherapeutic agent by the cell.

Gene conversion: Gene conversion is an event in DNA genetic recombination, which occurs at high frequencies during meiotic division but which also occurs in somatic cells.

Gene expression: Gene expression is the process by which information from a gene is used in the synthesis of a functional gene product. These products are often proteins, but in nonprotein coding genes such as ribosomal RNA (rRNA), transfer RNA (tRNA), or small nuclear RNA (snRNA) genes, the product is a functional RNA.

Gene flow: In population genetics, gene flow (also known as gene migration) is the transfer of alleles of genes from one population to another.

Gene imprinting: Genomic imprinting is a genetic phenomenon by which certain genes are expressed in a parent-of-origin-specific manner. It is an inheritance process independent of the classical Mendelian inheritance. Imprinted alleles are silenced such that the genes are either expressed only from the nonimprinted allele inherited from the mother (e.g., H19 or CDKN1C), or in other instances from the nonimprinted allele inherited from the father (e.g., IGF-2). Forms of genomic imprinting have been demonstrated in insects, mammals, and flowering plants.

Gene insertion: The process by which one or more genes from one organism are incorporated into the genetic makeup of a second organism.

Gene interaction: The collaboration of several different genes in the production of one phenotypic character (or related group of characters).

Gene library: A genomic library is a population of host bacteria, each of which carries a DNA molecule that was inserted into a cloning vector, such that the collection of cloned DNA molecules represents the entire genome of the source organism. This term also represents the collection of all of the vector molecules, each carrying a piece of the chromosomal DNA of the organism, prior to the insertion of these molecules into the host cells.

Gene pool: The total number of genes of every individual in an interbreeding population.

Gene probe: A gene probe is a specific segment of single-strand DNA that is complementary to a desired gene. For example, if the gene of interest contains the sequence AATGGCACA, then the probe will contain the complementary sequence TTACCGTGT. When added to the appropriate solution, the probe will match and then bind to the gene of interest. To facilitate locating the probe, scientists usually label it with a radioisotope or a fluorescent dye so that it can be visualized and identified.

Gene recombination: Genetic recombination is a process by which a molecule of nucleic acid (usually DNA, but can also be RNA) is broken and then joined to a different one. Recombination can occur between similar molecules of DNA, as in homologous recombination, or dissimilar molecules, as in nonhomologous end joining. Recombination is a common method of DNA repair in both bacteria and eukaryotes. In eukaryotes, recombination also occurs in meiosis, where it facilitates chromosomal crossover.

Gene sequencing: Gene sequencing includes several methods and technologies that are used for determining the order of the nucleotide bases adenine, guanine, cytosine, and thymine in a molecule of DNA.

Gene splicing: The process in which fragments of DNA from one or more different organisms are combined to form recombinant DNA.

Gene therapy: Gene therapy is the insertion, alteration, or removal of genes within an individual's cells and biological tissues to treat disease. It is a technique for correcting defective genes that are responsible for disease development.

Genetically engineered organism: Genetically modified organism (GMO) or genetically engineered organism (GEO) is an organism whose genetic material has been altered using genetic engineering techniques. These techniques, generally known as recombinant DNA technology, use DNA molecules from different sources, which are combined into one molecule to create a new set of genes.

Genetically modified food: Genetically modified foods (or GM foods) are foods derived from genetically modified organisms. Genetically modified organisms have had specific changes introduced into their DNA by genetic engineering techniques.

Genetic code: The genetic code is the set of rules by which information encoded in genetic material (DNA or mRNA sequences) is translated into proteins (amino acid sequences) by living cells.

Genetic complementation: In genetics, complementation refers to a relationship between two different strains of an organism which both have homozygous recessive mutations that produce the same phenotype (e.g., a change in wing structure in flies).

Genetic disease: A genetic disease is an illness caused by abnormalities in genes or chromosomes. While some diseases, such as cancer, are due in part to genetic disorders, they can also be caused by environmental factors. Most disorders are quite rare and affect one person in every several thousands or millions. Some types of recessive gene disorders confer an advantage in the heterozygous state in certain environments.

Genetic diversity: Genetic diversity, the level of biodiversity, refers to the total number of genetic characteristics in the genetic makeup of a species. It is distinguished from genetic variability, which describes the tendency of genetic characteristics to vary.

Genetic drift: Genetic drift or allelic drift is the change in the frequency of a gene variant (allele) in a population due to random sampling. The alleles in the offspring are a sample of those in the parents, and chance has a role in determining whether a given individual survives and reproduces.

Genetic engineering: Genetic engineering, also called genetic modification, is the direct human manipulation of an organism's genome using modern DNA technology. It involves the introduction of foreign DNA or synthetic genes into the organism of interest. The introduction of new DNA does not require the use of classical genetic methods; however, traditional breeding methods are typically used for the propagation of recombinant organisms.

Genetic equilibrium: A genetic equilibrium is at hand for an allele in a gene pool when the frequency of that allele is not changing (i.e., when it is not evolving). For this to be the case, evolutionary forces acting upon the allele must be equal and opposite.

Genetic heterogeneity: The phenomenon that a single phenotype or genetic disorder may be caused by any one of a multiple number of alleles or nonallele (locus) mutations.

Genetic linkage: Genetic linkage is the tendency of certain loci or alleles to be inherited together. Genetic loci that are physically close to one another on the same chromosome tend to stay together during meiosis, and are thus genetically linked.

Genetic mapping: Gene mapping, also called genome mapping is the creation of a genetic map assigning DNA fragments to chromosomes. When a genome is first investigated, this map is nonexistent. The map improves with the scientific progress and is perfect when the genomic DNA sequencing of the species has been completed.

Genetic marker: A gene or DNA sequence having a known location on a chromosome and associated with a particular gene or trait. Genetic markers associated with certain diseases can be detected in the blood and used to determine whether an individual is at risk for developing a disease.

Genetic polymorphism: The existence together of many forms of DNA sequences at a locus within the population. Genetic polymorphism promotes diversity within a population. It often persists over many generations because no single form has an overall advantage or disadvantage over the others regarding natural selection. A common example is the different allelic forms that give rise to different blood types in humans.

Genetic selection: The process of determining genetic attributes.

Genetic transformation: A process by which the genetic material carried by an individual cell is altered by the incorporation of foreign (exogenous) DNA into its genome.

Genetic variation: Genetic variation, variation in alleles of genes, occurs both within and among populations. Genetic variation is important because it provides the "raw material" for natural selection. Genetic variation is brought about by mutation, a change in a chemical structure of a gene.

Gene tracking: Gene tracking is the method used to trace throughout a family the inheritance of a gene such as those causing cystic fibrosis or Huntington's chorea, in order to diagnose and predict genetic disorders.

Gene translocation: The movement of a gene fragment from one chromosomal location to another, which often alters or abolishes expression.

Genome: In modern molecular biology and genetics, the genome is the entirety of an organism's hereditary information. It is encoded either in DNA or, for many types of virus, in RNA. The genome includes both the genes and the noncoding sequences of the DNA/RNA.

Genomic DNA library: A genomic library is a population of host bacteria, each of which carries a DNA molecule that was inserted into a cloning vector, such that the collection of cloned DNA molecules represents the entire genome of the source organism. This term also represents the collection of all of the vector molecules, each carrying a piece of the chromosomal DNA of the organism, prior to the insertion of these molecules into the host cells.

Genotype: The genetic makeup, as distinguished from the physical appearance, of an organism or a group of organisms.

Germ cell gene therapy: Germline gene therapy involves altering the genetic makeup of either an egg or sperm cell before fertilization, or altering the genetic makeup of the blastomere when it is in a very early stage of division. The goal of germline gene therapy is to effect changes in the genetic code of an organism that will be passed on to future generations

Germicide: An agent that kills germs, especially pathogenic microorganisms; a disinfectant.

Gestation: Gestation is the carrying of an embryo or fetus inside a female viviparous animal.

Glucocorticoid: Glucocorticoids (GC) are a class of steroid hormones that bind to the glucocorticoid receptor (GR), which is present in almost every vertebrate animal cell.

Glycolysis: Glycolysis is the metabolic pathway that converts glucose into pyruvate.

Glycosylation: Glycosylation is the enzymatic process that attaches glycans to proteins, lipids, or other organic molecules. This enzymatic process produces one of the fundamental biopolymers found in cells (along with DNA, RNA, and proteins).

Good laboratory practice: In the experimental research arena, the laboratory practice or GLP specifically refers to a quality system of management controls for research laboratories and organizations to try to ensure the uniformity, consistency, reliability, reproducibility, quality, and integrity of chemical (including pharmaceuticals) safety and efficacy tests.

Gram-negative bacteria: Gram-negative bacteria are bacteria that do not retain crystal violet dye in the Gram staining protocol. In a Gram stain test, a counterstain (commonly safranin) is added after the crystal violet, coloring all Gram-negative bacteria with a red or pink color. The test itself is useful in classifying two distinct types of bacteria based on the structural differences of their bacterial cell walls. Gram-positive bacteria will retain the crystal violet dye when washed in a decolorizing solution.

Gram-positive bacteria: Gram-positive bacteria are those that are stained dark blue or violet by Gram staining. This is in contrast to Gram-negative bacteria, which cannot retain the crystal violet stain, instead taking up the counterstain (safranin or fuchsine) and appearing red or pink. Gram-positive organisms are able to retain the crystal violet stain because of the high amount of peptidoglycan in the cell wall. Gram-positive cell walls typically lack the outer membrane found in Gram-negative bacteria.

Green Revolution: Green Revolution refers to a series of research, development, and technology transfer initiatives, occurring between the 1940s and the late 1970s, that increased agriculture production around the world, beginning most markedly in the late 1960s.

Growth curve: A growth curve is an empirical model of the evolution of a quantity over time. Growth curves are widely used in biology for quantities such as population size, body height, or biomass. Values for the measured property can be plotted on a graph as a function of time.

Growth factor: A growth factor is a naturally occurring substance capable of stimulating cellular growth proliferation and cellular differentiation. Usually it is a protein or a steroid hormone. Growth factors are important for regulating a variety of cellular processes.

Growth hormone: Growth hormone (GH) is a protein-based peptide hormone. It stimulates growth, cell reproduction and regeneration in humans and other animals.

Guide RNA: Guide RNA (gRNA) is the RNA that guides the insertion or deletion of uridine residues into mitochondrial mRNAs in kinetoplastid protists in a process known as RNA editing.

Guide sequence: An RNA molecule (or a part of it) which hybridizes with eukaryotic mRNA and aids in the splicing of intron sequences. Guide sequences may be either external (EGS) or internal (IGS) to the RNA being processed and may hybridize with either intron or exon sequences close to the splice junction.

Hemoglobin: Hemoglobin is the iron-containing oxygen-transport metalloprotein in the red blood cells of all vertebrates with the exception of the fish family Channichthyidae, as well as the tissues of some invertebrates.

Hemolymph: Hemolymph is a fluid in the circulatory system of some arthropods (including spiders, crustaceans such as crabs and shrimp, and even some insects such as stoneflies) and is analogous to the fluids and cells making up both blood and interstitial fluid (including water, proteins, fats, sugars, hormones, etc.) in vertebrates such as birds and mammals.

Haploid cell: A haploid cell is a cell that contains one complete set of chromosomes. Gametes are haploid cells that are produced by meiosis.

Haplotype: Haplotype in genetics is a combination of alleles (DNA sequences) at different places (loci) on the chromosome that are transmitted together.

Hardy–Weinberg equilibrium: The Hardy–Weinberg equilibrium states that both allele and genotype frequencies in a population remain constant that is, they are in equilibrium from generation to generation unless specific disturbing influences are introduced.

Helper cells: Any of the T cells that when stimulated by a specific antigen release lymphokines that promote the activation and function of B cells and killer T cells. Also called T-helper cell.

Helper plasmid: In the context of genetic transformation of plants, a helper plasmid is a plasmid present in *Agrobacterium* that provides functions required by the bacteria for transferring foreign DNA to a plant cell. They have been extremely important in plant genetic engineering. Generally, helper plasmids are derivatives of the Ti plasmid that contain an active virulence region, but from which the T-DNA has been removed.

Hemicellulose: A hemicellulose is any of several heteropolymers (matrix polysaccharides), such as arabinoxylans, present along with cellulose in almost all plant cell walls. While cellulose is crystalline, strong, and resistant to hydrolysis, hemicellulose has a random, amorphous structure with little strength.

Herbicide: An herbicide, commonly known as a weed killer, is a type of pesticide used to kill unwanted plants.

Herbicide resistance: Herbicide resistance in weeds occurs as a result of changes that prevent the herbicide from effectively inhibiting the target.

Heredity: Heredity is the passing of traits to offspring (from its parent or ancestors). This is the process by which an offspring cell or organism acquires or becomes predisposed to the characteristics of its parent cell or organism.

Heterochromatin: Heterochromatin is a tightly packed form of DNA, which comes in different varieties. These varieties lie on a continuum between the two extremes of constitutive and facultative heterochromatin.

Heterogeneous nuclear RNA: Heterogeneous nuclear RNA (hnRNA) a diverse group of long primary transcripts formed in the eukaryotic nucleus, many of which will be processed to mRNA molecules by splicing.

High efficiency particulate air: A high efficiency particulate air (HEPA) filter is a type of air filter that satisfies certain standards of efficiency such as those set by the United States Department of Energy (DOE).

Histocompatibility: Histocompatibility is the property of having the same, or mostly the same, alleles of a set of genes called the major histocompatibility complex (MHC). These genes are expressed in most tissues as antigens, to which the immune system makes antibodies.

Histology: Histology is the study of the microscopic anatomy of cells and tissues of plants and animals.

Homeobox: A homeobox is a DNA sequence found within genes that are involved in the regulation of patterns of anatomical development (morphogenesis) in animals, fungi, and plants.

Homeotic mutation: A mutation that causes tissues to alter their normal differentiation pattern, producing integrated structures but in unusual locations. For example, a homeotic mutation in the fruit fly, *Drosophila*, causes legs to develop where antennae normally form.

Homodimer: A protein composed of two identical polypeptide chains.

Homokaryon: A bi- or multinucleate cell having nuclei all of the same kind.

Homologous: Having the same alleles or genes in the same order of arrangement: homologous chromosomes.

Homologous recombination: Homologous recombination is a type of genetic recombination in which nucleotide sequences are exchanged between two similar or identical molecules of DNA.

Human immunodeficiency virus: Human immunodeficiency virus (HIV) is a lent virus (a member of the retrovirus family) that causes acquired immunodeficiency syndrome (AIDS), a condition in humans in which progressive failure of the immune system allows life-threatening opportunistic infections and cancers to thrive.

Human leukocyte antigen system: Human leukocyte antigen system (HLA) is the name of the major histocompatibility complex (MHC) in humans. The super locus contains a large number of genes related to immune system function in humans.

Humoral immune response: The humoral immune response (HIR) is the aspect of immunity that is mediated by secreted antibodies (as opposed to cell-mediated immunity, which involves T lymphocytes) produced in the cells of the B lymphocyte lineage (B cell).

Hybrid: A genetic hybrid carries two different alleles of the same gene.

Hybridization: Hybridization is the process of establishing a noncovalent, sequence-specific interaction between two or more complementary strands of nucleic acids into a single hybrid, which in the case of two strands is referred to as a duplex.

Hybridoma: A cell hybrid produced *in vitro* by the fusion of a lymphocyte that produces antibodies and a myeloma tumor cell. It proliferates into clones that produce a continuous supply of a specific antibody.

Hydrolysis: Hydrolysis is a chemical reaction during which molecules of water are split into hydrogen cations and hydroxide anions in the process of a chemical mechanism.

Ideogram: An ideogram is a graphic symbol that represents an idea or concept. Some ideograms are comprehensible only by familiarity with prior convention; others convey their meaning through pictorial resemblance to a physical object, and thus may also be referred to as pictograms.

Immediate-early gene: Immediate-early genes (IEGs) are genes which are activated transiently and rapidly in response to a wide variety of cellular stimuli. They represent a standing response mechanism that is activated at the transcription level in the first round of response to stimuli, before any new proteins are synthesized.

Immobilized cells: The immobilized whole cell system is an alternative to enzyme immobilization. Unlike enzyme immobilization, where the enzyme is attached to a substrate (such as calcium alginate), in immobilized whole cell systems, the target cell is immobilized.

Immortalization: Biological immortality refers to a stable rate of mortality as a function of chronological age. Some individual cells and entire organisms in some species achieve this state either throughout their existence or after living long enough.

Immune response: The immune response is how your body recognizes and defends itself against bacteria, viruses, and substances that appear foreign and harmful.

Immunoassay: An immunoassay is a biochemical test that measures the presence or concentration of a substance in solutions that frequently contain a complex mixture of substances. Analytes in biological liquids such as serum or urine are frequently assayed using immunoassay methods.

Immunodiagnostics: Immunodiagnostics is a diagnostic methodology that uses an antigen–antibody reaction as their primary means of detection. The concept of using immunology as a diagnostic tool was introduced in 1960 as a test for serum insulin. A second test was developed in 1970 as a test for thyroxine in the 1970s.

Immunogenicity: Immunogenicity is the ability of a particular substance, such as an antigen or epitope, to provoke an immune response in the body of a human or animal.

Immunoglobulin: A protein produced by plasma cells and lymphocytes and characteristic of these types of cells. Immunoglobulins play an essential role in the body's immune system. They attach to foreign substances, such as bacteria, and assist in destroying them. Immunoglobulin is abbreviated Ig. The classes of immunoglobulins are termed immunoglobulin A (IgA), immunoglobulin G (IgG), immunoglobulin M (IgM), immunoglobulin D (IgD), and immunoglobulin E (IgE).

Immunosensor: Immunosensors act on the principle that the immune response of certain biological species (usually bacteria) to contaminants will produce antibodies, which in turn can be measured.

Immunosuppression: Immunosuppression involves an act that reduces the activation or efficacy of the immune system. Some portions of the immune system itself have immunosuppressive effects on other parts of the immune system, and immunosuppression may occur as an adverse reaction to treatment of other conditions.

Immunosuppressor: Immunosuppression involves an act that reduces the activation or efficacy of the immune system. Some portions of the immune system itself have immunosuppressive effects on other parts of the immune system, and immunosuppression may occur as an adverse reaction to treatment of other conditions.

Immunotherapy: Immunotherapy is a medical term defined as the "treatment of disease by inducing, enhancing, or suppressing an immune response."

Immunotoxin: An immunotoxin is a human-made protein that consists of a targeting portion linked to a toxin. When the protein binds to that cell, it is taken in through endocytosis, and the toxin kills the cell. They are used for the treatment of some kinds of cancer and a few viral infections.

Inactivated agent: A virus, bacterium, or other organism that has been treated to prevent it from causing a disease. See attenuated vaccine.

Inbred line: Produced by inbreeding.

Inbreeding: Inbreeding is the reproduction from the mating of two genetically related parents, which can increase the chances of offspring being affected by recessive or deleterious traits.

Inclusion body: Inclusion bodies are nuclear or cytoplasmic aggregates of stainable substances, usually proteins. They typically represent sites of viral multiplication in a bacterium or a eukaryotic cell and usually consist of viral capsid proteins.

Incubator: A device for maintaining a bacterial culture at a particular temperature for a set length of time, in order to measure bacterial growth.

Indirect embryogenesis: Plant embryo formation on callus tissues derived from explants, including zygotic or somatic embryos and seedlings.

Indirect organogenesis: Plant organ formation on callus tissues derived from explants.

Inducer: In molecular biology, an inducer is a molecule that starts gene expression.

Inducible enzyme: An enzyme that is normally present in minute quantities within a cell, but whose concentration increases dramatically when a substrate compound is added.

Induction: A process in which a molecule (e.g., a drug) induces (i.e., initiates or enhances) or inhibits the expression of an enzyme.

Induction media: Media used to induce the formation of organs.

Infection: An infection is the colonization of a host organism by parasite species. Infecting parasites seek to use the host's resources to reproduce, often resulting in disease. Colloquially, infections are usually considered to be caused by microscopic organisms or microparasites such as viruses, prions, bacteria, and viroids, though larger organisms like macroparasites and fungi can also infect.

Infectious agent: An agent capable of producing infection.

Inhibitor: A substance that binds to an enzyme and decreases the enzyme's activity.

Inheritance: Inheritance is the practice of passing on property, titles, debts, and obligations upon the death of an individual. It has long played an important role in human societies. The rules of inheritance differ between societies and have changed over time.

Initiation codon: The mRNA sequence AUG, which specifies methionine, the first amino acid used in the translation process. (Occasionally GUG, valine, is recognized as an initiation codon.

Initiation factors: Initiation factors are proteins that bind to the small subunit of the ribosome during the initiation of translation, a part of protein biosynthesis.

Inoculate: To implant microorganisms or infectious material into a culture medium.

Inositol: Inositol is a chemical compound with formula $C_6H_{12}O_6$ or $(\text{-CHOH-})_6$, a sixfold alcohol (polyol) of cyclohexane.

Insecticide: An insecticide is a pesticide used against insects. They include ovicides and larvicides used against the eggs and larvae of insects, respectively. Insecticides are used in agriculture, medicine, industry, and the household.

Insertion element: A section of DNA that is capable of becoming inserted into another chromosome.

Insertion mutations: A type of mutation resulting from the addition of extra nucleotides in a DNA sequence or chromosome.

Insertion sequence: An insertion sequence (also known as an IS, an insertion sequence element, or an IS element) is a short DNA sequence that acts as a simple transposable element. Insertion sequences have two major characteristics: they are small relative to other transposable elements (generally around 700–2500 bp in length) and only code for proteins implicated in the transposition activity (they are thus different from other transposons, which also carry accessory genes such as antibiotic-resistance genes).

Insertion site: The point in a vein where a needle or catheter is inserted.

***In situ* colony:** A procedure for screening bacterial colonies or plaques growing on plates or membranes for the presence of specific DNA sequences by the hybridization of nucleic acid probes to the DNA molecules present in these colonies or plaques.

Insulin: Insulin is a hormone central to regulating carbohydrate and fat metabolism in the body. Insulin causes cells in the liver, muscle, and fat tissue to take up glucose from the blood, storing it as glycogen in the liver and muscle.

Intercalating agent: A chemical that can insert itself between the stacked bases at the center of the DNA double helix, possibly causing a frame-shift mutation.

Interferon: Interferons (IFNs) are proteins made and released by host cells in response to the presence of pathogens such as viruses, bacteria, or parasites or tumor cells. They allow communication between cells to trigger the protective defenses of the immune system that eradicate pathogens or tumors.

Intergeneric: A very rare type of hybrid formed between plants of two different genera. It is indicated by the symbol × before the genus name. For example, the Leyland cypress, × *Cupressocyparis leylandii*, is a cross between *Cupressus macrocarpa* and *Chamaecyparis nootkatensis*.

Intergenic regions: An intergenic region (IGR) is a stretch of DNA sequences located between clusters of genes that contain few or no genes. Occasionally some intergenic DNA acts to control genes nearby, but most of it has no currently known function.

Interleukin: Interleukins are a group of cytokines (secreted proteins/signaling molecules) that were first seen to be expressed by white blood cells (leukocytes).

Internal guide sequence: A polynucleotide sequence near the 5′-end of group I introns that pairs with sequences of the upstream exon in an intermediate of the self-splicing process (see also self-splicing).

Interphase: Interphase is the phase of the cell cycle in which the cell spends the majority of its time and performs the majority of its purposes including preparation for cell division. In preparation for cell division, it increases its size and makes a copy of its DNA.

Intracellular: In cell biology, molecular biology, and related fields, the word intracellular means "inside the cell."

Intracytoplasmic sperm injection: Intracytoplasmic sperm injection (ICSI) is an *in vitro* fertilization procedure in which a single sperm is injected directly into an egg.

Intraspecific: Intraspecific is a term used in biology to describe behaviors, biochemical variations, and other issues within individuals of a single species, thereby contrasting with interspecific.

Introgression: Introgression, also known as introgressive hybridization, in genetics (particularly plant genetics), is the movement of a gene (gene flow) from one species into the gene pool of another by repeated backcrossing of an interspecific hybrid with one of its parent species. Purposeful introgression is a long-term process; it may take many hybrid generations before the backcrossing occurs.

Inverted repeat: An inverted repeat (or IR) is a sequence of nucleotides that is the reversed complement of another sequence further downstream.

***In vitro* fertilization:** *In vitro* fertilization (IVF) is a process by which egg cells are fertilized by sperm outside the body—*in vitro*. IVF is a major treatment in infertility when other methods of assisted reproductive technology have failed. The process involves hormonally controlling the ovulatory process, removing ova (eggs) from the woman's ovaries and letting sperm fertilize them in a fluid medium.

***In vitro* maturation:** *In vitro* maturation (IVM) is the technique of letting ovarian follicles to mature *in vitro*.

***In vitro* mutagenesis:** The production of either random or specific mutations in a piece of cloned DNA. Typically, the DNA will then be reintroduced into a cell or an organism to assess the results of the mutagenesis.

***In vivo* gene therapy:** The gene therapy carried out in the living organism.

Ion channel: Ion channels are pore-forming proteins that help establish and control the small voltage gradient across the plasma membrane of cells (see cell potential) by allowing the flow of ions down their electrochemical gradient.

Ionizing radiation: Ionizing radiation consists of particles or electromagnetic waves that are energetic enough to detach electrons from atoms or molecules, therefore ionizing them. Direct ionization from the effects of single particles or single photons produces free radicals, which are atoms or molecules containing unpaired electrons, that tend to be especially chemically reactive due to their electronic structure.

Irradiation: Irradiation is the process by which an item is exposed to radiation. The exposure can originate from any of various sources, including those occurring naturally, or as part of a mechanical process, or otherwise.

Isochromosome: An isochromosome is a chromosome that has lost one of its arms and replaced it with an exact copy of the other arm. This is sometimes seen in some female individuals with Turner syndrome or in tumor cells.

Isoelectric focusing: Isoelectric focusing (IEF), also known as electrofocusing, is a technique for separating different molecules by their electric charge differences. It is a type of zone electrophoresis, usually performed on proteins in a gel, which takes advantage of the fact that overall charge on the molecule of interest is a function of the pH of its surroundings.

Isoenzyme: Isozymes are enzymes that differ in amino acid sequence but catalyze the same chemical reaction. These enzymes usually display different kinetic parameters or different regulatory properties.

Isoform: A protein that has the same functions as another protein but which is encoded by a different gene and may have small differences in its sequence. For example, transforming factor beta (TGF-B) exists in three versions, or isoforms (TGF-B1, TGF-B2, and TGF-B3), each of which can set off a signaling cascade that starts in the cytoplasm and terminates in the nucleus of the cell.

Isomerase: In biochemistry, an isomerase is an enzyme that catalyzes the structural rearrangement of isomers. Isomerases thus catalyze reactions of the form $A \rightarrow B$, where B is an isomer of A.

Isotonic: Isotonic solutions have equal osmotic pressure.

Isotope: Isotopes are variants of atoms of a particular chemical element, which have differing numbers of neutrons. Atoms of a particular element by definition must contain the same number of protons but may have a distinct number of neutrons which differs from atom to atom, without changing the designation of the atom as a particular element.

Isozyme: Isozyme is one of the multiple forms in which an enzyme may exist in an organism or in different species, the various forms differing chemically, physically, or immunologically, but catalyzing the same reaction.

Jumping genes: A fragment of nucleic acid, such as a plasmid or a transposon, that can become incorporated into the DNA of a cell.

Juvenile *in vitro* embryo technology: Juvenile *in vitro* embryo technology (JIVET) is a technology involving collection of immature eggs from young animals, *in vitro* maturation and fertilization, and the transfer of the resultant embryos into recipient females. The method is designed to achieve rapid generation turnover.

Kanamycin: Kanamycin sulfate is an aminoglycoside antibiotic, available in oral, intravenous, and intramuscular forms, and used to treat a wide variety of infections. Kanamycin is isolated from *Streptomyces kanamyceticus*.

Kappa chain: A polypeptide chain of one of the two types of light chain that is found in antibodies and can be distinguished antigenically and by the sequence of amino acids in the chain.

Karyogamy: Karyogamy is the fusion of pronuclei of two cells, as part of syngamy, fertilization, or true bacterial conjugation.

Karyogram: The complete set of chromosomes of a cell or organism. Used especially for the display prepared from photographs of mitotic chromosomes arranged in homologous pairs.

Karyokinesis: During cell division, the process of partition of a cell's nucleus into the daughter cells.

Karyotype: A karyotype is the number and appearance of chromosomes in the nucleus of a eukaryotic cell. The term is also used for the complete set of chromosomes in a species, or an individual organism.

Kilo base pair: Kilo base pair (kb) is a length of DNA or double-stranded RNA equal to 1000 base pairs.

Kilodalton: Kilodalton (kDa) is a unit of molecular mass equal to 1000 Da.

Kinase: In chemistry and biochemistry, a kinase, alternatively known as a phosphotransferase, is a type of enzyme that transfers phosphate groups from high-energy donor molecules, such as ATP, to specific substrates.

Kinetics: The study of biochemical reaction rates catalyzed by an enzyme.

Knockout mouse: A knockout mouse is a genetically engineered mouse in which researchers have inactivated, or "knocked out," an existing gene by replacing it or disrupting it with an artificial piece of DNA. The loss of gene activity often causes changes in a mouse's phenotype, which includes appearance, behavior, and other observable physical and biochemical characteristics.

Lactose: Lactose is a disaccharide sugar that is found most notably in milk and is formed from galactose and glucose. Lactose makes up around 2–8% of milk (by weight), although the amount varies among species and individuals.

Lagging strand: In DNA replication, the strand that is synthesized apparently in the 3′–5′ direction, but actually in the 5′–3′ direction by ligating short fragments synthesized individually. Strand of DNA being replicated discontinuously.

Lag phase: The initial growth phase, during which the cell number remains relatively constant prior to rapid growth.

Lambda chain: A polypeptide chain of one of the two types of light chain that are found in antibodies and can be distinguished antigenically.

Laminar flow cabinet: A laminar flow cabinet or laminar flow closet or tissue culture hood is a carefully enclosed bench designed to prevent contamination of semiconductor wafers, biological samples, or any particle-sensitive device. Air is drawn through a HEPA filter and blown in a very smooth, laminar flow toward the user. The cabinet is usually made of stainless steel with no gaps or joints where spores might collect.

Lampbrush chromosomes: Lampbrush chromosomes are a special form of chromosomes that are found in the growing oocytes (immature eggs) of most animals, except mammals.

Landrace: A landrace is a local variety of a domesticated animal or plant species which has developed largely by natural processes, by adaptation to the natural and cultural environment in which it lives. It differs from a formal breed which has been bred deliberately to conform to a particular standard type.

Leader sequence: The sequence at the 5′ end of an mRNA that is not translated into protein. The length of untranslated mRNA from the 5′ end to the initiation codon AUG.

Leading strand: Strand of DNA being replicated continuously. In DNA replication, the strand that is made in the 5′ to 3′ direction by continuous polymerization at the 3′ growing tip. See also lagging strand.

Lectin: Lectins are sugar-binding proteins (not to be confused with glycoproteins, which are proteins containing sugar chains or residues) that are highly specific for their sugar moieties.

Lethal dose 50: A dose at which 50% of subjects will die.

Lethal gene: A gene whose expression results in the death of the organism, usually during embryogenesis.

Lethal mutation: A type of mutation in which the effect(s) can result in the death or reduce significantly the expected longevity of an organism carrying the mutation.

Ligand: In coordination chemistry, a ligand is an ion or molecule (see also functional group) that binds to a central metal atom to form a coordination complex. The bonding between metal and ligand generally involves formal donation of one or more of the ligand's electron pairs.

Ligation: In molecular biology, the covalent linking of two ends of DNA molecules using DNA ligase.

Lineage genetics: Genetic lineage is a series of mutations which connect an ancestral genetic type (allele, haplotype, or haplogroup) to derivative type.

Linkage: Genetic linkage is the tendency of certain loci or alleles to be inherited together. Genetic loci that are physically close to one another on the same chromosome tend to stay together during meiosis, and are thus genetically linked.

Linker DNA: Linker DNA is double-stranded DNA in between two nucleosome cores that, in association with histone H1, holds the cores together. Linker DNA is seen as the string in the "beads and string model," which is made by using an ionic solution on the chromatin. Linker DNA connects to histone H1 and histone H1 sits on the nucleosome core.

Lipases: A lipase is a water-soluble enzyme that catalyzes the hydrolysis of ester chemical bonds in water-insoluble lipid substrates. Lipases are a subclass of the esterases.

Lipid: Lipids are a broad group of naturally occurring molecules which includes fats, waxes, sterols, fat-soluble vitamins (such as vitamins A, D, E, and K), monoglycerides, diglycerides, phospholipids, and others.

Lipofection: Lipofection (or liposome transfection) is a technique used to inject genetic material into a cell by means of liposomes, which are vesicles that can easily merge with the cell membrane since they are both made of a phospholipid bilayer. Lipofection generally uses a positively charged (cationic) lipid to form an aggregate with the negatively charged (anionic) genetic material.

Liposome: Liposomes are artificially prepared vesicles made of lipid bilayer. Liposomes can be filled with drugs, and used to deliver drugs for cancer and other diseases.

Liquid nitrogen: Liquid nitrogen is nitrogen in a liquid state at a very low temperature. It is produced industrially by fractional distillation of liquid air. Liquid nitrogen is a compact and readily transported source of nitrogen gas without pressurization. Further, its ability to maintain temperatures far below the freezing point of water makes it extremely useful in a wide range of applications, primarily as an open-cycle refrigerant, including for the cryopreservation of blood, reproductive cells (sperm and egg), and other biological samples and materials.

Litmus test: A test for chemical acidity or basicity using litmus paper.

Live vaccine: One prepared from live microorganisms that have been attenuated but that retain their immunogenic properties.

Logarithmic phase: The steepest slope of the growth curve of a culture—the phase of vigorous growth during which cell number doubles every 20–30 min.

Long terminal repeat: Long terminal repeats (LTRs) are sequences of DNA that repeat hundreds or thousands of times. They are found in retroviral DNA and in retrotransposons, flanking functional genes. They are used by viruses to insert their genetic sequences into the host genomes.

Loop bioreactors: Bioreactors in which the fermenting material is cycled between a bulk tank and a smaller tank or loop of pipes.

Luteinizing hormone: Luteinizing hormone (LH) is a hormone produced by the anterior pituitary gland.

Lux: The lux (symbol: lx) is the SI unit of illuminance and luminous emittance measuring luminous power per area. It is used in photometry as a measure of the intensity, as perceived by the human eye.

Lyase: In biochemistry, a lyase is an enzyme that catalyzes the breaking of various chemical bonds by means other than hydrolysis and oxidation, often forming a new double bond or a new ring structure.

Lymphocyte: A lymphocyte is a type of white blood cell in the vertebrate immune system.

Lymphokine: Lymphokines are a subset of cytokines that are produced by a type of immune cell known as a lymphocyte. They are protein mediators typically produced by T cells to direct the immune system response by signaling between its cells.

Lymphoma: Lymphoma is a cancer in the lymphatic cells of the immune system. Typically, lymphomas present as a solid tumor of lymphoid cells.

Lyophilize: To freeze-dry. The material is rapidly frozen and dehydrated under high vacuum. The process is termed lyophilization.

Lysis: Lysis refers to the breaking down of a cell, often by viral, enzyme, or osmotic mechanisms that compromise its integrity. A fluid containing the contents of lysed cells is called a "lysate."

Lysogenic bacteria: A bacterium which contains in its genome the DNA of a virus which is lying dormant, passively letting itself be replicated by the bacterium whenever the bacterium replicates its own genome (a lysogenic virus), but able to reactivate and destroy the bacterium at a time of the virus's choosing (becomes a lytic virus).

Lysosome: Lysosomes are cellular organelles that contain acid hydrolase enzymes to break down waste materials and cellular debris. They are found in animal cells, while in yeast and plants the same roles are performed by lytic vacuoles.

Lytic cycle: The lytic cycle is one of the two cycles of viral reproduction, the other being the lysogenic cycle.

M13: M13 is a filamentous bacteriophage composed of circular single-stranded DNA (ssDNA), which is 6407 nucleotides long encapsulated in approximately 2700 copies of the major coat protein P8, and capped with 5 copies of two different minor coat proteins (P9, P6, P3) on the ends.

Macromolecule: A macromolecule is a very large molecule commonly created by some form of polymerization. In biochemistry, the term is applied to the four conventional biopolymers (nucleic acids, proteins, carbohydrates, and lipids), as well as nonpolymeric molecules with large molecular mass such as macrocycles.

Macronutrient: Nutrients that the body uses in relatively large amounts—proteins, carbohydrates, and fats. This is as opposed to micronutrients, which the body requires in smaller amounts, such as vitamins and minerals. Macronutrients provide calories to the body as well as performing other functions.

Macrophages: Type of white blood that ingests (takes in) foreign material. Macrophages are key players in the immune response to foreign invaders such as infectious microorganisms.

Macropropagation: Production of plant clones from growing parts.

Major histocompatibility complex: The major histocompatibility complex (MHC) is a large genomic region or gene family found in most vertebrates that encodes MHC molecules. MHC molecules play an important role in the immune system and autoimmunity.

Malignant: Tending to be severe and become progressively worse, as in malignant hypertension.

Marker-assisted introgression: The use of DNA markers to increase the speed and efficiency of introgression of a new allele(s) or gene(s) into a breeding population.

Marker-assisted selection: Marker-assisted selection or marker-aided selection (MAS) is a process whereby a marker (morphological, biochemical, or one based on DNA/RNA variation) is used for indirect selection of a genetic determinant or determinants of a trait of interest (i.e., productivity, disease resistance, abiotic stress tolerance, and/or quality). This process is used in plant and animal breeding.

Marker gene: Detectable genetic trait or segment of DNA that can be identified and tracked. A marker gene can serve as a flag for another gene, sometimes called the target gene. A marker gene must be on the same chromosome as the target gene and near enough to it so that the two genes (the marker gene and the target gene) are genetically linked and are usually inherited together.

Marker peptide: A portion of fusion protein that facilitates its identification or purification.

Mean: The mean is the arithmetic average of a set of values, or distribution; however, for skewed distributions, the mean is not necessarily the same as the middle value (median), or the most likely (mode).

Median: In probability theory and statistics, a median is described as the numerical value separating the higher half of a sample, a population, or a probability distribution, from the lower half.

Megabase cloning: The cloning of very large DNA fragments.

Megadalton (MDa): A unit of mass equal to 1 million atomic mass units.

Meiosis: Meiosis is a special type of cell division necessary for sexual reproduction. In animals, meiosis produces gametes (sperm and egg cells), while in other organisms, such as fungi, it generates spores.

Melanin: Melanin is a pigment that is ubiquitous in nature, being found in most organisms (spiders are one of the few groups in which it has not been detected). In animals melanin pigments are derivatives of the amino acid tyrosine.

Melting temperature for DNA: Nucleic acid thermodynamics is the study of the thermodynamics of nucleic acid molecules, or how temperature affects nucleic acid structure. For multiple copies of DNA molecules, the melting temperature (T_m) is defined as the temperature at which half of the DNA strands are in the double-helical state and half are in the random coil states. The melting temperature depends on both the length of the molecule, and the specific nucleotide sequence composition of that molecule.

Membrane bioreactors: Membrane bioreactor (MBR) is the combination of a membrane process like microfiltration or ultrafiltration with a suspended growth bioreactor, and is now widely used for municipal and industrial wastewater treatment with plant sizes up to 80,000 population equivalent.

Memory cells: Memory B cells are a B cell subtype that are formed following primary infection.

Mendelian population: A group of interbreeding individuals; the total allelic gene content of the group is called their gene pool.

Mendel's laws: Mendel discovered that when crossing white flowered and purple flowered plants, the result is not a blend. Rather than being a mix of the two, the offspring was purple flowered. He then conceived the idea of heredity units, which he called "factors," one of which is a recessive characteristic and the other dominant. Mendel said that factors, later called genes, normally occur in pairs in ordinary body cells, yet segregate during the formation of sex cells.

Mesoderm: In all bilaterian animals, the mesoderm is one of the three primary germ cell layers in the very early embryo.

Messenger RNA: Messenger RNA (mRNA) is a molecule of RNA encoding a chemical "blueprint" for a protein product. mRNA is transcribed from a DNA template, and carries coding information to the sites of protein synthesis: the ribosomes. Here, the nucleic acid polymer is translated into a polymer of amino acids: a protein.

Metabolic cell: Undivided cell.

Metabolism: Metabolism is the set of chemical reactions that occur in living organisms to maintain life. These processes allow organisms to grow and reproduce, maintain their structures, and respond to their environments. Metabolism is usually divided into two categories. Catabolism breaks down organic matter, for example, to harvest energy in cellular respiration. Anabolism uses energy to construct components of cells such as proteins and nucleic acids.

Metabolite: Metabolites are the intermediates and products of metabolism. The term metabolite is usually restricted to small molecules.

Metaphase: Metaphase is a stage of mitosis in the eukaryotic cell cycle in which condensed and highly coiled chromosomes, carrying genetic information, align in the middle of the cell before being separated into each of the two daughter cells.

Metastasis: Metastasis or metastatic disease is the spread of a disease from one organ or part to another nonadjacent organ or part.

Methylation: In the chemical sciences, methylation denotes the addition of a methyl group to a substrate or the substitution of an atom or group by a methyl group. Methylation is a form of alkylation with, to be specific, a methyl group, rather than a larger carbon chain, replacing a hydrogen atom. These terms are commonly used in chemistry, biochemistry, soil science, and the biological sciences.

Michaelis constant: In biochemistry, Michaelis–Menten kinetics is one of the simplest and best-known models of enzyme kinetics. It is named after American biochemist Leonor Michaelis and Canadian physician Maud Menten.

Microarray: A DNA microarray (also commonly known as gene chip, DNA chip, or biochip) is a collection of microscopic DNA spots attached to a solid surface. Scientists use DNA microarrays to measure the expression levels of large numbers of genes simultaneously or to genotype multiple regions of a genome.

Microbe: A microscopic living organism, such as a bacterium, fungus, protozoan, or virus.

Microdroplet array: Microdroplet is a technique to use to simultaneously evaluate large numbers of media modifications, employing small quantities of medium into which are placed small numbers of cells or protoplasts.

Microencapsulation: Microencapsulation is a process in which tiny particles or droplets are surrounded by a coating to give small capsules many useful properties. In a relatively simplistic form, a microcapsule is a small sphere with a uniform wall around it. The material inside the microcapsule is referred to as the core, internal phase, or fill, whereas the wall is sometimes called a shell, coating, or membrane. Most microcapsules have diameters between a few micrometers and a few millimeters.

Microinjection: Microinjection refers to the process of using a glass micropipette to insert substances at a microscopic or borderline macroscopic level into a single living cell. It is a simple mechanical process in which a needle roughly 0.5–5 μm in diameter penetrates the cell membrane and/or the nuclear envelope.

Micron: A micrometer is one-millionth of a meter (1/1000 of a millimeter, or 0.001 mm). Its unit symbol in the International System of Units (SI) is μm.

Micronutrient: Micronutrients are nutrients required by humans and other living things throughout life in small quantities to orchestrate a whole range of physiological functions, but which the organism itself cannot produce.

Microsatellite: Microsatellite (genetics), a repeating sequence in DNA.

Microspore: In botany, microspores develop into male gametophytes, whereas megaspores develop into female gametophytes. The combination of megaspores and microspores is found only in heterosporous organisms. In seed plants the microspores give rise to the pollen grains, and the megaspores are formed within the developing seed.

Microtubules: Microtubules are one of the active matter components of the cytoskeleton. They have a diameter of 25 nm and length varying from 200 nm to 25 μm. Microtubules serve as structural components within cells and are involved in many cellular processes, including mitosis, cytokinesis, and vesicular transport.

Miniprep: Minipreparation of plasmid DNA is a rapid, small-scale isolation of plasmid DNA from bacteria. It is based on the alkaline lysis method invented by the researchers Birnboim and Doly in 1979. The extracted plasmid DNA resulting from performing a miniprep is itself often called a "miniprep." Minipreps are used in the process of molecular cloning to analyze bacterial clones. A typical plasmid DNA yield of a miniprep is 20–30 μg depending on the cell strain.

Minisatellite: A minisatellite (also referred as VNTR) is a section of DNA that consists of a short series of bases 10–60 bp. These occur at more than 1000 locations in the human genome. Some minisatellites contain a central (or "core") sequence of letters "GGGCAGGANG" (where N can be any base) or more generally a strand bias with purines (adenosine (A) and guanine (G)) on one strand and pyrimidines (cytosine (C) and thymine (T)) on the other.

Mismatch repair: DNA mismatch repair is a system for recognizing and repairing erroneous insertion, deletion and mis-incorporation of bases that can arise during DNA replication and recombination, as well as repairing some forms of DNA damage.

Missense mutation: In genetics, a missense mutation (a type of nonsynonymous mutation) is a point mutation in which a single nucleotide is changed, resulting in a codon those codes for a different amino acid (mutations that change an amino acid to a stop codon are considered nonsense mutations, rather than missense mutations).

Mitochondrial DNA: Mitochondrial DNA (mtDNA) is the DNA located in organelles called mitochondria, structures within eukaryotic cells that convert the chemical energy from food into a form that cells can use, adenosine triphosphate (ATP). Most other DNA present in eukaryotic organisms is found in the cell nucleus.

Mitosis: Mitosis is the process by which a eukaryotic cell separates the chromosomes in its cell nucleus into two identical sets in two nuclei. It is generally followed immediately by cytokinesis, which divides the nuclei, cytoplasm, organelles, and cell membrane into two cells containing roughly equal shares of these cellular components.

Modifying gene: A gene that alters or influences the expression function of another gene, including the suppression or reduction of the usual function of the modified gene.

Molarity: The molar concentration of a solution, usually expressed as the number of moles of solute per liter of solution.

Molecular cloning: Molecular cloning refers to a set of experimental methods in molecular biology that are used to assemble recombinant DNA molecules and to direct their replication within host organisms.

Molecular genetics: Molecular genetics is the field of biology and genetics that studies the structure and function of genes at a molecular level. The field studies how the genes are transferred from generation to generation.

Monoclonal antibody: Monoclonal antibodies (mAb or moAb) are monospecific antibodies that are the same because they are made by identical immune cells that are all clones of a unique parent cell.

Monocotyledon: Any of various flowering plants, such as grasses, orchids, and lilies, having a single cotyledon in the seed.

Monoculture: Monoculture is the agricultural practice of producing or growing one single crop over a wide area. It is also known as a way of farming practice of growing large stands of a single species.

Monosaccharide: Monosaccharides (from Greek monos: single, sacchar: sugar) are the most basic units of biologically important carbohydrates. They are the simplest form of sugar and are usually colorless, water-soluble, crystalline solids. Some monosaccharides have a sweet taste.

Morphogenesis: Morphogenesis is the biological process that causes an organism to develop its shape. It is one of three fundamental aspects of developmental biology along with the control of cell growth and cellular differentiation.

Multigene family: A set of genes descended by duplication and variation from some ancestral gene. Such genes may be clustered together on the same chromosome or dispersed on different chromosomes.

Mutagen: In genetics, a mutagen is a physical or chemical agent that changes the genetic material, usually DNA, of an organism and thus increases the frequency of mutations above the natural background level. As many mutations cause cancer, mutagens are typically also carcinogens.

Mutagenesis: Mutagenesis is a process by which the genetic information of an organism is changed in a stable manner, either in nature or experimentally by the use of chemicals or radiation. Mutagenesis as a science was developed especially by Charlotte Auerbach in the first half of the twentieth century.

Mutant: In biology and especially genetics, a mutant is an individual, organism, or new genetic character, arising or resulting from an instance of mutation, which is a base-pair sequence change within the DNA of a gene or chromosome of an organism resulting in the creation of a new character or trait not found in the wild type.

Mutation: In molecular biology and genetics, mutations are changes in a genomic sequence: the DNA sequence of a cell's genome or the DNA or RNA sequence of a virus. They can be defined as sudden and spontaneous changes in the cell.

Mycoprotein: Mycoprotein means protein from fungi. It can be used as part of any meal, particularly vegetarian.

Mycotoxin: A mycotoxin is a toxic secondary metabolite produced by organisms of the fungus kingdom, commonly known as molds. The term "mycotoxin" is usually reserved for the toxic chemical products produced by fungi that readily colonize crops. One mold species may produce many different mycotoxins and/or the same mycotoxin as another species.

Myosin: Myosins comprise a family of ATP-dependent motor proteins and are best known for their role in muscle contraction and their involvement in a wide range of other eukaryotic motility processes.

Nanometer: A nanometer is a unit of length in the metric system, equal to 1 billionth of a meter.

Native protein: The protein inside the cell that is in its native or natural state and unaltered by denaturing agents, such as heat, chemical, enzyme action, or the exigencies of extraction.

Natural selection: Natural selection is the nonrandom process by which biologic traits become more or less common in a population as a function of differential reproduction of their bearers. It is a key mechanism of evolution.

Necrosis: Necrosis is the premature death of cells and living tissue. Necrosis is caused by factors external to the cell or tissue, such as infection, toxins, or trauma.

Negative autogenous regulation: Inhibition of the expression of a gene or set of coordinately regulated genes by the product of the gene or the product of one of the genes.

Nematodes: The nematodes are the most diverse phylum of pseudocoelomates, and one of the most diverse of all animals.

Neo-formation: A new and abnormal growth of tissue; tumor; neoplasm.

Neoplasm: Neoplasm is an abnormal mass of tissue as a result of neoplasia. Neoplasia is the abnormal proliferation of cells. The growth of neoplastic cells exceeds and is not coordinated with that of the normal tissues around it.

Neoteny: Neoteny is the retention, by adults in a species, of traits previously seen only in juveniles, and is a subject studied in the field of developmental biology.

Neutral mutation: In genetics, a neutral mutation is a mutation that has no effect on fitness. In other words, it is neutral with respect to natural selection. For example, some mutations in a DNA triplet or codon do not change which amino acid is introduced: this is known as a synonymous substitution. Unless the mutation also has a regulatory effect, synonymous substitutions are usually neutral.

Neutral theory: The neutral theory of molecular evolution states that the vast majority of evolutionary changes at the molecular level are caused by random drift of selectively neutral mutants.

Nick translation: Nick translation (or head translation) is a tagging technique in molecular biology in which DNA polymerase I is used to replace some of the nucleotides of a DNA sequence with their labeled analogues, creating a tagged DNA sequence which can be used as a probe in fluorescent in situ hybridization or blotting techniques.

Nitrification: Nitrification is the biological oxidation of ammonia with oxygen into nitrite followed by the oxidation of these nitrites into nitrates. Degradation of ammonia to nitrite is usually the rate-limiting step of nitrification. Nitrification is an important step in the nitrogen cycle in soil. This process was discovered by the Russian microbiologist, Sergei Winogradsky.

Nitrocellulose: Nitrocellulose (also: cellulose nitrate, flash paper) is a highly flammable compound formed by nitrating cellulose through exposure to nitric acid or another powerful nitrating agent.

Nitrogen fixation: Nitrogen fixation is the natural process, either biological or abiotic, by which nitrogen (N_2) in the atmosphere is converted into ammonia (NH_3). This process is essential for life because fixed nitrogen is required to biosynthesize the basic building blocks of life, for example, nucleotides for DNA and RNA and amino acids for proteins. Nitrogen fixation also refers to other biological conversions of nitrogen, such as its conversion to nitrogen dioxide.

Nitrogenous bases: The purines (adenine and guanine) and pyrimidines (thymine, cytosine, and uracil) that form DNA and RNA molecules.

Nonhistone chromosomal proteins: Chromatin consists of DNA, histones, and a very heterogeneous group of other proteins that include DNA polymerases, regulator proteins, and so on. They are often lumped together terminologically as nonhistone proteins or acidic proteins, to distinguish them from the basic histones.

Northern blotting: The northern blot is a technique used in molecular biology research to study gene expression by detection of RNA (or isolated mRNA) in a sample.

Northern hybridization: A procedure in which RNA fragments are transferred from an agarose gel to a nitrocellulose filter, where the RNA is then hybridized to a radioactive probe.

Nuclear transfer: Nuclear transfer is a form of cloning. The steps involve removing the DNA from an oocyte (unfertilized egg), and injecting the nucleus which contains the DNA to be cloned.

Nuclease: A nuclease is an enzyme capable of cleaving the phosphodiester bonds between the nucleotide subunits of nucleic acids. Earlier publications may use terms such as "polynucleotidase" or "nucleodepolymerase."

Nucleic acid: Nucleic acids are biological molecules essential for life, and include DNA (deoxyribonucleic acid) and RNA (ribonucleic acid). Together with proteins, nucleic acids make up the most important macromolecules; each is found in abundance in all living things, where they function in encoding, transmitting, and expressing genetic information.

Nuclein: Any of the substances present in the nucleus of a cell, consisting chiefly of proteins, phosphoric acids, and nucleic acids.

Nucleo-cytoplasmic ratio: The ratio of the volume of a nucleus of a cell to the volume of the cytoplasm. The proportion is usually constant for a specific cell type, and an increase is indicative of malignant neoplasms.

Nucleolar organizer: The chromosomal region around which the nucleolus forms, a site of tandem repeats of the rRNA gene. A region (or regions) of the chromosome set.

Nucleolus: The nucleolus is a nonmembrane-bound structure composed of proteins and nucleic acids found within the nucleus. Ribosomal RNA (rRNA) is transcribed and assembled within the nucleolus.

Nucleoplasm: Similar to the cytoplasm of a cell, the nucleus contains nucleoplasm (nucleus sap) or karyoplasm. The nucleoplasm is one of the types of protoplasm, and it is enveloped by the nuclear membrane or nuclear envelope. The nucleoplasm is a highly viscous liquid that surrounds the chromosomes and nucleoli.

Nucleoprotein: A nucleoprotein is any protein which is structurally associated with nucleic acid (either DNA or RNA). Many viruses harness this protein, and they are known for being host specific, that is they find it difficult to infect species besides the ones they normally infect.

Nucleoside: Nucleosides are glycosylamines consisting of a nucleobase (often referred to as simply base) bound to a ribose or deoxyribose sugar via a beta-glycosidic linkage. Examples of nucleosides include cytidine, uridine, adenosine, guanosine, thymidine, and inosine.

Nucleoside analogue: Nucleoside analogues are a range of antiviral products used to prevent viral replication in infected cells. The most commonly used is Aciclovir, although its inclusion in this category is uncertain, as it contains only a partial nucleoside structure, as the sugar ring is replaced by an open-chain structure.

Nucleosome: Nucleosomes are the basic unit of DNA packaging in eukaryotes, consisting of a segment of DNA wound around a histone protein core. This structure is often compared to thread wrapped around a spool.

Nucleotide: Nucleotides are molecules that, when joined together, make up the structural units of RNA and DNA. In addition, nucleotides play central roles in metabolism, in which capacity they serve as sources of chemical energy (adenosine triphosphate and guanosine triphosphate), participate in cellular signaling (cyclic guanosine monophosphate and cyclic adenosine monophosphate), and are incorporated into important cofactors of enzymatic reactions (coenzyme A, flavin adenine dinucleotide, flavin mononucleotide, and nicotinamide adenine dinucleotide phosphate).

Nucleus: In cell biology, the nucleus is a membrane-enclosed organelle found in eukaryotic cells. It contains most of the cell's genetic material, organized as multiple long linear DNA molecules in complex with a large variety of proteins, such as histones, to form chromosomes.

Null mutation: A mutation (a change) in a gene that leads to its not being transcribed into RNA and/or translated into a functional protein product. For example, a null mutation in a gene that usually encodes a specific enzyme leads to the production of a nonfunctional enzyme or no enzyme at all.

Nullisomy: A type of genome mutation in which a pair of chromosomes that are normally present in the genome is missing. Organisms that exhibit nullisomy are called nullisomes. Nullisomy, especially in higher animals, usually results in death. Viable nullisomes can be found among polyploid plants; these nullisomes are used for nullisomic analysis and for establishing new, commercially valuable strains. Nullisomic analysis is used to determine genetic linkage groups and to study the traits that are controlled by these groups. The method is also applied to tissue-culture studies of human nullisomic cells.

Nutrient film technique: Nutrient film technique or NFT is a hydroponic technique wherein a very shallow stream of water containing all the dissolved nutrients required for plant growth is recirculated past the bare roots of plants in a watertight gully, also known as channels.

Nutrient gradient: A diffusion gradient of nutrients and gases that develops in tissues where only a portion of the tissue is in contact with the medium. Gradients are less likely to form in liquid media than in callus cultures.

Nutrient medium: A culture medium to which nutrient materials have been added.

Offspring: In biology, offspring is the product of reproduction, of a new organism produced by one or more parents.

Okazaki fragments: Okazaki fragments are short molecules of single-stranded DNA that are formed on the lagging strand during DNA replication. They are between 1000 and 2000 nucleotides long in *Escherichia coli* and are between 100 and 200 nucleotides long in eukaryotes.

Oligomer: In chemistry, an oligomer is a molecule that consists of a few monomer units in contrast to a polymer that, at least in principle, consists of an unlimited number of monomers. Dimers, trimers, and tetramers are oligomers. Many oils are oligomeric, such as liquid paraffin.

Oligonucleotide: An oligonucleotide is a short nucleic acid polymer, typically with 50 or fewer bases. Although they can be formed by bond cleavage of longer segments, they are now more commonly synthesized, in a sequence-specific manner, from individual nucleoside phosphoramidites. Automated synthesizers allow the synthesis of oligonucleotides up to about 200 bases.

Oligonucleotide ligation assay: Oligonucleotide ligation assay (OLA) is a rapid, sensitive, and specific method for the detection of known single-nucleotide polymorphisms (SNPs). This method is based on the joining of two adjacent oligonucleotide probes (Capture and Reporter Oligos) using a DNA ligase while they are annealed to a complementary DNA target (e.g., PCR product).

Oncogene: An oncogene is a gene that has the potential to cause cancer. In tumor cells, they are often mutated or expressed at high levels. Most normal cells undergo a programmed form of death (apoptosis). Activated oncogenes can cause those cells that ought to die to survive and proliferate instead.

Oncogenesis: The progression of cytological, genetic, and cellular changes that culminate in a malignant tumor.

Oncogenic: Oncogenic giving rise to tumors or causing tumor formation; said especially of tumor-inducing viruses.

Oncomouse: The Oncomouse or Harvard mouse is a type of laboratory mouse that has been genetically modified using modifications designed by Philip Leder and Timothy A. Stewart of Harvard University to carry a specific gene called an activated oncogene.

Ontogeny: Ontogeny describes the origin and the development of an organism, for example, from the fertilized egg to mature form.

Oocyte: An oocyte, ovocyte, or rarely ocyte, is a female gametocyte or germ cell involved in reproduction. In other words, it is an immature ovum, or egg cell. An oocyte is produced in the ovary during female gametogenesis.

Oogenesis: Oogenesis is the creation of an ovum (egg cell). It is the female form of gametogenesis. The male equivalent is spermatogenesis. It involves the development of the various stages of the immature ovum.

Oogonium: An oogonium is an immature ovum. It is a female gametogonium. They are formed in large numbers by mitosis early in fetal life from primordial germ cells, which are present in the fetus between weeks 4 and 8.

Oospore: An oospore is a thick-walled sexual spore that develops from a fertilized oosphere in some algae and fungi.

Open continuous culture: A continuous culture system, in which inflow of fresh medium is balanced by outflow of a corresponding volume of spent medium plus cells. In the steady state, the rate of cell wash-out equals the rate of formation of new cells in the system.

Open pollination: Open pollination is pollination by insects, birds, wind, or other natural mechanisms, and contrasts with cleistogamy, closed pollination, which is one of the many types of self-pollination. Open pollination also contrasts with controlled pollination, which is controlled so that all seeds of a crop are descended from parents with known traits, and are therefore more likely to have the desired traits.

Open reading frame: In molecular genetics, an open reading frame (ORF) is a DNA sequence that does not contain a stop codon in a given reading frame.

Operon: In genetics, an operon is a functioning unit of genomic DNA containing a cluster of genes under the control of a single regulatory signal or promoter. The genes are transcribed together into an mRNA strand and either translated together in the cytoplasm, or undergo *trans*-splicing to create monocistronic mRNAs that are translated separately, that is, several strands of mRNA that each encode a single gene product.

Organ culture: Organ culture is a development from tissue culture methods of research, the organ culture is able to accurately model functions of an organ in various states and conditions by the use of the actual *in vitro* organ itself.

Organic chemistry: Organic chemistry is a subdiscipline within chemistry involving the scientific study of the structure, properties, composition, reactions, and preparation (by synthesis or by other means) of carbon-based compounds, hydrocarbons, and their derivatives.

Organic complex: An organic compound is any member of a large class of gaseous, liquid, or solid chemical compounds whose molecules contain carbon. For historical reasons discussed below, a few types of carbon-containing compounds such as carbides, carbonates, simple oxides of carbon and cyanides, as well as the allotropes of carbon such as diamond and graphite, are considered inorganic.

Organogenesis: In animal development, organogenesis is the process by which the ectoderm, endoderm, and mesoderm develop into the internal organs of the organism.

Organoid: A structure that resembles an organ.

Organoleptic: Organoleptic relating to the senses (taste, sight, smell, touch) is a term also used to describe traditional USDA meat and poultry inspection techniques, because inspectors perform a variety of such procedures (involving visually examining, feeling, and smelling animal parts) to detect signs of disease or contamination. These inspection techniques alone are not adequate to detect invisible foodborne pathogens that now are the leading causes of food poisoning.

Origin of replication: The origin of replication (also called the replication origin) is a particular sequence in a genome at which replication is initiated. This can either be DNA replication in living organisms such as prokaryotes and eukaryotes, or RNA replication in RNA viruses, such as double-stranded RNA viruses. DNA replication may proceed from this point bidirectionally or unidirectionally.

Ortet: The plant from which a clone is obtained.

Osmolarity: Osmolarity is the measure of solute concentration, defined as the number of osmoles (Osm) of solute per liter (L) of solution (osmol/L or Osm/L).

Osmosis: Osmosis is the movement of solvent molecules through a selectively permeable membrane into a region of higher solute concentration, aiming to equalize the solute concentrations on the two sides. It may also be used to describe a physical process in which any solvent moves, without input of energy.

Osmotic potential: The potential of water molecules to move from a hypotonic solution (more water, less solutes) to a hypertonic solution (less water, more solutes) across a semipermeable membrane.

Outbreeding: The breeding of distantly related or unrelated individuals, often producing a hybrid of superior quality.

Ovary: The ovary is an ovum-producing reproductive organ, often found in pairs as part of the vertebrate female reproductive system. Ovaries in anatomically female individuals are analogous to testes in anatomically male individuals, in that they are both gonads and endocrine glands.

Overdominance: Overdominance is a condition in genetics where the phenotype of the heterozygote lies outside of the phenotypical range of both homozygote parents. Overdominance can also be described as heterozygote advantage, wherein heterozygous individuals have a higher fitness than homozygous individuals.

Overlapping reading frames: Start codons in different reading frames generate different polypeptides from the same DNA sequence.

Ovulation: Ovulation is the process in a female's menstrual cycle by which a mature ovarian follicle ruptures and discharges an ovum (also known as an oocyte, female gamete, or casually, an egg). Ovulation also occurs in the estrous cycle of other mammals, which differs in many fundamental ways from the menstrual cycle. The time immediately surrounding ovulation is referred to as the ovulatory phase or the periovulatory period.

Oxygen-electrode-based sensor: Sensor in which an oxygen electrode, which measures the amount of oxygen in a solution, is coated with a biological material such as an enzyme which generates or absorbs oxygen when the appropriate substrate is present.

Packed cell volume: The ratio of the volume occupied by packed red blood cells to the volume of the whole blood as measured by a hematocrit.

Pairing gene: The two copies of a particular gene present in a diploid cell (one in each chromosome set).

Pair-rule gene: A pair-rule gene is a type of gene involved in the development of the segmented embryos of insects. Pair-rule genes are defined by the effect of a mutation in that gene, which causes the loss of the normal developmental pattern in alternating segments.

Palaeontology: Palaeontology is the study of prehistoric life, including organisms' evolution and interactions with each other and their environments (their paleoecology).

Palindrome: A palindrome is a word, phrase, number, or other sequence of units that can be read the same way in either direction (the adjustment of punctuation and spaces between words is generally permitted).

Palindromic sequence: A palindromic sequence is a nucleic acid sequence (DNA or RNA) that is the same whether read 5′ (five-prime) to 3′ (three prime) on one strand or 5′ to 3′ on the complementary strand with which it forms a double helix.

Panicle culture: Aseptic culture of immature panicle explants to induce microspore germination and development.

Panmictic population: A population in which mating occurs at random.

Paracentric inversion: An inversion not involving the centromere. A chromosomal inversion that does not include the centromere.

Paraffin wax: In chemistry, paraffin is a term that can be used synonymously with "alkane," indicating hydrocarbons with the general formula C_nH_{2n+2}. Paraffin wax refers to a mixture of alkanes that falls within the $20 \le n \le 40$ range; they are found in the solid state at room temperature and begin to enter the liquid phase past approximately 37°C.

Parafilm: Parafilm is a plastic paraffin film with a paper backing produced by Pechiney Plastic Packaging Company, based in Chicago, Illinois primarily used in laboratories. It is commonly used for sealing or protecting vessels (such as flasks or cuvettes). It is ductile, malleable, waterproof, odorless, thermoplastic, semi-transparent, and cohesive.

Parahormone: Parahormone is a substance, not a true hormone, which has a hormone-like action in controlling the functioning of some distant organ.

Parallel evolution: Parallel evolution is the development of a similar trait in related, but distinct, species descending from the same ancestor, but from different clades.

Parasite: Traditionally parasite referred to organisms with lifestages that went beyond one host (e.g., *Taenia solium*), which are now called macroparasites (typically protozoa and helminths). Parasites can now also refer to microparasites, which are typically smaller, such as viruses and bacteria and can be directly transmitted between hosts of one species.

Parasitism: Parasitism is a type of symbiotic relationship between organisms of different species where one organism, the parasite, benefits at the expense of the other, the host.

Parasporal crystal: Tightly packaged insect pro-toxin molecules that are produced by strains of *Bacillus thuringiensis* during the formation of resting spores.

Parental generation: The first set of parents crossed in which their genotype is the basis for predicting the genotype of their offspring, which in turn, may be crossed (filial generation). In parental generation, two individuals are mated or crossed to determine or predict the genotypes of their offspring, called first filial generation (or F1 generation).

Par gene: One of a class of genes required for faithful plasmid segregation at cell division. Initially, par loci were identified on plasmids, but have also been found on bacterial chromosomes.

Parthenocarpy: In botany and horticulture, parthenocarpy (literally meaning virgin fruit) is the natural or artificially induced production of fruit without fertilization of ovules. The fruit is therefore seedless. It may also produce apparently seedless fruit, but the seeds are actually aborted while still small. Parthenocarpy occasionally occurs as a mutation in nature, but if it affects every flower, then the plant can no longer sexually reproduce but might be able to propagate by vegetative means.

Parthenogenesis: Parthenogenesis is a form of asexual reproduction found in females, where growth and development of embryos occurs without fertilization by a male. In plants, parthenogenesis means development of an embryo from an unfertilized egg cell, and is a component process of apomixis.

Partial digest: A restriction digest that has not been allowed to go to completion and thus contains pieces of DNA with some restriction endonuclease sites that have not yet been cleaved.

Particle radiation: Particle radiation is the radiation of energy by means of fast-moving subatomic particles. Particle radiation is referred to as a particle beam if the particles are all moving in the same direction, similar to a light beam.

Parturition: Childbirth, the process of delivering the baby and placenta from the uterus to the vagina to the outside world.

Passage: Passage is the number of times cells are being multiplied under culture condition.

Passage number: The passage number simply refers to the number of times the cells in the culture have been subcultured, often without consideration of the inoculation densities or recoveries involved. The population doubling level (PDL) refers to the total number of times the cells in the population have doubled since their primary isolation *in vitro*.

Passive immunity: Passive immunity is the transfer of active humoral immunity in the form of readymade antibodies, from one individual to another. Passive immunity can occur naturally, when maternal antibodies are transferred to the fetus through the placenta, and can also be induced artificially, when high levels of human (or horse) antibodies specific for a pathogen or toxin are transferred to nonimmune individuals. Passive immunization is used when there is a high risk of infection and insufficient time for the body to develop its own immune response, or to reduce the symptoms of ongoing or immunosuppressive diseases.

Patent: A patent is a set of exclusive rights granted by a state (national government) to an inventor or their assignee for a limited period of time in exchange for the public disclosure of an invention.

Pathogen: A pathogen is a microbe or microorganism such as a virus, bacterium, prion, or fungus that causes disease in its animal or plant host. A pathogen introduced by deliberate human agency as in bioterrorism is termed a biological agent, or bioagent. There are several substrates including pathways whereby pathogens can invade a host; the principal pathways have different episodic time frames, but soil contamination has the longest or most persistent potential for harboring a pathogen.

Pathogen free: A term applied to animals reared for experimentation or to commence new herds or flocks of disease-free animals. Animals usually obtained as for axenic animals but are then placed into a nonsterile environment in which they become infected with a range of microorganisms, many colonizing as so-called normal flora.

Pathovar: A pathovar is a bacterial strain or set of strains with the same or similar characteristics, that is differentiated at infra-subspecific level from other strains of the same species or subspecies on the basis of distinctive pathogenicity to one or more plant hosts.

pBR322: pBR322 is a plasmid and for a time was one of the most commonly used *E. coli* cloning vectors. Created in 1977, it was named eponymously after its Mexican creators, p standing for plasmid, and BR for Bolivar and Rodriguez.

Pectin: Pectin is a structural heteropolysaccharide contained in the primary cell walls of terrestrial plants.

Pectinase: Pectinase is a general term for enzymes, such as pectolyase, pectozyme, and polygalacturonase, commonly referred to in brewing as pectic enzymes. These break down pectin, a polysaccharide substrate that is found in the cell walls of plants. One of the most studied and widely used commercial pectinases is polygalacturonase.

Pedigree: Pedigree can refer to the lineage or genealogical descent of people, whether documented or not, or of animals, whether purebred or not.

Penetrance: Penetrance the frequency with which a heritable trait is manifested by individuals carrying the principal gene or genes conditioning it.

Peptide: Peptides are short polymers of amino acids linked by peptide bonds. They have the same peptide bonds as those in proteins, but are commonly shorter in length.

Peptide bond: A peptide bond (amide bond) is a covalent chemical bond formed between two molecules when the carboxyl group of one molecule reacts with the amino group of the other molecule, causing the release of a molecule of water (H_2O), hence the process is a dehydration synthesis reaction (also known as a condensation reaction), and usually occurs between amino acids.

Peptide vaccine: A peptide vaccine is a type of subunit vaccine in which a peptide of the original pathogen is used to immunize an organism.

Peptidyl transferase: Peptidyl transferase is an aminoacyltransferase as well as the primary enzymatic function of the ribosome, which forms peptide links between adjacent amino acids using tRNAs during the translation process of protein biosynthesis.

Periplasm: The region near or immediately within a bacterial or other cell wall, outside the plasma membrane.

Permanent wilting point: Permanent wilting point (PWP) or wilting point (WP) is defined as the minimal point of soil moisture the plant requires not to wilt. If moisture decreases to this or any lower point a plant wilts and can no longer recover its turgidity when placed in a saturated atmosphere for 12 h.

Permeable: That can be permeated or penetrated, especially by liquids or gases.

Pesticide: Pesticides are substances or mixture of substances intended for preventing, destroying, repelling, or mitigating any pest. A pesticide may be a chemical substance, biological agent (such as a virus or bacterium), antimicrobial, disinfectant, or device used against any pest. Pests include insects, plant pathogens, weeds, molluscs, birds, mammals, fish, nematodes (roundworms), and microbes that destroy property, spread disease, or are a vector for disease or cause a nuisance.

Petal: Petals are modified leaves that surround the reproductive parts of flowers. They often are brightly colored or unusually shaped to attract pollinators.

Petiole: In botany, the petiole is the small stalk attaching the leaf blade to the stem. The petiole usually has the same internal structure as the stem. Outgrowths appearing on each side of the petiole are called stipules.

Petite mutant: Petite is a mutant first discovered in the yeast *Saccharomyces cerevisiae*. The "petite" yeast has little or no mitochondrial DNA, and forms small anaerobic colonies when grown on media. A neutral petite produces all wild-type progeny when crossed with wild type. Petite mutations can be induced using a variety of mutagens, including DNA intercalating agents, as well as chemicals that can interfere with DNA synthesis in growing cells. Mutagens that create petites are implicated in increased rates of degenerative diseases and in the aging process.

Petri dish: A Petri dish (or Petri plate or cell culture dish) is a shallow glass or plastic cylindrical lidded dish that biologists use to culture cells or small moss plants. It was named after German bacteriologist, Julius Richard Petri.

pH: In chemistry, pH is a measure of the acidity or basicity of an aqueous solution. Pure water is said to be neutral, with a pH close to 7.0°C at 25°C (77°F). Solutions with a pH less than 7 are said to be acidic and solutions with a pH greater than 7 are basic or alkaline. pH measurements are important in medicine, biology, chemistry, agriculture, forestry, food science, environmental science, oceanography, civil engineering, and many other applications.

Phage: A bacteriophage.

Phagemids: A phagemid or phasmid is a type of cloning vector developed as a hybrid of the filamentous phage M13 and plasmids to produce a vector that can grow as a plasmid, and also be packaged as single-stranded DNA in viral particles. Phagemids contain an origin of replication (ori) for double-stranded replication, as well as an f1 ori to enable single-stranded replication and packaging into phage particles.

Phagocytes: Phagocytes are the white blood cells that protect the body by ingesting (phagocytosing) harmful foreign particles, bacteria, and dead or dying cells.

Phagocytosis: Phagocytosis is the cellular process of engulfing solid particles by the cell membrane to form an internal phagosome by phagocytes and protists. Phagocytosis is a specific form of endocytosis involving the vesicular internalization of solid particles, such as bacteria, and is, therefore, distinct from other forms of endocytosis such as the vesicular internalization of various liquids.

Pharmaceutical drug: A pharmaceutical drug, also referred to as medicine, medication or medicament, can be loosely defined as any chemical substance intended for use in the medical diagnosis, cure, treatment, or prevention of disease.

pH-electrode-based sensor: Sensor in which a standard pH electrode is coated with a biological material. Many biological processes raise or lower pH, and the changes can be detected by the pH electrode.

Phenocopy: A phenocopy is an individual whose phenotype (generally referring to a single trait), under a particular environmental condition, is identical to the one of another individual whose phenotype is determined by the genotype. In other words, the phenocopy environmental condition mimics the phenotype produced by a gene.

Phenols: In organic chemistry, phenols, sometimes called phenolics, are a class of chemical compounds consisting of a hydroxyl group (-OH) bonded directly to an aromatic hydrocarbon group. The simplest of the class is phenol (C_6H_5OH).

Phenotype: A phenotype is an organism's observable characteristics or traits: such as its morphology, development, biochemical or physiological properties, behavior, and products of behavior (such as a bird's nest). Phenotypes result from the expression of an organism's genes as well as the influence of environmental factors and the interactions between the two.

Phenylalanine: Phenylalanine is an α-amino acid with the formula $C_6H_5CH_2CH(NH_2)COOH$. This essential amino acid is classified as nonpolar because of the hydrophobic nature of the benzyl side chain. L-Phenylalanine (LPA) is an electrically neutral amino acid, one of the 20 common amino acids used to biochemically form proteins, coded for by DNA.

Pheromone: Pheromone is a secreted or excreted chemical factor that triggers a social response in members of the same species. Pheromones are chemicals capable of acting outside the body of the secreting individual to impact the behavior of the receiving individual.

Phosphatase: A phosphatase is an enzyme that removes a phosphate group from its substrate by hydrolyzing phosphoric acid monoesters into a phosphate ion and a molecule with a free hydroxyl group (see dephosphorylation). This action is directly opposite to that of phosphorylases and kinases, which attach phosphate groups to their substrates by using energetic molecules like ATP. A common phosphatase in many organisms is alkaline phosphatase.

Phosphodiester bond: A phosphodiester bond is a group of strong covalent bonds between a phosphate group and two 5-carbon ring carbohydrates (pentoses) over two ester bonds. Phosphodiester bonds are central to most life on Earth, as they make up the backbone of each helical strand of DNA.

Phospholipase: A phospholipase is an enzyme that hydrolyzes phospholipids into fatty acids and other lipophilic substances.

Phospholipid: Phospholipids are a class of lipids and are a major component of all cell membranes as they can form lipid bilayers. Most phospholipids contain a diglyceride, a phosphate group, and a simple organic molecule such as choline; one exception to this rule is sphingomyelin, which is derived from sphingosine instead of glycerol.

Phosphorolysis: Phosphorolysis is the cleavage of a compound in which inorganic phosphate is the attacking group. It is analogous to hydrolysis. An example of this is glycogen breakdown by glycogen phosphorylase, which catalyzes attack by inorganic phosphate on the terminal glycosyl residue at the nonreducing end of a glycogen molecule. The result is glucose 1-phosphate and glycogen (or starch) (*n*–1) glucose units.

Phosphorylation: Phosphorylation is the addition of a phosphate (PO_4^{3-}) group to a protein or other organic molecule. Phosphorylation activates or deactivates many protein enzymes.

Photoperiod: The duration of an organism's daily exposure to light, considered especially with regard to the effect of the exposure on growth and development.

Photoperiodism: Photoperiodism can be defined as the developmental responses of plants to the relative lengths of the light and dark periods. Here it should be emphasized that photoperiodic effects relate directly to the timing of both the light and dark periods.

Photophosphorylation: The production of ATP using the energy of sunlight is called photophosphorylation. Only two sources of energy are available to living organisms: sunlight and oxidation–reduction (redox) reactions. All organisms produce ATP, which is the universal energy currency of life.

Photoreactivation: The process whereby dimerized pyrimidines (usually thymines) in DNA are restored by an enzyme (deoxyribodipyrimidine photolyase) that requires light energy.

Photosynthate: A chemical product of photosynthesis.

Photosynthesis: Photosynthesis is a chemical process that converts carbon dioxide into organic compounds, especially sugars, using the energy from sunlight. Photosynthesis occurs in plants, algae, and many species of bacteria, but not in archaea. Photosynthetic organisms are called photoautotrophs, since they can create their own food.

Photosynthetically active radiation: Photosynthetically active radiation, often abbreviated PAR, designates the spectral range (wave band) of solar radiation from 400 to 700 nm that photosynthetic organisms are able to use in the process of photosynthesis. This spectral region corresponds more or less with the range of light visible to the human eye.

Phototropism: Phototropism is directional growth in which the direction of growth is determined by the direction of the light source. In other words, it is the growth and response to a light stimulus. Phototropism is most often observed in plants, but can also occur in other organisms such as fungi. The cells on the plant that are farthest from the light have a chemical called auxin that reacts when phototropism occurs.

Phylogeny: Phylogeny, the history of the evolution of a species or group, especially in reference to lines of descent and relationships among broad groups of organisms.

Phytochrome: Phytochrome is a photoreceptor, a pigment that plants use to detect light. It is sensitive to light in the red and far-red region of the visible spectrum. Many flowering plants use it to regulate the time of flowering based on the length of day and night (photoperiodism) and to set circadian rhythms.

Phytohormone: It is a plant hormone.

Phytoparasite: Any plant parasitic organism.

Pinocytosis: In cellular biology, pinocytosis ("cell-drinking," "bulk-phase pinocytosis," "nonspecific, nonabsorptive pinocytosis," "fluid endocytosis") is a form of endocytosis in which small particles are brought into the cell suspended within small vesicles that subsequently fuse with lysosomes to hydrolyze, or to break down, the particles.

Pipette: A pipette (also called a pipettor or chemical dropper) is a laboratory instrument used to transport a measured volume of liquid.

Plant cell culture: Plant tissue culture is a practice used to propagate plants under sterile conditions, often to produce clones of a plant. Different techniques in plant tissue culture may offer certain advantages over traditional methods of propagation.

Plantlet: Plantlets are young or small plants used as propagules. They are usually grown from clippings of mature plants.

Plasma cells: Plasma cells, also called plasma B cells, plasmocytes, and effector B cells, are white blood cells which produce large volumes of antibodies. They are transported by the blood plasma and the lymphatic system. Like all blood cells, plasma cells ultimately originate in the bone marrow; however, these cells leave the bone marrow as B cells, before terminal differentiation into plasma cells, normally in lymph nodes.

Plasma membrane: In animals the plasma membrane is the outermost covering of the cell whereas in plants, fungi, and some bacteria it is located beneath the cell wall.

Plasmid: In microbiology and genetics, a plasmid is a DNA molecule that is separate from, and can replicate independently of, the chromosomal DNA. They are double stranded and, in many cases, circular.

Plasmolysis: Plasmolysis is the process in plant cells where the plasma membrane pulls away from the cell wall due to the loss of water through osmosis. The reverse process, cytolysis, can occur if the cell is in a hypotonic solution resulting in a higher external osmotic pressure and a net flow of water into the cell. Through observation of plasmolysis and deplasmolysis it is possible to determine the tonicity of the cell's environment as well as the rate solute molecules cross the cellular membrane.

Plastid: Plastids are major organelles found in the cells of plants and algae. Plastids are the site of manufacture and storage of important chemical compounds used by the cell. Plastids often contain pigments used in photosynthesis, and the types of pigments present can change or determine the cell's color.

Pleiotropy: Pleiotropy occurs when a single gene influences multiple phenotypic traits. Consequently, a mutation in a pleiotropic gene may have an effect on some or all traits simultaneously. This can become a problem when selection on one trait favors one specific version of the gene (allele), while the selection on the other trait favors another allele.

Ploidy: Ploidy is the number of sets of chromosomes in a biological cell.

Pluripotent: Not fixed as to developmental potentialities; especially: capable of differentiating into one of many cell types.

Point mutation: A point mutation, or single base substitution, is a type of mutation that causes the replacement of a single base nucleotide with another nucleotide of the genetic material, DNA or RNA.

Polar auxin transport: Polar auxin transport is the regulated transport of the plant hormone, auxin, in plants. It is suggested that it involves the components of the cytoskeleton, plasma membrane, and cell wall.

Polar body: A polar body is a cell structure found inside an ovum. Both animal and plant ova possess it. It is also known as a polar cell.

Polar mutation: A polar mutation affects expression of downstream genes or operons. It can also affect the expression of the gene in which it occurs, if it occurs in a transcribed region. These mutations tend to occur early within the sequence of genes and can be nonsense, frame shift, or insertion mutations.

Polar nuclei: The two haploid nuclei found in the center of the embryo sac after division of the megaspore. They may fuse to form a diploid definitive nucleus before fusing with the male gamete to form the triploid primary endosperm nucleus.

Pole cells: In early Drosophila development, the 13 first mitosis are nuclear divisions without cell division, resulting in a multinucleate cell (a syncytium). The first mononucleate cells are created at the posterior pole, where the polar granules are tethered. These cells are called pole cells, and they will form the fly's germ line.

Pollen: Pollen is a fine-to-coarse powder containing the microgametophytes of seed plants, which produce the male gametes (sperm cells). Pollen grains have a hard coat that protects the sperm cells during the process of their movement between the stamens to the pistil of flowering plants or from the male cone to the female cone of coniferous plants.

Pollen grain: A structure produced by plants containing the male haploid gamete to be used in reproduction. The gamete is covered by protective layers which perform their role until the pollen grain is capable of fertilizing when reaching the female stigma.

Pollination: Pollination is the process by which pollen is transferred in plants, thereby enabling fertilization and sexual reproduction. Pollen grains, which contain the male gametes (sperm) to where the female gamete(s) are contained within the carpel; in gymnosperms the pollen is directly applied to the ovule itself. The receptive part of the carpel is called a stigma in the flowers of angiosperms.

Poly (A) polymerase: Poly (A) polymerase catalyzes the addition of adenine residues to the 3′ end of pre-mRNAs to form the poly(A) tail.

Polyacrylamide gel electrophoresis (PAGE): In PAGE, proteins charged negatively by the binding of the anionic detergent SDS (sodium dodecyl sulfate) separate within a matrix of polyacrylamide gel in an electric field according to their molecular weights. Polyacrylamide is formed by the polymerization of the monomer molecule-acrylamide crosslinked by *N,N′*-methylene-bis-acrylamide (abbreviated BIS). Free radicals generated by ammonium persulfate (APS) and a catalyst acting as an oxygen scavenger (-*N,N,N′,N′*-tetramethylethylene diamine [TEMED]) are required to start the polymerization since acrylamide and BIS are nonreactive by themselves or when mixed together.

Polyadenylation: Polyadenylation is the addition of a poly(A) tail to an RNA molecule. The poly(A) tail consists of multiple adenosine monophosphates; in other words, it is a stretch of RNA which only has adenine bases. In eukaryotes, polyadenylation is part of the process that produces mature messenger RNA (mRNA) for translation. It therefore forms part of the larger process of gene expression.

Polyclonal antibodies: Polyclonal antibodies (or antisera) are antibodies that are obtained from different B cell resources. They are a combination of immunoglobulin molecules secreted against a specific antigen, each identifying a different epitope.

Polyethylene glycol: Polyethylene glycol (PEG) is a polyether compound with many applications from industrial manufacturing to medicine. It has also been known as polyethylene oxide (PEO) or polyoxyethylene (POE), depending on its molecular weight, and under the trade name Carbowax.

Polymerase: A polymerase is an enzyme whose central function is associated with polymers of nucleic acids such as RNA and DNA. The primary function of a polymerase is the polymerization of new DNA or RNA against an existing DNA or RNA template in the processes of replication and transcription. In association with a cluster of other enzymes and proteins, they take nucleotides from solvent, and catalyze the synthesis of a polynucleotide sequence against a nucleotide template strand using base-pairing interactions.

Polymerase chain reaction: The polymerase chain reaction (PCR) is a scientific technique in molecular biology to amplify a single or a few copies of a piece of DNA across several orders of magnitude, generating thousands to millions of copies of a particular DNA sequence.

Polymerization: In polymer chemistry, polymerization is a process of reacting monomer molecules together in a chemical reaction to form three-dimensional networks or polymer chains.

Polymorphism: Polymorphism in biology occurs when two or more clearly different phenotypes exist in the same population of a species in other words, the occurrence of more than one form or morph.

Polynucleotide: A polynucleotide molecule is a biopolymer composed of 13 or more nucleotide monomers covalently bonded in a chain. DNA (deoxyribonucleic acid) and RNA (ribonucleic acid) are examples of polynucleotides with distinct biological function.

Polypeptide: A peptide consisting of two or more amino acids. Amino acids make up polypeptides which, in turn, make up proteins.

Polyploidy: Polyploidy is a term used to describe cells and organisms containing more than two paired (homologous) sets of chromosomes. Most eukaryotic species are diploid, meaning they have two sets of chromosomes one set inherited from each parent. However, polyploidy is found in some organisms and is especially common in plants.

Polysaccharide: Polysaccharides are polymeric carbohydrate structures, formed of repeating units (either mono- or di-saccharides) joined together by glycosidic bonds. These structures are often linear, but may contain various degrees of branching.

Polytene chromosomes: To increase cell volume, some specialized cells undergo repeated rounds of DNA replication without cell division (endomitosis), forming a giant polytene chromosome. Polytene chromosomes form when multiple rounds of replication produce many sister chromatids that remain synapsed together.

Polyvalent vaccine: Vaccine which is prepared from cultures or antigens of more than one strain or species.

Polyvinylpyrrolidone: Polyvinylpyrrolidone (PVP), also commonly called polyvidone or povidone, is a water-soluble polymer made from the monomer *N*-vinylpyrrolidone.

Population genetics: Population genetics is the study of allele frequency distribution and change under the influence of the four main evolutionary processes: natural selection, genetic drift, mutation, and gene flow. It also takes into account the factors of recombination, population subdivision, and population structure. It attempts to explain such phenomena as adaptation and speciation.

Positional cloning: Positional cloning is a technique which is used in genetic screening to identify specific areas of interest in the genome, and then determine what they do. This type of genetic screening is sometimes referred to as reverse genetics, because researchers start by figuring out where a gene is, and then they determine what it does, in contrast with methods which start by determining the function of a gene and then finding it in the genome. Genes related to conditions such as Huntington's disease and cystic fibrosis have been identified with this technique.

Postreplication repair: Postreplication repair is the repair of damage to the DNA that takes place after replication. DNA damage prevents the normal enzymatic synthesis of DNA by the replication fork. At damaged sites in the genome, both prokaryotic and eukaryotic cells utilize a number of postreplication repair (PRR) mechanisms to complete DNA replication.

Posttranslational modification: Posttranslational modification (PTM) is the chemical modification of a protein after its translation. It is one of the later steps in protein biosynthesis, and thus gene expression, for many proteins.

PPM: parts-per-million, 10^{-6}.

Primary antibody: Primary antibodies are antibodies raised against an antigenic target of interest (a protein, peptide, carbohydrate, or other small molecule) and are typically unconjugated (unlabeled). Primary antibodies that recognize and bind with high affinity and specificity to unique epitopes across a broad spectrum of biomolecules are available as high specificity monoclonal antibodies and/or as polyclonal antibodies. These antibodies are useful not only to detect specific biomolecules but also to measure changes in their level and specificity of modification by processes such as phosphorylation, methylation, or glycosylation. A primary antibody can be very useful for the detection of biomarkers for diseases such as cancer, diabetes, Parkinson's, and Alzheimer's disease and they are used for the study of ADME and multi-drug resistance (MDR) of therapeutic agents.

Primary cell wall: The primary cell wall is the part or layer of cell wall in which cell growth is permitted. Compared to secondary cell wall, this layer contains more pectin and lignin is absent until a secondary wall has formed on top of it.

Primary culture: A cell or tissue culture started from material taken directly from an organism, as opposed to that from an explant from an organism.

Primary transcript: A primary transcript is an RNA molecule that has not yet undergone any modification after its synthesis. For example, a precursor messenger RNA (pre-mRNA) is a primary transcript that becomes a messenger RNA (mRNA) after processing, and a primary microRNA (pri-miRNA) precursor becomes microRNA (miRNA) after processing.

Primer: A primer is a strand of nucleic acid that serves as a starting point for DNA synthesis. They are required for DNA replication because the enzymes that catalyze this process, DNA polymerases, can only add new nucleotides to an existing strand of DNA. The polymerase starts replication at the 3′-end of the primer, and copies the opposite strand.

Primer DNA polymerase: A DNA polymerase is an enzyme that helps catalyze in the polymerization of deoxyribonucleotides into a DNA strand. DNA polymerases are best known for their feedback role in DNA replication, in which the polymerase "reads" an intact DNA strand as a template and uses it to synthesize the new strand.

Primer walking: Primer walking is a sequencing method of choice for sequencing DNA fragments between 1.3 and 7 kb. Such fragments are too long to be sequenced in a single sequence read using the chain termination method.

Primordium: In embryology, organ or tissue in its earliest recognizable stage of development.

Primosome: In molecular biology, a primosome is a protein complex responsible for creating RNA primers on single-stranded DNA during DNA replication.

Prion: Prion is an infectious agent composed of protein in a misfolded form. This is in contrast to all other known infectious agents, which must contain nucleic acids (DNA, RNA, or both). The word prion, coined in 1982 by Stanley B. Prusiner, is a portmanteau derived from the words protein and infection.

Probability: Probability is a way of expressing knowledge or belief that an event will occur or has occurred. The concept has an exact mathematical meaning in probability theory, which is used extensively in such areas of study as mathematics, statistics, finance, gambling, science, artificial intelligence/machine learning, and philosophy to draw conclusions about the likelihood of potential events and the underlying mechanics of complex systems.

Probe DNA: A single-stranded DNA molecule used in laboratory experiments to detect the presence of a complementary sequence among a mixture of other single-stranded DNA molecules.

Progeny testing: Progeny testing is a test of the value for selective breeding of an individual's genotype by looking at the progeny produced by different matings.

Progesterone: Progesterone also known as P4 (pregn-4-ene-3,20-dione) is a C-21 steroid hormone involved in the female menstrual cycle, pregnancy (supports gestation) and embryogenesis of humans and other species. Progesterone belongs to a class of hormones called progestogens, and is the major naturally occurring human progestogen.

Prokaryote: The prokaryotes are a group of organisms that lack a cell nucleus, or any other membrane-bound organelles.

Prolactin: Prolactin (PRL) also known as luteotropic hormone (LTH) is a protein that in humans is encoded by the PRL gene. Prolactin is a peptide hormone discovered by Henry Friesen, primarily associated with lactation. In breastfeeding, the act of an infant suckling the nipple stimulates the production of oxytocin, which stimulates the "milk let-down" reflex, which fills the breast with milk via a process called lactogenesis, in preparation for the next feed.

Proliferation cell: The term cell proliferation or growth is used in the contexts of cell development and cell division (reproduction). When used in the context of cell division, it refers to growth of cell populations, where one cell (the "mother cell") grows and divides to produce two "daughter cells" (M phase). When used in the context of cell development, the term refers to increase in cytoplasmic and organelle volume (G1 phase), as well as increase in genetic material before replication (G2 phase).

Promoter: In genetics, a promoter is a region of DNA that facilitates the transcription of a particular gene. Promoters are located near the genes they regulate, on the same strand and typically upstream (toward the 5′ region of the sense strand).

Pronucleus: A pronucleus is the nucleus of a sperm or an egg cell during the process of fertilization, after the sperm enters the ovum, but before they fuse.

Propagation: Plant propagation is the process of creating new plants from a variety of sources: seeds, cuttings, bulbs, and other plant parts. Plant propagation can also refer to the artificial or natural dispersal of plants.

Prophage: A prophage is a phage (viral) genome inserted and integrated into the circular bacterial DNA chromosome. A prophage, also known as a temperate phage, is any virus in the lysogenic cycle; it is integrated into the host chromosome or exists as an extra-chromosomal plasmid. Technically, a virus may be called a prophage only while the viral DNA remains incorporated in the host DNA. This is a latent form of a bacteriophage, in which the viral genes are incorporated into the bacterial chromosome without causing disruption of the bacterial cell.

Protamines: Protamines are small, arginine-rich, nuclear proteins that replace histones late in the haploid phase of spermatogenesis and are believed essential for sperm head condensation and DNA stabilization.

Protease: A protease (also termed peptidase or proteinase) is any enzyme that conducts proteolysis, that is, begins protein catabolism by hydrolysis of the peptide bonds that link amino acids together in the polypeptide chain forming the protein.

Protein: Proteins are biochemical compounds consisting of one or more polypeptides typically folded into a globular or fibrous form, facilitating a biological function. A polypeptide is a single linear polymer chain of amino acids bonded together by peptide bonds between the carboxyl and amino groups of adjacent amino acid residues. The sequence of amino acids in a protein is defined by the sequence of a gene, which is encoded in the genetic code.

Protein crystallization: Proteins, like many molecules, can be prompted to form crystals when placed in the appropriate conditions. To crystallize a protein, the purified protein undergoes slow precipitation from an aqueous solution. As a result, individual protein molecules align themselves in a repeating series of unit cells by adopting a consistent orientation.

Protein engineering: Protein engineering is the process of developing useful or valuable proteins. It is a young discipline, with much research taking place into the understanding of protein folding and recognition for protein design principles.

Protein kinase: A protein kinase is a kinase enzyme that modifies other proteins by chemically adding phosphate groups to them (phosphorylation). Phosphorylation usually results in a functional change of the target protein (substrate) by changing enzyme activity, cellular location, or association with other proteins.

Protein sequencing: Protein sequencing is a technique to determine the amino acid sequence of a protein, as well as which conformation the protein adopts and the extent to which it is complexed with any nonpeptide molecules. Discovering the structures and functions of proteins in living organisms is an important tool for understanding cellular processes, and allows drugs that target specific metabolic pathways to be invented more easily.

Protein synthesis: Protein synthesis is the process in which cells build proteins. The term is sometimes used to refer only to protein translation but more often it refers to a multi-step process, beginning with amino acid synthesis and transcription of nuclear DNA into messenger RNA, which is then used as input to translation.

Proteolysis: Proteolysis is the directed degradation (digestion) of proteins by cellular enzymes called proteases or by intramolecular digestion.

Protoclone: Regenerated plant derived from protoplast culture or a single colony derived from protoplasts in culture.

Protocol: In the natural sciences a protocol is a predefined written procedural method in the design and implementation of experiments. Protocols are written whenever it is desirable to standardize a laboratory method to ensure successful replication of results by others in the same laboratory or by other laboratories. Detailed protocols also facilitate the assessment of results through peer review.

Proto-oncogene: A normal gene which, when altered by mutation, becomes an oncogene that can contribute to cancer. Proto-oncogenes may have many different functions in the cell. Some proto-oncogenes provide signals that lead to cell division. Other proto-oncogenes regulate programmed cell death (apoptosis).

Protoplasm: Protoplasm is the living content of a cell that is surrounded by a plasma membrane (cell membrane). Protoplasm is composed of a mixture of small molecules such as ions, amino acids, monosaccharides and water, and macromolecules such as nucleic acids, proteins, lipids and polysaccharides.

Protoplast: A protoplast is a plant, bacterial, or fungal cell that had its cell wall completely or partially removed using either mechanical or enzymatic means.

Protoplast fusion: Protoplast fusion, is a type of genetic modification in plants by which two distinct species of plants are fused together to form a new hybrid plant with the characteristics of both, a somatic hybrid.

Protozoan: Any of a large group of single-celled, usually microscopic, eukaryotic organisms, such as amoebas, ciliates, flagellates, and protozoans.

Pseudoautosomal region: The pseudoautosomal regions, PAR1 and PAR2 are homologous sequences of nucleotides on the X and Y chromosomes. The pseudoautosomal regions get their name because any genes located within them (so far at least 29 have been found) are inherited just like any autosomal genes. PAR1 comprises 2.6 Mbp of the short-arm tips of both X and Y chromosomes in humans and other great apes (X and Y are 155 and 59 Mbp in total). PAR2 is located at the tips of the long arms, spanning 320 kbp.

Pseudogene: Pseudogenes are dysfunctional relatives of known genes that have lost their protein-coding ability or are otherwise no longer expressed in the cell. Although some do not have introns or promoters (these pseudogenes are copied from mRNA and incorporated into the chromosome and are called processed pseudogenes), most have some gene-like features (such as promoters, CpG islands, and splice sites), they are nonetheless considered nonfunctional, due to their lack of protein-coding ability resulting from various genetic disablements (stop codons, frameshifts, or a lack of transcription) or their inability to encode RNA (such as with rRNA pseudogenes).

PUC: pUC19 is a plasmid cloning vector created by Messing and coworkers in the University of California. p stands for plasmid and UC represents the University in which it was created. It is a circular double-stranded DNA and has 2686 base pairs. pUC19 is one of the most widely used vector molecules as the recombinants, or the cells into which foreign DNA has been introduced, can be easily distinguished from the nonrecombinants based on color differences of colonies on growth media. pUC18 is similar to pUC19, but the MCS region is reversed.

Pulsed-field gel electrophoresis: Pulsed-field gel electrophoresis is a technique used for the separation of large deoxyribonucleic acid (DNA) molecules by applying an electric field that periodically changes direction to a gel matrix.

Pure culture: In microbiology, a laboratory culture containing a single species of organism. A pure culture is usually derived from a mixed culture (one containing many species) by transferring a small sample into new, sterile growth medium in such a manner as to disperse the individual cells across the medium surface or by thinning the sample manifold before inoculating the new medium.

Purine: A purine is a heterocyclic aromatic organic compound, consisting of a pyrimidine ring fused to an imidazole ring. Purines, including substituted purines and their tautomer's, are the most widely distributed kind of nitrogen-containing heterocycle in nature.

Pyrimidine: Pyrimidine is a heterocyclic aromatic organic compound similar to benzene and pyridine, containing two nitrogen atoms at positions 1 and 3 of the six-member ring. It is isomeric with two other forms of diazine.

Quantitative genetics: Quantitative genetics is the study of continuous traits (such as height or weight) and their underlying mechanisms. It is effectively an extension of simple Mendelian inheritance in that the combined effect of the many underlying genes results in a continuous distribution of phenotypic values.

Quantitative PCR: In molecular biology, real-time polymerase chain reaction, also called quantitative real-time polymerase chain reaction (Q-PCR/qPCR/qrt-PCR) or kinetic polymerase chain reaction (KPCR), is a laboratory technique based on the PCR, which is used to amplify and simultaneously quantify a targeted DNA molecule. For one or more specific sequences in a DNA sample, real time-PCR enables both detection and quantification. The quantity can be either an absolute number of copies or a relative amount when normalized to DNA input or additional normalizing genes.

Quantitative traits: Quantitative traits refer to phenotypes (characteristics) that vary in degree and can be attributed to polygenic effects, that is, product of two or more genes, and their environment. Quantitative trait loci (QTLs) are stretches of DNA containing or linked to the genes that underlie a quantitative trait. Mapping regions of the genome that contain genes involved in specifying a quantitative trait is done using molecular tags such as AFLP or, more commonly SNPs. This is an early step in identifying and sequencing the actual genes underlying trait variation.

Quantum: In physics, a quantum is the minimum amount of any physical entity involved in an interaction. Behind this, one finds the fundamental notion that a physical property may be "quantized," referred to as "the hypothesis of quantization."

Quarantine: Quarantine is compulsory isolation, typically to contain the spread of something considered dangerous, often but not always disease. The word comes from the Italian (seventeenth century Venetian) quarantena, meaning 40-day period. Quarantine can be applied to humans, but also to animals of various kinds.

Race: In biology, races are distinct genetically divergent populations within the same species with relatively small morphological and genetic differences. The populations can be described as ecological races if they arise from adaptation to different local habitats or geographic races when they are geographically isolated. If sufficiently different, two or more races can be identified as subspecies, which is an official biological taxonomy unit subordinate to species.

Radioisotope: A version of a chemical element that has an unstable nucleus and emits radiation during its decay to a stable form. Radioisotopes have important uses in medical diagnosis, treatment, and research. A radioisotope is so-named because it is a radioactive isotope, an isotope being an alternate version of a chemical element that has a different atomic mass.

Random amplified polymorphic DNA: RAPD (pronounced "rapid") stands for random amplification of polymorphic DNA. It is a type of PCR reaction, but the segments of DNA that are amplified are random. The scientist performing RAPD creates several arbitrary, short primers (8–12 nucleotides), then proceeds with the PCR using a large template of genomic DNA, hoping that fragments will amplify. By resolving the resulting patterns, a semi-unique profile can be gleaned from a RAPD reaction.

Random genetic drift: Changes in allelic frequency due to sampling error. Changes in allele frequency that result because the genes appearing in offspring are not a perfectly representative sampling of the parental genes.

Random primer method: A method for labeling DNA probes, mainly for Southern hybridization experiments. A mixture of short oligonucleotides is hybridized to a single-stranded DNA probe. In the presence of DNA polymerase and deoxyribonucleotides—one of which is labeled—DNA synthesis then generates labeled copies of probe DNA.

RecA: RecA is a 38 kDa *Escherichia coli* protein essential for the repair and maintenance of DNA. RecA has a structural and functional homolog in every species in which it has been seriously sought and serves as an archetype for this class of homologous DNA repair proteins. The homologous protein in *Homo sapiens* is called RAD51.

Receptor: A receptor is a molecule found on the surface of a cell, which receives specific chemical signals from neighboring cells or the wider environment within an organism. These signals tell a cell to do something—for example, to divide or die, or to allow certain molecules to enter or exit the cell.

Recessive: In genetics, the term "recessive gene" refers to an allele that causes a phenotype (visible or detectable characteristic) that is only seen in a homozygous genotype (an organism that has two copies of the same allele) and never in a heterozygous genotype.

Recessive oncogene*:* A single copy of this gene is sufficient to suppress cell proliferation; the loss of both copies of the gene contributes to cancer formation.

Reciprocal crosses: In genetics, a reciprocal cross is a breeding experiment designed to test the role of parental sex on a given inheritance pattern. All parent organisms must be true breeding to properly carry out such an experiment. In one cross, a male expressing the trait of interest will be crossed with a female not expressing the trait. In the other, a female expressing the trait of interest will be crossed with a male not expressing the trait.

Recognition site: The recognition sequence, sometimes also referred to as recognition site, of any DNA-binding protein motif that exhibits binding specificity, refers to the DNA sequence (or subset thereof), to which the domain is specific. Recognition sequences are palindromes. The transcription factor Sp1, for example, binds the sequences 5′-(G/T) GGGCGG (G/A) (G/A)(C/T)-3′, where (G/T) indicates that the domain will bind a guanine or thymine at this position.

Recombinant DNA: Recombinant DNA (rDNA) molecules are DNA sequences that result from the use of laboratory methods (molecular cloning) to bring together genetic material from multiple sources, creating sequences that would not otherwise be found in biological organisms. Recombinant DNA is possible because DNA molecules from all organisms share the same chemical structure; they differ only in the sequence of nucleotides within that identical overall structure. Consequently, when DNA from a foreign source is linked to host sequences that can drive DNA replication and then introduced into a host organism, the foreign DNA is replicated along with the host DNA.

Recombinant DNA technology: Recombinant technology begins with the isolation of a gene of interest. The gene is then inserted into a vector and cloned. A vector is a piece of DNA that is capable of independent growth; commonly used vectors are bacterial plasmids and viral phages. The gene of interest (foreign DNA) is integrated into the plasmid or phage, and this is referred to as recombinant DNA.

Recombinant protein: Recombinant protein is a protein that its code was carried by a recombinant DNA.

Recombinant toxin: A hybrid cytotoxic protein made by recombinant DNA technology, designed to selectively kill malignant cells.

Recombinant vaccine: Recombinant hepatitis B vaccine is the only recombinant vaccine licensed at present.

Recombination: Genetic recombination is a process by which a molecule of nucleic acid (usually DNA, but can also be RNA) is broken and then joined to a different one. Recombination can occur between similar molecules of DNA, as in homologous recombination, or dissimilar molecules, as in nonhomologous end joining. Recombination is a common method of DNA repair in both bacteria and eukaryotes. In eukaryotes, recombination also occurs in meiosis, where it facilitates chromosomal crossover. The crossover process leads to offspring's having different combinations of genes from those of their parents, and can occasionally produce new chimeric alleles. In organisms with an adaptive immune system, a type of genetic recombination called V(D)J recombination helps immune cells rapidly diversify to recognize and adapt to new pathogens. The shuffling of genes brought about by genetic recombination is thought to have many advantages, as it is a major engine of genetic variation and also allows sexually reproducing organisms to avoid Muller's ratchet, in which the genomes of an asexual population accumulate deleterious mutations in an irreversible manner.

Regeneration: In biology, regeneration is the process of renewal, restoration, and growth that makes genomes, cells, organs, organisms, and ecosystems resilient to natural fluctuations or events that cause disturbance or damage. Every species is capable of regeneration, from bacteria to humans. At its most elementary level, regeneration is mediated by the molecular processes of DNA synthesis.

Regulatory gene: A regulator gene, regulator, or regulatory gene is a gene involved in controlling the expression of one or more than one gene. A regulator gene may encode a protein, or it may work at the level of RNA, as in the case of genes encoding microRNAs.

Relaxed plasmid: A circular, double-stranded unit of DNA that replicates within a cell independently of the chromosomal DNA. Plasmids are most often found in bacteria and are used in recombinant DNA research to transfer genes between cells.

Replication: DNA replication is a biological process that occurs in all living organisms and copies their DNA; it is the basis for biological inheritance. The process starts with one double-stranded DNA molecule and produces two identical copies of the molecule. Each strand of the original double-stranded DNA molecule serves as template for the production of the complementary strand. Cellular proofreading and error toe-checking mechanisms ensure near-perfect fidelity for DNA replication.

Replicative form: An intermediate stage in the replication of either dNA or rNA viral genomes that is usually double stranded, the altered, double-stranded form to which single-stranded coli phage DNA is converted after infection of a susceptible bacterium, formation of the complementary (minus) strand being mediated by enzymes that were present in the bacterium before entrance of the viral (plus) strand.

Replicon: A replicon is a DNA molecule or RNA molecule, or a region of DNA or RNA that replicates from a single origin of replication.

Replisome: The replisome is a complex molecular machine that carries out replication of DNA. It is made up of a number of subcomponents that each provides a specific function during the process of replication.

Reporter gene: In molecular biology, a reporter gene (often simply reporter) is a gene that researchers attach to a regulatory sequence of another gene of interest in cell culture, animals, or plants.

Repressible enzyme: One whose rate of production is decreased as the concentration of certain metabolites is increased.

Repressor: In molecular genetics, a repressor is a DNA-binding protein that regulates the expression of one or more genes by binding to the operator and blocking the attachment of RNA polymerase to the promoter, thus preventing transcription of the genes. This blocking of expression is called repression.

Repulsion: The tendency of some linked genetic characters to be inherited separately because a dominant allele for each character occurs on the same chromosome as a recessive allele of the other.

Residues: In biochemistry and molecular biology, a residue refers to a specific monomer within the polymeric chain of a polysaccharide, protein, or nucleic acid.

Restriction endonuclease: A restriction enzyme (or restriction endonuclease) is an enzyme that cuts double-stranded or single-stranded DNA at specific recognition nucleotide sequences known as restriction sites. Such enzymes, found in bacteria and archaea, are thought to have evolved to provide a defense mechanism against invading viruses. Inside a bacterial host, the restriction enzymes selectively cut up foreign DNA in a process called restriction; host DNA is methylated by a modification enzyme (a methylase) to protect it from the restriction enzyme's activity. Collectively, these two processes form the restriction modification system. To cut the DNA, a restriction enzyme makes two incisions, once through each sugar–phosphate backbone (i.e., each strand) of the DNA double helix.

Restriction exonuclease: Exonucleases are enzymes that work by cleaving nucleotides one at a time from the end (exo) of a polynucleotide chain. A hydrolyzing reaction that breaks phosphodiester bonds at either the 3′ or the 5′ end occurs. Its close relative is the endonuclease, which cleaves phosphodiester bonds in the middle (endo) of a polynucleotide chain. Eukaryotes and prokaryotes have three types of exonucleases involved in the normal turnover of mRNA: 5′–3′ exonuclease, which is a dependent decapping protein, 3′–5′ exonuclease, an independent protein, and poly(A)-specific 3′–5′ exonuclease.

Restriction fragment: A restriction fragment is a DNA fragment resulting from the cutting of a DNA strand by a restriction enzyme (restriction endonucleases), a process called restriction. Each restriction enzyme is highly specific, recognizing a particular short DNA sequence, or restriction site, and cutting both DNA strands at specific points within this site. Most restriction sites are palindromic, (the sequence of nucleotides is the same on both strands when read in the 5′–3′ direction), and are four to eight nucleotides long. Many cuts are made by one restriction enzyme because of the chance repetition of these sequences in a long DNA molecule, yielding a set of restriction fragments. A particular DNA molecule will always yield the same set of restriction fragments when exposed to the same restriction enzyme. Restriction fragments can be analyzed using techniques such as gel electrophoresis or used in recombinant DNA technology.

Restriction fragment-length polymorphism: In molecular biology, restriction fragment-length polymorphism, or RFLP (commonly pronounced "rif-lip"), is a technique that exploits variations in homologous DNA sequences. It refers to a difference between samples of homologous DNA molecules that come from differing locations of restriction enzyme sites, and to a related laboratory technique by which these segments can be illustrated. In RFLP analysis, the DNA sample is broken into pieces (digested) by restriction enzymes and the resulting restriction fragments are separated according to their lengths by gel electrophoresis. Although now largely obsolete due to the rise of inexpensive DNA sequencing technologies, RFLP analysis was the first DNA profiling technique inexpensive enough to see widespread application. In addition to genetic fingerprinting, RFLP was an important tool in genome mapping, localization of genes for genetic disorders, determination of risk for disease, and paternity testing.

Restriction map: A restriction map is a map of known restriction sites within a sequence of DNA. Restriction mapping requires the use of restriction enzymes. In molecular biology, restriction maps are used as a reference to engineer plasmids or other relatively short pieces of DNA, and sometimes for longer genomic DNA.

Restriction nuclease: Restriction nuclease cuts nucleic acid at specific restriction sites and produce restriction fragments; obtained from bacteria (where they cripple viral invaders); used in recombinant DNA technology.

Retrovirus: A retrovirus is an RNA virus that is duplicated in a host cell using the reverse transcriptase enzyme to produce DNA from its RNA genome. The DNA is then incorporated into the host's genome by an integrase enzyme. The virus thereafter replicates as part of the host cell's DNA. Retroviruses are enveloped viruses that belong to the viral family Retroviridae.

Reverse genetics: Reverse genetics is an approach to discovering the function of a gene by analyzing the phenotypic effects of specific gene sequences obtained by DNA sequencing. This investigative process proceeds in the opposite direction of the so-called forward genetic screens of classical genetics. Simply put, while forward genetics seeks to find the genetic basis of a phenotype or trait, reverse genetics seeks to find what phenotypes arise as a result of particular genes.

Reverse transcriptase: In the fields of molecular biology and biochemistry, a reverse transcriptase, also known as RNA-dependent DNA polymerase, is a DNA polymerase enzyme that transcribes single-stranded RNA into double-stranded DNA. It also helps in the formation of a double-helix DNA once the RNA has been reverse transcribed into a single-strand cDNA. Normal transcription involves the synthesis of RNA from DNA; hence, reverse transcription is the reverse of this.

Rhizobacteria: Rhizobacteria are root-colonizing bacteria that form a symbiotic relationship with many plants. The name is derived from Greek "rhiza" meaning root. Though parasitic varieties of rhizobacteria exist, the term usually refers to bacteria that form a relationship beneficial for both parties (mutualism). Such bacteria are often referred to as plant growth-promoting rhizobacteria, or PGPRs.

Ribonuclease: Ribonuclease (commonly abbreviated RNase) is a type of nuclease that catalyzes the degradation of RNA into smaller components. Ribonucleases can be divided into endoribonucleases and exoribonucleases.

Ribosomal binding site: A ribosomal binding site (RBS) is a sequence on mRNA that is bound by the ribosome when initiating protein translation. It can be either the 5′ cap of a messenger RNA in eukaryotes, a region 6–7 nucleotides upstream of the start codon AUG in prokaryotes (called the Shine–Dalgarno sequence), or an internal ribosome entry site (IRES) in viruses. The sequence is complementary to the 3′ end of the rRNA. The ribosome searches for this site and binds to it through base pairing of nucleotides. Then, the ribosome begins the translation process and recruits initiation factors. After finding the ribosome binding site in eukaryotes, the ribosome recognizes the Kozak consensus sequence and begins translation at the +1 AUG codon.

Ribosomal RNA: Ribosomal ribonucleic acid (rRNA) is the RNA component of the ribosome, the organelle that is the site of protein synthesis in all living cells. Ribosomal RNA provides a mechanism for decoding mRNA into amino acids and interacts with tRNAs during translation by providing peptidyl transferase activity. The tRNAs bring the necessary amino acids corresponding to the appropriate mRNA codon.

Ribosome: A ribosome is an organelle (an internal component of a biological cell) the function of which is to assemble the 20 specific amino acid molecules to form the particular protein molecule determined by the nucleotide sequence of an RNA molecule.

Ribozyme: A ribozyme is an RNA molecule with a well-defined tertiary structure that enables it to catalyze a chemical reaction. Ribozyme means ribonucleic acid enzyme.

Ribulose biphosphate: Ribulose-1,5-bisphosphate (RuBP) is an organic substance that is involved in photosynthesis. The anion is a double phosphate ester of the ketose (ketone-containing sugar) called ribulose. Salts of this species can be isolated, but its crucial biological function involves this colorless anion in solution.

R-loops: A single-stranded loop section of dNA formed by the association of a section of ssRNA with the other strand of the DNA in this region whereby one DNA strand is displaced as the loop.

RNA: Ribonucleic acid or RNA, is one of the three major macromolecules (along with DNA and proteins) that are essential for all known forms of life.

RNAase: Ribonuclease A (RNase A) is a pancreatic ribonuclease that cleaves single-stranded RNA. Bovine pancreatic RNase A is one of the classic model systems of protein science.

RNA editing: The term RNA editing describes those molecular processes in which the information content in an RNA molecule is altered through a chemical change in the base makeup. To date, such changes have been observed in tRNA, rRNA, mRNA, and microRNA molecules of eukaryotes but not prokaryotes. RNA editing occurs in the cell nucleus and cytosol, as well as in mitochondria and plastids, which are thought to have evolved from prokaryotic-like endosymbionts.

RNA polymerase: RNA polymerase (RNAP or RNApol) is an enzyme that produces RNA. In cells, RNAP is needed for constructing RNA chains from DNA genes as templates, a process called transcription. RNA polymerase enzymes are essential to life and are found in all organisms and many viruses. In chemical terms, RNAP is a nucleotidyl transferase that polymerizes ribonucleotides at the 3′ end of an RNA transcript.

Root apex: The tip of a tooth root, the part farthest from the incisal or occlusal side.

Root cap: The root cap is a section of tissue at the tip of a plant root. It is also called calyptra. Root caps contain statoliths which are involved in gravity perception in plants. If the cap is carefully removed the root will grow randomly.

Ruminant animals: A ruminant is a mammal of the order Artiodactyla that digests plant-based food by initially softening it within the animal's first stomach, then regurgitating the semi-digested mass, now known as cud, and chewing it again. The process of rechewing the cud to further break down plant matter and stimulate digestion is called "ruminating."

S phase: S phase (synthesis phase) is the part of the cell cycle in which DNA is replicated, occurring between G1 phase and G2 phase. Precise and accurate DNA replication is necessary to prevent genetic abnormalities which often lead to cell death or disease. Owing to the importance, the regulatory pathways that govern this event in eukaryotes are highly conserved. This conservation makes the study of S phase in model organisms such as *Xenopus laevis* embryos and budding yeast relevant to higher organisms.

S_1 mapping: A method for mapping precursor or mature mRNA to particular DNA sequences using the enzyme S_1 nuclease.

S_1 nuclease: S_1 nuclease is an endonuclease that is active against single-stranded DNA and RNA molecules. It is five times more active on DNA than RNA. Its reaction products are oligonucleotides or single nucleotides with 5′ phosphoryl groups. Although its primary substrate is single stranded, it can also occasionally introduce single-stranded breaks in double-stranded DNA or RNA, or DNA–RNA hybrids. It is used in the laboratory as a reagent in nuclease protection assays. In molecular biology, it is used in removing single-stranded tails from DNA molecules to create blunt-ended molecules and opening hairpin loops generated during synthesis of double-stranded cDNA.

Salmonella: *Salmonella* is a genus of rod-shaped, Gram-negative, nonspore forming, predominantly motile enterobacteria with diameters around 0.7–1.5 µm, length from 2 to 5 µm, and flagella which grade in all directions.

Salt tolerance plant: The plant which withstands or survives at very high salt concentrations is called a salt tolerance plant.

Satellite DNA: Satellite DNA consists of very large arrays of tandemly repeating, noncoding DNA. Satellite DNA is the main component of functional centromeres, and form the main structural constituent of heterochromatin.

Satellite RNA: A small, self-splicing RNA molecule that accompanies several plant viruses, including tobacco ringspot virus.

Scaffold protein: In biology, scaffold proteins are crucial regulators of many key signaling pathways. Although scaffolds are not strictly defined in function, they are known to interact and/or bind with multiple members of a signaling pathway, tethering them into complexes.

Scanning electron microscope: A scanning electron microscope (SEM) is a type of electron microscope that images a sample by scanning it with a high-energy beam of electrons in a raster scan pattern. The electrons interact with the atoms that make up the sample producing signals that contain information about the sample's surface topography, composition, and other properties such as electrical conductivity.

Screen drug candidate: Two main approaches exist for the finding of new bioactive chemical entities from natural sources: random collection and screening of material; and exploitation of ethno-pharmacological knowledge in the selection. The former approach is based on the fact that only a small part of Earth's biodiversity has ever been tested for pharmaceutical activity, and organisms living in a species-rich environment need to evolve defensive and competitive mechanisms to survive.

Secondary antibody: A secondary antibody is an antibody that binds to primary antibodies or antibody fragments. They are typically labeled with probes that make them useful for detection, purification, or cell sorting applications.

Secondary cell wall: The secondary cell wall is a structure found in many plant cells, located between the primary cell wall and the plasma membrane. The cell starts producing the secondary cell wall after the primary cell wall is complete and the cell has stopped expanding.

Secondary growth: In many vascular plants, secondary growth is the result of the activity of the vascular cambium. The latter is a meristem that divides to produce secondary xylem cells on the inside of the meristem (the adaxial side) and secondary phloem cells on the outside (the abaxial side).

Secondary metabolite: Secondary metabolites are organic compounds that are not directly involved in the normal growth, development, or reproduction of an organism. Unlike primary metabolites, absence of secondary metabolites does not result in immediate death, but rather in long-term impairment of the organism's survivability, fecundity, or aesthetics, or perhaps in no significant change at all. Secondary metabolites are often restricted to a narrow set of species within a phylogenetic group. Secondary metabolites often play an important role in plant defense against herbivory and other interspecies defenses. Humans use secondary metabolites as medicines, flavorings, and recreational drugs.

Secondary messenger: Second messengers are molecules that relay signals from receptors on the cell surface to target molecules inside the cell, in the cytoplasm or nucleus. They relay the signals of hormones like epinephrine (adrenalin), growth factors, and others, and cause some kind of change in the activity of the cell. They greatly amplify the strength of the signal. Secondary messengers are a component of signal transduction cascades.

Secondary plant products: Plant secondary metabolites are a generic term used for more than 30,000 different substances that are exclusively produced by plants. The plants form secondary metabolites, for example, for protection against pests, as coloring, scent, or attractants and as the plant's own hormones. It used to be believed that secondary metabolites were irrelevant for the human diet.

Secondary root: A branch or lateral root.

Secretion: Secretion is the process of elaborating, releasing, and oozing chemicals, or a secreted chemical substance from a cell or gland. In contrast to excretion, the substance may have a certain function, rather than being a waste product. Many cells contain this such as glaucoma cells.

Segment-polarity gene: A segmentation gene is a generic term for a gene whose function is to specify tissue pattern in each repeated unit of a segmented organism. In the fruit fly *Drosophila melanogaster*, segment polarity genes help to define the anterior and posterior polarities within each embryonic para-segment by regulating the transmission of signals via the Wnt signaling pathway and Hedgehog signaling pathway. Segment polarity genes are expressed in the embryo following expression of the gap genes and pair-rule genes. The most commonly cited examples of these genes are engrailed and gooseberry in *Drosophila*.

Selectable marker: A selectable marker is a gene introduced into a cell, especially a bacterium or to cells in culture that confers a trait suitable for artificial selection. They are a type of reporter gene used in laboratory microbiology, molecular biology, and genetic engineering to indicate the success of a transfection or other procedure meant to introduce foreign DNA into a cell. Selectable markers are often antibiotic-resistance genes; bacteria that have been subjected to a procedure to introduce foreign DNA are grown on a medium containing an antibiotic, and those bacterial colonies that can grow have successfully taken up and expressed the introduced genetic material.

Selection coefficient: In population genetics, the selection coefficient is a measure of the relative fitness of a phenotype. Usually denoted by the letter s, it compares the fitness of a phenotype to another favored phenotype, and is the proportional amount that the considered phenotype is less fit as measured by fertile progeny.

Self-fertilization: Self-fertilization, fusion of male and female gametes (sex cells) produced by the same individual. Self-fertilization occurs in bisexual organisms, including most flowering plants, numerous protozoans, and many invertebrates. Autogamy, the production of gametes by the division of a single parent cell, is frequently found in unicellular organisms such as the protozoan Paramecium.

Self-pollination: The pollen grains can be carried from an anther to the stigma of the same flower is known as self-pollination.

Semi-conservative replication: Semiconservative replication describes the mechanism by which DNA is replicated in all known cells.

Sense RNA: In virology, the genome of an RNA virus can be said to be either positive sense, also known as a "plus-strand," or negative sense, also known as a "minus-strand." In most cases, the terms sense and strand are used interchangeably, making such terms as positive strand equivalent to positive sense, and plus strand equivalent to plus sense. Whether a virus genome is positive sense or negative sense can be used as a basis for classifying viruses.

Sepsis: Sepsis is a potentially deadly medical condition that is characterized by a whole-body inflammatory state (called a systemic inflammatory response syndrome or SIRS) and the presence of a known or suspected infection.

Sequence hypothesis: The sequence hypothesis was first formally proposed in a review *On Protein Synthesis* by Francis Crick in 1958. It states that the sequence of bases in the genetic material (DNA or RNA) determines the sequence of amino acids for which that segment of nucleic acid codes, and this amino acid sequence determines the three-dimensional structure into which the protein folds.

Sequence-tagged site: A sequence-tagged site (or STS) is a short (200–500 base pair) DNA sequence that has a single occurrence in the genome and whose location and base sequence are known.

Sequencing DNA: DNA sequencing includes several methods and technologies that are used for determining the order of the nucleotide bases adenine, guanine, cytosine, and thymine in a molecule of DNA.

Serology: Serology is the scientific study of blood serum and other bodily fluids. In practice, the term usually refers to the diagnostic identification of antibodies in the serum. Such antibodies are typically formed in response to an infection (against a given microorganism), against other foreign proteins (in response, e.g., to a mismatched blood transfusion), or to one's own proteins (in instances of autoimmune disease).

Serum albumin: Serum albumin, often referred to simply as albumin is a protein that in humans is encoded by the ALB gene.

Sewage treatment: Sewage treatment, or domestic wastewater treatment, is the process of removing contaminants from wastewater and household sewage, both runoff (effluents) and domestic. It includes physical, chemical, and biological processes to remove physical, chemical, and biological contaminants.

Sex chromosomes: Sex chromosome, either of a pair of chromosomes that determine whether an individual is male or female. The sex chromosomes of human beings and other mammals are designated by scientists as X and Y. In humans the sex chromosomes comprise one pair of the total of 23 pairs of chromosomes. The other 22 pairs of chromosomes are called autosomes.

Sex determination: A sex-determination system is a biological system that determines the development of sexual characteristics in an organism. Most sexual organisms have two sexes. In many cases, sex determination is genetic: males and females have different alleles or even different genes that specify their sexual morphology. In animals, this is often accompanied by chromosomal differences. In other cases, sex is determined by environmental variables (such as temperature) or social variables (the size of an organism relative to other members of its population). The details of some sex-determination systems are not yet fully understood.

Sex hormones: Any of various hormones, such as estrogen and androgen, affecting the growth or function of the reproductive organs, the development of secondary sex characteristics, and the behavioral patterns of animals.

Sex-influenced dominance: Sex-influenced dominance is the phenomenon in which the manifestation of a phenotype of a gene in heterozygosity depends on the sex of the individual.

Sex-limited genes: Sex-limited genes are genes which are present in both sexes of sexually reproducing species but turned on in only one sex. In other words, sex-limited genes cause the two sexes to show different traits or phenotypes. An example of sex-limited genes are genes which instructs male elephant seal to grow big and fight, at the same time instructing female seals to grow small and avoid fights. These genes are responsible for sexual dimorphism.

Sex linkage: Sex linkage is the phenotypic expression of an allele related to the chromosomal sex of the individual. This mode of inheritance is in contrast to the inheritance of traits on autosomal chromosomes, where both sexes have the same probability of inheritance. Since humans have many more genes on the X than the Y, there are many more X-linked traits than Y-linked traits.

Sexual reproduction: Sexual reproduction is the creation of a new organism by combining the genetic material of two organisms. The two main processes are: meiosis, involving the halving of the number of chromosomes; and fertilization, involving the fusion of two gametes and the restoration of the original number of chromosomes. During meiosis, the chromosomes of each pair usually cross over to achieve homologous recombination.

Shake culture: A method for isolating anaerobic bacteria by shaking a deep liquid culture of an agar or gelatin to distribute the inoculum before solidification of the medium. A liquid medium in a flask that has been inoculated with an aerobic microorganism and placed on a shaking machine; action of the machine continually aerates the culture.

Shine–Dalgarno sequence: The Shine–Dalgarno sequence (or Shine–Dalgarno box), proposed by Australian scientists John Shine (1946–present) and Lynn Dalgarno

(1935–present), is a ribosomal binding site in the mRNA, generally located 8 base pairs upstream of the start codon AUG. The Shine–Dalgarno sequence exists only in prokaryotes.

Short-day plant: A plant requiring less than 12 h of daylight in order for flowering to occur.

Short interspersed nuclear elements: Short interspersed elements (SINE) are short DNA sequences (<500 bases) that represent reverse-transcribed RNA molecules originally transcribed by RNA polymerase III into tRNA, rRNA, and other small nuclear RNAs. SINEs do not encode a functional reverse transcriptase protein and rely on other mobile elements for transposition.

Shuttle vector: A shuttle vector is a vector (usually a plasmid) constructed so that it can propagate in two different host species. Therefore, DNA inserted into a shuttle vector can be tested or manipulated in two different cell types. The main advantage of these vectors is they can be manipulated in *E. coli* then used in a system which is more difficult or slower to use (e.g., yeast, other bacteria).

Sieve cell: An elongated cell whose walls contain perforations (sieve pores) that are arranged in circumscribed areas (sieve plates) and that afford communication with similar adjacent cells.

Sigma factor: A sigma factor (σ factor) is a prokaryotic transcription initiation factor that enables specific binding of RNA polymerase to gene promoters. Different sigma factors are activated in response to different environmental conditions. Every molecule of RNA polymerase contains exactly one sigma factor subunit, which in the model bacterium *Escherichia coli* is one of those listed below. *E. coli* has seven sigma factors; the number of sigma factors varies between bacterial species. Sigma factors are distinguished by their characteristic molecular weights. For example, $\sigma70$ refers to the sigma factor with a molecular weight of 70 kDa.

Signal sequence: A peptide present on proteins that are destined either to be secreted or to be membrane components. It is usually at the N terminus and normally absent from the mature protein.

Signal transduction: Signal transduction is the process by which an extracellular signaling molecule activates a membrane receptor that in turn alters intracellular molecules creating a response. There are two stages in this process: a signaling molecule activates a certain receptor on the cell membrane, causing a second messenger to continue the signal into the cell and elicit a physiological response. In either step, the signal can be amplified, meaning that one signaling molecule can cause many responses.

Silencer DNA: In genetics a silencer is a DNA sequence capable of binding transcription regulation factors termed repressors. Upon binding, RNA polymerase is prevented from initiating transcription thus decreasing or fully suppressing RNA synthesis.

Simple sequence repeats: Simple sequence repeats (SSR), also called microsatellites, are becoming the most important molecular markers in both animals and plants.

Single-cell protein: Single-cell protein (SCP) typically refers to sources of mixed protein extracted from pure or mixed cultures of algae, yeasts, fungi, or bacteria (grown on agricultural wastes) used as a substitute for protein-rich foods, in human and animal feeds.

Single-nucleotide polymorphism: Single-nucleotide polymorphism (SNP, pronounced snip) is a DNA sequence variation occurring when a single nucleotide A, T, C, or G—in the genome (or other shared sequence) differs between members of a biological species or paired chromosomes in an individual. For example, two sequenced DNA fragments from different individuals, AAGCCTA to AAGCTTA, contain a difference in a single nucleotide. In this case we say that there are two alleles: C and T. Almost all common SNPs have only two alleles.

Single-strand-DNA-binding protein: Single-strand binding protein, also known as SSB or SSBP, binds to single-stranded regions of DNA to prevent premature annealing. The strands have a natural tendency to revert to the duplex form, but SSB binds to the single strands, keeping them separate and allowing the DNA replication machinery to perform its function.

Site-directed mutagenesis: Site-directed mutagenesis, also called site-specific mutagenesis or oligonucleotide-directed mutagenesis, is a molecular biology technique in which a mutation is created at a defined site in a DNA molecule. In general, this form of mutagenesis requires that the wild-type gene sequence be known.

Small nuclear ribonucleoprotein: Small nuclear ribonucleoprotein (snRNPs) (pronounced "snurps"), or small nuclear ribonucleoproteins, are RNA–protein complexes that combine with unmodified pre-mRNA and various other proteins to form a spliceosome, a large RNA–protein molecular complex upon which splicing of pre-mRNA occurs. The action of snRNPs is essential to the removal of introns from pre-mRNA, a critical aspect of posttranscriptional modification of RNA, occurring only in the nucleus of eukaryotic cells.

Small nuclear RNA: Small nuclear ribonucleic acid (snRNA) is a class of small RNA molecules that are found within the nucleus of eukaryotic cells. They are transcribed by RNA polymerase II or RNA polymerase III and are involved in a variety of important processes such as RNA splicing (removal of introns from hnRNA), regulation of transcription factors (7SK RNA) or RNA polymerase II (B2 RNA), and maintaining the telomeres.

Sodium dodecyl sulfate: Sodium dodecyl sulfate (SDS or NaDS), sodium laurylsulfate or sodium lauryl sulfate (SLS) ($C_{12}H_25SO_4Na$) is an anionic surfactant used in many cleaning and hygiene products. The salt consists of an anionic organosulfate consisting of a 12-carbon tail attached to a sulfate group, giving the material the amphiphilic properties required of a detergent.

Somaclonal variation: Somaclonal variation is the term used to describe the variation seen in plants that have been produced by plant tissue culture. Chromosomal rearrangements are an important source of this variation.

Somatic cell embryogenesis: Plant embryogenesis is the process that produces a plant embryo from a fertilized ovule by asymmetric cell division and the differentiation of undifferentiated cells into tissues and organs. It occurs during seed development, when the single-celled zygote undergoes a programmed pattern of cell division resulting in a mature embryo. A similar process continues during the plant's life within the meristems of the stems and roots.

Somatic hybridization: The production of cells, tissues, or organisms by fusion of nongametic nuclei. The phenomenon may be induced under laboratory conditions in cells that never normally fuse together and used as a plant breeding or genetic tool. It may also occur naturally, especially in fungi.

Somatostatin: Somatostatin (also known as growth hormone-inhibiting hormone [GHIH] or somatotropin release-inhibiting factor [SRIF]) is a peptide hormone that regulates the endocrine system and affects neurotransmission and cell proliferation via interaction with G-protein-coupled somatostatin receptors and inhibition of the release of numerous secondary hormones.

Somatotrophin: Growth hormone, a polypeptide containing 191 amino acids, produced by the anterior pituitary, the front section of the pituitary gland. It acts by stimulating the release of another hormone called somatomedin by the liver, thereby causing growth. Somatotropin is also known as somatropin.

Sonication: Sonication is the act of applying sound (usually ultrasound) energy to agitate particles in a sample, for various purposes. In the laboratory, it is usually applied using an ultrasonic bath or an ultrasonic probe, colloquially known as a sonicator. In a paper machine, an ultrasonic foil can distribute cellulose fibres more uniformly and strengthen the paper.

SOS response: The SOS response is a global response to DNA damage in which the cell cycle is arrested and DNA repair and mutagenesis are induced. The SOS uses the RecA protein (Rad51 in eukaryotes). The RecA protein, stimulated by single-stranded DNA, is involved in the inactivation of the LexA repressor thereby inducing the response. It is an error-prone repair system.

Southern blotting: A Southern blot is a method routinely used in molecular biology for detection of a specific DNA sequence in DNA samples. Southern blotting combines transfer of electrophoresis-separated DNA fragments to a filter membrane and subsequent fragment detection by probe hybridization.

Spermatid: The spermatid is the haploid male gamete that results from division of secondary spermatocytes. As a result of meiosis, each spermatid contains only half of the genetic material present in the original primary spermatocyte.

Spermatocyte: A spermatocyte is a male gametocyte, derived from a spermatogonium, which is in the developmental stage of spermatogenesis during which meiosis occurs. It is located in the seminiferous tubules of the testis.

Spermatogenesis: Spermatogenesis is the process by which male primary germ cells undergo division, and produce a number of cells termed spermatogonia, from which the primary spermatocytes are derived.

Spliceosomes: A spliceosome is a complex of snRNA and protein subunits that removes introns from a transcribed pre-mRNA (hnRNA) segment. This process is generally referred to as splicing.

Split genes: Genes where the genomic sequences are interrupted by intervening sequences (introns) that are spliced out of the mRNA prior to translation.

Staggered cuts: The cleavage of two opposite strands of duplex DNA at points near one another.

Standard deviation: Standard deviation is a widely used measurement of variability or diversity used in statistics and probability theory. It shows how much variation or "dispersion" there is from the average (mean, or expected value).

Standard error: The standard error is a method of measurement or estimation of the standard deviation of the sampling distribution associated with the estimation method.

Starch: Starch or amylum is a carbohydrate consisting of a large number of glucose units joined together by glycosidic bonds. This polysaccharide is produced by all green plants as an energy store.

Start codon: The start codon is generally defined as the point, sequence, at which a ribosome begins to translate a sequence of RNA into amino acids.

Stationary culture: *In vitro* cell culture without agitation.

Stem cell: Stem cells are biological cells found in all multicellular organisms that can divide through mitosis and differentiate into diverse specialized cell types and can self-renew to produce more stem cells.

Sterile room: Hygienic or bacteria-free room.

Sterilization: The process of making bacteria free.

Sticky ends: DNA end or sticky end refers to the properties of the end of a molecule of DNA or a recombinant DNA molecule. The concept is important in molecular biology, especially in cloning or when sub-cloning inserts DNA into vector DNA. All the terms can also be used in reference to RNA.

Stigma: The stigma is the receptive tip of a carpel, or of several fused carpels, in the gynoecium of a flower. The stigma receives pollen at pollination and it is on the stigma that the pollen grain germinates.

Stock solutions: In chemistry, a stock solution is a large volume of a common reagent, such as hydrochloric acid or sodium hydroxide, at a standardized concentration. This term is commonly used in analytical chemistry for procedures such as titrations, where it is important that exact concentrations of solutions are used.

Stop codon: In the genetic code, a stop codon (or termination codon) is a nucleotide triplet within messenger RNA that signals a termination of translation. Proteins are based on polypeptides, which are unique sequences of amino acids. Most codons in messenger RNA correspond to the addition of an amino acid to a growing polypeptide chain, which may ultimately become a protein. Stop codons signal the termination of this process by binding release factors, which cause the ribosomal subunits to disassociate, releasing the amino acid chain.

Stringent plasmid: A plasmid that only replicates along with the main bacterial chromosome and is present as a single copy, or at most several copies, per cell.

Stroma: In animal tissue, stroma refers to the connective, supportive framework of a biological cell, tissue, or organ.

Structural gene: A structural gene is a gene that codes for any RNA or protein product other than a regulatory factor (i.e., regulatory protein). It may code for a structural protein, an enzyme, or an RNA molecule not involved in regulation. Structural genes represent an enormous variety of protein structures and functions, including structural proteins, enzymes with catalytic activities, and so on.

Subcloning: In molecular biology, subcloning is a technique used to move a particular gene of interest from a parent vector to a destination vector in order to further study its functionality.

Sub-culture: In sociology, anthropology, and cultural studies, a subculture is a group of people with a culture (whether distinct or hidden) which differentiates them from the larger culture to which they belong.

Subspecies: Subspecies (commonly abbreviated subsp. or ssp.) in biological classification is either a taxonomic rank subordinate to species or a taxonomic unit in that rank (plural: subspecies). A subspecies cannot be recognized in isolation: a species will either be recognized as having no subspecies at all or two or more, never just one.

Subunit vaccine: a vaccine produced from specific protein subunits of a virus and thus having less risk of adverse reactions than whole virus vaccines.

Superbug: Antibiotic resistance is a type of drug resistance where a microorganism is able to survive exposure to an antibiotic. Genes can be transferred between bacteria in a horizontal fashion by conjugation, transduction, or transformation. Thus, a gene for antibiotic resistance which had evolved via natural selection may be shared. Evolutionary stress such as exposure to antibiotics then selects for the antibiotic-resistant trait. Many antibiotic-resistance genes reside on plasmids, facilitating their transfer. If a bacterium carries several resistance genes, it is called multi-resistant or, informally, a superbug or super bacterium.

Supercoiled DNA: DNA supercoiling refers to the over- or under-winding of a DNA strand, and is an expression of the strain on the polymer. Supercoiling is important in a number of biological processes, such as compacting DNA. Additionally, certain enzymes such as topoisomerases are able to change DNA topology to facilitate functions such as DNA replication or transcription. Mathematical expressions are used to describe supercoiling by comparing different coiled states to relaxed B-form DNA.

Supergene: A supergene is a group of neighboring genes on a chromosome which are inherited together because of close genetic linkage and are functionally related in an evolutionary sense, although they are rarely co-regulated genetically.

Supernatant: The usually clear liquid overlying material deposited by settling, precipitation, or centrifugation.

Suppressor: A suppressor, sound suppressor, sound moderator, or silencer, is a device attached to or part of the barrel of a firearm which reduces the amount of noise and flash generated by firing the weapon.

Suppressor mutation: A suppressor mutation is a mutation that counteracts the phenotypic effects of another mutation.

Susceptible: In epidemiology a susceptible individual (sometimes known simply as a susceptible) is a member of a population who is at risk of becoming infected by a disease, or cannot take a certain medicine, antibiotic, and so on if he or she is exposed to the infectious agent.

Suspension culture: The cultivation of cells suspended in the medium rather than adhering to a surface. Suspension culture is common for microorganisms but less so for the culture of the cells of most multicellular organisms. When referring to mammalian cells, suspension culture is used for the maintenance of cell types, which do not adhere, including some types of blood cells, or in order to have cells express characteristics, which are not seen in the adherent form.

Symbiotic association: Symbiotic relationships include those associations in which one organism lives on another or where one partner lives inside the other endosymbiosis, such as lactobacilli and other bacteria in humans.

Synaptonemal complex: The synaptonemal complex is a protein structure that forms between homologous chromosomes (two pairs of sister chromatids) during meiosis and that is thought to mediate chromosome pairing, synapsis, and recombination (crossing-over). It is now evident that the synaptonemal complex is not required for genetic recombination.

Synchronous culture: A synchronous or synchronized culture is a microbiological culture or a cell culture that contains cells that are all in the same growth stage.

Syndrome: In medicine and psychology, a syndrome is the association of several clinically recognizable features, signs (observed by a physician), symptoms (reported by the patient), phenomena or characteristics that often occur together, so that the presence of one or more features alerts the physician to the possible presence of the others.

Syngamy: The process of union of two gametes to form a zygote. It involves both plasmogamy and karyogamy.

Synkaryon: The nucleus of a fertilized egg immediately after the male and female nuclei has fused.

Tandem array: Repetitive DNA, where the repeating units are contiguous. Some genes of high copy number occur in tandem arrays, for example, ribosomal DNA.

Taq polymerase: Taq polymerase is a thermostable DNA polymerase named after the thermophilic bacterium *Thermus aquaticus* from which it was originally isolated by Thomas D. Brock in 1965. It is often abbreviated to "Taq Pol" (or simply "Taq"), and is frequently used in polymerase chain reaction (PCR), a method for greatly amplifying short segments of DNA.

Targeted drug delivery: Targeted drug delivery, sometimes called smart drug delivery, is a method of delivering medication to a patient in a manner that increases the concentration of the medication in some parts of the body relative to others. The goal of a targeted drug delivery system is to prolong, localize, target, and have a protected drug interaction with the diseased tissue. The conventional drug delivery system is the absorption of the drug across a biological membrane, whereas the targeted release system is when the drug is released in a dosage form. The advantages to the targeted release system is the reduction in the frequency of the dosages taken by the patient, having a more uniform effect of the drug, reduction of drug side effects, and reduced fluctuation in circulating drug levels. The disadvantage of the system is high cost which makes productivity more difficult and the reduced ability to adjust the dosages.

TATA box: The TATA box (also called Goldberg–Hogness box) is a DNA sequence (*cis*-regulatory element) found in the promoter region of genes in archaea and eukaryotes; approximately 24% of human genes contain a TATA box within the core promoter.

Tautomerism: Tautomerism, the existence of two or more chemical compounds that are capable of facile interconversion, in many cases merely exchanging a hydrogen atom between two other atoms, to either of which it forms a covalent bond. Unlike other classes of isomers, tautomeric compounds exist in mobile equilibrium with each other, so that attempts to prepare the separate substances usually result in the formation of a mixture that shows all the chemical and physical properties to be expected on the basis of the structures of the components.

T cells: T cells or T lymphocytes belong to a group of white blood cells known as lymphocytes, and play a central role in cell-mediated immunity. They can be distinguished from other lymphocyte types, such as B cells and natural killer cells (NK cells) by the presence of a special receptor on their cell surface called T cell receptors (TCR).

T-cell-mediated (cellular) immune response: Cell-mediated immunity is an immune response that does not involve antibodies or complement but rather involves the activation of macrophages, natural killer cells (NK), antigen-specific cytotoxic T-lymphocytes, and the release of various cytokines in response to an antigen. Historically, the immune system was separated into two branches: humoral immunity, for which the protective function of immunization could be found in the humor (cell-free bodily fluid or serum) and cellular immunity, for which the protective function of immunization was associated with cells. CD4 cells or helper T cells provide protection against different pathogens.

T-DNA: The transfer DNA (abbreviated T-DNA) is the transferred DNA of the tumor-inducing (Ti) plasmid of some species of bacteria such as *Agrobacterium tumefaciens* and *Agrobacterium rhizogenes*. It derives its name from the fact that the bacterium transfers this DNA fragment into the host plant's nuclear DNA genome.

T4 DNA ligase: In molecular biology, DNA ligase is a specific type of enzyme, a ligase) that repairs single-stranded discontinuities in double-stranded DNA molecules, in simple words strands that have double-strand break (a break in both complementary strands of DNA).

Telomerase: Telomerase is an enzyme that adds DNA sequence repeats ("TTAGGG" in all vertebrates) to the 3′ end of DNA strands in the telomere regions, which are found at the ends of eukaryotic chromosomes.

Telophase: Telophase is a stage in both meiosis and mitosis in a eukaryotic cell. During telophase, the effects of prophase and prometaphase events are reversed. Two daughter nuclei form in the cell. The nuclear envelopes of the daughter cells are formed from the fragments of the nuclear envelope of the parent cell.

Template strand: When referring to DNA transcription, the coding strand is the DNA strand which has the same base sequence as the RNA transcript produced (although with thymine replaced by uracil). It is this strand which contains codons, while the noncoding strand contains anticodons.

Terminal deoxynucleotidyl transferase: Terminal deoxynucleotidyl transferase (TDT), also known as DNA nucleotidylexotransferase (DNTT) or terminal transferase, is a specialized DNA polymerase expressed in immature, pre-B, pre-T lymphoid cells, and acute lymphoblastic leukemia/lymphoma cells.

Tetracycline: Tetracycline is a broad-spectrum polyketide antibiotic produced by the *Streptomyces* genus of Actinobacteria, indicated for use against many bacterial infections. It is a protein synthesis inhibitor.

Tetraploid: An individual or cell having four sets of chromosomes.

Thermophile: A thermophile is an organism a type of extremophile that thrives at relatively high temperatures, between 45°C and 80°C (113°F and 176°F). Many thermophiles are archaea. It has been suggested that thermophilic eubacteria are among the earliest bacteria.

Thermosensitivity: The central perception of temperature is located in the anterior hypothalamus (preoptic region) and in the spinal cord. The preoptic sensitivity is more important in mammals and in the spinal cord center in birds.

Thermostability: Thermostability is the quality of a substance to resist irreversible change in its chemical or physical structure at a high relative temperature.

Thymidine: Thymidine (more precisely called deoxythymidine; can also be labeled deoxyribosylthymine, and thymine deoxyriboside) is a chemical compound, more precisely a pyrimidine deoxynucleoside. Deoxythymidine is the DNA nucleoside T, which pairs with deoxyadenosine (A) in double-stranded DNA. In cell biology it is used to synchronize the cells in S phase.

Thymidine kinase: Thymidine kinase is an enzyme, a phosphotransferase (a kinase): 2′-deoxythymidine kinase, ATP-thymidine 5′-phosphotransferase. It can be found in most living cells. It is present in two forms in mammalian cells, TK1 and TK2. Certain viruses also have genetic information for expression of viral thymidine kinases.

Thymine: Thymine (T, Thy) is one of the four nucleobases in the nucleic acid of DNA that are represented by the letters G–C–A–T. The others are adenine, guanine, and cytosine. Thymine is also known as 5-methyluracil, a pyrimidine nucleobase.

Topoisomerase: Topoisomerases are enzymes that unwind and wind DNA, in order for DNA to control the synthesis of proteins, and to facilitate DNA replication. The enzyme is necessary due to inherent problems caused by the DNA's double helix.

Totipotency: The ability of a cell, such as an egg, to give rise to unlike cells and thus to develop into or generate a new organism or part.

Toxicity: Toxicity is the degree to which a substance can damage an organism. Toxicity can refer to the effect on a whole organism, such as an animal, bacterium, or plant, as well as the effect on a substructure of the organism, such as a cell (cytotoxicity) or an organ (organotoxicity), such as the liver (hepatotoxicity). By extension, the word may be metaphorically used to describe toxic effects on larger and more complex groups, such as the family unit or society at large.

Transcription: Transcription is the process of creating a complementary RNA copy of a sequence of DNA. Both RNA and DNA are nucleic acids, which use base pairs of nucleotides as a complementary language that can be converted back and forth from DNA to RNA by the action of the correct enzymes. During transcription, a DNA sequence is read by RNA polymerase, which produces a complementary, antiparallel RNA strand.

Transcription factor: In molecular biology and genetics, a transcription factor (sometimes called a sequence-specific DNA-binding factor) is a protein that binds to specific DNA sequences, thereby controlling the flow (or transcription) of genetic information from DNA to mRNA. Transcription factors perform this function alone or with other proteins in a complex, by promoting (as an activator), or blocking (as a repressor) the recruitment of RNA polymerase (the enzyme that performs the transcription of genetic information from DNA to RNA) to specific genes.

Transcription unit: A stretch of DNA being transcribed into an RNA molecule.

Transduction: Transduction is the process by which DNA is transferred from one bacterium to another by a virus. It also refers to the process whereby foreign DNA is introduced into another cell via a viral vector. This is a common tool used by molecular biologists to stably introduce a foreign gene into a host cell's genome.

Transfection: Transfection is the process of deliberately introducing nucleic acids into cells. The term is used notably for nonviral methods in eukaryotic cells. It may also refer to other methods and cell types, although other terms are preferred: "transformation" is more often used to describe nonviral DNA transfer in bacteria, non-animal eukaryotic cells and plant cells—a distinctive sense of transformation refers to spontaneous genetic modifications (mutations to cancerous cells [carcinogenesis], or under stress [UV irradiation]). "Transduction" is often used to describe virus-mediated DNA transfer.

Transferase: In biochemistry, a transferase is an enzyme that catalyzes the transfer of a functional group (e.g., a methyl or phosphate group) from one molecule (called the donor) to another (called the acceptor).

Transfer RNA: Transfer RNA (tRNA) is an adaptor molecule composed of RNA, typically 73–93 nucleotides in length that is used in biology to bridge the three-letter genetic code in messenger RNA (mRNA) with the 20-letter code of amino acids in proteins.

Transformation: In molecular biology transformation is the genetic alteration of a cell resulting from the direct uptake, incorporation, and expression of exogenous genetic material (exogenous DNA) from its surrounding and taken up through the cell membrane(s). Transformation occurs most commonly in bacteria and in some species occurs naturally. Transformation can also be effected by artificial means. Bacteria that are capable of being transformed, whether naturally or artificially, are called competent. Transformation is one of three processes by which exogenous genetic material may be introduced into a bacterial cell, the other two being conjugation (transfer of genetic material between two bacterial cells in direct contact), and transduction (injection of foreign DNA by a bacteriophage virus into the host bacterium).

Transforming oncogene: A gene that upon transfection, converts an immortalized cell, into malignant phenotype.

Transgene: A transgene is a gene or genetic material that has been transferred naturally or by any of a number of genetic engineering techniques from one organism to another.

Transgenesis: Transgenesis is the process of introducing an exogenous gene—called a transgene—into a living organism so that the organism will exhibit a new property and transmit that property to its offspring. Transgenesis can be facilitated by liposomes, plasmid vectors, viral vectors, pronuclear injection, protoplast fusion, and ballistic DNA injection.

Transgenic animal: The term transgenic animal refers to an animal in which there has been a deliberate modification of the genome. Foreign DNA is introduced into the animal, using recombinant DNA technology, and then must be transmitted through the germ line so that every cell, including germ cells, of the animal contains the same modified genetic material.

Translation DNA: In molecular biology and genetics, translation is the third stage of protein biosynthesis (part of the overall process of gene expression). In translation, messenger RNA (mRNA) produced by transcription is decoded by the ribosome to produce a specific amino acid chain, or polypeptide, that will later fold into an active protein. In bacteria, translation occurs in the cell's cytoplasm, where the large and small subunits of the ribosome are located, and bind to the mRNA.

Transmission electron microscope: Transmission electron microscopy (TEM) is a microscopy technique whereby a beam of electrons is transmitted through an ultra-thin specimen, interacting with the specimen as it passes through. An image is formed from the interaction of the electrons transmitted through the specimen; the image is magnified and focused onto an imaging device, such as a fluorescent screen, on a layer of photographic film, or to be detected by a sensor such as a CCD camera.

Transposable genetic element: Transposons are only one of several types of mobile genetic elements. Transposons themselves are assigned to one of two classes according to their mechanism of transposition, which can be described as either "copy or paste" (class I) or "cut and paste" (class II).

Transposase: Transposase is an enzyme that binds to the ends of a transposon and catalyzes the movement of the transposon to another part of the genome by a cut and paste mechanism or a replicative transposition mechanism.

Transposon: Transposons are sequences of DNA that can move or transpose themselves to new positions within the genome of a single cell.

Transposon tagging: The term "transposon tagging" refers to a process in genetic engineering where transposons (transposable elements) are amplified inside a biological cell by a tagging techique. Transposon tagging has been used with several species to isolate genes. Even without knowing the nature of the specific genes, the process can still be used.

Trinucleotide repeat disorder: Trinucleotide repeat disorders (also known as trinucleotide repeat expansion disorders, triplet repeat expansion disorders or codon reiteration disorders) are a set of genetic disorders caused by trinucleotide repeat expansion, a kind of mutation where trinucleotide repeats in certain genes exceeding the normal, stable, threshold, which differs per gene. The mutation is a subset of unstable microsatellite repeats that occur throughout all genomic sequences. If the repeat is present in a healthy gene, a dynamic mutation may increase the repeat count and result in a defective gene.

Trisomy: A trisomy is a genetic abnormality in which there are three copies, instead of the normal two, of a particular chromosome. A trisomy is a type of aneuploidy (an abnormal number of chromosomes).

Trypsin: Trypsin is a serine protease found in the digestive system of many vertebrates, where it hydrolyzes proteins. Trypsin is produced in the pancreas as the inactive proenzyme trypsinogen.

Trypsin inhibitor: Trypsin inhibitors are chemicals that reduce the availability of trypsin, an enzyme essential to nutrition of many animals, including humans.

Tubulin: Tubulin is one of several members of a small family of globular proteins. The most common members of the tubulin family are α-tubulin and β-tubulin, the proteins that make up microtubules. Each has a molecular weight of approximately 55 kDa. Microtubules are assembled from dimers of α- and β-tubulin.

Tumor-inducing plasmid: A giant plasmid of *Agrobacterium tumefaciens* that is responsible for tumor formation in infected plants. Ti plasmids are used as vectors to introduce foreign DNA into plant cells.

Twins: A twin is one of two offspring produced in the same pregnancy. Twins can either be identical (in scientific usage, "monozygotic"), meaning that they develop from one zygote that splits and forms two embryos, or fraternal ("dizygotic") because they develop from two separate eggs that are fertilized by two separate sperms.

Ultra-sonication: In biological applications, ultra-sonication is used to disrupt or deactivate a biological material. For example, ultra-sonication is often used to disrupt cell membranes and release cellular contents.

Ultraviolet radiation: Ultraviolet (UV) light is electromagnetic radiation with a wavelength shorter than that of visible light, but longer than x-rays, in the range 10–400 nm. It is named because the spectrum consists of electromagnetic waves with frequencies higher than those that humans identify as the color violet.

Upstream processing: The manufacture of human proteins by the methods of modern biotechnology is separated into two stages: upstream processing during which proteins are produced by cells genetically engineered to contain the human gene, which will express the protein of interest and downstream processing during which the produced proteins are isolated and purified. Following purification of the protein of interest, the final product is formulated (meaning excipients are added to the protein), filter sterilized, filled aseptically, lyophilized, sealed, inspected, and labeled. Upstream processing, downstream processing, final drug production, and the general environment of the facility are monitored by the quality control division of the manufacturing facility.

Uracil: Uracil is one of the four nucleo-bases in the nucleic acid of RNA that are represented by the letters A, C, G, and U. The others are adenine, cytosine, and guanine. In RNA, uracil (U) binds to adenine (A) via two hydrogen bonds. In DNA, the uracil nucleobase is replaced by thymine.

Variable number tandem repeat: A variable number tandem repeat (or VNTR) is a location in a genome where a short nucleotide sequence is organized as a tandem repeat. These can be found on many chromosomes, and often show variations in length between individuals. Each variant acts as an inherited allele, allowing them to be used for personal or parental identification. Their analysis is useful in genetics and biology research, forensics, and DNA fingerprinting.

Variance: In probability theory and statistics, the variance is used as a measure of how far a set of numbers are spread out from each other. It is one of several descriptors of a probability distribution, describing how far the numbers lie from the mean (expected value). In particular, the variance is one of the moments of a distribution. In that context, it forms part of a systematic approach to distinguishing between probability distributions. While other such approaches have been developed, those based on moments are advantageous in terms of mathematical and computational simplicity.

Vascular: Vascular in zoology and medicine means "related to blood vessels," which are part of the circulatory system. An organ or tissue that is vascularized is heavily endowed with blood vessels and thus richly supplied with blood.

Vegetative propagation: Vegetative reproduction (vegetative propagation, vegetative multiplication, vegetative cloning) is a form of asexual reproduction in plants. It is a process by which new individuals arise without production of seeds or spores. It can occur naturally or be induced by horticulturists.

Vernalization: Vernalization is the acquisition of a plant's ability to flower or germinate in the spring by exposure to the prolonged cold of winter. After vernalization, plants have acquired the ability to flower, but they may require additional seasonal cues or weeks of growth before they will actually flower.

Viability cell: Cell viability is a determination of living or dead cells, based on a total cell sample. Cell viability measurements may be used to evaluate the death or life of cancerous cells and the rejection of implanted organs. In other applications cell viability tests might calculate the effectiveness of a pesticide or insecticide, or evaluate environmental damage due to toxins.

Viability test: Test to determine the proportion of living individuals, cells or organisms, in a sample. Viability tests are most commonly performed on cultured cells and usually depend on the ability of living cells to exclude a dye.

Viral oncogene: Any virus that promotes cancer.

Viral vaccines: A vaccine is a biological preparation that improves immunity to a particular disease. A vaccine typically contains an agent that resembles a disease-causing microorganism, and is often made from weakened or killed forms of the microbe or its toxins. The agent stimulates the body's immune system to recognize the agent as foreign, destroy it, and "remember" it, so that the immune system can more easily recognize and destroy any of these microorganisms that it later encounters.

Virion: An entire virus particle, consisting of an outer protein shell called a capsid and an inner core of nucleic acid (either ribonucleic or deoxyribonucleic acid RNA or DNA). The core confers infectivity, and the capsid provides specificity to the virus. In some virions the capsid is further enveloped by a fatty membrane, in which case the virion can be inactivated by exposure to fat solvents such as ether and chloroform.

Viroid: Viroids are plant pathogens that consist of a short stretch (a few hundred nucleobases) of highly complementary, circular, single-stranded RNA without the protein coat that is typical for viruses.

Western blot: The western blot (sometimes called the protein immunoblot) is a widely used analytical technique used to detect specific proteins in the given sample of tissue homogenate or extract. It uses gel electrophoresis to separate native or denatured proteins by the length of the polypeptide (denaturing conditions) or by the 3-D structure of the protein (native/nondenaturing conditions). The proteins are then transferred to a membrane (typically nitrocellulose or PVDF), where they are probed (detected) using antibodies specific to the target protein.

Wild type: Wild type refers to the phenotype of the typical form of a species as it occurs in nature. Originally, the wild type was conceptualized as a product of the standard, "normal" allele at a locus, in contrast to that produced by a nonstandard, "mutant" allele.

X-chromosome: The X chromosome is one of the two sex-determining chromosomes in many animal species, including mammals (the other is the Y chromosome). It is a part of the XY sex-determination system and X0 sex-determination system. The X chromosome was named for its unique properties by early researchers, which resulted in the naming of its counterpart Y chromosome, for the next letter in the alphabet, after it was discovered later.

Xenobiotic: A xenobiotic is a chemical which is found in an organism but which is not normally produced or expected to be present in it. It can also cover substances which are present in much higher concentrations than are usual. Specifically, drugs such as antibiotics are xenobiotics in humans because the human body does not produce them, nor are they part of a normal diet.

Xenotransplantation: Xenotransplantation is the transplantation of living cells, tissues, or organs from one species to another, such as from pigs to humans. Such cells, tissues, or organs are called xenografts or xenotransplants. In contrast, the term allotransplantation refers to a same-species transplant. Human xenotransplantation offers a potential treatment for end-stage organ failure, a significant health problem in parts of the industrialized world. It also raises many novel medical, legal, and ethical issues. There are few published cases of successful xenotransplantation.

X-linked disease: Genetic disease associated with X chromosome.

X-ray crystallography: X-ray crystallography is a method of determining the arrangement of atoms within a crystal, in which a beam of X-rays strikes a crystal and diffracts into many specific directions. From the angles and intensities of these diffracted beams, a crystallographer can produce a three-dimensional picture of the density of electrons within the crystal.

Y-chromosome: The Y chromosome is one of the two sex-determining chromosomes in most mammals, including humans. In mammals, it contains the gene SRY, which triggers testis development if present. The human Y chromosome is composed of about 60 million base pairs. DNA in the Y chromosome is passed from father to son, and Y-DNA analysis may thus be used in genealogy research.

Yeast: Yeasts are eukaryotic microorganisms classified in the kingdom Fungi, with 1500 species currently described estimated to be only 1% of all fungal species. Most reproduce asexually by mitosis, and many do so via an asymmetric division process called budding.

Yeast artificial chromosome: A yeast artificial chromosome (YAC) is a vector used to clone DNA fragments larger than 100 kb and up to 3000 kb. YACs are useful for the physical mapping of complex genomes and for the cloning of large genes. First described in 1983 by Murray and Szostak, a YAC is an artificially constructed chromosome and contains the telomeric, centromeric, and replication origin sequences needed for replication and preservation in yeast cells.

Z-DNA: Z-DNA is one of the many possible double helical structures of DNA. It is a left-handed double helical structure in which the double helix winds to the left in a zig-zag pattern (instead of to the right, like the more common B-DNA form). Z-DNA is thought to be one of three biologically active double helical structures along with A- and B-DNA.

Zoo blot: A zoo blot or garden blot is a type of Southern blot that demonstrates the similarity between specific, usually protein coding, DNA sequences of different species. A zoo blot compares animal species while a garden blot compares plant species.

Zygonema: The synaptic chromosome formation that occurs in the zygotene stage of the first meiotic prophase of gametogenesis.

Zygote: A zygote is the initial cell formed when two gamete cells are joined by means of sexual reproduction. It is the earliest developmental stage of the embryo. A zygote is always synthesized from the union of two gametes, and constitutes the first stage in a unique organism's development.

Zymogen: A zymogen (or proenzyme) is an inactive enzyme precursor. A zymogen requires a biochemical change (such as a hydrolysis reaction revealing the active site, or changing the configuration to reveal the active site) for it to become an active enzyme. The biochemical change usually occurs in a lysosome where a specific part of the precursor enzyme is cleaved in order to activate it. The amino acid chain that is released upon activation is called the activation peptide.

Index

C

D

F

G

H

J

K

L

M

S

T

U